A Beginner's Guide to

Total Knee Replacement

A Beginner's Guide to
Total Knee Replacement

L Prakash MS (Orth), MCh (Orth) (Liverpool)
Institute for Special Orthopaedics
Chennai, Tamil Nadu

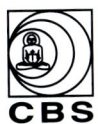

CBS

CBS Publishers & Distributors Pvt Ltd

New Delhi • Bengaluru • Chennai • Kochi • Kolkata • Mumbai
Hyderabad • Nagpur • Patna • Pune • Vijayawada

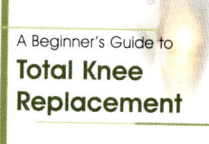

A Beginner's Guide to
Total Knee Replacement

ISBN: 978-93-86217-48-6

First Edition: 2017

Published by Satish Kumar Jain and produced by Varun Jain for

CBS Publishers & Distributors Pvt Ltd

4819/XI Prahlad Street, 24 Ansari Road, Daryaganj, New Delhi 110 002, India.
Ph: 23289259, 23266861, 23266867 Website: www.cbspd.com
Fax: 011-23243014   e-mail: delhi@cbspd.com; cbspubs@airtelmail.in.
Corporate Office: 204 FIE, Industrial Area, Patparganj, Delhi 110 092
Ph: 4934 4934   Fax: 4934 4935   e-mail: publishing@cbspd.com; publicity@cbspd.com

Branches

- **Bengaluru:** Seema House 2975, 17th Cross, K.R. Road, Banasankari 2nd Stage, Bengaluru 560 070, Karnataka
  Ph: +91-80-26771678/79   Fax: +91-80-26771680   e-mail: bangalore@cbspd.com
- **Chennai:** 7, Subbaraya Street, Shenoy Nagar, Chennai 600 030, Tamil Nadu
  Ph: +91-44-26680620, 26681266   Fax: +91-44-42032115   e-mail: chennai@cbspd.com
- **Kochi:** Ashana House, No. 39/1904, AM Thomas Road, Valanjambalam, Ernakulam 682 016, Kochi, Kerala
  Ph: +91-484-4059061-65   Fax: +91-484-4059065   e-mail: kochi@cbspd.com
- **Kolkata:** 6/B, Ground Floor, Rameswar Shaw Road, Kolkata-700 014, West Bengal
  Ph: +91-33-22891126, 22891127, 22891128   e-mail: kolkata@cbspd.com
- **Mumbai:** 83-C, Dr E Moses Road, Worli, Mumbai-400018, Maharashtra
  Ph: +91-22-24902340/41   Fax: +91-22-24902342   e-mail: mumbai@cbspd.com

Representatives

- **Hyderabad** 0-9885175004
- **Nagpur** 0-9021734563
- **Patna** 0-9334159340
- **Pune** 0-9623451994
- **Vijayawada** 0-9000660880

Printed at : Rashtriya Printers Delhi-110095

to

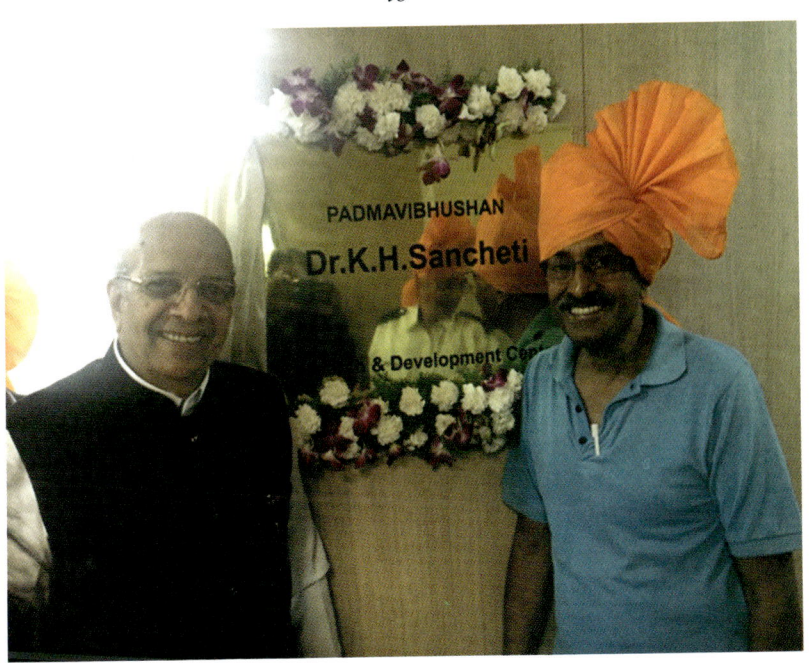

Dr KH Sancheti
The inventor of Indus Knee, my knee Guru and the person who
taught me many things about knee joint.

to

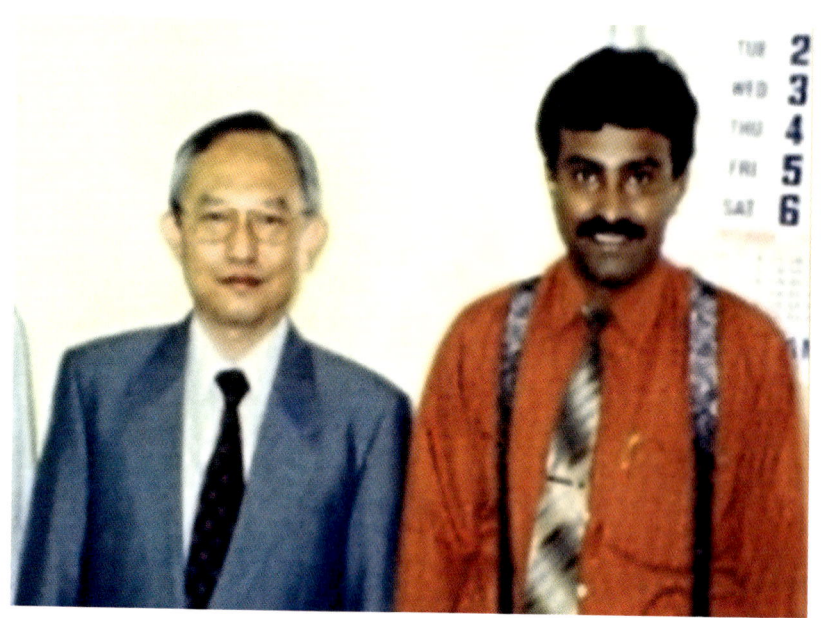

Dr Raymon Gustilo, MD
The inventor of Genesis Knee, my old friend and a brilliant
orthopaedic teacher.

Foreword

I first met Dr L Prakash around twenty-seven years back, when he was doing a live demonstration of a cemented total knee replacement and I was moderating the session in the hall with a live video broadcast before over a hundred surgeons. There was no doubt that he was an exceptional surgeon, because few dare to operate on a complex case in the presence of a live audience. The surgery went off well; he was almost an artist, the tissues seemed to part before his fingers. Despite not using a tourniquet, everything was clear and the audience gave a standing ovation.

The interesting part was that the surgery was completed in forty minutes even while he was explaining each step in detail and performing the knee replacement in an unhurried manner. I still remember it was a complex rheumatoid knee with gross fixed flexion and varus deformities. That evening in the banquet we had an interesting conversation.

"Prakash! You must write a book. An atlas rather. Explain your master techniques in detail."

"Well Venkat! You know my workload. Where do I have the time? So many patients and such a long list of patients waiting for surgery."

"And Prakash, when you do the book, it should have excellent drawings. Not black and white ones. Proper colour ones like FH Netter illustrations."

"Venkat! That is the main difficulty. Where will I find an artist like that? I need an artist who is a surgeon himself and can illustrate things better than a photograph. May be if I get a proper artist, I'll do it. Probably after my retirement!"

Last week when I visited him in Chennai, I got a wonderful surprise. This book was almost ready, and I was given the pleasant task of writing its foreword. The illustrations were really good, the operative pictures exceptionally clear, and the multimedia videos really educative.

I have great pleasure in presenting this book to orthopaedic surgeons of the world. Written like a graphic novel, with 90%

pictures and 10% text, this book is a pleasure to read, while full of knowledge. Dr L Prakash has himself painted water colours for all pictures and the photos are from his own cases taken by his assistant. He has himself edited the videos, and done part of the formatting and design of the book. I was envious that one man could do so many different things!!

This book is a must-read for a surgeon planning to embark on the arduous but fascinating journey of becoming a primary knee arthroplasty surgeon. It is also an essential read for those doing knee replacements, sporadically or occasionally. For those doing it regularly, this will be an exceptional refresher, while it will be an invaluable addition to any operation theatre library. Even an experienced arthroplasty surgeon like me could glean many valuable tips from this fascinating book. Combining illustrations, photographs, videos and multimedia content is a brilliant idea and this book shows years of hard work and ceaseless toil to write.

It is with pride and pleasure that I write this foreword and dedicate the book to the orthopaedic fraternity.

S Venkateswaran
Consultant Orthopaedic Surgeon
North East London NHS Treatment Centre,
King George Hospital, Ilford, Essex.IG3 8YY.
Ph: 0208 598 4600.
Consulting Rooms in London & Birmingham
10 Harley Street, London, W1G 9PF. Phone 02074678301
Guildhall Back Care Centre, Navigation Street,
Birmingham B24BT. Phone: 0121632 5332

Acknowledgements

My parents Mr TS Lakshmanan, and Radha Lakshman. I owe my existence to them.

Dr TS Ramaswamy and Dr Pramila Ramaswamy, who made my life worth living, and because of whom I am now a medical teacher and scientist.

Dr Mayil, my best friend, and more importantly, my foul weather friend.

TG Seshadri, my medical assistant who learnt photography, designed a sterilizable camera sleeve, and who scrubbed up in every case to take the brilliant close up photos and the excellent videos in this book.

Dr Vijay Sharma, Dr Simon Thomas, Dr Mithin Aachi, Dr Vivek Mahajan, and Dr Anuj Agrawal, the new generation of arthroplasty surgeons from our country, who have taught me new tricks, shared their clinical cases with me, and have agreed to be the co-authors of the second part of this book, 'Master Tips and Tricks: Total Knee Replacement Made Easy'.

Jagga—my biomedical engineer, Puliarasi—my orthopaedic nurse, and Babu—my man Friday who helped me to stretch my day beyond twenty-four hours.

Mr LR Ashok, my editor who has rendered the book flawless as far as the language and grammar is concerned.

My patients, who placed their trust in me from the time I began implanting locally forged and machined implants twenty-five years ago.

L Prakash

Contents

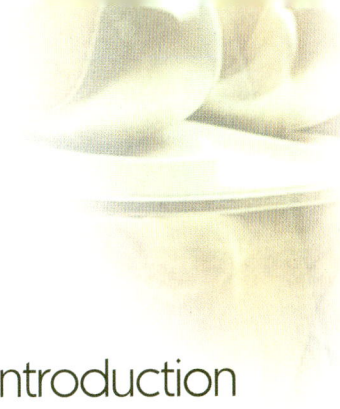

Introduction

Knee replacements have now come of age. In the Asian continent, the importance of this method of treatment is paramount, because the incidence of knee arthritis in our parts is much more than that in the western world.

As opposed to the hip joint, which is hidden and camouflaged by layers of muscle and fat, the knee is an exhibitionist that the patient sees and feels each day. Globally there is a tremendous difference between the epidemiology of primary osteoarthritis of the knee and the hip. John Goodfellow of Oxford and former editor of the JBJS always used to remark, *"I am surprised that primary osteoarthritis of the hip is practically unknown amongst the Asians. I suppose that this is very well compensated by the extremely prevalent primary knee arthritis. I suppose that the extremes of flexion during squatting somehow protects the hip at the cost of the knee joint."*

Primary knee arthritis is nine times as common as hip arthritis in our country. Most of us have seen an elderly granny in the house with a pair of painful knees.

With the new generation modular knees providing over 130° of flexion, and the average lifespan of knee replacements approaching that of second generation Charnley's hips, this procedure is no doubt unsurpassed amongst other transient and temporary surgical methods for the cure of knee arthritis.

Knee replacement surgery has now been established as a definite method of relieving painful and crippling knee joint arthritis. Over the last 55 years, acceptable results from this procedure have been published in the literature.

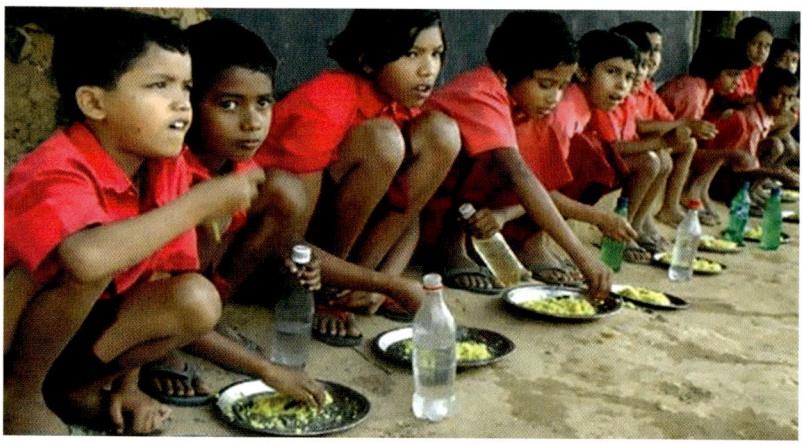

Squatting probably causes a higher incidence of osteoarthritis of the knee while sparing the hips.

On a review of the literature, one fact that emerges very clearly is that long-term success of knee replacement is dependent upon four factors:

1. Proper soft tissue releases
2. Correct balancing of ligaments
3. Precise bone cuts
4. Perfect component placements

Irrespective of the knee design used, it is imperative that the biomechanical principles are clearly understood and correct operative steps followed to achieve consistent long-lasting and reproducible results.

This surgery is not devoid of its demerits. Prohibitive cost of the imported knees, innumerable designs, a plethora of instrumentation, lack of basic knowledge of arthroplasty, poor operation theatre facilities, and long-lasting crippling complications (when they occur) bring diffidence and hesitation in the minds of our Indian surgeons when they embark upon this procedure.

This book is an attempt to clear a few of these confusions and challenge many prevailing myths. The facts mentioned in subsequent chapters may well be unconventional and may not all be in conformity with established norms described in conventional textbooks, but one fact lends weight to all that is said. Whatever is written here is **tried and tested**.

An Indian patient may well want to squat pain-free more than want to walk a mile. An Indian male may well be more concerned about his postoperative ability to use an Indian toilet rather than to play golf.

However, once the standards of the femoral and tibial dimensions of an average accidental patient are defined either by a pioneer in knee surgery or a highly powerful multinational surgical firm, these dimensions tend to become Hammurabi codes chiseled in stone, which no Indian surgeon has the courage to challenge. Rather than fit a shoe to the foot it fits, we are advised to either trim the foot or use too many paddings to make it fit. This attitude has gone unchallenged for many many decades. Now a time has come to question these 'Hammurabi codes'!

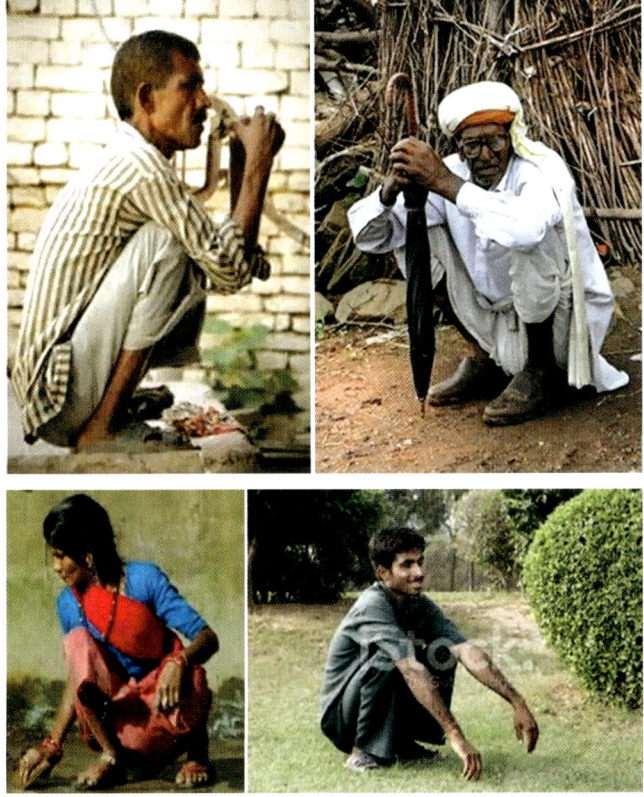

Asian patients have their own special needs.

We have come to realize that Asian patients are different. They have a different average national height; they have different social habits needing entirely different degrees of motion; they are financially constrained, with most of them not covered by insurance and have different demands from the surgical procedure and implants. The facilities available for the average surgeon are all too different, as are the skills, exposure and training in arthroplasty.

Initially, knee replacements were performed only in specialist centres with exceptional theatre and back-up facilities. However, with increasing commercialisation, half trained or even untrained surgeons began performing knee replacements in operating rooms not having adequate infrastructure. This led to numerous complications, and things have deteriorated to such an extent that (a) I am currently doing more revisions than primary and (b) most knees I currently revise are less than 10 years old, and symptomatic enough to demand revision.

Something has gone wrong or is still going wrong!

I have identified a few reasons for these avoidable complications, and principal amongst them are:

1. Non-standardisation of sizes, of implants or designs of instruments. You cannot use instruments from company A to implant B knees.

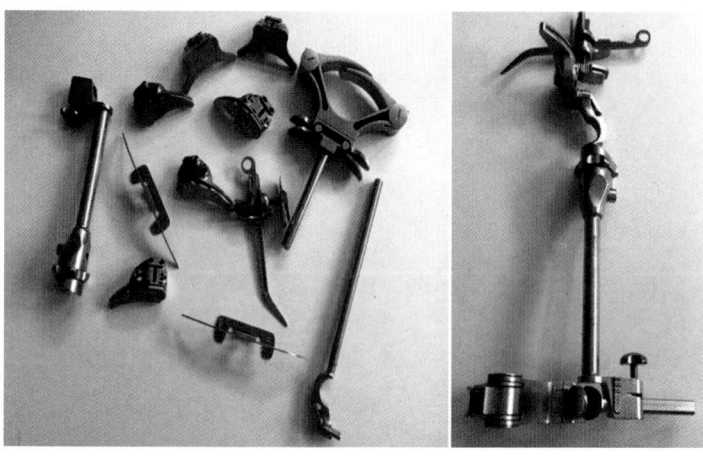

Modern knees are accompanied with an excess baggage of a plethora of instrumentation and jigs, each specific to one implant.

2. Companies insisting on sending non-doctors as surgical scrub assistants, who end up doing most of the surgery.

3. Shift of the TKR paradigm from gardening to carpentry. Now all that is considered important is the precision of bone cuts. Nobody bothers about mid flexion gaps, and for that matter, no instruments are available to measure this important parameter.

4. The knee that fits perfectly in AP overhangs or is undersized in lateral or vice versa.

5. The current mantra seems to be bone cuts, bone cuts and bone cuts. The current belief is that soft tissues will balance automatically with time. But the most important point is forgotten. HDPE is forgiving for the first five years. Imbalance caused wear is symptomatic or radiologically apparent only between six to eight years.

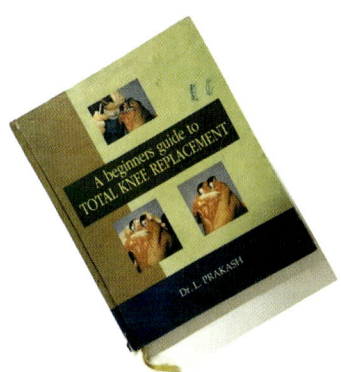

The book, originally written in 1991, which helped a generation of Indian surgeons to embark upon their career as arthroplasty surgeons.

The first edition of the book was primarily based on a single author's experience. This (second edition) is completely rewritten; though a single author's opinionated treatise, it includes all that I have learned in the 25 years that elapsed after the first edition.

At the end of this volume, I have listed some excellent works on this subject that will constitute further reading for serious students. I would consider my ambitions fulfilled if readers get at least a tenth of the pleasure from reading this book as I have had writing it.

Historical Aspects and Design Criteria of Total Knee Arthroplasty

Arthroplasty arrived on the orthopaedic scene in the mid-nineteenth century. when surgeons started their attempts to improve mobility of ankylosed joints by resection of the joint itself. But as is apparent, simple resections do not give long-lasting pain-free mobility and there is a definite tendency for the joint surfaces to rejoin. It has been always been bewildering to surgeons that bones and joints seem to have minds of their own. When we attempt to produce a pseudoarthrosis, nature tends to glue up the ends. And where we desire union, we frequently end up with pseudoarthrosis. Thus attempts were made to interpose substances between the resected surfaces, first biological, then man-made.

Resection arthroplasty of the knee was first reported by Fergusson in 1861 and interposition arthroplasty by Verneuil in 1863. The latter used the knee joint capsule to prevent the bone ends from fusing. Later, various materials like fascia, skin, muscle, chromatized pig's bladder, glass, bakelite and ivory were tried without significant long term success.

The concept on which total joint replacement is based can be traced only after 1880, when Thermestocles Gluck gave a series of lectures describing a system of joint replacement by a unit made of ivory. He stabilized it in bone with cement made of colophony, pumice and plaster of Paris.

In the early 1940s, Boyd and Campbell and Smith-Peterson tried a metallic hemi-arthroplasty for the knee, which predictably failed after a short while. Likewise, tibial sided hemi-arthroplasty designs by Maceever and Macintosh also suffered from early loss of fixation and painful loosening.

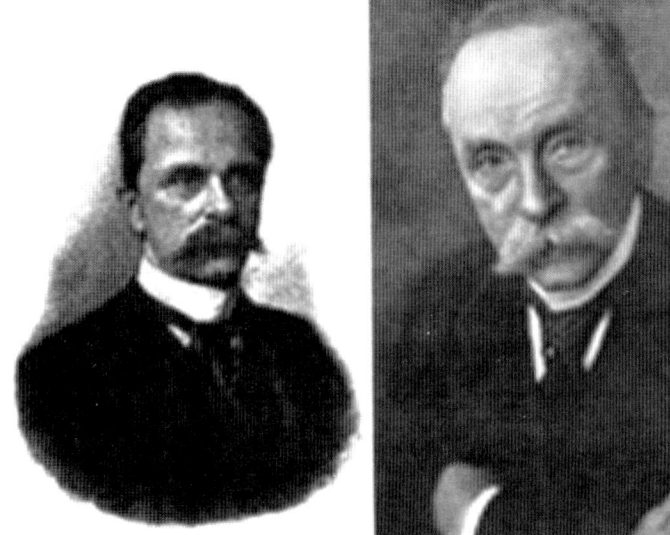

Thermestocles Gluck, first surgeon to perform a "Total Knee Replacement".

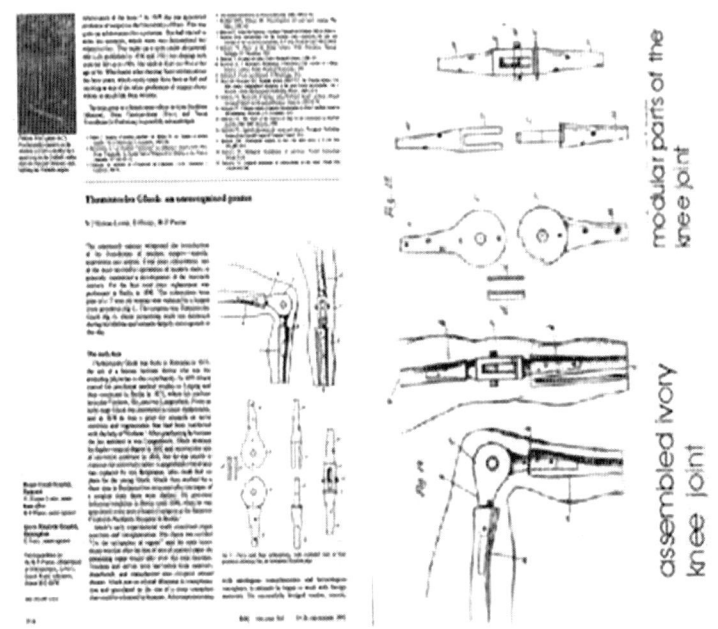

Gluck's classic paper describing his ivory hinge fixed with pumice and POP as cement.

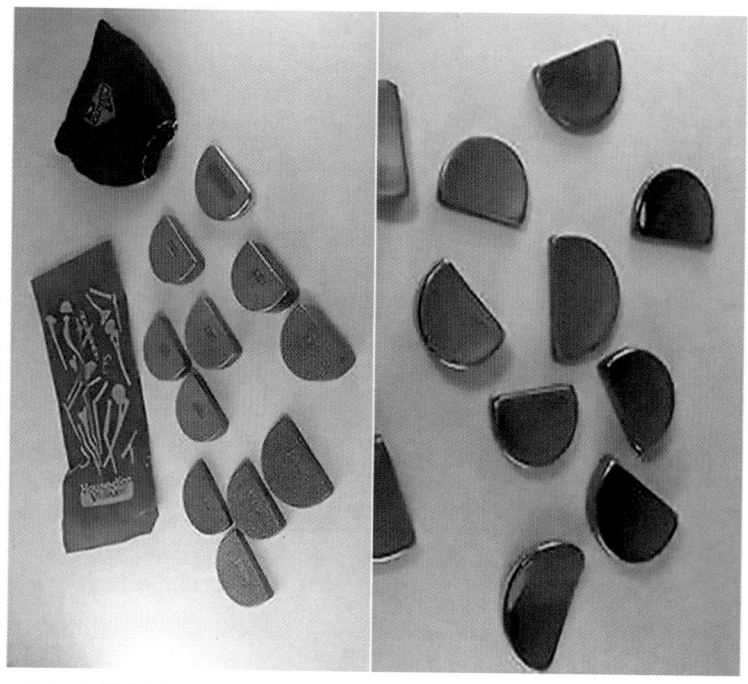

Macintosh tibial buttons. Original implants from Dr Prakash's collection.

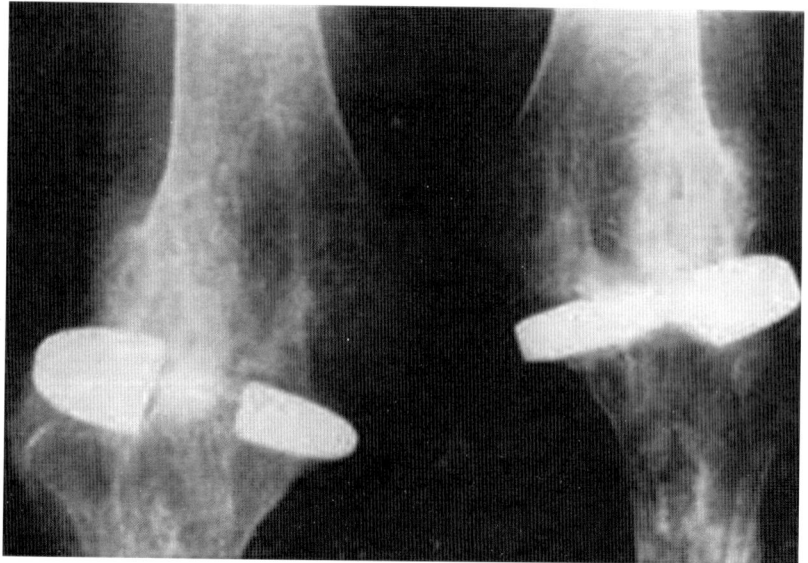

Failure of Macintosh buttons at six years. Surprising that it lasted for six years.

In the early 1950s, Walldius, Shiers, Guiepar, etc. developed hinges to replace both the femoral and tibial surfaces simultaneously and achieved limited success. These and their modifications are even now being regularly used in tertiary revisions, tumour resections, and customized mega prosthesis surgeries.

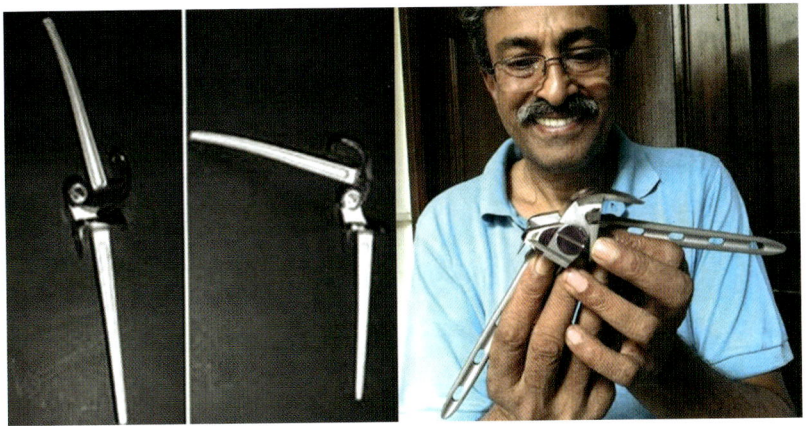

Walldius hinge prosthesis from the author's collection.

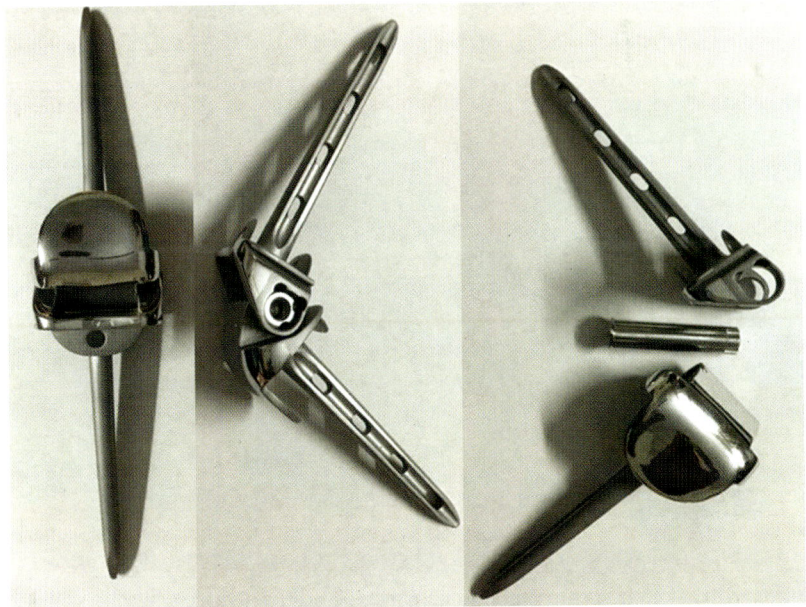

In condylar replacement knee prostheses, the femoral and tibial hemiarthroplasty surfaces are replaced with non-connected artificial components. Work on the design of an implant that resurfaced the distal femur and proximal tibia without any direct

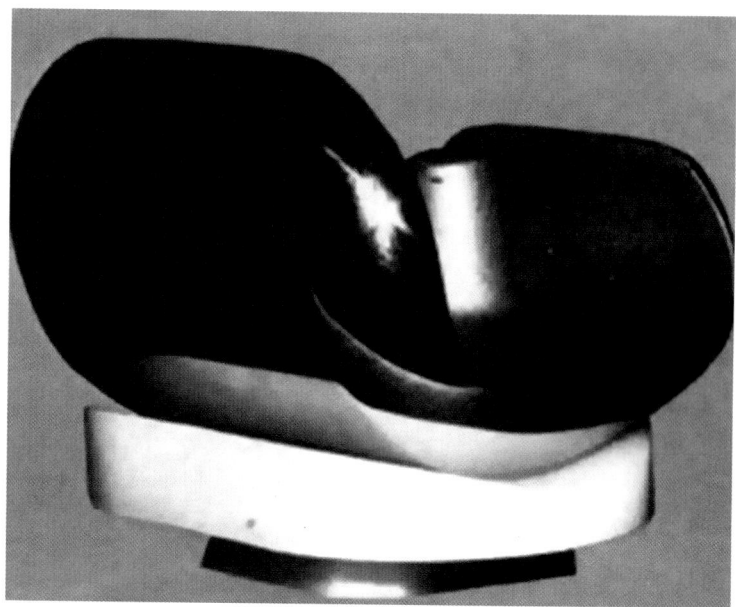

The original Freeman Swanson total knee replacement.

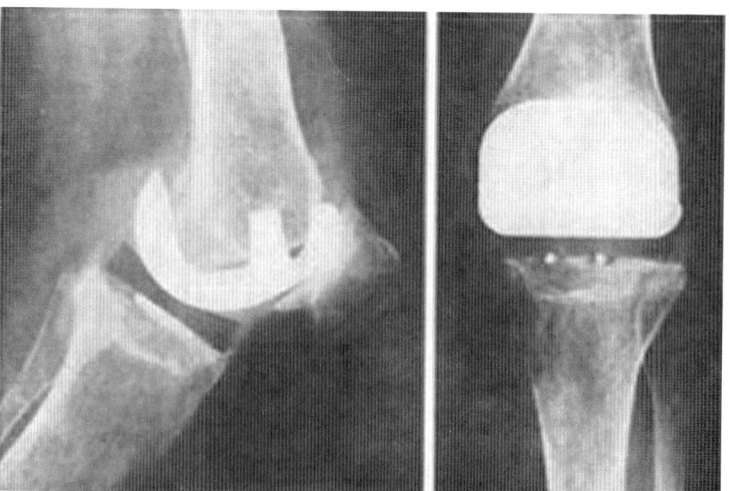

A Freeman Swanson knee surviving for 17 years. Remarkable indeed!

mechanical link between the components began at the end of the 1960s at the Imperial College, London. The original design, known as Freeman-Swanson prosthesis, consisted of a metal "roller" placed on the distal femur that articulated with a polyethylene tibial tray and required resection of both cruciate ligaments.

Gunston can be really called the father of modern knee replacements. In 1971, he developed minimally constrained cemented surface replacements with plastic articulating with metal based on Charnley's concepts. These met with generous success and heralded the start of a new era of knee replacements.

With the success of the Gunston model in a limited way and with increasing knowledge of the mode of its failure, newer models were developed.

Increasing research into bio-mechanics, modern computer controlled design applications, advances in metallurgical and plastic technology and an evidence-based assessment of the performance and failure pattern of the implanted knees studied over a period of years gave an insight into the modern design of knee replacements.

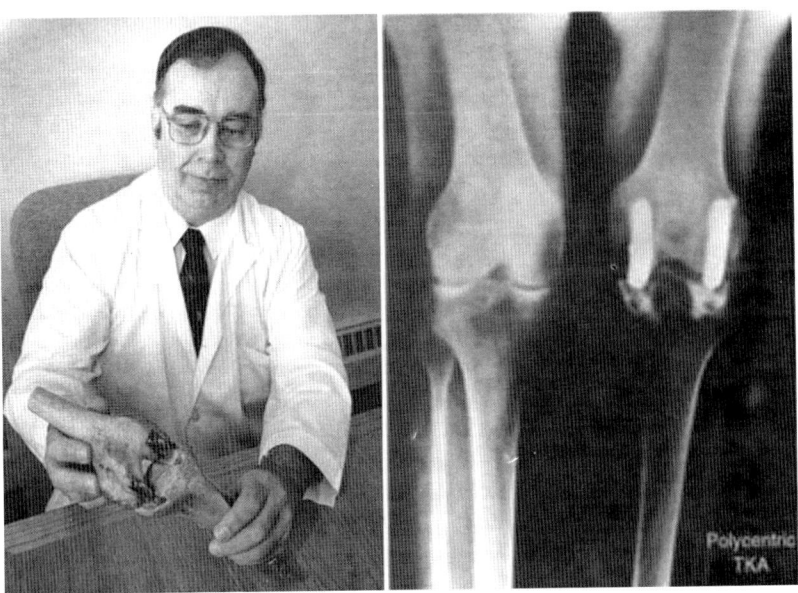

Gunston is considered the father of modern knee replacements.

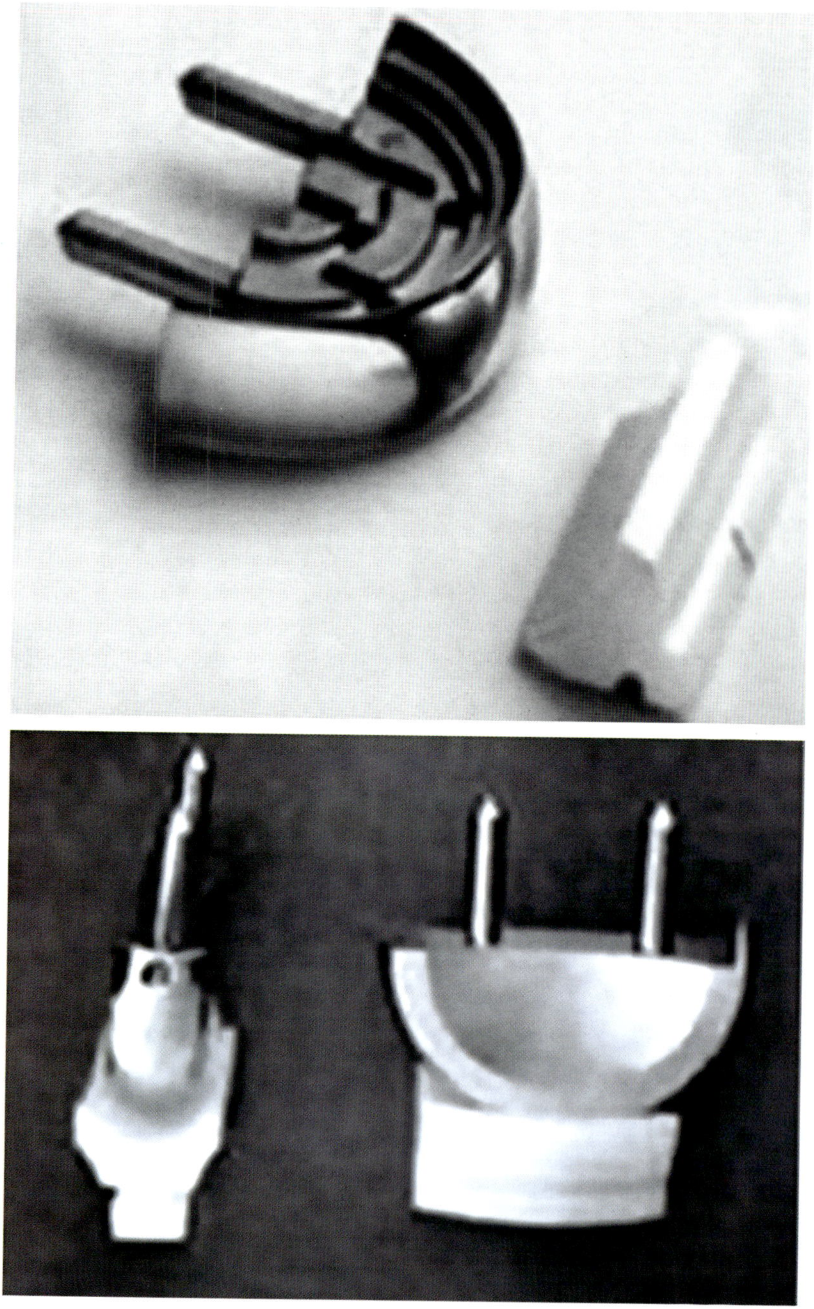

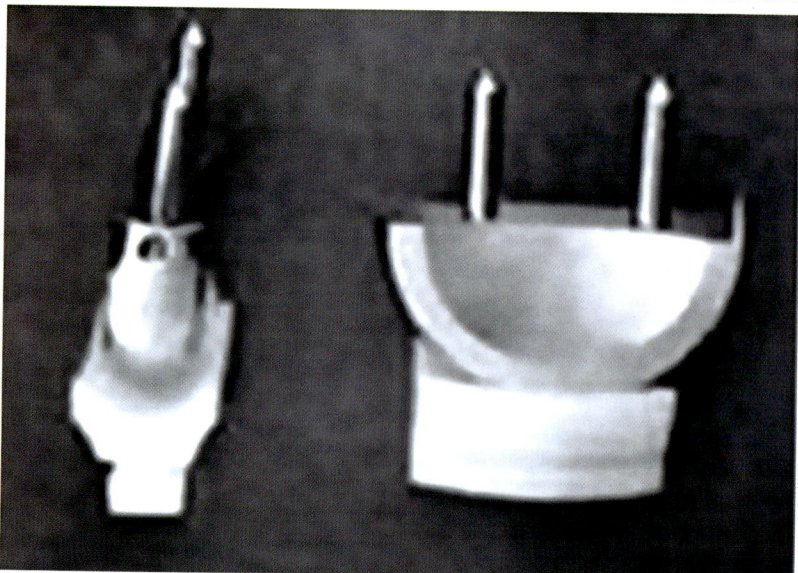

The original Gunston Knee. Copied from the internet and not from the author's personal collection.

The following chart chronicles the development of knee replacements from 1940 till now (2016).

Hemiarthroplasties of the knee, femoral replacements	
1940, Willis Campbell: Vitallium prosthesis for the distal end of femur	Four cases. Early satisfactory results. Abandoned because of poor medium term results. In hindsight, cause of failure fully attributable to complete resection of cruciates.
1952, Lachertez: Acrylic femoral endo prosthesis	Described as the treatment of ankylosed knees!
1954. Kraft and Levinthall: Acrylic prosthesis	Good short term results. Initially for Giant cell tumour.
1967, Jones: Vitallium distal femoral prosthesis	Few publications with good 3- to 5-year results
1954, DePalma: Tibial plateau replacement	One of the earliest reported tibial replacements.
1955, Maceever	Tibial plateau replacement with a metallic ledge polished on one surface and a flange for fixation into the cancellous tibia.
1958, McIntosh	Uni- or bi-compartmental tibial replacement with a D shaped plate with rough underside and polished upper side for femoral articulation.
1964, Townley	Tibial replacement anchored with screws

Total knee replacements	
1950, Majnoni d'Intignano	Hinged acrylic knee prosthesis, which for the first time replaced both femoral and tibial surfaces. Unsuccessful in outcome.
1954, Moeys	Experimental study of hinged prosthesis on dogs. Limited success, but his efforts were the forerunner for later models of hinged prostheses.
1957, Walldius	Hinged acrylic prosthesis, later changed to hinged VITALLIUM prosthesis. Good short-term results and poor long-term results.

(Contd.)

Total knee replacements (*Contd.*)

1961, Shiers	Hinged prosthesis with a long intramedullary stem for cementless fixation. Same problems as Walldius hinge.
1963, Young	Hinge prosthesis.
1973, Maza	The Guepar hinge knee prosthesis.
1973, Gunston	Father of modern total knee replacements. He described a cemented non constrained knee arthroplasty: Two independent polycentric metallic runners cemented to the lower part of femur that articulated with two plastic tibial bearings. He published the results of his first 224 cases. This was by far the most successful knee to be designed till that date.
1973–1978, Marmor, Savastano, Cavendish, Shaw and Chaterlee	Modifications of the Gunston knee! More anatomic femoral components and better fitting tibial runners. Both cruciates were retained. Better instrumentation was designed for a more anatomic insertion of the prosthesis. Some of these knees did very well for short to medium term follow-up, whereas others failed fairly rapidly. The complexity of insertion, with retention of both cruciates, and the practical difficulties in restoration of the knee alignment resulted in some knees implanted perfectly and others not in a correct axis. The former survived for considerable periods giving good to excellent results.
1973, Ranawat and Shin	Moved from four components to three, by linking both the femoral condyles, but retaining the tibial bearings as separate units.
1973–1976, Coventry, Skolnick	First modern knee with a metal bridge between the femoral components and a ledge between the tibial components. Better instrumentation and operative principles towards alignment.

(*Contd.*)

Total knee replacements (*Contd.*)	
1973, Waugh	Designed the UCI prosthesis; the shapes were a bit more anatomic with a horseshoe shaped tibial component. This implant allowed some degree of rotation and roll back.
1978, Freeman and Swanson	An essential departure from the existing designs. The roller trough design with a thick tibial component. Possibly one of the first knees to have an anterior flange to the femoral component for accommodating the patellar articulation. Finned HDPE pegs for immediate weight bearing in a cementless situation without depending on bone ingrowth.
1979, Insall and colleagues	First total condylar knee design with a patellar resurfacing button; the generic knee on which most knee designs are based somewhat roughly.
1980–1990	Kenna and Hungerford describe universal instrumentation. Cementless designs, porous coating, hydroxyapatite coating, meniscal bearing, revision stems, etc.
1990–2000	Kyocera Bisurface knee, Medial pivot knee, 3D knee, LCS knee
2000–2010	High flex knee, Biphasic knee, Ceramic femoral components
2010 to the present	Oxidized zirconium coating, oxinium ceramic coating, mobile bearing posterior stabilized, single medial pivot knees, single radius high flex knees.

HEMIARTHROPLASTIES: FEMORAL REPLACEMENTS

In 1940, Willis Campbell introduced Vitallium prosthesis for the distal end of femur. He did four cases with early satisfactory results, but the procedure was abandoned because of poor medium term results. In hindsight, cause of failure was fully attributable to complete resection of cruciates.

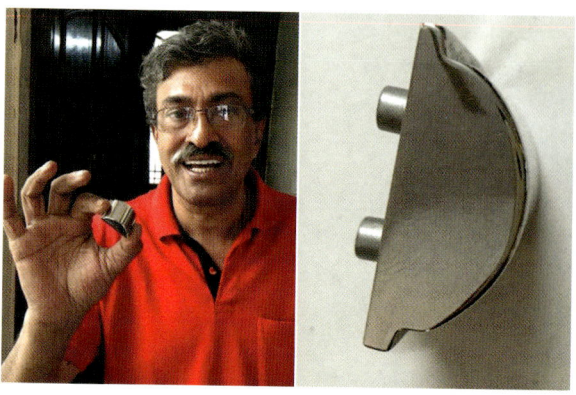

Campbell's original prosthesis made by Howmedica in 1940s. One of my prized collectibles.

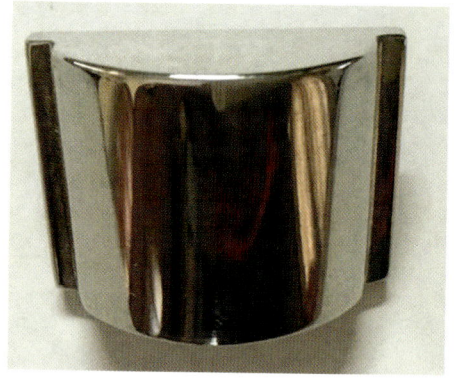

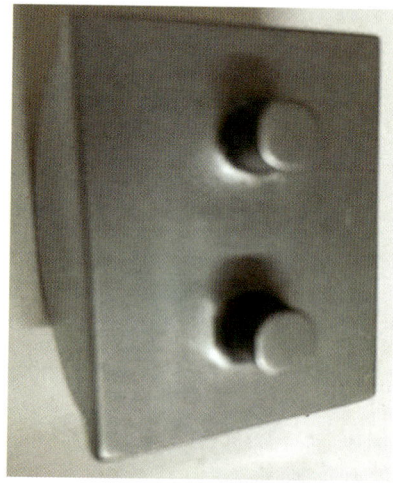

Campbell's Vitallium prosthesis.

Vitallium was just then introduced in orthopaedic surgery; his concept and design were far ahead of his time.

In 1952, Lachertez introduced an acrylic femoral endoprosthesis. He described it for the treatment of ankylosed knees! Just like Judet hips, these too met with spectacular initial success and disastrous consequences in 12 to 18 months.

In 1954, Kraft and Levinthall devised an acrylic prosthesis which was first used for a Giant cell tumour of the lower end of femur. They then expanded the indications to include fused knees, with results similar to those of Lachertez.

In 1967, Jones introduced a Vitallium distal femoral prosthesis. A few publications showed good 3- to 5-year results. This was one of the earliest successful total knees of those times.

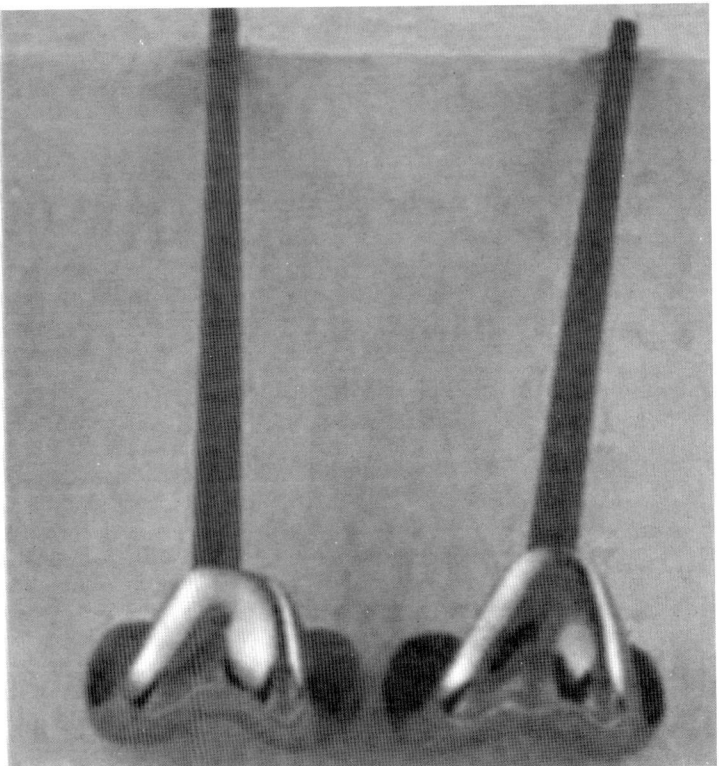

Jones's Cobalt chrome femoral hemiarthroplasty. Surprisingly the component looks very much like a modern TKR.

HEMIARTHROPLASTIES: TIBIAL REPLACEMENTS

In 1954, DePalma replaced the tibial plateau. This was one of the earliest reported tibial surface replacements.

In 1955, McKeever described a tibial plateau replacement with a metallic ledge polished on one surface and a flange for fixation into the cancellous tibia on the other.

In 1958, MacIntosh described both uni- and bi-compartmental tibial replacement with a D-shaped stainless steel plate having a rough underside and polished upper side for femoral articulation. This met with limited success and provided pain relief for 5 to 7 years, especially for varus knees.

In 1964, Townley invented a tibial replacement anchored with screws. This too met with initial limited success.

However, by now it was understood that hemi replacements for knee were bound to fail, and the need for designs replacing both femoral and tibial surfaces was understood.

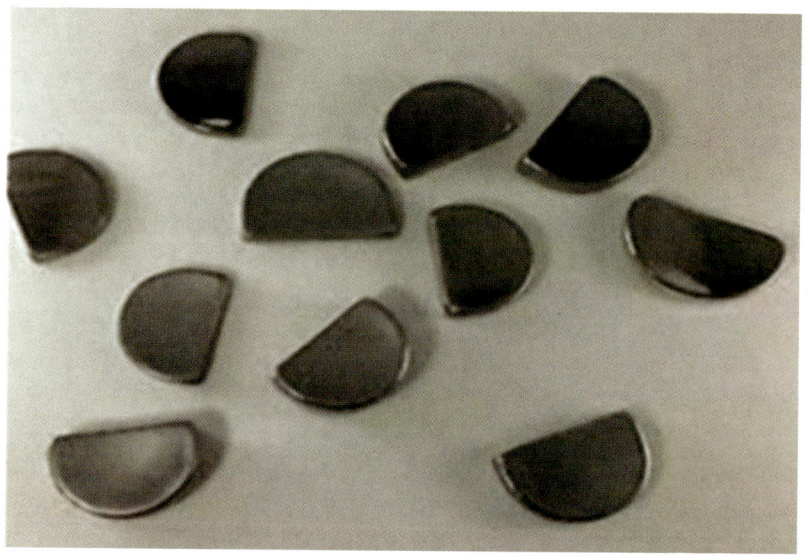

MacIntosh buttons.

TOTAL KNEE REPLACEMENTS

In 1950, Mainoni d'Intignano described his hinged acrylic knee prosthesis which, for the first time, replaced both femoral and tibial surfaces. However, this was a failure and abandoned.

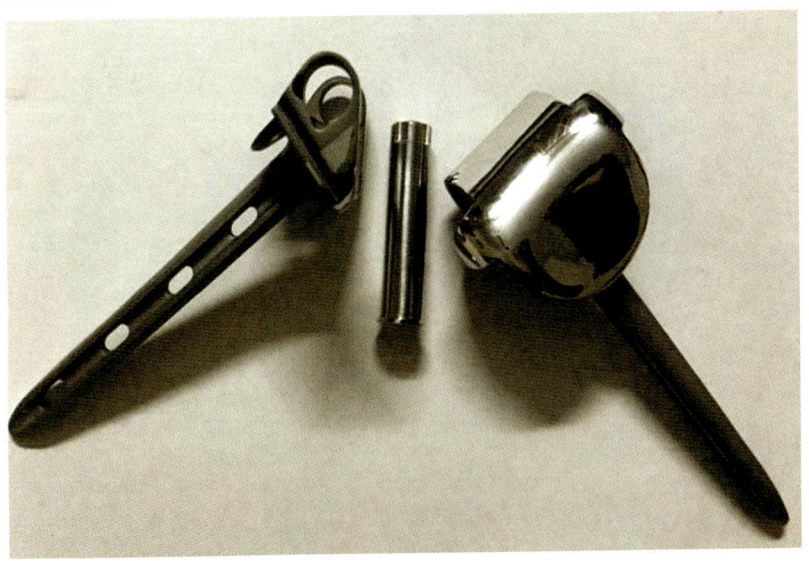

The original Walldius hinge.

In 1954, Moeys published results of his animal experiments and probably produced the first prototype (which was a simple hinge) of a working total knee. His meticulously documented study on hinge prostheses in dogs was the forerunner of modern knee replacements.

Between 1957 and 1963, Walldius, Shiers and Young independently devised almost similar designs of Vitallium hinge prostheses with intramedullary stems. These knees enjoyed limited success in some patients, while they lasted for as long as 20 years in others!

In 1973, Maza described his hinge with good medium term results. The constrained hinge thus became an acceptable design and is in use even today.

Again, in 1973, Gunston described a cemented non constrained knee arthroplasty. His design had two independent polycentric polished runners cemented to the lower femur, articulating with two cemented tibial bearings.

He retained both cruciates. Though not successful in all cases, in most it provided sustained pain relief without significant loss of motion. Gunston should thus be rightly called the father of modern knee replacements.

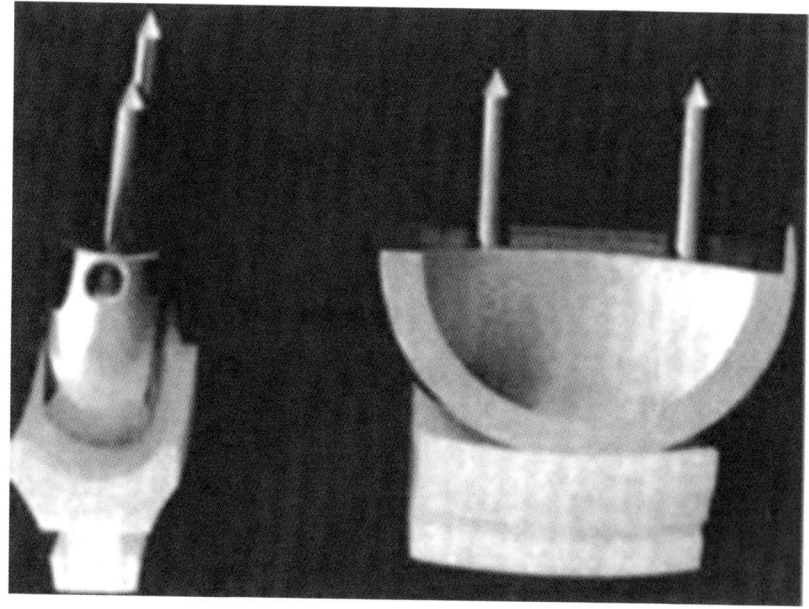

The original Gunston knee prosthesis.

From 1973 to 1978 came modifications by Marmor, Savastano, Cavendish, Shaw and Chaterlee. They designed more anatomically accurate femoral components and better fitting tibial runners. Both cruciates were retained. Better instrumentation was designed for a more anatomic insertion of the prosthesis. Some of these knees did very well for short to medium term follow-up, whereas others failed fairly rapidly.

The complexity of insertion with retention of both cruciates, and the practical difficulties in restoration of the knee alignment resulted in some implants placed perfectly and others not in a correct axis. The former survived for considerable periods, giving good to excellent results at 10 to 20 years.

The anatomical approach uses prostheses that preserve both cruciate ligaments, allowing the femur to roll back on the tibia. Yamamoto, from the Okayama University Medical School in Japan, was the first to report implanting an anatomical femoral component with a minimally constrained single-piece polyethylene tibial component in 1970.

Called the Kodama-Yamamoto knee, it consisted of an anatomical femoral mold component, including an anterior

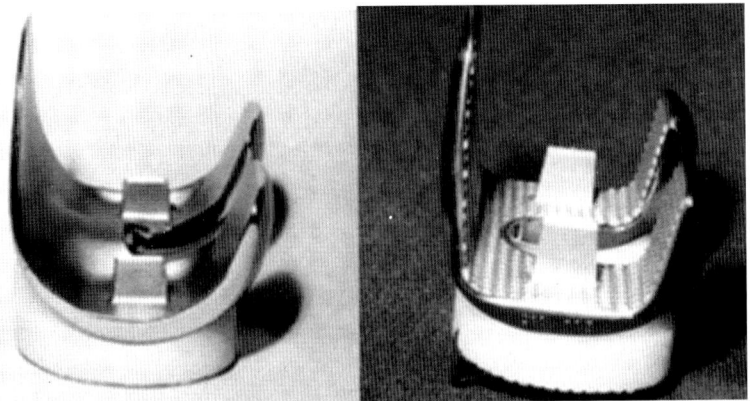

The Kodama-Yamamoto mark one and two knees.

femoral flange, made of COP alloy (Co, Cr, Ni, Mo, C, and P). There was a one-piece, mildly dished polyethylene tibial component with a central cutout for preservation of both cruciate ligaments. He also designed an instrumentation set to give perfect reproducible cuts.

Others authors who followed the same approach were Waugh (in 1973 at the University of California UCI), Townley (in 1974 with the cemented anatomical knee) and Sheedom (who designed the Leeds knee around the same time).

Each of these prostheses had a horseshoe shaped tibial component with a space behind and centrally for the retention of both anterior and posterior cruciate ligaments.

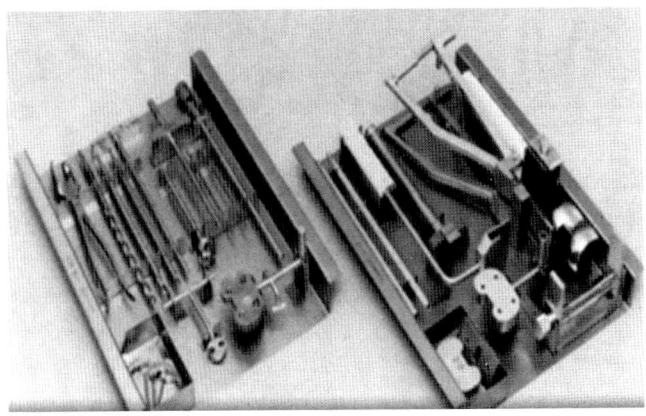

The original Kodama-Yamamoto knee instrumentation set.

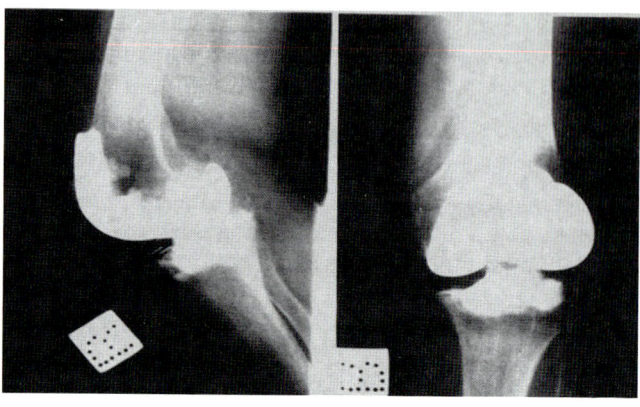

X-ray of a Townley total knee.

During the early 1970s, the Duocondylar knee was redesigned at the HSS with an anatomical and symmetrical design and renamed Duopatellar.

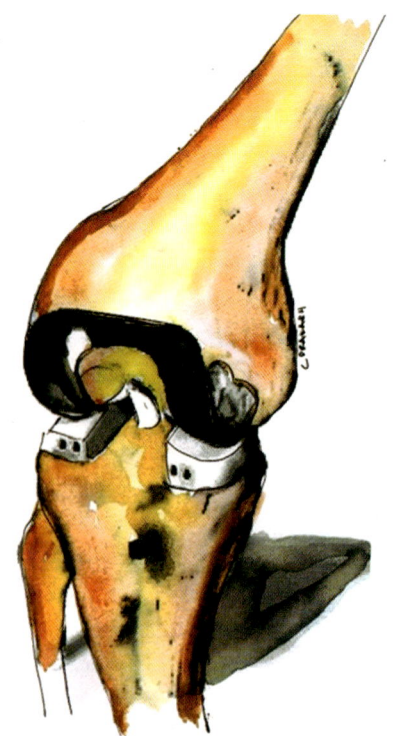

The Duocondylar knee.

An anterior femoral flange, patellar button, and a more dished tibial surface were added. The tibial component had a fixation peg, identical to the Total Condylar, the archetype of the functional approach, and, for the first time, a posterior rectangular cutout, specifically designed for the preserved posterior cruciate ligament.

Meanwhile in Boston, Robert Breck developed his own design of posterior cruciate sparing knee implant in which the medial tip of the femoral trochlear flange was removed, creating right and left designs based on the asymmetry of the proximal femoral flange. This was done to reduce the medial overhang seen in small female rheumatoid patients. The posterior cruciate-sparing version of the Robert Brigham Hospital would later evolve into the PFC knee (Cintor Division of Codman; later, Depuy, Johnson & Johnson).

In 1973, Ranawat and Shin simplified the design by reducing the components from four to three. They linked both femoral condyles, while tibial bearings were separate for medial and lateral compartments.

By 1976, Coventry and Skolnick had introduced the two component design, the father of the current day condylar designs. Waugh too devised a similar two component arthroplasty system.

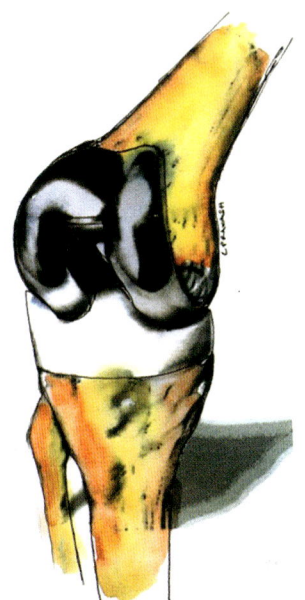

The Coventry knee, father of modern knee design.

In 1978, Mike Freeman introduced a design which was a tangential shift from earlier designs. A roller trough single radius femoral articulation, a thick tibial bearing and some sort of tibial midline constraint were combined with a deep patellar flange. His components were uncemented and depended on exact bone cuts for maximum surface contact. In addition, the components were affixed to the cancellous bone by self-locking finned HDPE pegs, screwed into the components.

These knees have an 80% survival at 20 to 25 years. I had the good fortune of learning my knee replacement from Mr. Freeman himself.

In 1979, the modern knee was born. John Insall and his colleagues designed a total condylar knee and a patellar button for resurfacing the under surface of patella. This met with spectacular success. Later, they introduced a tibial constraint, with introduction of a posterior stabilized knee. This is the design on which most current knees are based.

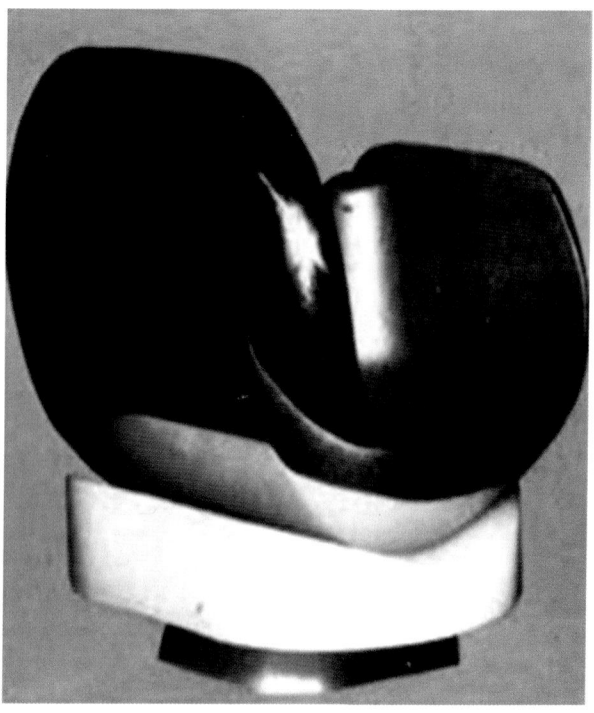

Freeman Swanson knee replacement.

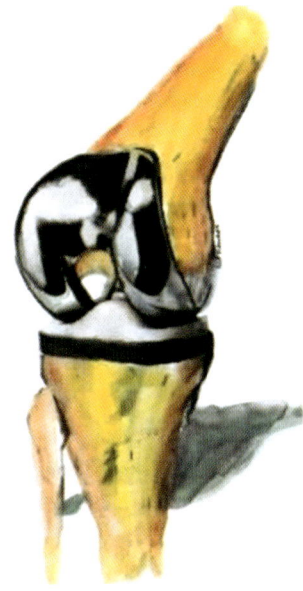

The total condylar knee.

At the same time, Peter Walker, Clement Sledge and Fred Ewald continued the Duo-patella concept in the posterior cruciate retaining version of the Kinematic knee (Howmedica),

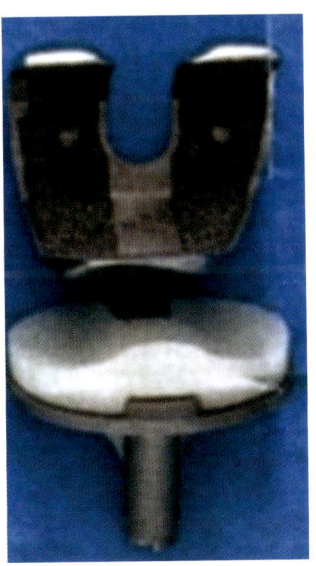

Kinemax Plus systems from Howmedica.

which was introduced by Ewald in June 1978. This later evolved into the posterior cruciate sparing version of the Kinematic II, Kinemax, and Kinemax Plus systems (Howmedica).

The 1980s saw significant advances in knee arthroplasty, particularly in the area of surgical technique and instrumentation. Kenna, Hungerford, and Krackow participated in the design of instruments that were later called Universal Instruments. Their instruments were based on the anatomical concept of measured resection rather than the more functional approach of creating equal and parallel flexion and extension gaps which were being used until then.

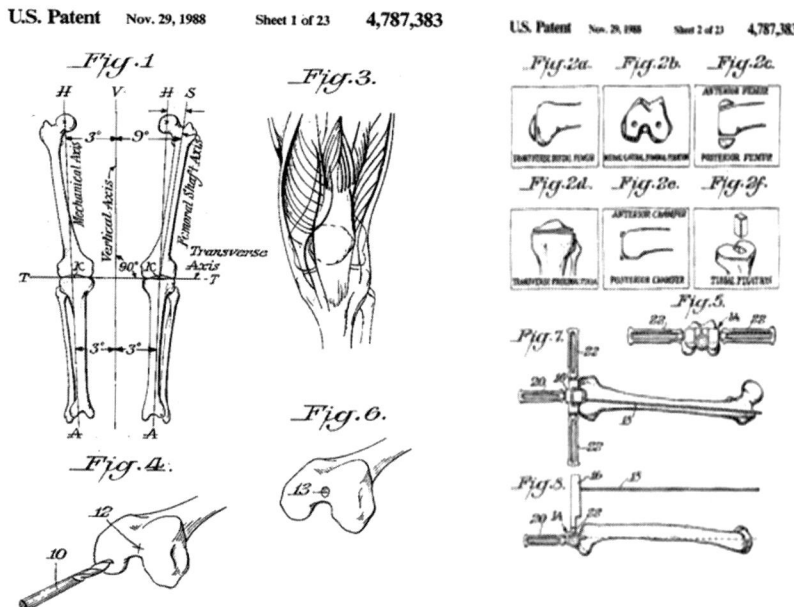

Drawings from Kenna's US Patent application.

The principal aspect of this new concept was that the bone and cartilage removed were to equal the thickness of the prosthetic material replacing them.

The drawings submitted by Dr Kenna for his US Patent are extremely interesting are reproduced below.

Until this time, fixation of the condylar total knee was primarily achieved with cement.

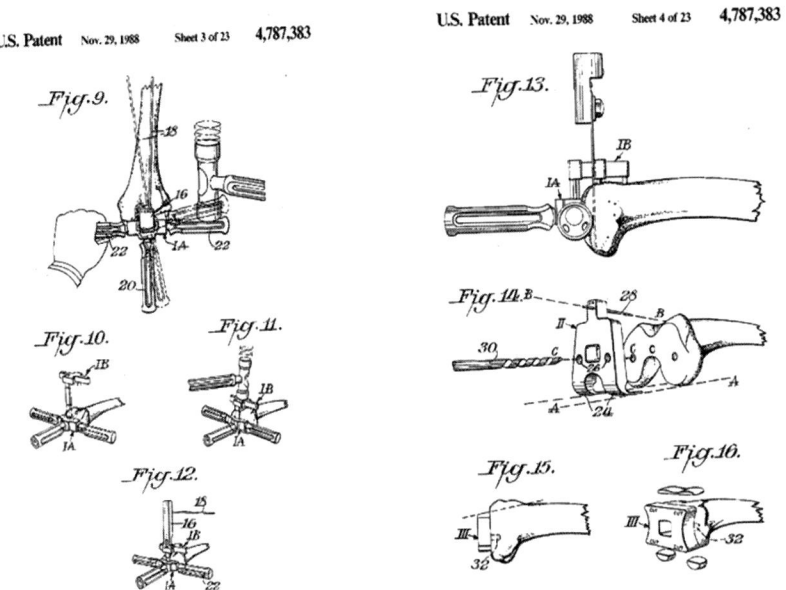

These universal instruments form the basis of most of today's instrumentation sets.

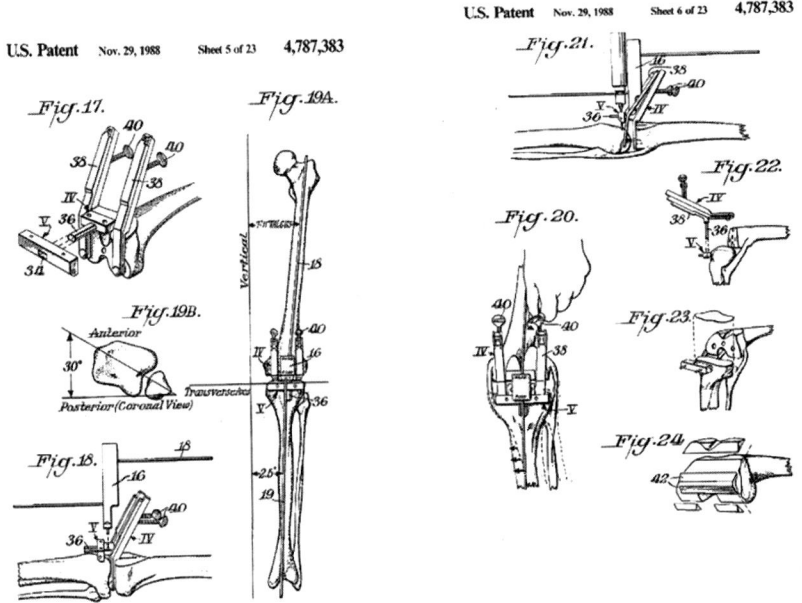

Instruments for distal, femoral and upper tibial cuts.

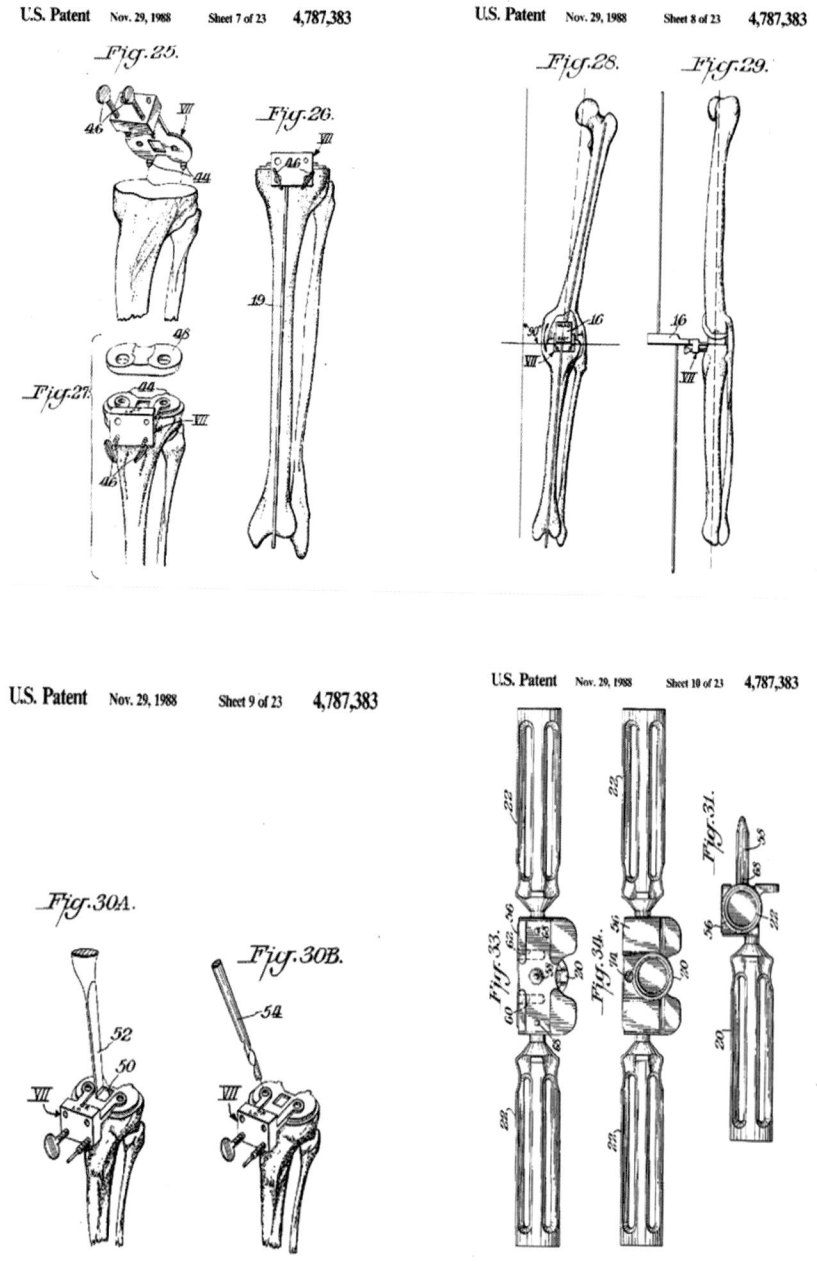

Various jigs and positioning devices.

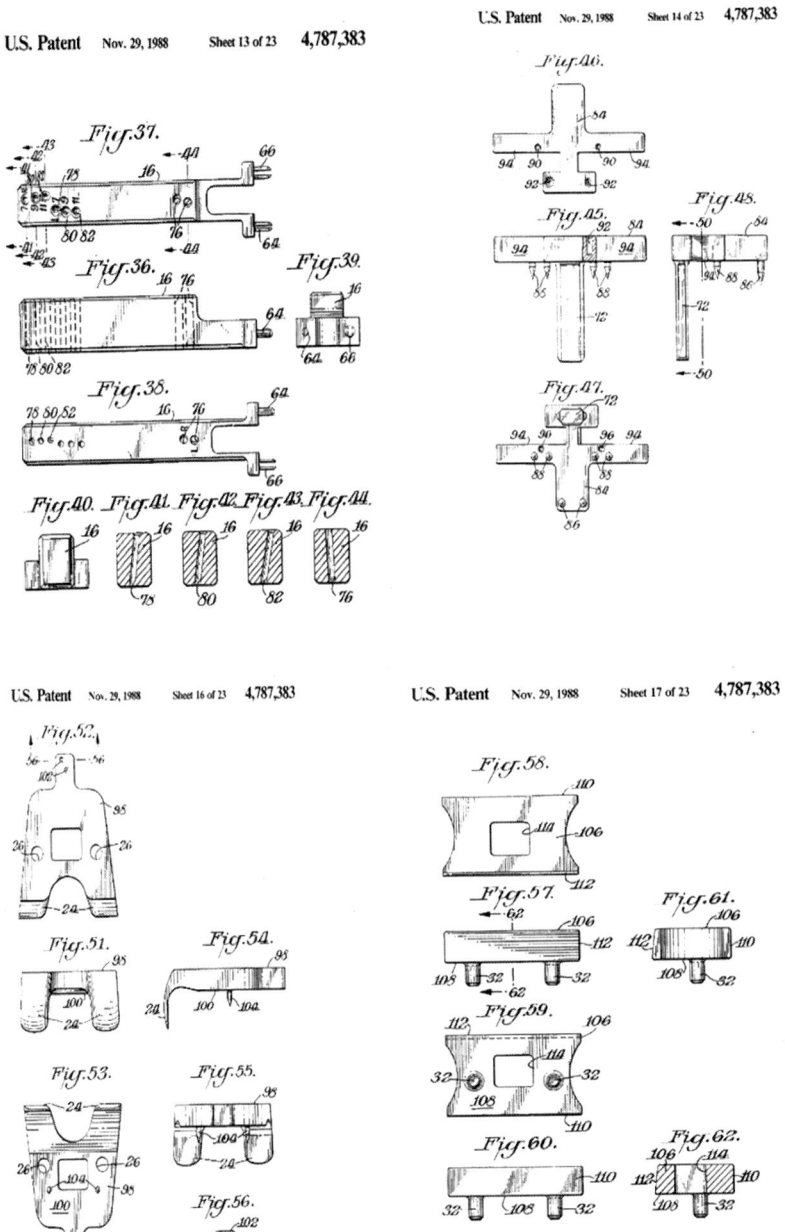

Trial prostheses and measuring jigs.

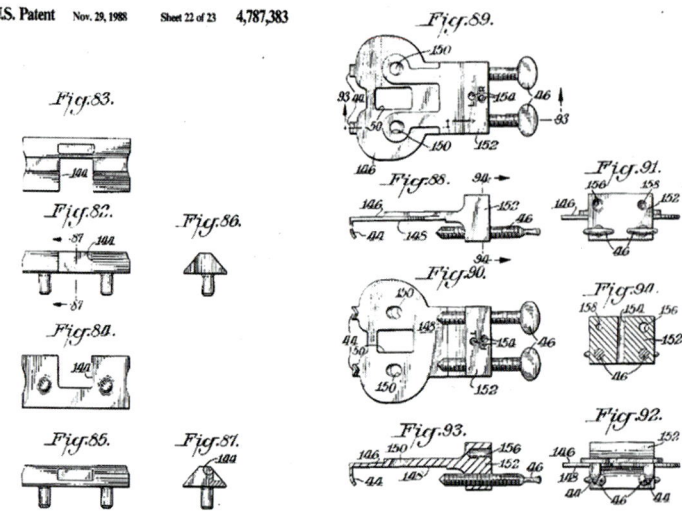

U.S. Patent   Nov. 29, 1988   Sheet 22 of 23   4,787,383

In January 1980, the first Porous-Coated Anatomical Knee (PCA) was implanted by Hungerford at Johns Hopkins. The implant was anatomical with asymmetric medial and lateral femoral condyles (similar to the Leeds and the original Townley designs). However, for the first time, it introduced porous coating in a total condylar knee for a cementless fixation.

Each of the three components was backed with metal and had a 1.5 mm thick sintered porous coating of cobalt chrome beads.

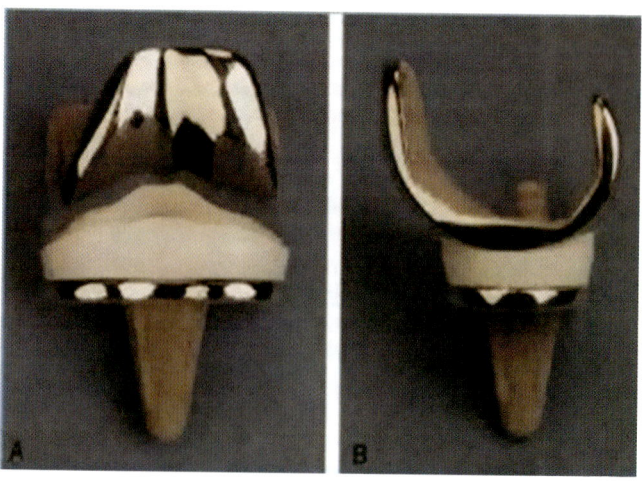

The porous coated anatomic knee.

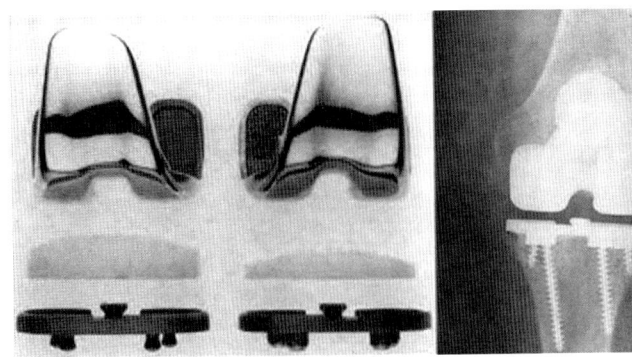

The Miller Galante knee.

The Miller-Galante total knee, one of the first knee replacements designed for use with cement or cementless fixation, was first implanted in 1986. The principal innovation of this implant was the choice of a titanium fibre composite for the bony ingrowth surface, because of its well-recognized biocompatibility, and the use of a Titanium, Aluminium and Vanadium alloy (Ti_6Al_4V).

The implant was fixed to the tibia with titanium screws and pegs. The uncemented version for patellar resurfacing consisted of a metal-backed patella fixed with fibre-mesh pegs. Modularity of tibial polyethylene inserts was introduced to allow better ligamentous tension and possibility of future isolated polyethylene replacement.

"Cruciate retaining" prostheses developed from the anatomical concept were all different; some consisted of a

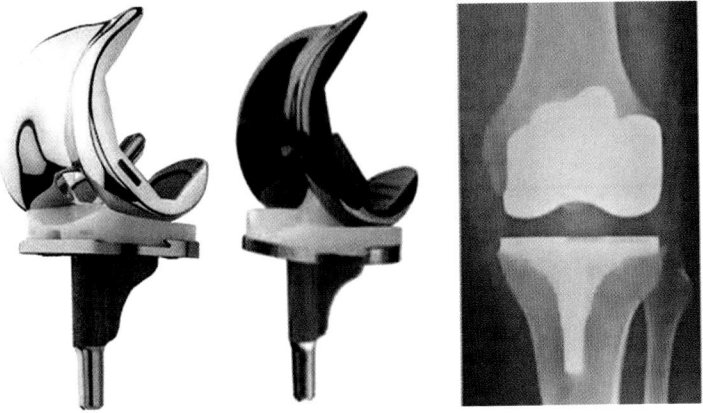

The Genesis II knee.

relatively flat surface on the sagittal and transversal plane (Kinemax, PCA) while others maintained a more congruent surface on the sagittal plane. Genesis II (Smith & Nephew), Duracon (Howmedica), Nexgen CR (Zimmer), PFC CR (Depuy) represent some actual examples of this conception.

The functional approach simplifies the knee biomechanics by removing both cruciate ligaments. The first system derived from the functional concept is represented by the Total Condylar prosthesis developed in 1973 at the Hospital for Special Surgery of New York.

The Total Condylar prosthesis consisted of two symmetric condylar surfaces with a posterior decreasing radius of curvature and an articular surface made of polyethylene, perfectly congruent in extension and partially congruent in flexion.

The Total Condylar Knee would prove to be highly successful, widely used, and would later demonstrate long survival. Two concerns, however, pointed out the early failures of its clinical use. The femoral component would shift forward, particularly in flexion. In rare cases, this would even result in tibial loosening or anterior dislocation. The second concern was the limited flexion achieved. Average knee flexion was about 90°.

In 1978, the Insall-Burstein prosthesis was designed to correct these problems by replacing the posterior cruciate ligament with a mechanical lock to reduce posterior translation of the femoral

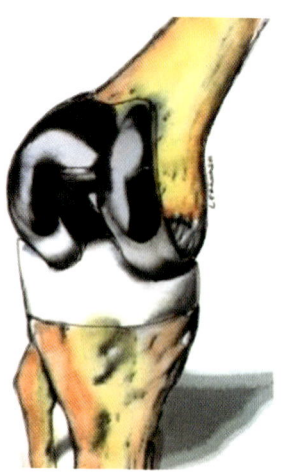 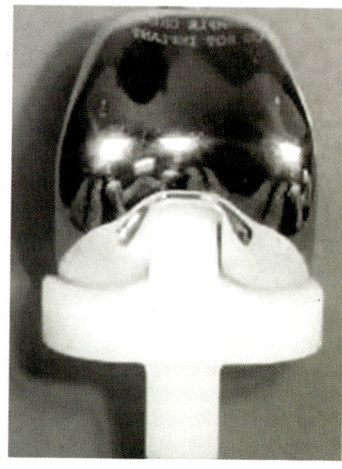

The IB II prosthesis.

component by using a mechanism of a cam articulated with a post on the tibial component.

The cam of the femoral component connected with the tibial central spine at about 70° of flexion and then the femur could roll-back so to increase flexion. The first Insall Burstein Posterior Stabilized knee, implanted in 1978 by Insall at the HSS, became one of the most successful total condylar knee designs. Anterior femoral subluxation was eliminated and average flexion reached up to 115°. A metal-backed monoblock tibial component with direct-molded polyethylene was introduced in November 1980: the Insall-Burstein Modular knee.

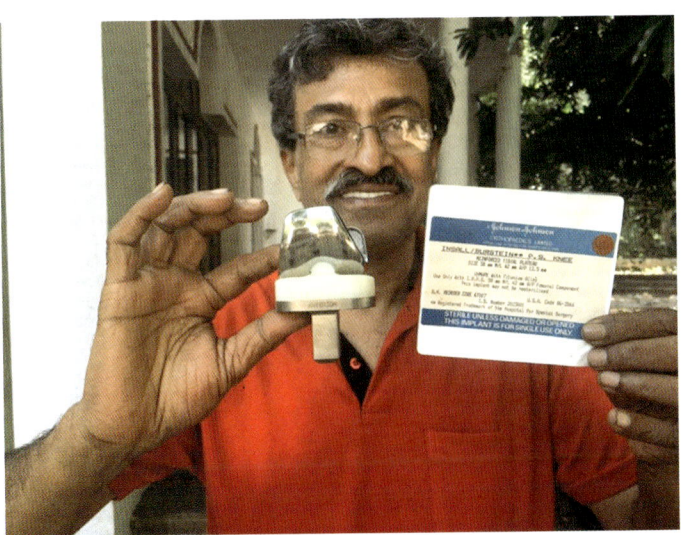

The Insall-Burstein two knee in its original packing.

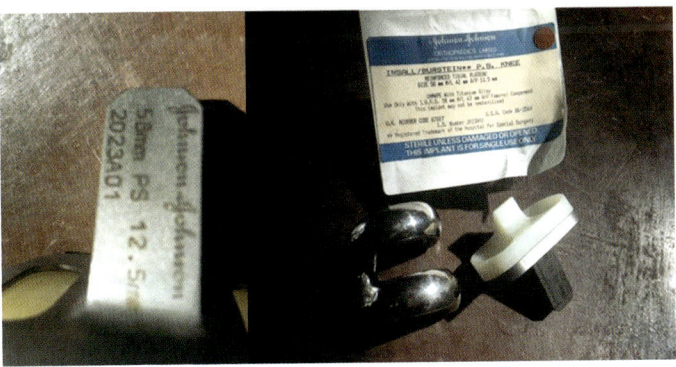

The HSS posterior-stabilized knee design would evolve into the Insall-Burstein Modular (IBPS II) knee in 1988, the Optetrak Posterior-Stabilized knee (Exactech) in 1994, and the Advance Posterior-Stabilized knee (Wright Medical) in 1994.

In the 1980s and 1990s, many variations of these functional designs were introduced by different manufacturers. All of them had features to produce their movements through a so-called *guided motion*, which means that some characteristics of the motion, such as rollback, were produced by mechanical interaction between the femoral and tibial components.

In the Kyocera Bi-Surface knee (Akagi et al., 2000), the knee behaves as a standard condylar replacement with moderately conforming bearing surfaces for the major part of the flexion range. Beyond that, the load is transferred to a spherical surface protruding behind from the femoral intercondylar region, contacting within a spherical depression at the posterior of the plastic tibial component.

Another example of guided motion knee is The Medial Pivot knee (Wright Mfg. Co.). In that prosthesis, the femoral component owns a single radius of femoral curvature and a high level of conformity in the medial compartment where a ball-and-socket configuration is present.

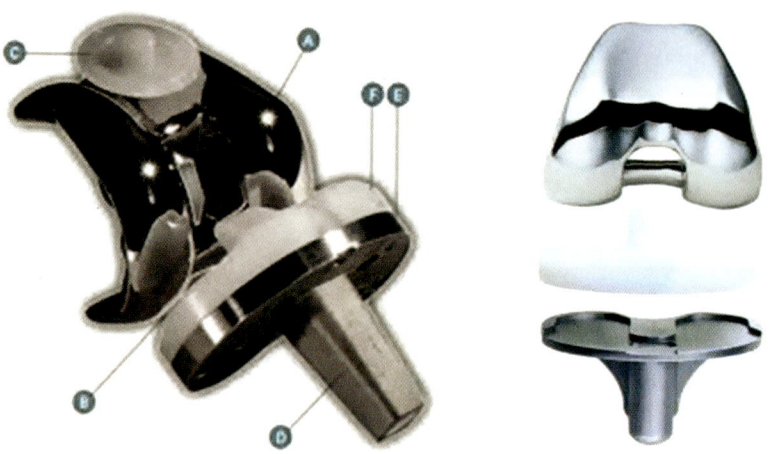

Optetrak and advance posterior stabilized knees.

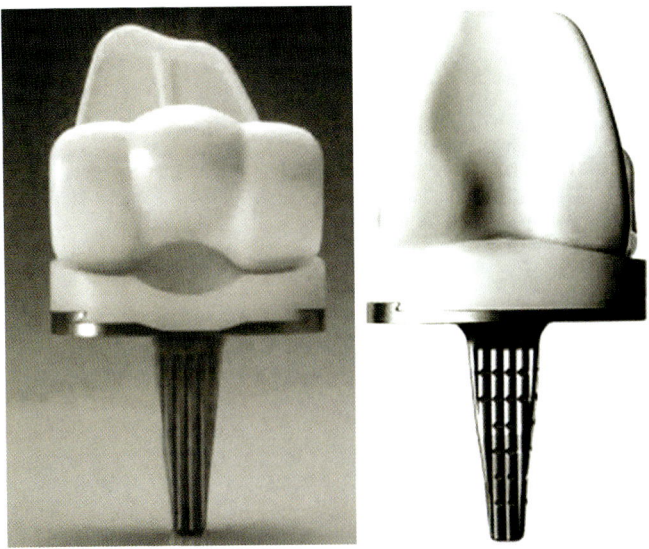

The Kyocera bi-surface knee.

Because of its configuration, the medial side remains in the same position during flexion, but the lateral femoral condyle can displace behind with flexion. The purpose of the medial pivot design is to reproduce a more physiological kinematics.

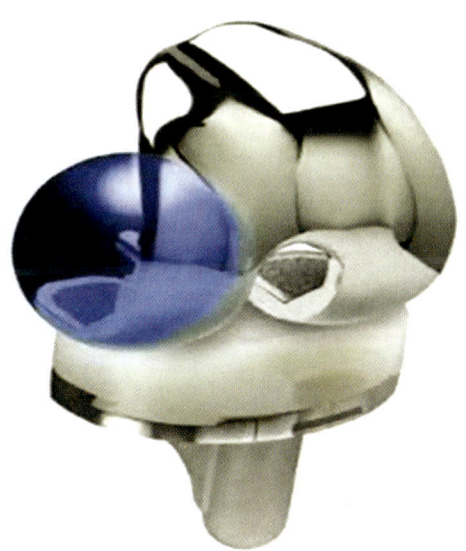

The medial pivot knee.

In contrast with this type of solution, a new design has recently been introduced in the market: the 3D knee which provides A/P stability similar to ACL deficient valgus knees through a concave lateral compartment. The lateral compartment is fully congruent in extension and allows 15° of axial rotation. As the knee flexes, a greater range of femoral motion is possible, but is controlled by the concave lateral compartment. The aim of the 3D knee is then to accommodate and control the cruciate deficient patterns of motion without constraint in shape to reproduce the normal kinematics of the knee.

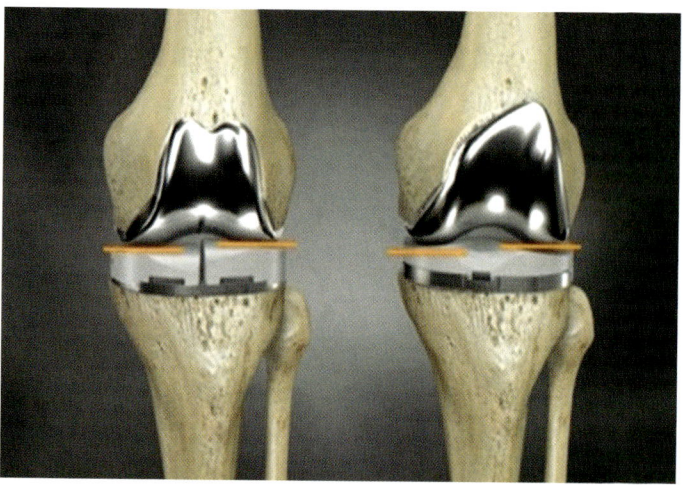

A 3D knee versus a conventional knee.

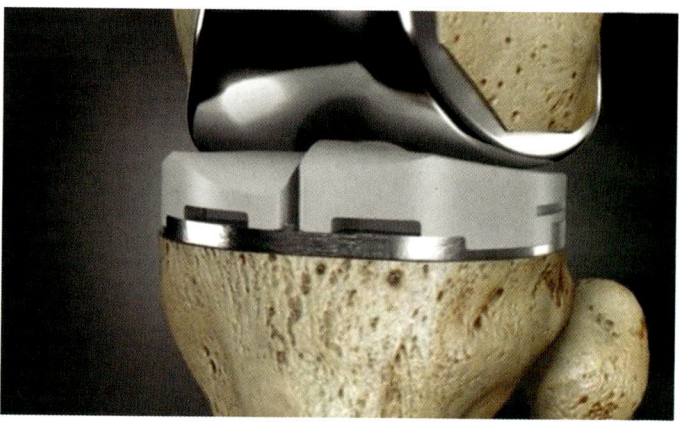

Implant design compensates cruciate deficiency.

One of the most innovative functional approaches to condylar total knee design evolved from a collaboration between Frederic Buechel, an orthopaedic surgeon at the New Jersey Medical School, and Michael Pappas, a professor of mechanical engineering. Their project to achieve low polyethylene contact stresses while maintaining knee flexion and avoiding overload of the implant bone interfaces started in 1977 (Buechel & Pappas, 1986) with the introduction of the Low Contact Stress (LCS) knee system.

It was the first complete systems approach to total knee replacement using meniscal bearing surfaces.

The principal characteristic of the femoral component was based on the same spherical surface on the mediolateral plane while a decreasing radius of curvature from extension to flexion was present on the lateral side. This shape maintained full area contact on the upper meniscal bearing from 0 to 45° (at which walking loads are encountered), and maintaining at least spherical line at deeper flexion angles.

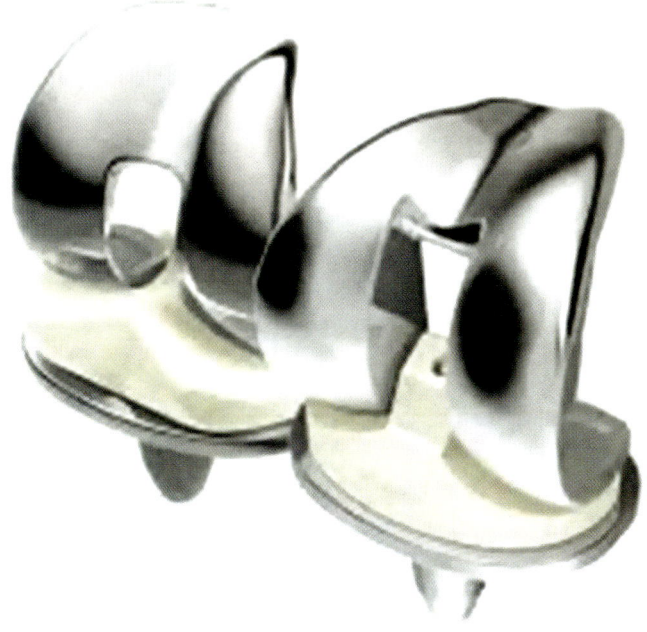

The LCS knee.

In its origin, the LCS was proposed as a system inclusive of both cruciate-sparing meniscal bearing and PCL-sacrificing rotating platform variant, with the latter gaining the majority of popular usage over time.

After the introduction of the LCS system, several types of mobile bearing knees were produced. They are categorized according to their conformity (partially or fully conforming), and a third group represented by the posterior stabilized MB.

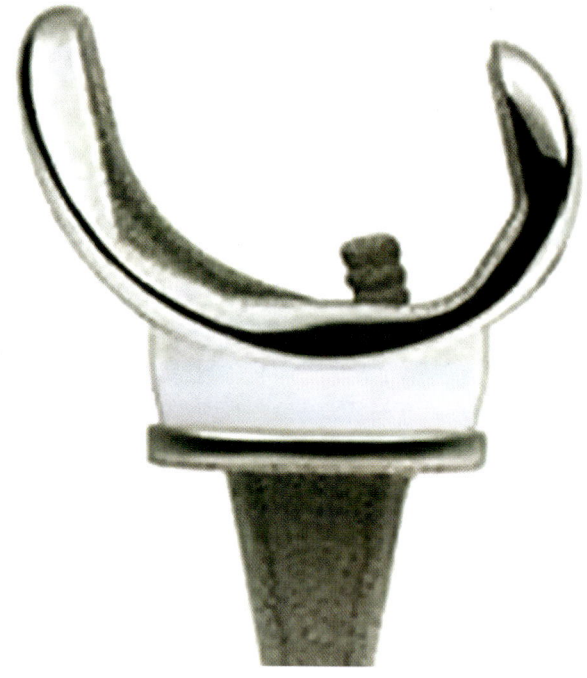

Full contact with the bearings during extension in LCS knees.

Partially conforming mobile bearing The LCS was the forerunner of all the MB prostheses that followed. Its second version (prototype of the partially conforming MB) had a single plastic bearing freely rotating about its post seated in a hole in the tibial tray.

The Self Aligning MB (Sulzer) designed by Bourne and Rorabeck in 1987 is also partially conforming. Its oval recess in the posterior aspect of the polyethylene allowed unlimited rotation and limited AP translation about a tibial tray peg.

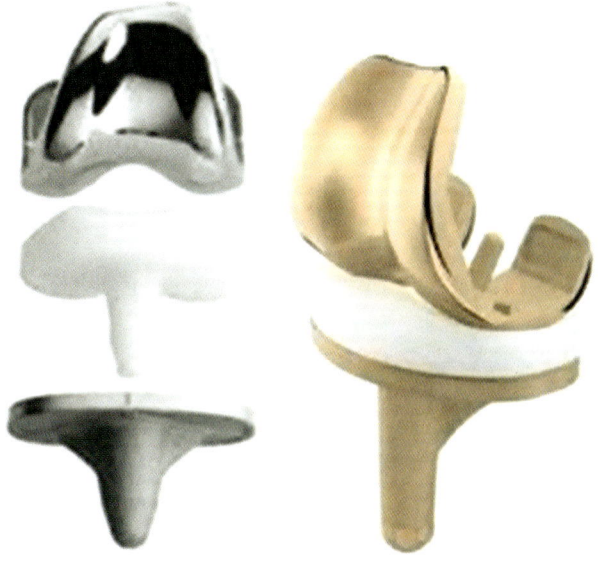

The self aligning rotating bearing.

The mobile bearing knee TACK (produced by Waldemar Link in Hamburg in 1990) is characterized by the tibial tray having two semicircular guides that engage circular tracks on both sides of the polyethylene platform, permitting wide rotational movement.

The Interax Integrated Secure Asymmetric (Howmedica) prosthesis has nearly fully conformity between femoral condyle and tibial surface in extension, but the conformity gradually decreases in flexion. The tibial base plate has two central posts that engage a curved, T-shaped guide track within the meniscal bearing.

In Italy, Prof. Ghisellini designed the Total Rotating Knee (TRK) (Cremascoli) characterized by a central tibia post projecting from the centre of the tibial tray.

Two types of plastic bearings were available: the R type (to allow freedom of rotation) was intended to be used in case of PCL excision, whereas the RS (allowing 10 mm of AP sliding and freedom of rotation) was indicated when PCL was retained.

Fully conforming mobile bearing The progenitor of fully conforming MB knees is certainly the Rotaglide total knee system

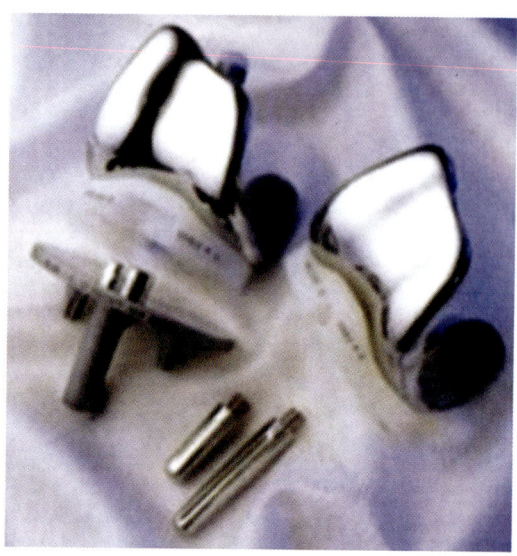

The Rotaglide TKR system.

(Corin, Cirencester, UK) designed in 1986 by Polyzoides and Tsakonas. The Rotaglide femoral component has a constant flexion radius of curvature in the femoro-meniscal articulation, each condyle being part of a sphere of diameter 24 mm. This design ensures that congruency is retained throughout the range of flexion. The mobile meniscal bearing has two undercuts which permit up to 5 mm of anteroposterior translation and 25° of rotation, 12.5° for each side.

The tibial plateau has an anterior bollard (that prevents anterior dislocation while restricting the rotation of the platform) and another bollard in the middle of the tray (that resists posterior dislocation).

The Medially Biased Kinematics (MBK) Knee was developed by J. Insall, P. Aglietti and P. Walker in 1992 (Fig. 10 a-b). The design concept of this prosthesis is complete conformity between the femoral component and the polyethylene insert at any degree of flexion and during rotation, and AP translation of the tibial insert on the tibial tray.

The prosthesis design allows a medially biased kinematics guided by the natural knee's stronger medial structures and greater lateral mobility. The polyethylene has approximately 20° of both internal and external rotation on the tibial base plate

Medial Rotation Knee™

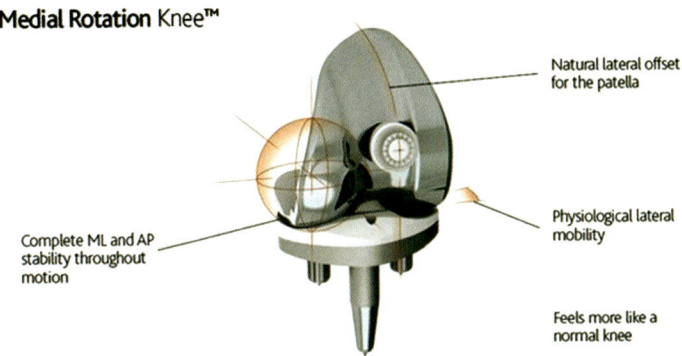

Natural lateral offset
for the patella

Physiological lateral
mobility

Complete ML and AP
stability throughout
motion

Feels more like a
normal knee

Natural Asymmetry, Complete Stability and Full Mobilisation

Catalogue description of MBK knee.

about a D-shaped "mushroom" post. The tibial base plate translates 4.5 mm in an AP direction. An anterior stop prevents the plastic bearing from sliding off the tibial tray.

Posterior stabilized mobile bearing These designs are based on the "cam and post" mechanism on a rotating polyethylene platform.

The common feature is the presence of a cam situated between the posterior femoral condyles that engages a post projecting from the mobile polyethylene platform. The "cam and post" mechanism acts as a third weight-bearing condyle to help

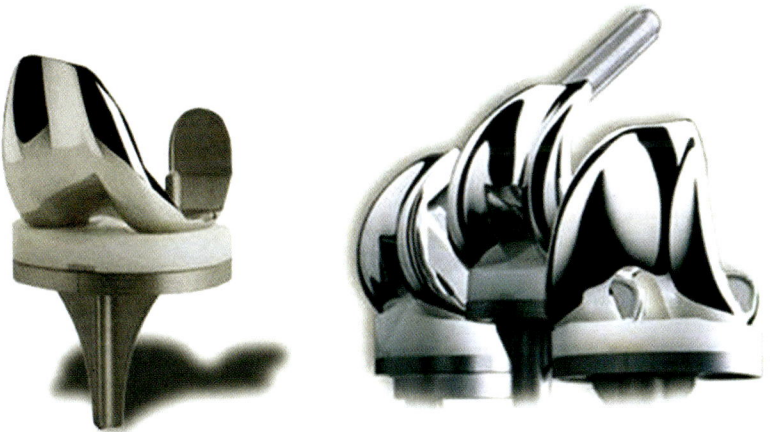

The PFC sigma PS mobile bearing knee.

improve, load transfer and minimize polyethylene stress. The Two Radii Area Contact (TRAC) Biomet, introduced in 1997, belongs to this category. More recent designs are the P.F.C. Sigma RPF (Deputy) and the LPS mobile Flex (Zimmer).

Patello-femoral joint Symptoms related to the patello-femoral joint have been reported to be a frequent cause of failure following total knee arthroplasty. During the 1980s, up to 30% of patients suffered complications associated with the patello-femoral joint (Rhoads et al., 1990). This disappointing feature of what was otherwise a successful procedure led to a debate between surgeons as to whether the articular surface of the patella should be replaced and if so, exactly how this should be performed. At the same time, various authors (Grace & Rand, 1988; Yoshii et al., 1992) pointed out the importance of prosthetic femoral and patella components.

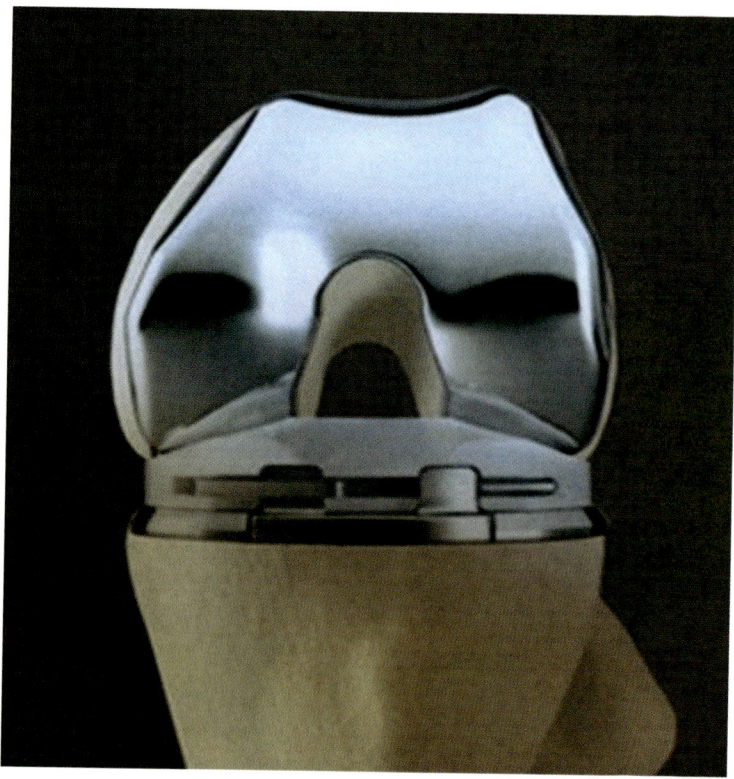

Two radii area contact (TRAC) knee from Biomet.

This problem started with the improvement of flexion allowed by the second generation of resurfacing condylar knee. Minimal patello-femoral problems were associated with the TC which permitted only about 90° flexion, but with increasing flexion achieved by newer designs, the principal concern of designers was to avoid patellar problems. Surgeons began to perform a deeper trochlea such that its floor could extend behind and cover the intercondylar notch to provide a surface for the patella to articulate against in full extension.

In an effort to obtain a suitably designed trochlea, Kulkarni and Freeman (Kulkarni et al., 2000) stressed the importance that the trochlear surface that would extend proximally sufficiently to enable even the highest patella to articulate with the femur in full extension.

In their philosophy, this part of the femoral prosthesis should be provided with a lateral wall and floor to ensure that the patella remains in contact with the floor of the trochlea from 0° to 20° of flexion. Lastly, the Kulkarni and Freeman trochlea surface should have a lateral wall of the trochlear groove sufficiently steep to provide a distinct resistance to lateral subluxation.

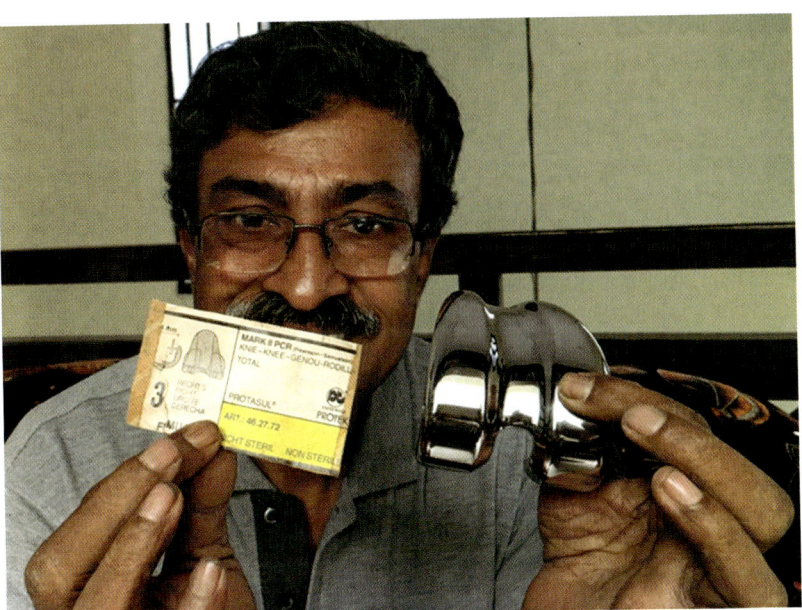

The Freeman mark II knee from the author's collection.

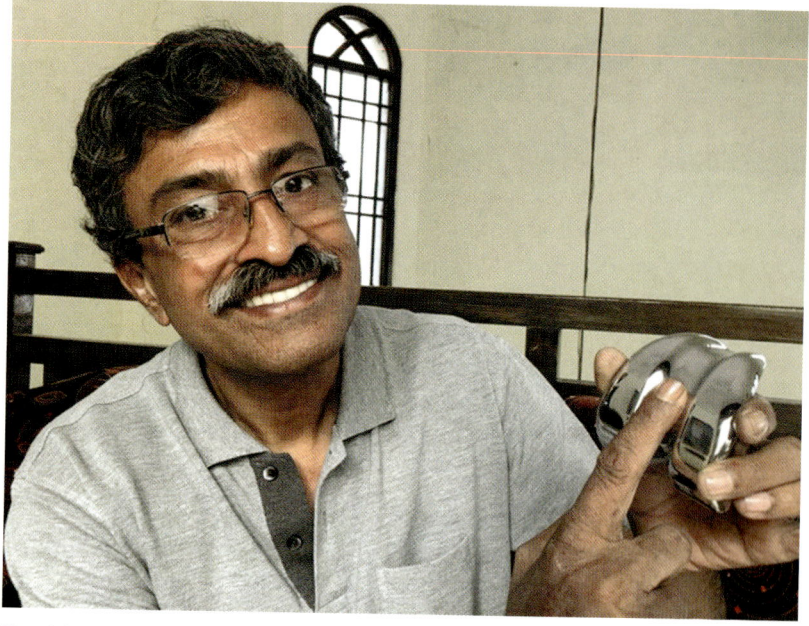

The high femur and a deep notch is friendly to all patellar situations.

According to these criteria, most of the designs introduced during the 1990s have incorporated multiple changes in the geometry of the trochlear groove, which have been shown to have a positive impact on the patellar complication rate (Bindelglass & Dorr, 1998; Kavolus et al., 2008; Mont et al., 1999).

The welcome reduction in patello-femoral complications over the years is undoubtedly due to these useful changes and attention to the rotational alignment of the femoral component.

Polyethylene In spite of designers' success in solving some of the above-mentioned problems, the 1990s marked a period of concern regarding the catastrophic failure of polyethylene. Polyethylene (UHMW) and its low friction properties makes it very resistant while articulating with metallic and extremely smooth surfaces of prostheses. The survival curves after 15 years is still over 94% for knee prostheses using UHMWHDPE (Insall & Scott, 2001).

Despite these characteristics, failure is a problem, especially among young active patients. The damage mechanisms of polyethylene are delamination, usually caused by adhesive and abrasive wear mechanism. Many factors can negatively affect the mechanical properties of polyethylene, some due to type of prosthesis and material, others by clinical conditions (post operative alignment, weight, age of patient, etc.).

Polyethylene properties can be modified by sterilization by radiation and by exposure to oxidative environment; the effects are increase in the material's density and elasticity.

Since 1995, virtually all manufacturers modified polyethylene sterilization procedures by eschewing gamma ray sterilization.

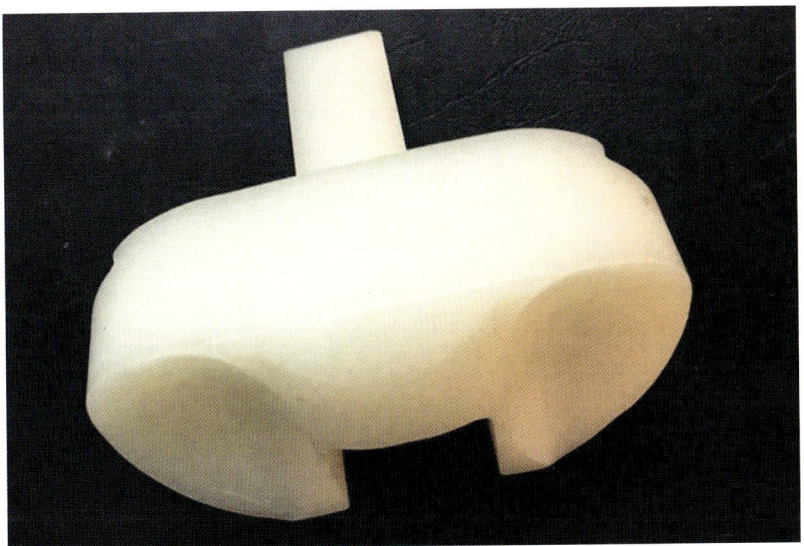

An all poly cruciate sparing tibial component.

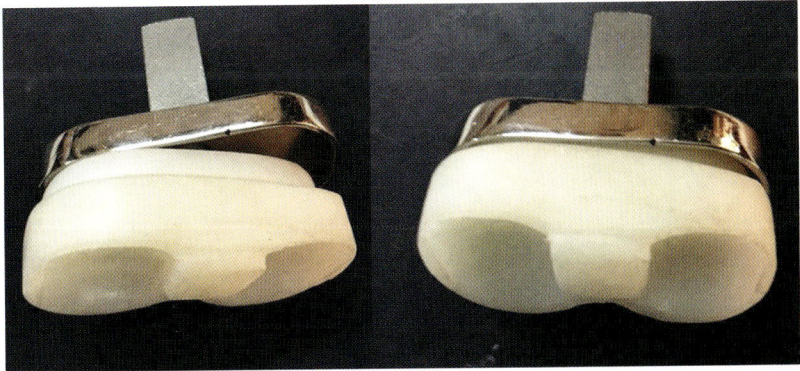

Author's design of a rotating bearing cruciate sparing design.

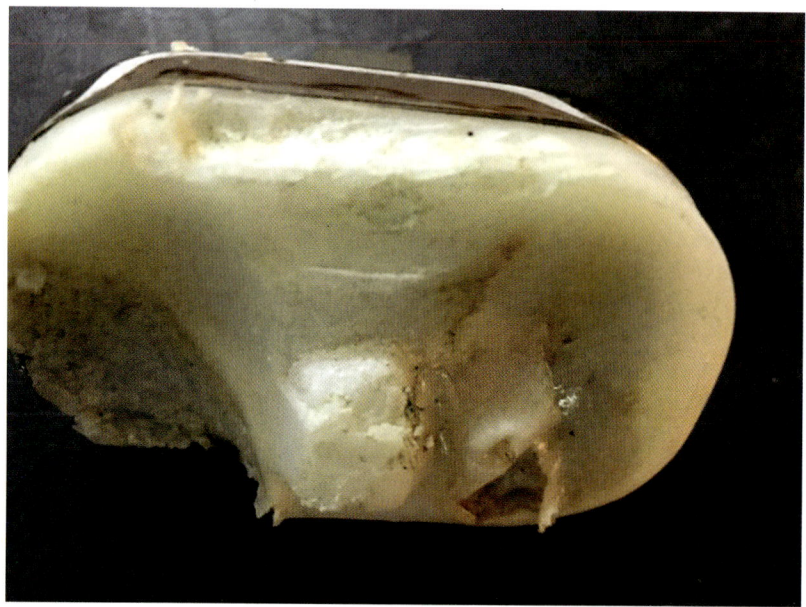

Five year wear of a gamma radiated polyethylene component.

Sterilization in inert environment, gas plasma, and ethylene oxide are the most common sterilization methods in current use. At the same time, packaging and conserving systems have been modified.

Radiation-induced cross-linking is not always beneficial, and though the same has been tried and used extensively in hip replacements, their role in knee bearings of a flatter architecture is limited. Having experienced the results of virgin, non-cross-linked, non-irradiated polyethylene for over twenty years, I am still skeptical of this step during manufacture of a knee prosthesis.

High flexion knee and new materials Some important issues have characterized the beginning of the new millennium in efforts to improve movement and research for new materials. Both these issues are directed for better performing prostheses for younger more active patients who wish to run, play tennis, and ski.

Range of Motion (ROM) after total knee arthroplasty is an important issue in determining clinical outcome and better patient satisfaction. In efforts to expand the indication of total knee arthroplasty to younger and more active patients, their demands and expectations have increased, including secondary goals other than pain relief, such as restoration of "normal-like" joint function, especially weight-bearing range of motion, to suit their desired lifestyles (Noble et al., 2006). Apart from being influenced by the condition of the patient and surgical technique, the final outcome, at least in part, depends on the implant design.

Therefore, implant manufacturers have strived and continue to strive to design TKAs that better accommodate knee mechanics in high flexion up to 155°. Since it has been shown that posterior cruciate ligament retaining designs generally have erratic motion (with potential for paradoxical roll forward), most new designs are posterior cruciate substituting prostheses (Dennis et al., 1998).

These new high-flexion designs are not radically different from their traditional (non high-flexion) counterparts, but incorporate subtle changes in the components' geometry to allow improved contact mechanics in the high-flexion ranges (compared to traditional designs).

Regarding the sagittal geometry of the femoral component, a reduction of the femoral condyles' radii in the mid- and high-flexion ranges has showed some advantage when compared with traditional implants.

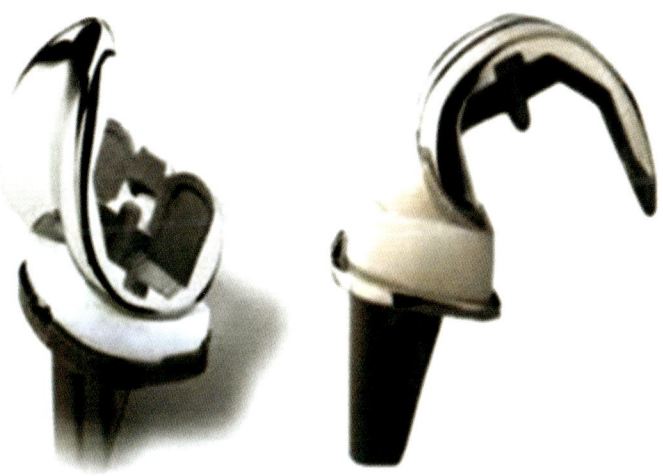

The high flex knee.

In order to eliminate edge loading on the femoral component on the posterior tibial articular surface, newer designs extend the posterior femoral condyles.

In addition, an extended posterior femoral condyle helps to restore the posterior condylar offset (Bellemans et al., 2002) as an important factor in achieving high flexion. In that study, the authors observed that for every 2 mm decrease in posterior condylar offset, the maximal obtainable flexion was reduced by a mean of 12.2°.

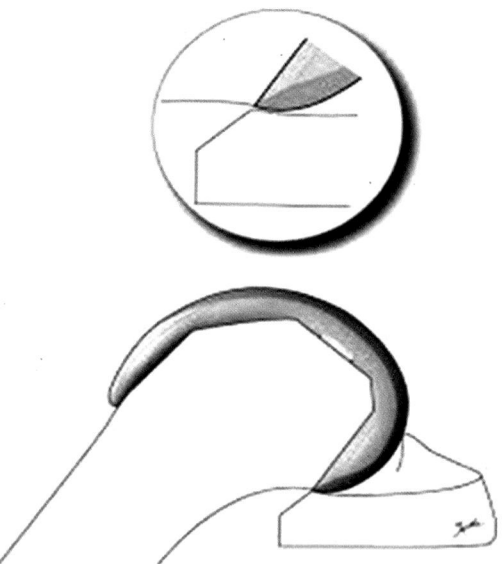

Reduction of the posterior condylar offset reduces final flexion achieved.

Some designers prefer mobile bearings with the opinion that a large internal rotation of the tibia is needed for achieving deep knee flexion, which occurs with extreme posterior shift of the lateral femoral condyle over the posterior tibial plateau in this state (Kurosaka et al. 2002; Nakagawa et al. 2000).

These changes are incorporated into a modified cam/post-mechanism which allows an increased jump distance and avoids dislocation at deep flexion angles.

Other characteristics of high flex design include the patello-femoral joint, which is designed to accommodate high angles of knee flexion.

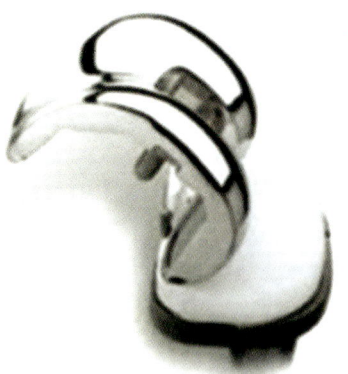
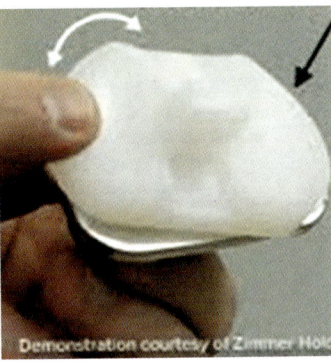

A high flex knee with a mobile bearing.

The femoral trochlear articulation is deep enough to reduce the contact stresses on the patella, which glides smoothly through a full range of motion. In such prostheses, the anterior margin of the tibial articular component has been recessed in order to reduce extensor mechanism impingement during deep flexion.

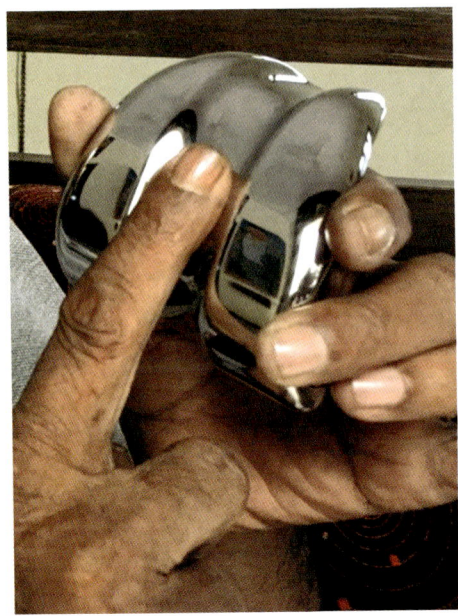

Deep patellar trough with high femur to prevent patellar problems during extreme flexion.

To accommodate the oriental lifestyle in Japan, where people sit more often on the floor than on chairs, a new design (originally called KU) was developed in 1989 (Kyoto University Knee). The most outstanding feature of this model is an auxiliary ball-and-socket joint at the centre of the posterior part, which not only facilitates a rollback movement, but also adds a rotational function.

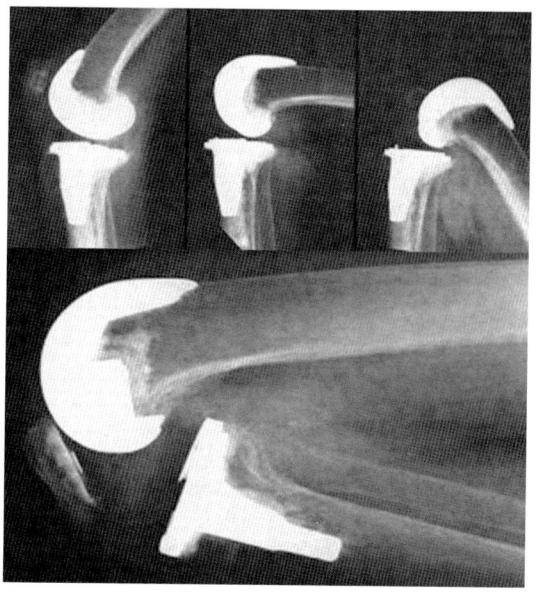

Almost full flexion with the Japanese knees.

During a gait under load, the femorotibial articular surface in a conventional design works as for the standard design, but when the flexion increases, the auxiliary joint functions as a rotation centre in the flexion motion. This auxiliary joint represents a certain type of posterior-stabilized knee and works to achieve a rollback; when in flexion, rotation of tibia is also achieved. Because this knee was unique in its biphasic surface structure for different purposes, weight bearing, and flexion movement, it was later called bisurface knee (BS knee). Another characteristic of this prosthesis is the presence of zirconia ceramics (ZrO_2) for the femoral component.

Others companies modified this design, incorporating a lateral compartment which is fully congruent in extension, but relatively lax in flexion (Mikashima et al., 2010).

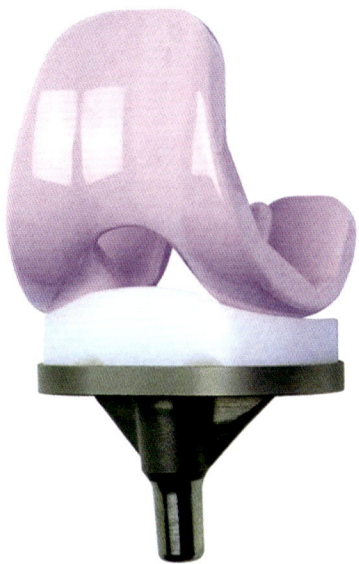

Biphasic knee replacement with ceramic femoral component.

This articular geometry provides anteroposterior stability and acts through the lateral femoral condyle in a manner similar to the function of the anterior cruciate ligament (ACL). In addition, the modified design has a more posterior tibial sulcus and the maximum femoral posterior condylar offset occurs later in the flexion arc.

However, further improvement in the longevity of the arthroplasty can be achieved with more durable bearing materials. Due to the nonconforming shape of the bearing surface, hard-on-hard articulations are unlikely to have a role in TKA, hence polyethylene (PE) will remain an important bearing surface material. Research and efforts are continuing towards development of femoral bearing surfaces which would wear out a minimal amount of polyethylene.

Previous studies have shown that roughening of the cobalt-chromium (CoCr) alloy surface can potentiate wear of the PE (Fisher et al. 2004; White et al. 1994). This wear can then lead to osteolysis, instability, and loosening of the implants from the underlying bone.

Designers are now concentrating on researching different alloys (as alternatives to the classic CoCrMo) for femoral components, in the form of both complete ceramic or metals coated with ceramic surfaces. A longer lasting prosthesis with ceramic femoral components should be useful for younger patients with higher functional demands. Moreover, ceramic is useful when dealing with patients affected by allergies to metallic ions.

The advantages of ceramic bearing surfaces in terms of superior lubrication, friction, and wear properties compared to cobalt-chrome alloy (CoCr) surfaces in total joint arthroplasty are well recognized (Greenwald et al., 2001; Jacobs et al., 1994).

Laboratory and clinical data have demonstrated that ceramic bearings are associated with fewer wear particles that incite a less intense inflammatory host-immune response than metal-on-polyethylene articulations that are the accepted standard in total hip arthroplasty and total knee arthroplasty (Mont et al., 2003; Spector et al. 2001).

The brittle nature of ceramics and their inability to withstand high-impact tensile forces is of concern in clinical applications. However, more than 10 years' long-term follow-up of different ceramic cemented knees from Japan showed satisfactory results with low rate fractures of ceramic component.

An important improvement has recently been introduced in Europe by CeramTec (AG, Polchingen, Germany) using BIOLOX

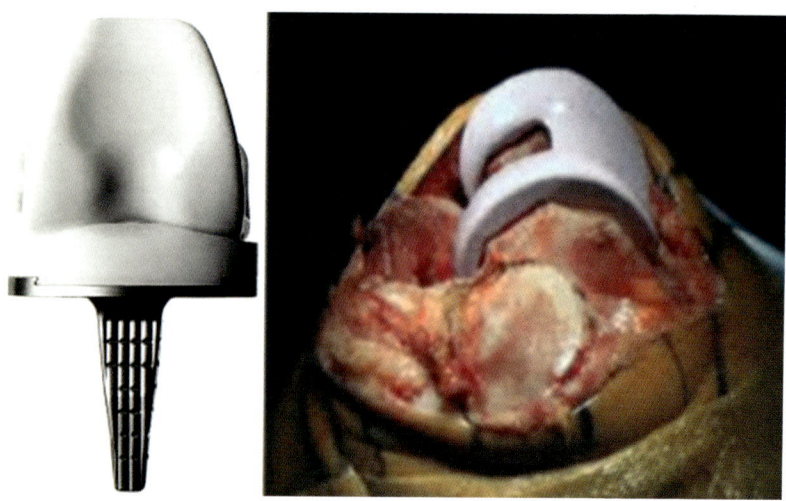

A ceramic femoral component.

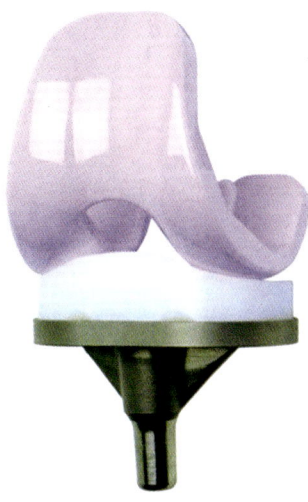

Ceramic femoral component.

Delta, a composite matrix material containing 82% vol. alumina (Al_2O_3) and 17% vol. zirconia (ZrO_2) providing good mechanical characteristics in terms of strength and resistance. Using this material, it was possible to develop a femoral component with a tensile strength that met the demands for application in TKR. A prospective international multicentre study was started in 2008 to evaluate the clinical and radiological outcomes of the unconstrained Multigen Plus total knee system (Lima-Lto) with the new BIOLOX Delta ceramic femoral component.

In USA, an alternative strategy has been followed to decrease PE wear in THA and TKA, by the surface transformation of metal to oxidized zirconium. A wrought zirconium alloy (Zr-2.5% Niobium) is oxidized by thermal diffusion to create a 5 mm oxidized zirconium layer (Oxinium, Smith & Nephew, Memphis, TN; Laskin, 2003). Although existing data are encouraging (Innocenti et al., 2010), further studies are needed with both strategies to define the precise indications and outcomes of ceramic surfaces in TKA.

From 2005 to the present, only cosmetic design changes have been made. In my opinion, nothing new which could be called a significant breakthrough has emerged in knee replacement design in the last decade. However, multinational companies

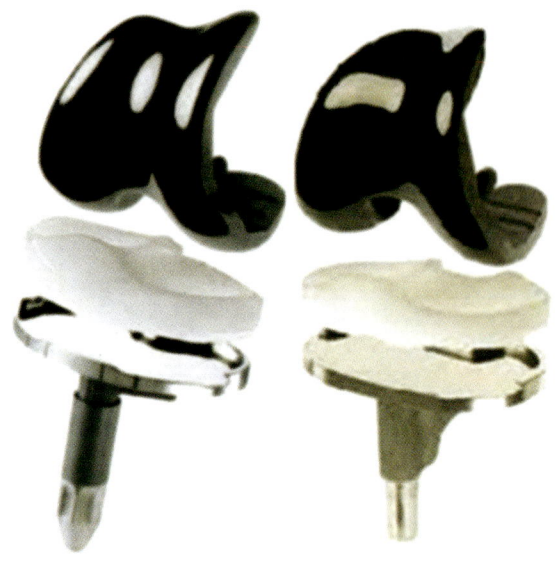

Oxidized zirconium-oxinium knee.

wax eloquent about various revolutionary changes, but whether any of these will stand the test of time will be only known after 25 years!

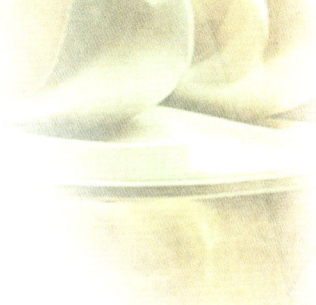

3

Biomaterials of the Artificial Knee

Materials

Metals, plastic and acrylic cement form the three common materials used in arthroplasty. Ceramics have now made their appearance on the scene. This chapter will give you enough knowledge not to be fooled by snake oil salesmen, the employees of multinational companies selling those exotic high priced knees at 50 plus times the manufacturing cost!

The materials for knee arthroplasty were based on the materials successfully used in total hip replacements, so let us begin with the common origins. In the beginning, when hemi-arthroplasties were done, the implant material varied from heat cured acrylic to resins, then to stainless steel. Stainless steel showed less wear than acrylic and soon replaced it. The fact that the non-replaced acetabulum showed significant wear prompted research into total joints. Charnley's work laid the foundation of modern arthroplasty. In spite of continuing research in implant materials, the time-honoured combination of metal articulating with ultra high molecular weight polyethylene is yet to be challenged. However, the choice of metal has changed from stainless steel of Charnley's time to stronger steel alloys, then to cobalt-chromium and titanium-aluminium-vanadium. Ceramics are also used because of their excellent frictional and wear characteristics, but have their own disadvantage of brittleness.

There is a lot of confusing terminology whilst describing materials, e.g. yield strength, toughness, ultimate tensile strength, ductility, elasticity, and fatigue strength. This book is

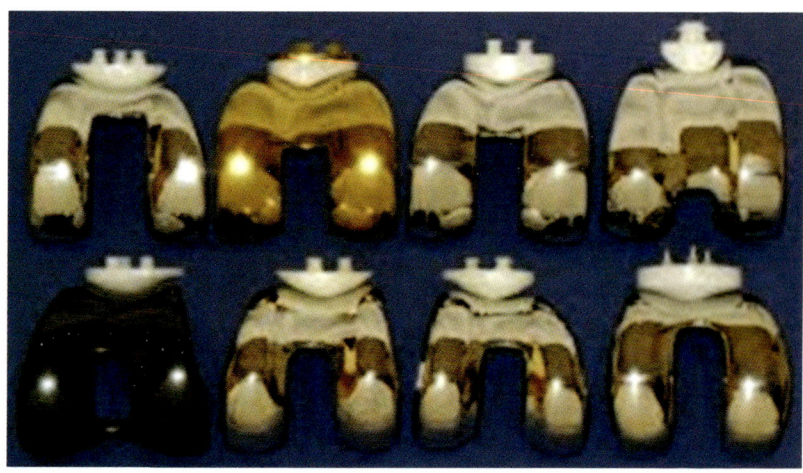

A very wide range of materials are used for knee replacements.

not a treatise on material science, hence the reader may have to read more advanced manuals for those details. I would however teach you enough about biomaterials and biomechanics, so that when a high flying scientist from a multinational implant manufacturing company tries to bamboozle you with highly cross-linked poly, or plasma coated surfaces, Chiruleen, Gur 10/50, titanium dinitride coatings, or alumina ceramics, you can ask him some questions, the answers to which he would probably not know!!

Metals

Stainless steel: This no doubt the cheapest material, tried and tested for a long period (since 1900). 316L stainless steel is popular for implants as it is the most corrosion resistant when in direct contact with biological fluids. What makes 316L ideal as an implant material is the lack of inclusion. Alloys with inclusion contain sulphur, which is a key ingredient in accelerating metallic corrosion.

Stainless steel is an iron alloy. By adding 16% chromium it becomes corrosion resistant stainless steel. The addition of 7% nickel helps stabilize the austenite to stainless steel. Type 316L stainless steel selected for surgical implants contains approximately 17–19% chromium and 14% nickel. Molybdenum added to the alloy forms a protective layer, sheltering the metal from exposure to an acidic environment. Corrosion resistance can also be achieved with the carbon element, but only when the carbon is in a solid solution state.

Stainless steel can be heat forged, cold worked, machined from blocks, or cast into complex shapes. Its final mechanical properties entirely depend on how it is made.

It has to be stressed that the ferrite element (which gives the alloy a magnetic property) should not be incorporated, as the magnetic property could interfere with Magnetic Resonance Imaging (MRI) equipment. One of the most apparent problems with using magnetic implants is their susceptibility to heating which could change their shape and/or structural composition.

If we evaluate all types of metallic implants that have gone into the human body since the 1900s, roughly 70% would be stainless steel, 20% cobalt chrome alloys and 10% titanium. However, among the currently available commercial knee implants, SS 316L is no longer used. Only the higher priced cobalt chrome alloys or titanium form the basic materials for most femoral and tibial components, the purported reason being their better strength and biocompatibility.

However, if the steels available today are compared with cobalt-chrome alloy, the steels are only marginally weaker. But cobalt-chrome alloys are heavier, and if cast, seldom approach the strength of forged virgin stainless steel. Cobalt chrome molybdenum alloy, most commonly used in knee implants, is

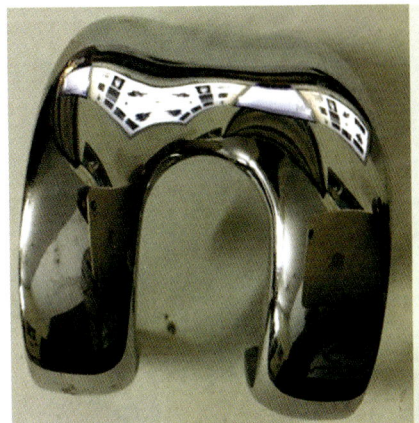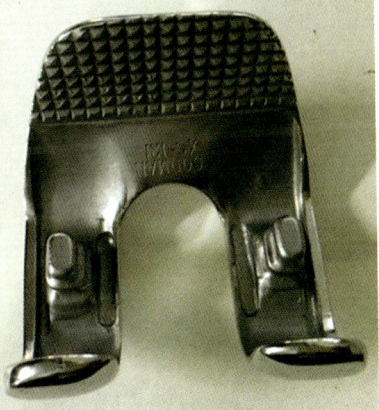

A cast stainless steel implant.

about three to four times as expensive as stainless steel. Total joints were initially made with stainless steel on HDPE constructs; the initial 100,000 plus hips made by Charnley and Thackeray were stainless steel have exhibited excellent mechanical properties and tolerances, Yet stainless steel is surprisingly no longer in current use as an implant material for knee replacements.

One would thus like to question the wisdom of generically moving away from stainless steel in implantable joints, though it is extensively used in most internal fixation and trauma products. Maybe commercial considerations outweigh patients' benefits!!

Cobalt Based Alloys

The material approved for orthopaedic use is ASTM F75. Though superior to stainless steel based alloys in corrosion resistance and fatigue failure, there is a tendency for the alloy grains to become non-homogenous, leading to different implant strengths in different batches. It is indeed surprising that in the United States, this is the most popular alloy for all endoprosthesis (and steel based alloys are almost out). From the surgeon's point of view, this assumption is a little biased, because Charnley's initial experience using simple stainless steel 316L is a definite landmark that is still to be equaled or excelled.

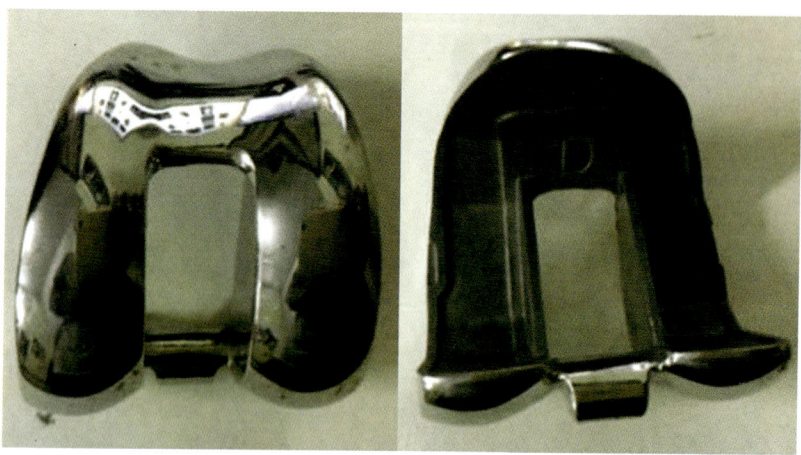

Cast cobalt chrome femoral component.

The ASTM F75 standard specifies that the alloy should contain cobalt as its principal element, with 27 to 30% chromium, 5 to 7% molybdenum, and limits on other important elements such as manganese and silicon, less than 1% iron, less than 0.75% nickel, less than 0.5% of nitrogen, tungsten, phosphorus, sulphur, boron, etc.

Besides cobalt-chromium-molybdenum (CoCrMo), cobalt-nickel-chromium-molybdenum (CoNiCrMo) is also used for implants. The possible toxicity of released Ni ions from CoNiCr alloys and also their limited frictional properties are a matter of concern in using these alloys as articulating components. Thus, CoCrMo is usually the dominant alloy for total joint arthroplasty.

Titanium Based Alloys

These are the best as far as modulus of elasticity, weight and corrosion resistance are concerned, but the adhesive and abrasive wear properties are much less than the above two. In addition, despite the low weight and good strength, titanium and its alloys suffer from a paradox of excellent bio-compatibility when fixed firmly and a very poor tissue response when loose (leading to particulate debris). Consequently, if a bearing surface is to be made of titanium, it is indeed imperative that it is either anodized or coated with a non degradable substance to allow for a high quality of abrasive resistant mirror polish. Added to this, the cost of the metal is very high. In many cases, especially in our country, its cost may deteriment it from being selected in implant manufacture.

Recent studies from the western world do show that the choice of titanium for an implant material is indeed not a wise one! The

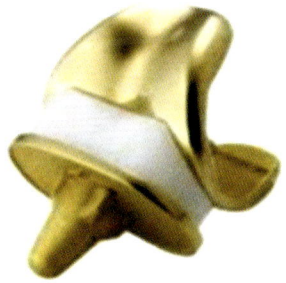

Titanium knee implants are still being evaluated and are not widely used.

bio-degradation of the implants fixed not too snugly has not only led to early loosening, but also to massive osteolysis, migration of the titanium particles, and even black stained lymph nodes at sites distant from the joint, which confirms that inertness may be a more important factor than higher elasticity and lower weight.

COMPARISON BETWEEN THE THREE COMMONLY USED METALS IN ARTHROPLASTY

1. Modulus of Elasticity

The modulus of elasticity is the ratio of applied stress to the resultant strain in the linear (elastic) portion of the stress–strain curve. This is also referred to as "Young's modulus 'E'". This parameter corresponds to the stiffness of a material; thus a high modulus of elasticity would mean a stiffer implant, while a low modulus of elasticity would mean a more elastic implant.

2. Specific Gravity or Density

Weight by volume is density, with water having a density of 1 gm/cc. A litre of water weighs a kilogram. Incidentally, when Archimedes jumped out of his bath tub and displayed his testicles to the whole of Athens, it was this discovery, his EUREKA moment. Thus materials with high density or specific gravity will be heavier than an identically sized implant of lower SG.

Cortical bone has a Young's modulus varying in the direction of deformation; for a tibia it is about 5 to 10 in transverse axis and 11 to 23 in longitudinal axis. Compared to this, 316L SS is 186, cobalt chrome is 241, and titanium 5 is 105.

The SG of human bone is between 1.7 and 2.3; that of titanium is 4.5, stainless steel 7.9 and cobalt chrome alloy 8.36.

3. Other Mechanical Properties

Metal	Ultimate tensile strength MPa	Yield strength MPa	Elongation %	Area reduction %
SS 316l	480	170	40	0
ASTM F75	890	517	20	20
Titanium 5	900	520	15	25

The four characteristics we look for in implantable materials are UTS (ultimate tensile strength), YS (yield strength), elongation and reduction. This is how the three metals compare:

What do these numbers mean? None of the three metals are as light or as elastic as human bones. What is the relevance? If you leave aside the commercially motivated research papers, the clear conclusion is that there is no significant difference between cobalt and SS except that the latter is about 25% the cost. Titanium, which is 15 times as expensive as SS, is lighter and more elastic. The elasticicity may be desirable in implants to avoid stress shielding. However in total knees, where a fairly rigid, noncorrosive, non deforming, cancellous contact flat implant is used, in my opinion titanium is a bad metal to use. The *50% lighter than SS* is a characteristic with questionable benefits.

Likewise, the ultimate tensile strength and yield strength might be relevant only in thin plates or hollow nails. With cast femoral and tibial components for the knee with such big dimensions, and no part is thinner than 6 mm; even deep thinking and repeated discussions with scientists in the field could not convince me about the advantages of using titanium as a knee implant. But if we look into emerging trends, almost all implant manufacturers are racing towards their own titanium models, which in my opinion is due to one solitary factor: COMMERCE.

I still believe that stainless steel 316L is one of the best materials for knee implants. Easily available, manufactured in India, capable of excellent finish, economical to invest cast, easy to machine and with proven 18 to 24 years of life! I am working on bringing a commercial model of a sub 200$ knee, and only time will tell if I will succeed.

Ultra High Molecular Weight Polyethylene: HDPE was an accident, but probably one of the luckiest accidents which has brought a wide smile to millions of patients suffering from pain and immobility due to crippling arthritis. It all began with Charnley's experiments in total hip arthroplasty! Charnley first began using Mckee Farar hips (highly polished metal-on-metal hips fixed with cement). While some failed soon, others lasted surprisingly long, some even up to 23 years. When Charnley, a keen observer and excellent clinician, examined a few Mckee Farar hips, he heard squeaks. His engineer friends told him that it was a friction squeak, and he became interested to know all about friction. Friction is resistance to two surfaces rubbing against each other. You do not need to learn complex physics to know logical, self explanatory facts about friction.

1. *Area:* Smaller the area, lesser the friction. It is easier to slide a rupee coin on a table than a dinner plate.

2. *Surface:* Smoother the surface, lesser the friction. Two sandpapers rubbing against one other will have more friction than two mirrors.

3. *Lubrication:* A good lubricant naturally reduces friction.

With these points in mind, John Charnley began his experiments with the bearing surface for his hips. Metal was out. He began experimenting with industrial plastics. Teflon or PTFE (polytetrafluroethylene), was a new plastic with wonderful properties. Lab tests showed that the friction in stainless steel rubbing against PTFE was practically zero.

Charnley, an engineer and surgeon, devised a prosthesis made of stainless steel which he machined himself on a lathe and implanted in a patient. He replaced the cup surface with one of Teflon. The initial results were very good; his patients were pain free immediately after the operation. People who had not walked for years started running. Charnley was thrilled. He went before the orthopaedic surgeons of England and announced that he had discovered an operation he would even do on his mother!! So spectacular were the results!

But unfortunately the results were shortlived. In his initial enthusiasm, Charnley miscalculated wear and tear. So engrossed was he with friction that he did not anticipate the possibility that Teflon can rub out after constant movement against metal. In a human body the hip is put through vigorous movements with sufficient load over prolonged periods, which causes a significant Teflon wear.

The Teflon material just wore away in a year's time and Charnley was left with a hundred failed hip joints.

Way back in the 1960s, you could get away with a hundred failed operations without a Consumer Protection Council above

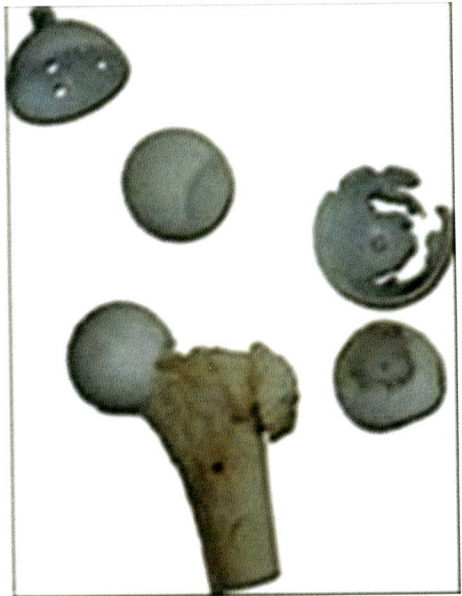

Rapid wear of Teflon cup in Charnley's initial experiments.

your head. Charnley was shattered. He went back before the same British orthopaedic surgeons and told them that the operation was no good, so he would not do it even on his own mother-in-law!

Then Charnley was given a piece of HDPE (High Density Polyethylene). He saw another plastic and was not impressed. A hundred failures had disillusioned him. But he did make a trial cup and put it on a machine which he used to test the wear. Someone forgot to switch off the machine that weekend and what was found on Monday was a spinning system which would have been in the human body for two years. Charnley measured the wear and found none! This amazed Charnley. He put it through further tests and the results were the same. Polyethylene did not wear out. At least in experiments its wear was not even a fraction of Teflon's. Further research resulted in the final UHMUHDPE being discovered. Ultra high density, ultra high molecular weight polyethylene to be precise.

UHMWPE is a member of the polyethylene family of polymers with the repeat unit $[C_2H_4]_n$, with n denoting the degree of polymerization. The International Standards Organization (ISO

11542) (ISO) defines UHMWPE as having a molecular weight of at least 1 million g/mole, resulting in a minimum degree of polymerization of n ≈ 36,000, while the American Society for Testing and Materials (ASTM D 4020) (ASTM) specifies that UHMWPE has a molecular weight greater than 3.1 million g/mole (n ≈ 110,000). The UHMWPEs used in orthopaedic applications typically have a molecular weight between 2–6 million with a degree of polymerization between 71,000–214,000.

UHMWPE is a linear (non-branching) semi-crystalline polymer which can be described as a two phase composite of crystalline and amorphous phases. The crystalline phase contains chains folded into highly oriented lamellae, with the crystals being orthorhombic in structure. The lamellae are 10–50 nm thick and 10–50 µm long. The lamellae are oriented randomly within the amorphous phase with tie molecules linking individual lamellae to one another.

The two resins of UHMWPE currently used in orthopaedics are GUR 1020 (3.5 million g/mole) and GUR 1050 (5.5–6 million g/mole). These resins can either be compression moulded into sheets or ram extruded into rods. Both resin and conversion methods are significant predictors of tensile mechanical

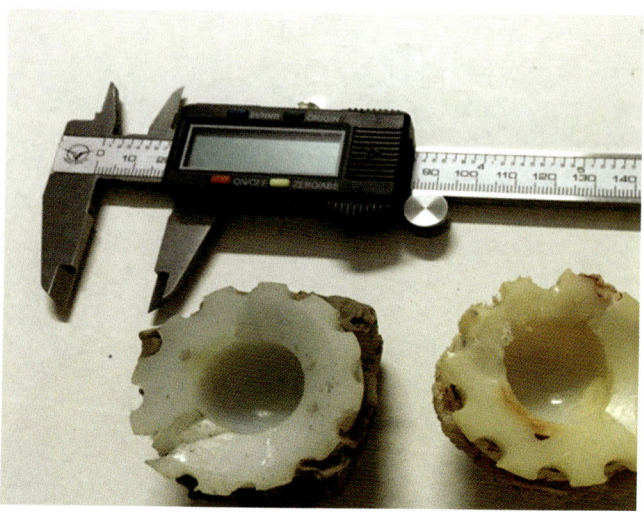

UHMWHDPE has exceptional wear properties. The cups retrieved by the author show minimal wear at 9 years (left) and wear at 19 years (right). This is noncross-linked virgin poly!

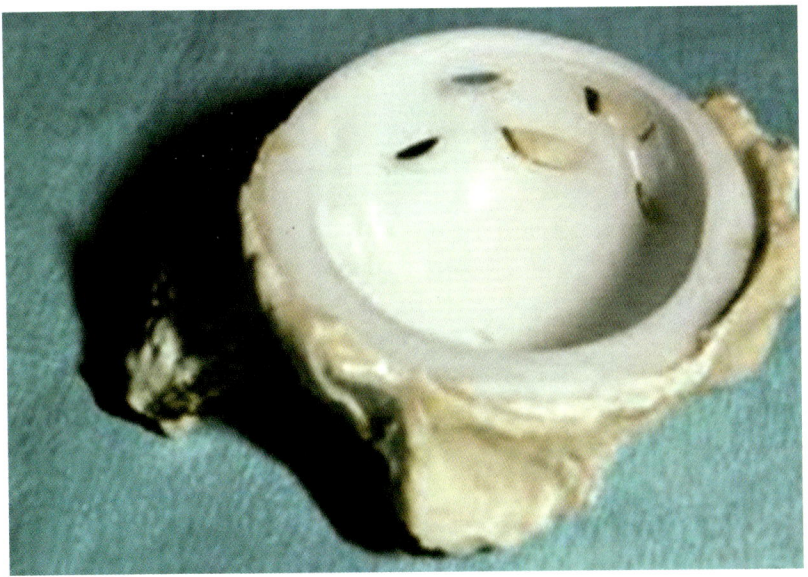

Early Muller cups showed much greater wear for two reasons. Thin cup due to large head and gamma radiation.

properties and impact strength. Virgin UHMWHDPE, a non-cross-linked, nongamma irradiated plastic, was first used in joint replacements. This is plastic with slight deformative properties, a reasonable modulus of elasticity and *return to shape* after deforming forces are removed.

Charnley autoclaved his femoral components, but gas sterilized (Ethylene Oxide) the HDPE cups. Around the same time, Maurice Muller of Switzerland began making larger head (32 mm) hips. He gamma radiated both the stems and cups. Initial results of the two systems were similar, but at five years, the wear rate of Muller's radiated cups was extremely high compared to Charnley's nonirradiated cups.

It was at this time that scientists began to worry about plastic wear. It was found that radiation produced cross-linking of the molecules and when gamma sterilized in the presence of air, the cups underwent oxidative degradation, making them brittle over the years, leading to progressive wear.

The German company Ruhrchemie AG first introduced a UHDPE for orthopaedic use: RCH 100 [(R)uhr (CH)emie 100]. This company then became Hoechst and the next gen

UHMWHDPE produced by them was named Chirulen. Now the company is called Tikona and the plastics are called GUR or (G)ranular (U)hmwhdpe (R)uhrchemie. The product is designated with a four digit number, e.g. GUR 1050, GUR 1020, etc. The first digit is the loose density, the second is presence or absence of calcium strerate, the third digit is molecular weight in million and the last digit is the resin grade.

Application of heat and pressure produces sheets or extruded rods, which are then machined to the correct component dimensions. Though some manufacturers directly moulded the granules to the desired component using a die, it was later found that these extra polished components wore out faster. The current concept is to use machined parts from stock blocks of larger size.

Virgin HDPE has stood the test of time, so long as it is not irradiated and the components are not too thin. However, the principal cause of knee revision was found to be wear. Scientists thus began experimenting with gilding the lily to produce *better* variants. Carbon reinforced polymer composite was one such disaster; Zimmer had to recall its entire stocks and discontinue the product seven years after release. Heat pressing was another disaster.

Cross-linking is currently being used in an attempt to improve the wear performance. Normally HDPE is linear linked with long molecular chains. It was assumed that this was the defect of the polymer, causing wear. By adding linking agents like peroxides or silanes, and gamma radiating the plastic to controlled levels, the molecular structure was reorganized to allow linking in both linear and transverse directions, producing what is known as a cross-linked polymer.

Though hip cups have shown some degree of wear resistance due to cross-linking, only commercial publications wax eloquent about cross-linking in knee replacements. Some studies have shown that cross-linking actually makes the plastic more rigid and brittle, more susceptible to fractures and early failure.

Cross-linking reduces crystallinity, and thereby makes the plastic more brittle, less elastic, stronger in one way but weaker in another. Whether it is actually beneficial in the long run is a matter to be seen with time.

Ceramics: Ceramics are non-metallic inorganic materials and vary in composition. They are made by mixing fine powders of the ingredient material with water and adhesive binder. This dough is then squeezed into a mould to obtain the desired shape, air dried, and the binder is then burned out by thermal treatment. Firing or sintering at this stage at a high temperature (over 100°C) makes the residual material extremely dense.

The final microscopic structure of the resultant ceramic is greatly dependent on the thermal process used, highest temperature reached and duration of furnace heat treatment.

Five types of ceramics are used in arthroplasty:

1. Glass
2. Plasma-sprayed polycrystalline ceramic
3. Vitrified ceramic
4. Solid state sintered ceramic
5. Polycrystalline glass-ceramic

Other factors determining the mechanical and biological properties are the purity of the powder, the size and distribution of the grains, and the porosity.

Ceramics used in orthopaedic surgery are classified as *bioactive* or *inert* according to the tissue response when implanted in an osseous environment.

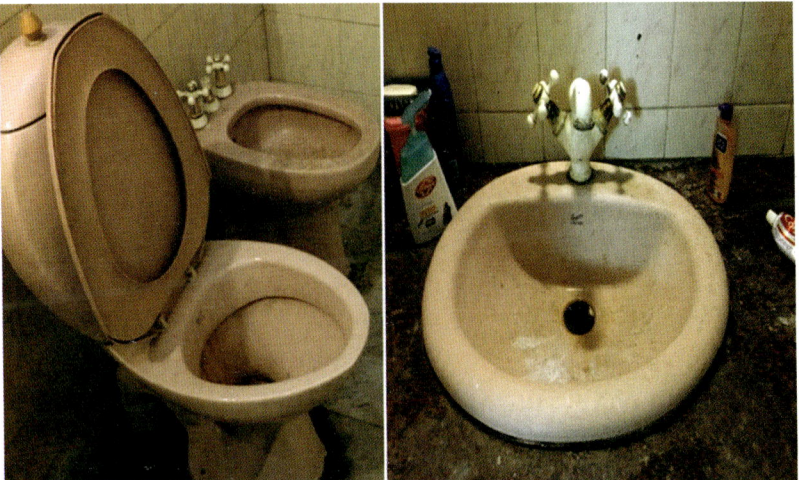

The ceramics, materials and technology used in hips are no different from those used in toilets and wash basins.

The *bioactivity* of a material can be defined as its ability to bond biologically to bone. An *inert* ceramic merely elicits a minor fibrous reaction. In clinical practice, inert fully-dense ceramics are used as bearings in total joint replacements because of their exceptional resistance to wear; bioactive ceramics are used as coatings to enhance the fixation of the femoral stems or acetabular shells.

Sliding ceramics: The most widely used bearing combination in total joint replacements is metal-on-polyethylene. The long-term survival of the artificial joint is dependent on the wear of its components. It is the poly wear which ultimately leads to osteolysis around the implant, leading to an inflammatory response induced by wear debris occurring from both the articulating and non-articulating surfaces.

Pierre Boutin first introduced ceramics in orthopaedics in the early 1970s to tackle complications related to polyethylene wear.

Ceramics are mainly used in total hip arthroplasty as femoral heads articulating against polyethylene, and as cups in the alumina-on-alumina combination. Because of their relatively brittle nature, fracture of ceramic femoral heads has been, along with cost, the main limitation to their expanded use worldwide.

The risk of fracture, however, has been virtually eliminated because of a great improvement in the manufacturing process

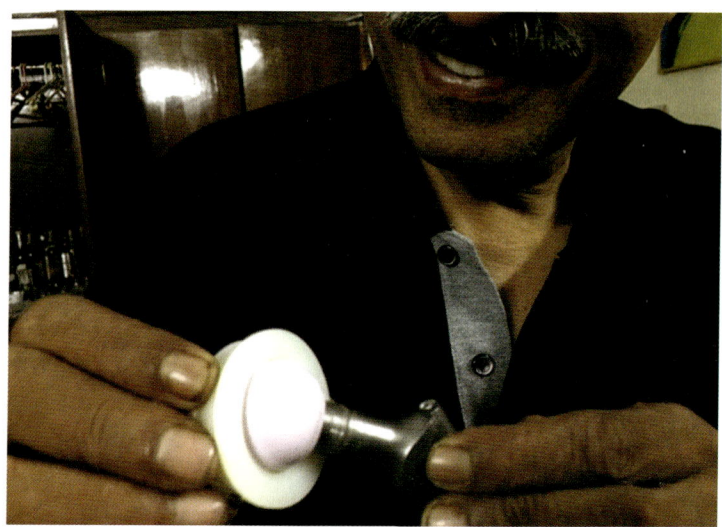

Currently the most popular use of ceramics is as a bearing with HDPE.

with increased purity and density, increase in the size and distribution of the grains and better quality control.

Accurate fixation of the ceramic ball to the femoral stem through a well-designed Morse taper avoids undesirable stresses in the head and improved surgical techniques augment the longevity of the implant.

The fracture rate of ceramic heads has been evaluated as 0.02% for alumina heads and 0.03% for zirconia heads, indicating that fracture of the ceramic head is no longer a constraint.

Alumina ceramic: Dense alumina of surgical grade is obtained by sintering alumina powder at temperatures between 1600 and 1800°C. The resultant material is in its highest state of oxidation, allowing thermodynamic stability, chemical inertness and excellent resistance to corrosion.

Improvement in the manufacturing process has lowered the size and distribution of the grains, which are major factors in avoiding cracks and fractures.

Alumina is a brittle material with excellent compression strength but the bending strength is limited. The Young's modulus is 300 times greater than that of cancellous bone, and 190 times higher than polymethylmethacrylate (PMMA).

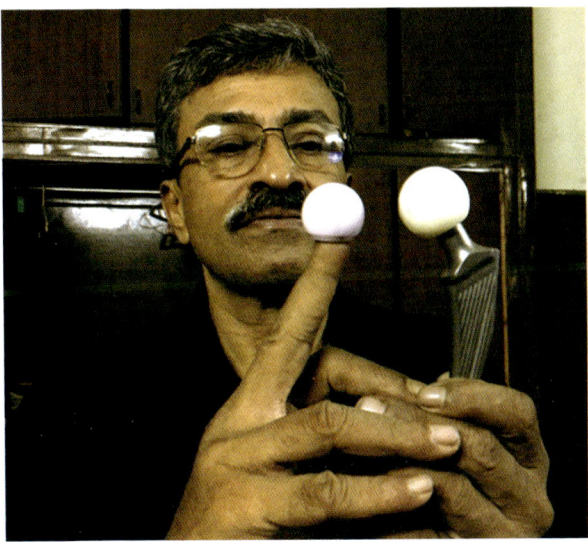

Alumina and zirconia ceramics are not too different in look and feel on the operating table.

Alumina has been a standardized material since 1984 (International Standard Organisation, ISO 6474). The tribological properties of alumina ceramic against itself are outstanding, with a linear wear rate 4000 times lower than that of metal-on-polyethylene.

The excellent frictional characteristics are due in part to a high wettability because of the hydrophilic surface and fluid film lubrification which minimizes adhesive wear.

These properties, demonstrated both *in vitro* and on analysis of retrieved implants, are responsible for the limited amount of wear particles produced and the subsequent moderate biological reaction to ceramic wear debris.

The clearance between the two components in the case of the alumina-on-alumina combination should be around 50 nm to avoid Hertz stresses at the surface of the alumina (which may result in detachment of grains and third-body wear). Hertz stress causes geometrically progressive wear, as the particles are produced exponentially.

Wroblewski, Siney and Fleming recently described the results of 22 mm alumina femoral heads articulating against cross-linked polyethylene in a ten-year follow-up. A running-in rate of penetration was noted, which then decreased to 0.022 mm/year after the first 18 months. It is difficult, however, to conclude from this study whether the alumina head, the small diameter of the femoral head, or the cross-linked nature of the polyethylene cups was responsible for the low rate of wear observed.

Comparative physical properties of alumina and zirconia ceramics of surgical grade:

Property	Alumina	Zirconia
Purity (%)	>99.8	>97.0
Density (g/cm^3)	3.98	6.05
Bending strength (MPa)	595	1000
Compressive strength (MPa)	4250	2000
Young's modulus (GPa)	380	210
Hardness (Vickers hardness no.)	2000	1200
Fracture toughness KIC (MN/m$^{3/2}$)	5	7
Grain size (m)	3.6	0.2 to 0.4
Surface finish (Ra, m)	0.02	XXX

Zirconia ceramic was introduced in the manufacture of femoral heads for total hip replacements because of its higher strength and toughness (which would reduce the risk of fracture). Pure zirconia is an unstable material showing three different crystalline phases: Monoclinic, tetragonal and cubic.

The phase changes result in a large variation in volume and significantly degrade its mechanical properties due to cracks produced. Zirconia is stabilized by adding oxides to maintain the tetragonal phase.

Yttrium-stabilized tetragonal polycrystalline zirconia (Y-TZP) has a fine grain size and offers the best mechanical properties (as shown in the table on the previous page).

This material was standardized in 1997 (International Standard Organisation, ISO 13356). Zirconia femoral heads should articulate only against polyethylene sockets since both zirconia against alumina and zirconia against zirconia 20 have been shown to produce catastrophic rates of wear *in vitro*. Zirconia-on-polyethylene has demonstrated similar rates of wear as alumina-on-polyethylene *in vitro*, but *in vivo*, the results have not been so favourable.

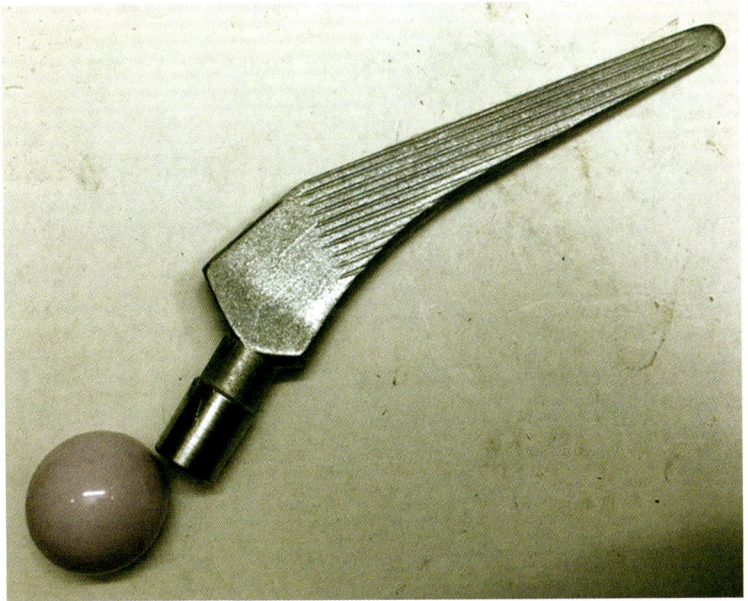

A zirconia ceramic head with a hydroxyappatite coated stem.

Allain et al. recently described a consecutive series of 78 hips using a zirconia femoral head and a polyethylene cup. Complete radiolucent lines were observed around the cup in 23% of the hips, and 17% of the femoral implants had radiolucency greater than 1 mm. Survival at 8 years was 63%. These worrying results were confirmed by Hernigou and Babrami in a study comparing wear of the cup and osteolysis in 40 hips over a period of 10 years.

2 comparable groups of 20 hips each had either a 32 mm alumina or a 28 mm zirconia femoral head. During the first 5 years, the zirconia group had a lower rate of wear of 0.04 mm/year compared with 0.08 mm/year, and osteolysis on the calcar measured in square millimetres was similar in both groups.

Between 5 and 10 years, however, the rate of wear increased dramatically in the zirconia group to 0.15 mm/year at 10 years as opposed to 0.07 mm/year in the alumina group. Osteolysis of the calcar was significantly greater in the zirconia group at 135 mm compared with 65 mm.

These results are of concern. The long-term performance of zirconia ceramic may well be altered by degradation *in vivo* with the material transforming into its monoclinic unstable phase.

Another explanation was suggested by Lu and McKellop, who measured the frictional heating of polyethylene cups in a hip joint simulator. The steady-state temperature of the polyethylene reached 99°C with heads of zirconia ceramic compared with 45°C with alumina prostheses.

This may account for the long-term wear because the consequent structural changes may also produce precipitation of lubricant proteins. Better results are apparent in current clinical trials.

Mixed-oxide ceramics: A new class of materials has been developed recently to combine the tribological properties of alumina and the mechanical characteristics of yttrium stabilized zirconia.

These mixed-oxide ceramics containing 40% to 80% zirconia have shown rates of wear *in vitro* comparable to those of alumina ceramic. Preliminary results in hip joint simulators have been promising, but further investigations are needed to assess their long-term performance.

Bioactive ceramics: These are osteoconductive, acting as scaffolds to enhance bone formation on their surface, and are used either as a coating on various substrates or to fill bone defects. An osteoconductive material can only elicit bone formation in an osseous environment, whereas an osteoinductive substance can promote bone formation even in an extraosseous situation.

Calcium phosphate ceramics: HA and tricalcium phosphate (TCP), two bioceramics belonging to the calcium phosphate family, have had extensive evaluation as orthopaedic implants. Stochiometric synthetic HA ($Ca_{10}(PO_4)_6(OH)_2$), with a calcium-to-phosphate atomic ratio of 1.67, was introduced as a bone-graft substitute because its formula is similar to that of the inorganic mineral phase of bone.

Biological HA, however, is Ca deficient and a carbonated apatite. The bonding mechanism of HA to bone, although not completely understood, seems to be due osteogenically-competent cells getting attached to the surface of the HA, and later differentiating into osteoblasts.

A cellular bone matrix is then formed at the surface of the HA. An amorphous area is present between the surface and the bone tissue containing thin apatite crystals. As maturation occurs, this bonding zone shrinks and HA becomes attached to

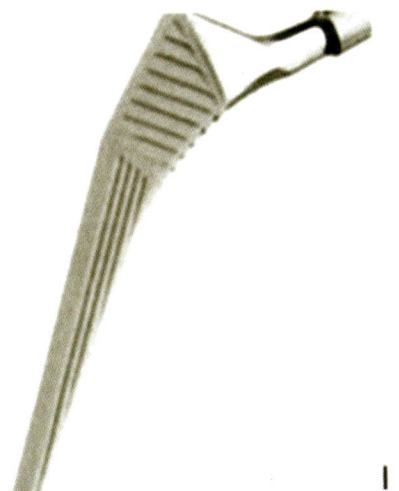

A hydroxy appatite coated stem.

bone through a thin epitaxial layer, resulting in a strong interface with no layer of fibrous tissue interposed between the bone and HA.

Bone formation grows from the surface of the HA towards the centre of the pores. HA coating (usually applied by plasma spray) is widely used on femoral prostheses and on sockets as a means of fixation in order to avoid complications related to the use of PMMA.

An American multicentre study has reported excellent results with a rate of femoral revision of 0.3% at a mean follow-up of 8.1 years, with 1 case of loosening out of 324 implants.

However, it has not yet been clearly shown that HA offers improved fixation when compared with bone cement. The thickness of the coating, the chemical composition of the material and the roughness and nature of the metal substrate seem to be key factors in ensuring good results.

The main disadvantages which have limited the clinical application of HA as a bone-graft substitute are related to its brittle nature and poor tensile strength. Consequently, information on the clinical use of ceramic bone-graft substitutes is scarce.

TCP has been evaluated in spinal fusion with results comparable to those with autogenous bone.

Bioactive glasses: Bioactive glasses, first developed by Hench and Wilson, have a vitreous structure. They bond chemically to bone. The model in this class of materials is Bioglass 45S5 of which the composition (by weight) is: 45% SiO_2, 24.5% CaO, 6% P_2O_5 and 24.5% Na_2O.

The bonding mechanism of silicate bioactive glasses to bone has been attributed to a series of surface reactions ultimately leading to the formation of a hydroxycarbonate apatite layer at the glass surface.

Greater production of bone has been demonstrated with Bioglass 45S5 when compared with HA, but due to its poor mechanical properties, this material has not been used in load-bearing applications.

Recently, in order to improve the reactivity of the material, sol-gel processed glasses, hydrolysed at ambient temperatures, have been developed to obtain bioactive gelglasses in the SiO_2-CaO-P_2O_5 system, with an initial high specific surface area.

These materials have osteoconductive properties similar to those of melt-derived glasses, but improved degradability.

The low temperatures used to produce sol-gel glasses allow them to be used as a coating on alumina substrates. When implanted in an animal model, sol-gel glass-coated alumina has demonstrated the ability to form an interface mainly composed of newly-formed bone by 24 weeks.

In this class of material, apatite wollastonite (CaO-SiO_2) glass ceramic developed by Kokubo et al. has osteoconductive properties similar to Bioglass 45S5 but increased mechanical strength. It has been used with favourable results as a spacer at the iliac crest, for vertebral prostheses and as a shelf in procedures about the shoulder.

Bioactive bone cements: Bioactive bone cements have been explored as an alternative to PMMA in order to avoid complications related to PMMA debris and to enhance fixation of the prosthesis. These materials, which have undergone extensive basic research, include calcium-phosphate based bone cement and glass-ceramic bone cement. A strong cement-bone interface is obtained by the formation of HA at the surface of the cement. Moreover, calcium phosphate cements are resorbable and are progressively replaced by newly-formed bone.

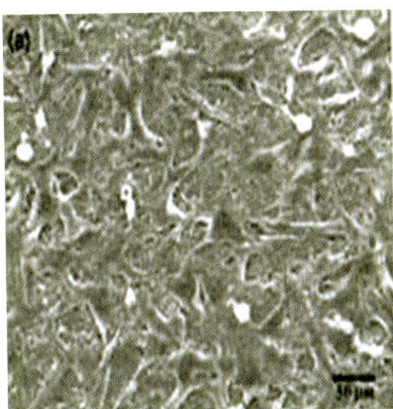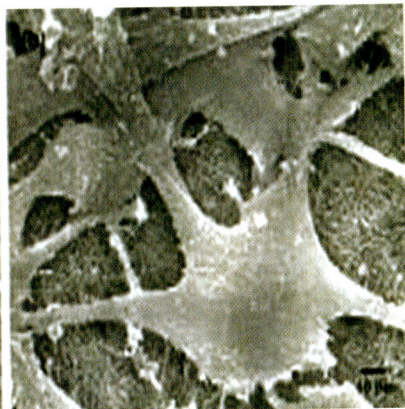

Bone, bioactive glass interface at 26 weeks.

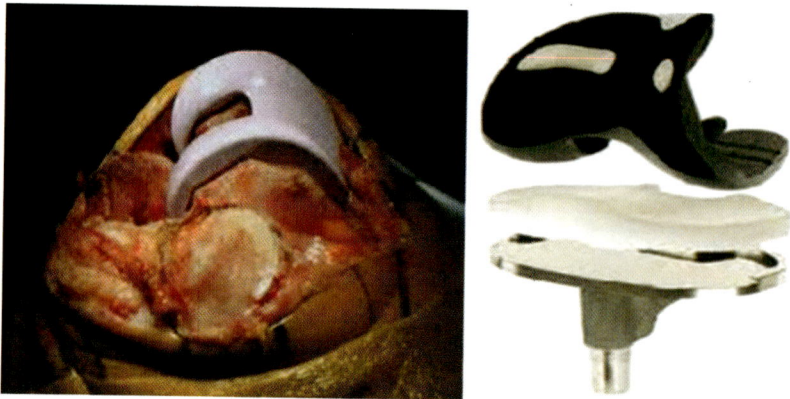

Ceramic or ceramic coated knees are still being evaluated.

Ceramic coatings provide an attractive alternative for biological fixation. In the near future, ceramic substitutes for bone grafts will probably be used in association with osteoinductive materials (such as bone morphogenetic proteins or mesenchymal stem cells) to further accelerate bone formation.

Polymethyl Methacralate: Polymethyl methacrylate remains one of the most enigmatic but enduring materials in orthopaedic surgery. With a central role in the success of total joint replacement, it is also used in newer techniques such as percutaneous vertebroplasty and kyphoplasty.

In reality, "cement" is a misnomer, because the word cement is used to describe a substance that bonds two things together. However, PMMA acts as a space-filler that creates a tight space and holds the implant against the bone, thus acting as a 'grout'. Bone cements have no intrinsic adhesive properties; instead, they rely on close mechanical interlock between the irregular bone surface and the prosthesis.

Polymethyl methacrylate (PMMA) was first employed by orthopaedic surgeons over 60 years ago and remains a key component of modern practice. The understanding of its properties has evolved and progressed alongside the advance of the specialty, and has indirectly helped improve implant design, particle science, cell biology and biomechanics. The use of acrylic by orthopaedic surgeons is likely to continue, and knowledge of the properties and applications of this material remains essential. Polymethylmethacrylate was unveiled by the chemical industry in 1843 and named 'acide acrylique' on account of the acrid smell of the monomer. In 1936, it was noted that mixing ground polymer with monomer produced a dough that could be manipulated and moulded; hence it became one of the earliest biomaterials.

Early applications were in dentistry. Its use as a grout to improve implant fixation was pioneered in 1953 by Haboush. However, the major breakthrough in the use of PMMA in total hip replacement (THR) was the work of Charnley in 1970, who used it to secure fixation of the acetabular and femoral components and to transfer loads to bone.

Sir John Charnley can well be credited with introducing bone cement in Orthopaedics. Working alone, constantly researching, improvising and improving, he invented what we can call the first modern total joint replacement. The early results were spectacular. And the results remained spectacular. Hundreds upon hundreds were relieved of pain and crippling. They remained pain free for a long period, so joint replacements had come to stay. Once the principles were established, replacement of other joints began to follow. Charnley, the meticulous and dedicated scientist, was working very hard on all aspects of this specialty. Theatre asepsis, lamellar air flows, antibiotic prophylaxis, deep vein thrombosis, cement polymerization, cement bone interaction—these were among the subjects on which Sir John conducted research.

The American surgeons at this time were keen to try out hip replacements on their own. And as was the custom, bone cement was sent to the FDA (the agency that monitors quality and standards of consumables in the US) for testing. They found that cement was carcinogenic in the mice they tested them in! Approval for use of bone cement was withheld, hence American surgeons could not use bone cement or perform hip replacements.

This was in the early 1960s. Plane loads of patients flew into England and got their hips replaced. Back in the US, they thumbed their nose at the FDA!!! This state of affairs persisted for a decade. Indignant US surgeons demanded a reevaluation of the facts. And it was found that the mice on which cement was tested and found carcinogenic were indeed carcinogen-

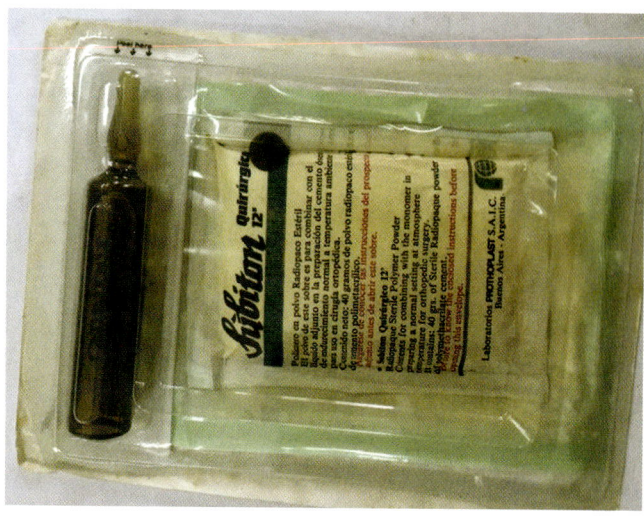

Argentinian black market cement used in USA when FDA had not yet approved the use of bone cement.

susceptible mice in the first place! The experiments were repeated; this time it was found to be reasonably safe, and only in the early 1970s was cement approved for use in the US. This gave a 10-year lead to the British in the field of hip surgery.

The use of bone cement was considered a weak link in the development process of joint replacements. Since early days, there have been efforts to design and develop a prosthesis that can be anchored without bone cement. As a matter of fact, Austin Moore's endoprosthesis depended on a self-locking mechanism as a result of bone ingrowth to help anchor the prosthesis in the hip.

Bone cement is available in two components: a polymer and a monomer. The polymer is a white powder (usually sold in 40 gm sachets), in a double or triple packing and sterilized by gamma irradiation. The monomer is a liquid (usually available in 20 ml ampoules), again double packed and sterilized by gamma irradiation.

PMMA is a self-curing acrylic polymer, unlike the heat cured version used in the original Judet hips. There is a catalyst in the powder and an accelerator in the liquid. Both act together in causing a polymerization, forming longer chains of the acrylate which changes its constituency with the passage of time. The

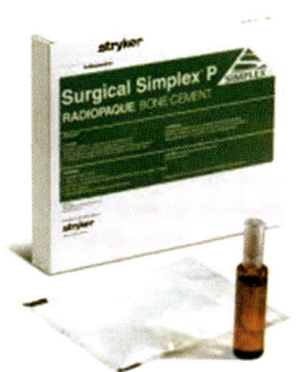
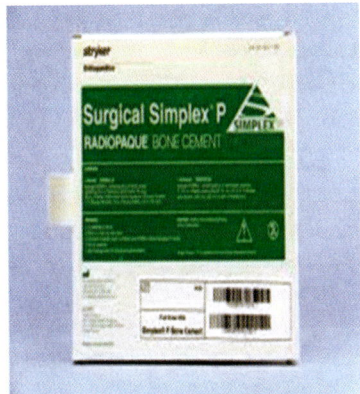

The original low viscosity cement, best for injection under pressure.

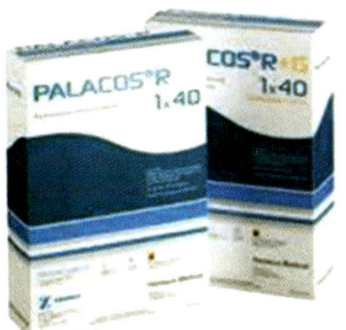
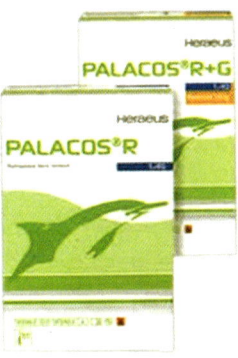

Antibiotic loaded bone cements are slightly less viscous.

cement is not glue and does not have any adhesive qualities. As a matter of fact, it is a grout or a filler to enable a more uniform transmission of forces.

As it sets and is mouldable, it is distributed uniformly all over the surfaces transmitting weight proportionately across all dimensions of the implant. Due to the absence of mechanical bonding properties, the cement does not adhere to the polished surfaces of the prosthesis. However, it does slightly bond to the rough metallic surfaces or the plastic tibia. Some manufacturers choose to precoat the surface of the implant with a thin coat of PMMA to enhance its bonding qualities. However, since the time of Sir John, cement was never intended to be glue; it was never intended to bond either the prosthesis or the cup to the body.

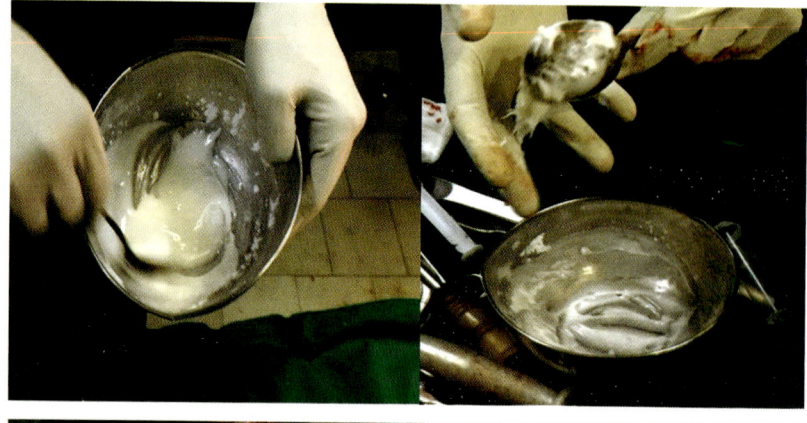

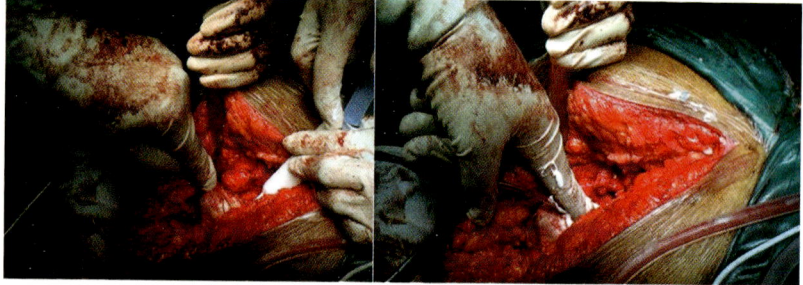

Cement can be hand pressurized or injected with a gun or syringe.

Especially with knee replacement, it is to be understood that it is a rigid and brittle structure; only when it fully conforms to the outer surface of the implant will it act as a uniform weight transmitter.

Recent studies have shown that bone cement is 3 times stronger in compression than with shear forces. Actually a good analogy would be the Portland cement between bricks. This supports a strong ceiling and a weight on the ceiling, but cannot withstand a blow from the side (as is used to demolish buildings). Thus in the long run, failure would often occur because the cement was not packed tightly enough and the crevices in it would fail due to the rotatory and bending movements (rather than compression).

Subsequent studies have shown that the properties of the cement implant bondage not only depend upon the stage at which it is introduced; they also depend upon constant pressure exertion at the time of setting and absence or diminution of air bubbles (which lead to porosity of the cement) in the mixture. Newer methods like vacuum stirring and pressure injection address this problem. A closed cavity onto which liquid cement is pushed with pressure will of course enhance the bondage between the walls and the cement; hence the newer techniques of syringe injection are currently used.

Many surgeons advocate adding antibiotics to bone cement. It has been found that less than 2 grams of heat stable antibiotics (powder) added to 40 grams of the cement powder does not significantly inhibit the tensile and compressive strength. Very recent studies do show that fatigue strength may be compromised by such addition; hence their routine use in primary arthroplasty is not recommended. Further, as the chances of infection are much less in a primary replacement arthroplasty than in revision, and as routine antibiotic-loaded cement usage in primary arthroplasties may cause resistant strains of organisms to develop, adding antibiotics in cement is not routinely recommended.

Radio-opaque substances like barium sulphate are now being routinely added. These are very important for an accurate correlation in follow-up radiographs. The use of cement without this is almost given up. After remaining in the body for a sufficient time, the cement tends to attain a light brown shade; in many revision cases, it may be difficult to distinguish this from cortical bone. To help identify cement in revision procedures, certain companies now add pigments like methylene blue and chlorophyll.

A word here about hypotension induced by cement. It has been found that between 3 and 4 minutes after femoral cementation, a transient hypotension is noticed. This is more marked with liquid preparations than with doughy masses. The reason for this is the absorption of the monomer into the blood. The absorbed monomer is subsequently metabolized as methacrylic acid and then to carbon dioxide. The anaesthetist should be forewarned and the blood pressure has to be kept a little high to avoid complications.

Almost all brands of cement are available in India. The shelf life of the monomer is less than that of the polymer and one must note the expiry date carefully while purchasing. There is

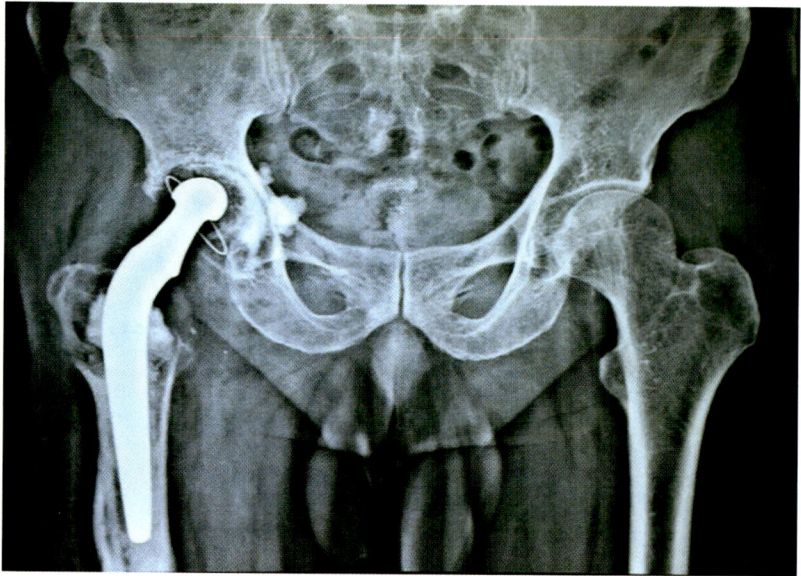

Mixing of radio-opaque substances with bone cement allows us to radiologically study the cement bone interface.

not much to choose between the various forms of cement, except when you are using pressurization techniques and the need to use a cement gun. Low viscosity cements available include Surgical Simplex and CMW. Doughy mixes include Zimmer, Palacos and Sulfix.

In conclusion, bone cement is a good thing, but only as long as one understands how to use it properly. Use it well and it will last for years; bad cementation will lead to early failures.

Even today, best results of cemented hips are superior to cementless knees, both in short and long term.

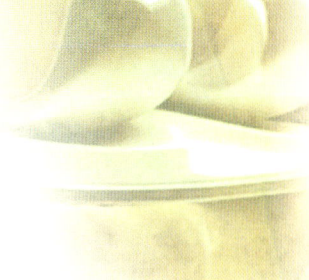

The Making of a Knee Prosthesis

Design, development and manufacturing of a total knee prosthesis is no rocket science. In engineering terms, despite the major hype generated by the big companies, the technology is fairly basic.

It is pertinent that Sir John Charnley made his initial 500 hips in his own lathe in his workshop. Mckee personally hand polished the head of his first hip. Our own Dr KH Sancheti, began making his Indus Knees in his basement workshop.

Throughout the world, surgeon innovators have participated in the process of manufacturing the total knee implants, and even if the reader doesn't intend to manufacture his/her own prosthesis, knowledge of the complete manufacturing process improves one's understanding of the product and procedure.

The first step is to do a dimensional analysis of bones, radiographs and CT scans to get the sizes of the knees of the population spread.

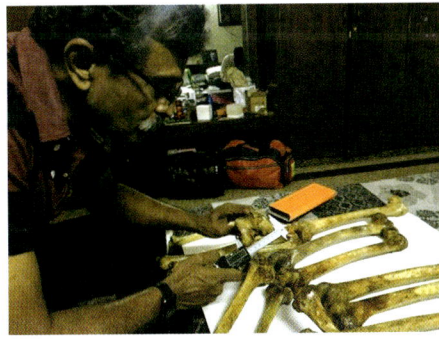
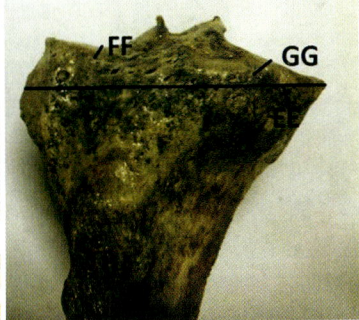

Skeletal measurements to get bone size spread.

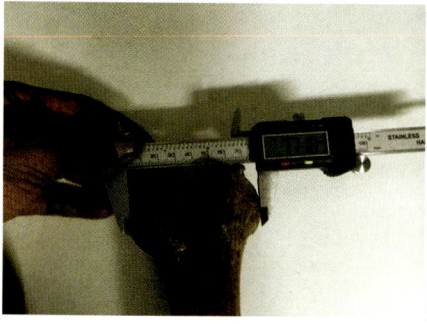 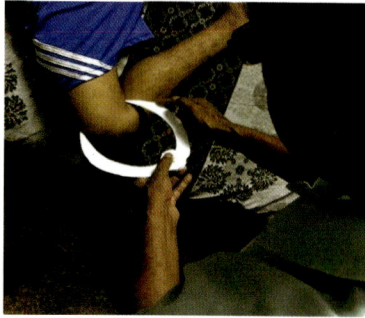

Anthropometric and cadaveric measurements for dimensional analysis.

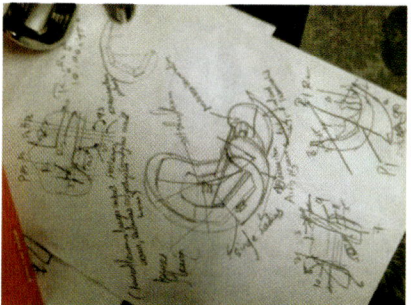 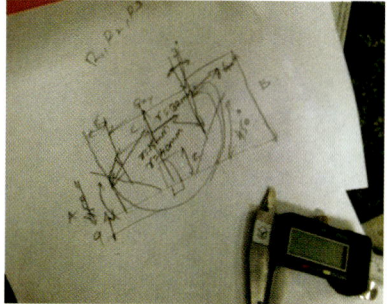

First raw design of shape and dimensions of the prosthesis.

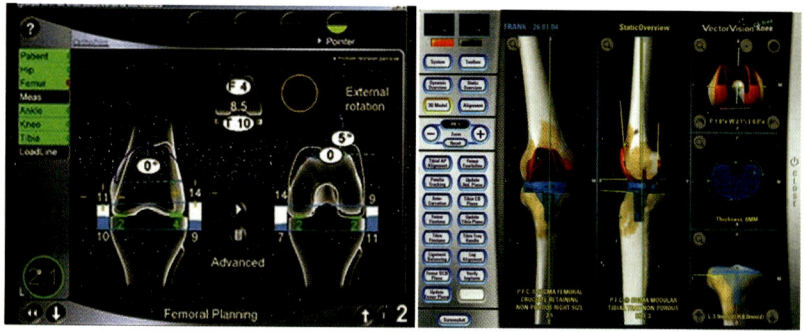

CAD design of the components.

The next step is designing the actual components. Most modern knees are very similar with minor differences. The basic design is made on a CAD programme, and the same is fed into a multi axis CNC machine to produce the first prototype components.

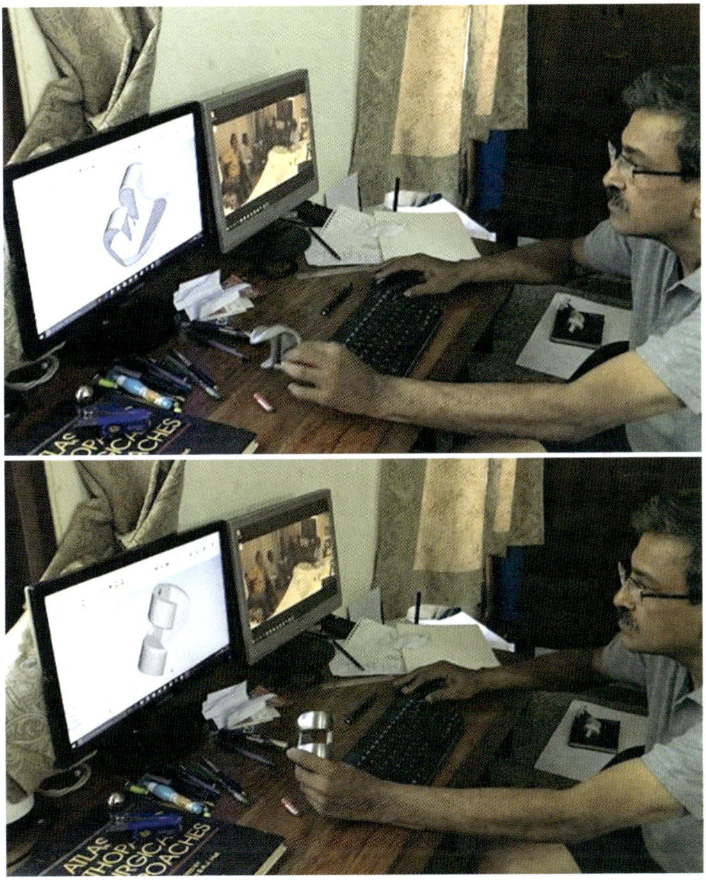

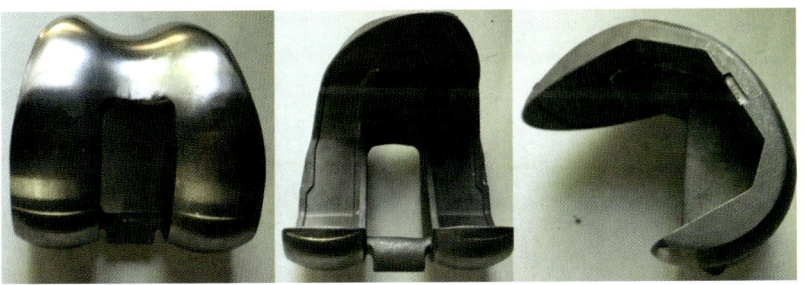

Output in the form of IGES or STEP file.

Component prototype for making the die.

The next step is making a die for wax patterns as the metallic components are going to be cast by investment casting or lost wax process.

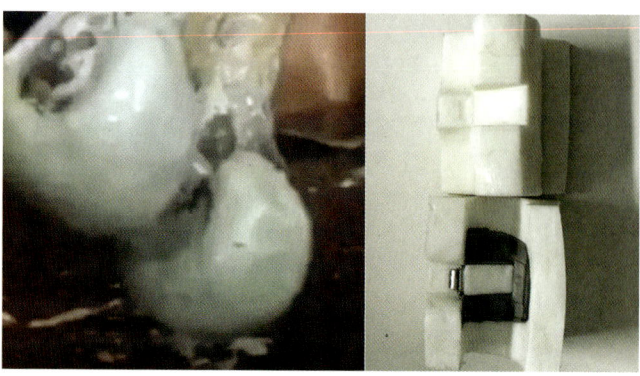

Silicone rubber dies for wax patterns.

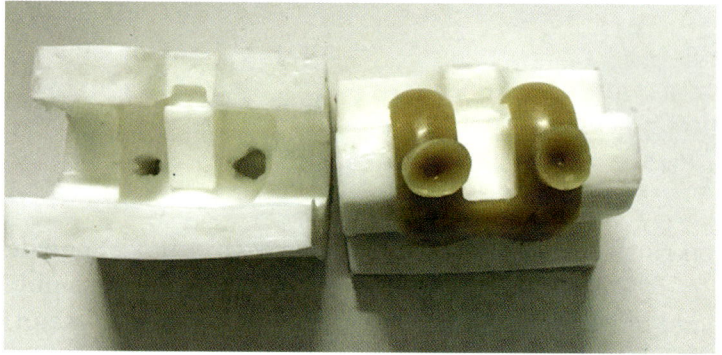

A wax pattern from the mould.

The dies can be made in metal or silicone rubber. Metal dies would give thousands of pieces while rubber dies have to be frequently replaced.

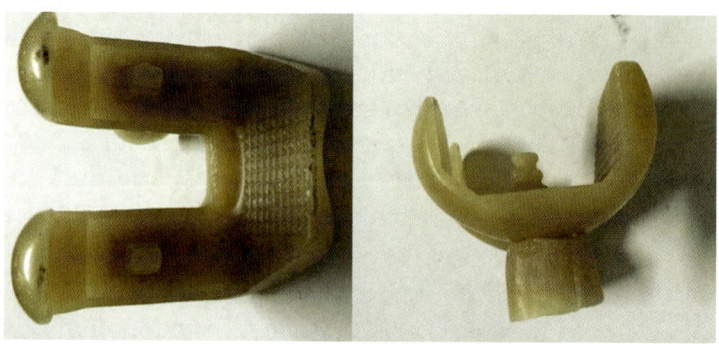

These wax patterns are coated with layers of fine ceramic clay and dried to form clay moulds with the pattern inside.

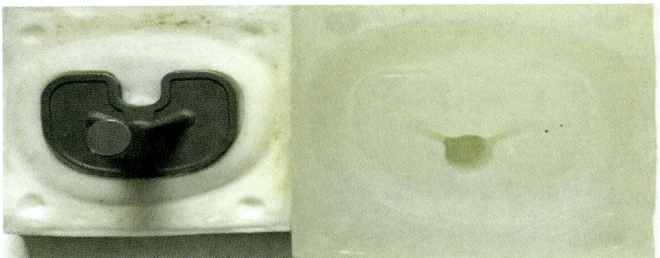

Irrespective or the metal used for casting, this step remains the same.

At this stage, we get the metallic component replicas in wax with dimensional tolerances accurate up to 0.2 mm. These are coated with fine ceramic clay by repeated dipping in a clay bath.

The dies are allowed to air dry to remove moisture, then oven fired to melt the wax and produce a single-use ceramic casting die into which molten metal is poured.

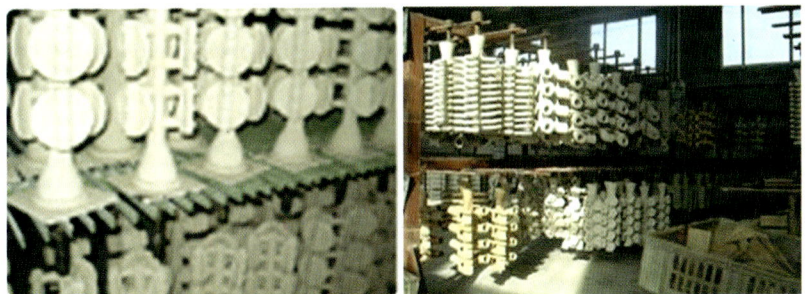

Ceramic shell trees being air dried and fired to make one time ceramic dies.

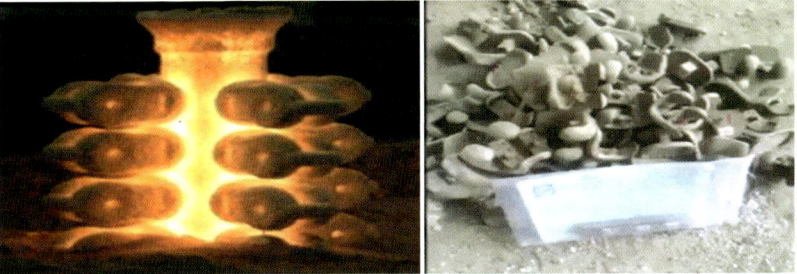

Molten metal, most often cobalt chrome molybdenum alloy, is poured into the dies. On cooling, the outer shells are broken open to extract the components.

The rough castings undergo radiographic testing, followed by metallurgical analysis and material testing, both destructive and non-destructive. Only components which pass the tests are taken up for the next stage.

The cast component is machined by a multi-axis vertical machine centre to match the drawings. VMC machines easily achieve tolerances up to 0.1 mm.

Repeated quality checks are conducted at each stage to ensure that every product is perfect.

UHMWHDPE comes in blocks or sheets. One metre square and fifty millimetre thick sheets are the standard. They are machined in a VMC and the CAD programme ensures dimensional accuracy of each component.

All that remains to be done now is polishing of the components. This can be done either by automatic tumbler

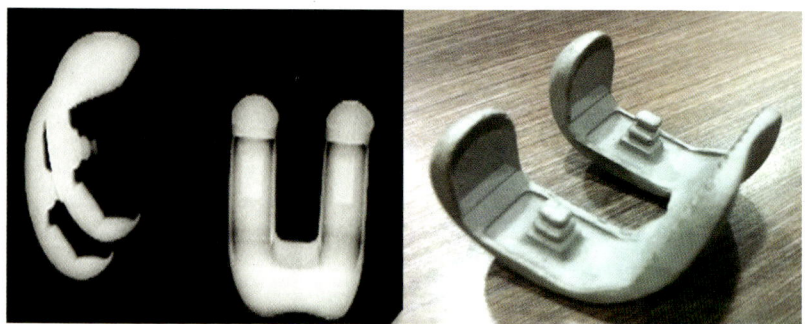

Radiological and other tests are done to choose the approved castings.

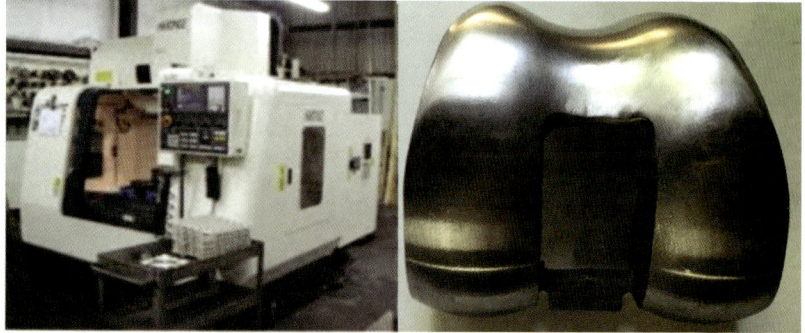

A 5-axis VMC is used to accurately machine the articular surfaces, which will be polished later.

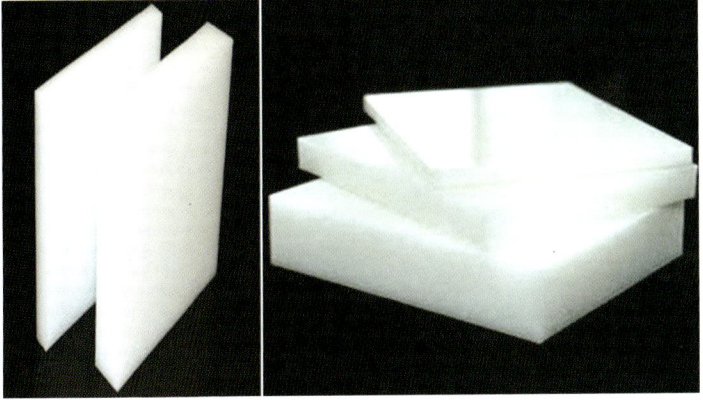

HDPE sheets for tibial inserts.

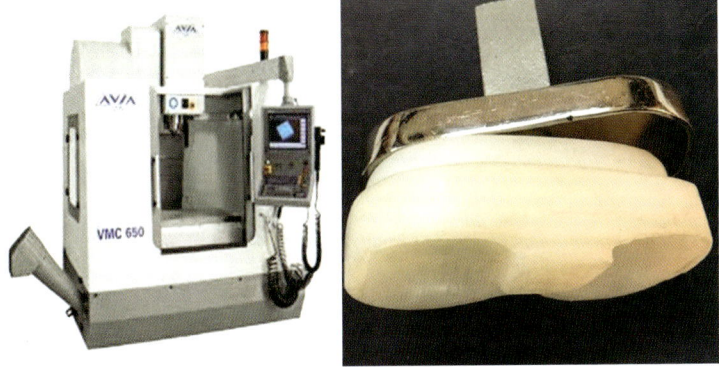

Machined in a VMC to appropriate shape.

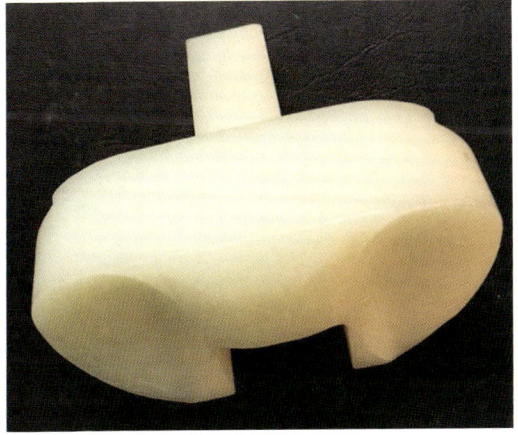

An all poly component machined in a VMC.

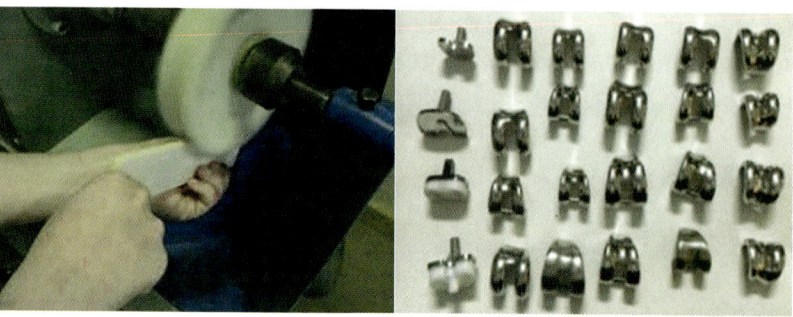

Polishing of the components to achieve mirror finish.

polishers which use ceramic grinding wedges, or manually using buffing wheels of increasing softness.

The aim is to achieve a mirror polish without any imperfections. The long-term success of a knee replacement certainly depends on the polish of the femoral articulating surface.

Finished components are laser marked with sizes and batch numbers. Each component bears a serial number essential for traceability and process control.

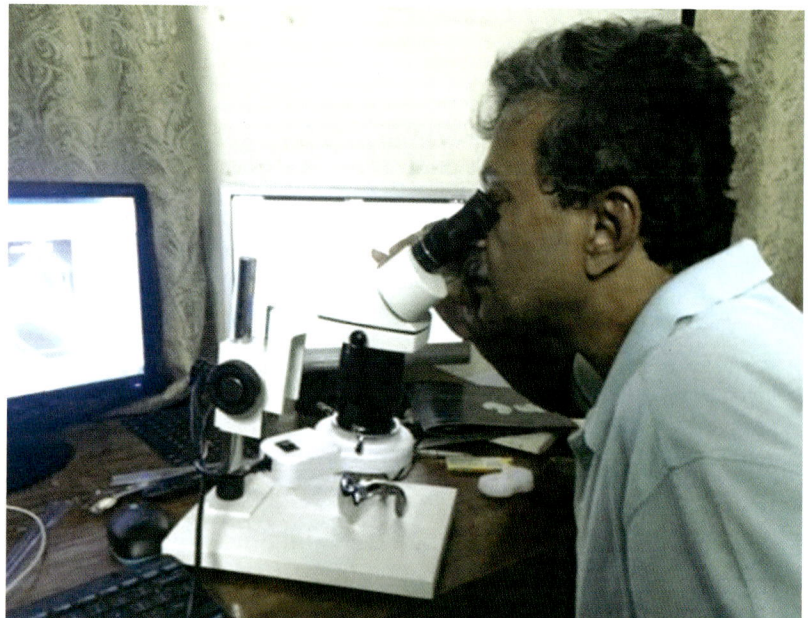

Inspection with metallurgical microscope for surface finish and absence of scratches or imperfections.

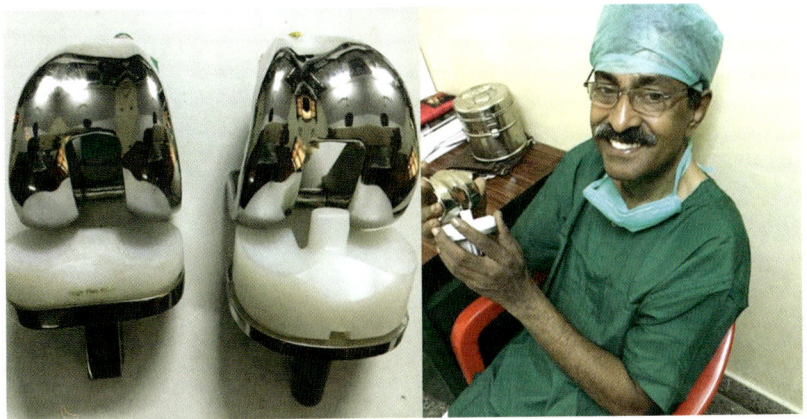

Prototype components of the Madras High Flex Knee designed by the author.

The components are repeatedly cleaned at each stage. Once complete and inspected, the entire operation shifts to a clean room with laminar air flow and restricted entry.

The components are packed appropriately and readied for sterilization. The metallic components are sterilized by Gamma radiation and two centres in India do this: RASHMI in Bengaluru and BARC in Mumbai.

The plastic components are sterilized by ethylene oxide sterilization. Certain companies use low dose radiation, with the components packed in vacuum or nitrogen. However, evidence currently supports non-radiation sterilization of plastic components for a longer in bio life and diminished brittleness and failure.

Biomechanical Considerations

The surgeon contemplating to start this procedure must bear in mind that a total joint significantly differs from other orthopaedic implants like plates and screws. The latter are used only as temporary supports until the bone heals but with a joint, it is for good. (At least we hope so.)

Thus, one has to consider the constant forces acting on the joint day in and out, the effects of cyclic loading of 2 to 10 times body weight on the implant, and the fact that technical flaws resulting from an improper understanding of the biomechanical problems will cause failure with disastrous consequences of marked pain and disability, which on occasions may be greater than the problems for which the surgery was performed in the first place.

By all standards, these implants are very expensive. Thus their use in an average patient is restricted not only by availability, but also by cost. Unlike a simple ball and socket joint of the hip, the knee is a complex diarthrodial joint with large joint surfaces. A human knee is not inherently or structurally stable by the bone shape congruity; rather, the joint depends considerably on the ligaments and soft tissue around it for stability, support and movement.

Thus if an artificial knee joint is expected to last long, its design should incorporate features that would ensure some stability based upon the available ligaments and soft tissues around the knee. Its surfaces should be congruent enough to spread the area of contact over large surfaces and at the same time, should not be too congruent to cause constraint amongst the joint surfaces, increasing friction dramatically.

The following parameters are important:
1. Knee biomechanics and loading
2. Alignment of the components
3. Congruency of the implant surfaces
4. Inbuilt implant constraints
5. Soft tissue balance

Knee Biomechanics and Loading

The human knee (according to the anatomist) is a diarthrodial ginglymus. However in the actual sense, the knee is not a simple hinge, and movements of flexion, extension, abduction, adduction, and rotation all occur in it!

In a normal knee, the cruciates form an important part to determine its functionality and competence. And as one or both are invariably sacrificed, the implant design has to compensate for it.

The above diagram displays this fact clearly. AB is the direction of neutral fibres of ACL. CD is the direction of neutral fibres of PCL. BD is the link between the tibial attachment sites, and CA is the femoral insertion point.

The points of insertion between links AB and CD make the flexion axis. Understanding this concept is very important in knee design. This is represented in a normal human knee by a

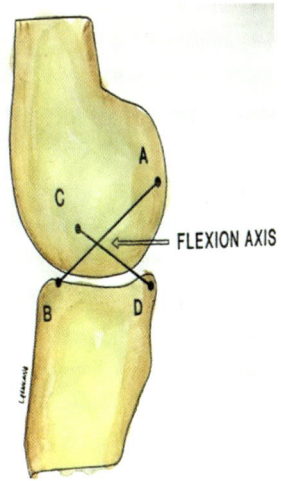

Flexion axis for a normal knee.

screwhome mechanism, wherein there is an external rotation of the tibia over the femur as the knee is straightened from a flexed position. The winding and unwinding of the cruciates accomplish this maneuvre; if one or both cruciates are removed during a knee replacement surgery, the implant design should contribute to compensate this deficiency and ensure stability by introducing sufficient constraint in the implant.

The knee has a constant changing centre of rotation from flexion to extension, with a polycentric curve comprised of a slide, glide and a roll-over motion. Thus with these diverse axes of motion, the knee's stability is dependant both on the anatomical shape of the joint as well as the ligaments and muscles.

The loads transmitted across the knee are tremendous; up to 3 times the body weight is transmitted in level walking and up to 4 times in stair climbing. Despite the knee being a large joint, all weight is not uniformly transmitted across the knee. Relatively small areas of the tibial surface transmit the loads, and menisci play a significant part in force dissipation. The medial compartment bears a greater load than the lateral!

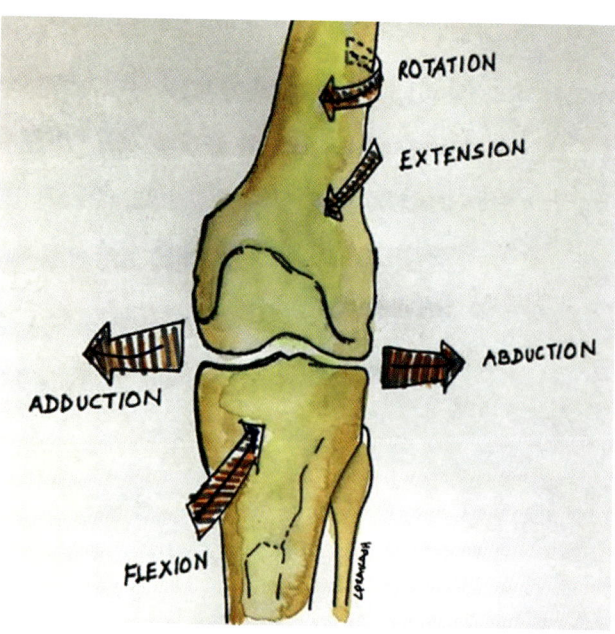

The knee is capable of motion in all 3 planes.

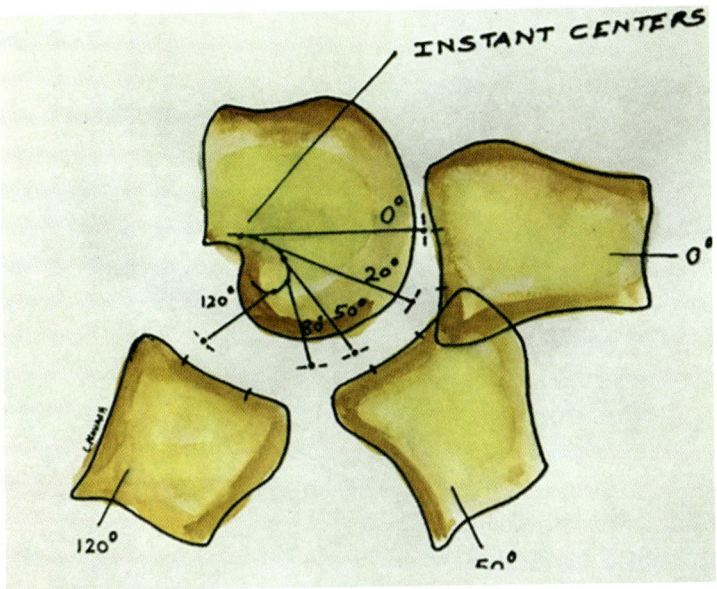

A knee has a constant changing centre of rotation from flexion to extension.

Alignment of the Components

Mediolateral Axis: The hip joints are fixed structures. When a person is standing or walking, the two relevant points of the plumb line that represent the line of weight transmission are the centre of the hip joint and the centre of ankle joint. If a straight line drawn through the two passes through the centre of the knee joint, then weight will be transmitted uniformly over the entire area of the joint surface. However, if the line passes through one compartment or the other, then it invariably follows that one-half of the joint will bear all the forces, will consequently suffer from unequal load distribution and also an early wear.

When a person stands on one leg (Trendelenburg stance), the partial body weight W is held by the lateral tension band T in equilibrium. The resultant force R thus passes through the centre of the knee joint.

Thus if the knee is in a neutral axis, we find that the line of weight bearing is passing through the medial compartment alone as shown in the following diagram. If the knee happens to be in a varus, then the line of weight transmission will pass through

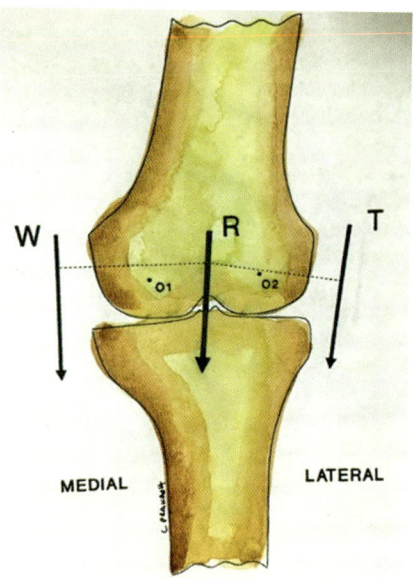

The forces generated in the knee while standing on one leg.

the space medial to the medial-most part of the joint, which is a disaster because the wear will be restricted to the most medial part of the medial compartment and there will be no weight transmission through the lateral half of the joint.

However, if the knee is in a valgus position, it is apparent that the weight is transmitted more or less through the centre of the knee joint; it hence follows that there will be a uniform distribution of the stresses, hence preferential loading of a single compartment of the knee is avoided. The importance of the above statements cannot be over emphasized!

Knee loading due to mechanical axis deviation

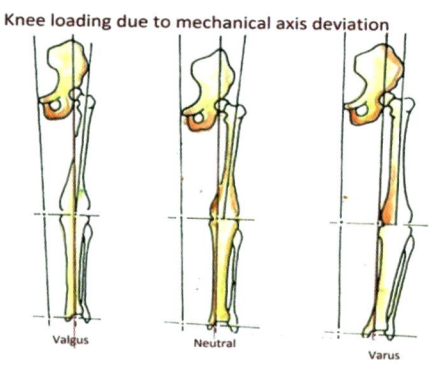

As most osteoarthritic knees are in varus, it follows that the medial compartment bears the major brunt of all forces and wears out first.

If there is one single lesson that the reader remembers from this book, it should be the above. In a physiological knee, if there is a varus, there is definite early medial compartment arthritis. However, a valgus knee of up to 7° or 9° can become a more global arthritis as the years pass by!

As a corollary, knees that are in gross valgus will suffer from lateral compartment arthritis. *Thus to repeat: A varus to rectus knee will have a medial arthritis, a moderate valgus will have a global arthritis and a markedly valgus knee will surely have a lateral compartment arthritis.*

The friction forces on a synovial cartilage/synovial cartilage articulation are very minimal and no man-made bearing surface ever matches this. The following chart shows the friction on various bearing surfaces!

With such excellent natural bearing surfaces, if misalignment causes wear within the life span of the individual, it necessarily follows that with man-made inferior material, a mal-alignment will cause a much more rapid wear and failure!

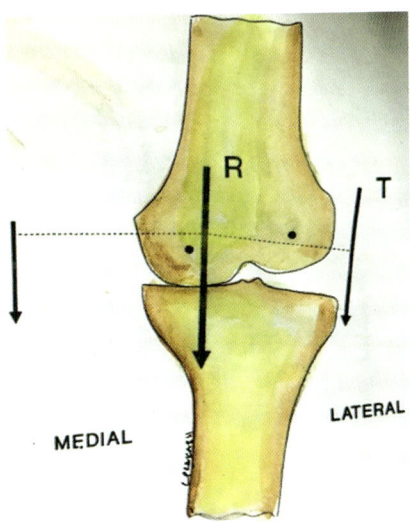

The resultant force R in a varus knee passes fully through the medial compartment.

Material	Lubrication	Coef. of friction
Metal on metal nonpolished	Dry	100.00
Tyre on road	Dry	1.00
Nylon on steel	Dry	0.20
PTFE on PTFE	Dry	0.07
PTFE on PTFE	Water	0.04
SS on SS	Water	0.36
CoCr on CoCr	Water	0.38
SS on HDPE	Water	0.04
CoCr on HDPE	Water	0.04
Human Knee Joint	Water	0.009

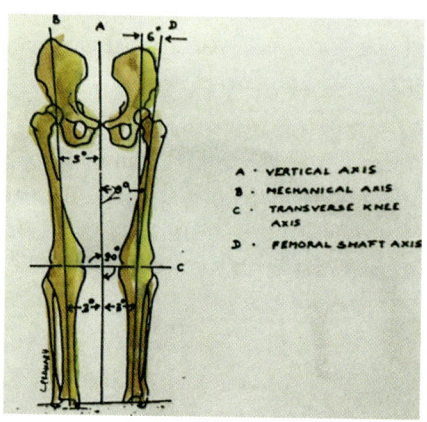

Alignment and axes of the knee.

Anterio-posterior axis: There should be a slight posterior slope to allow for a greater flexion. A slope from back to front is a mechanical disadvantage because on weight bearing and standing, the femoral component will have a tendency towards unrestricted forward fall, leading to rapid failure.

Based on the above logical inferences, one can conclude that the distal femur should be cut at 5° to 7° of valgus, the upper tibia should be parallel to the floor or up to 2° slope posteriorly.

Congruency of implant surfaces: When a person stands or walks, different loads are transmitted through various joints in different phases of activity like level walking, running, stair climbing, or jogging. Two logical assumptions can be made at this stage. Smaller the area, more the load transmitted per square mm. Just imagine sliding a brick on the table, first wide side down, and then on its edges. Naturally the same load distributed over a wider area will be lesser per square mm.

However, the exact opposite is true of friction-induced wear. Larger the contact area, greater the surfaces rubbing against one another, more the friction and more the wear. These points should receive very careful consideration while a knee implant is being designed.

In addition to the nature of the articulating surfaces, loading depends on the surface area. To give a simple example, it is easier to push a brick that lies flat, than when it is standing upright. As the material that is going to be used is a constant, the design of the knee must provide minimal contact surfaces to produce lowest friction possible.

Friction on the contrary depends on the area of contact; thus, a smaller contact area will have a lower friction than a larger area of contact, the bearing surfaces being constant! By these statements it is apparent that friction and wear are independent, and both are of concern to the surgeon.

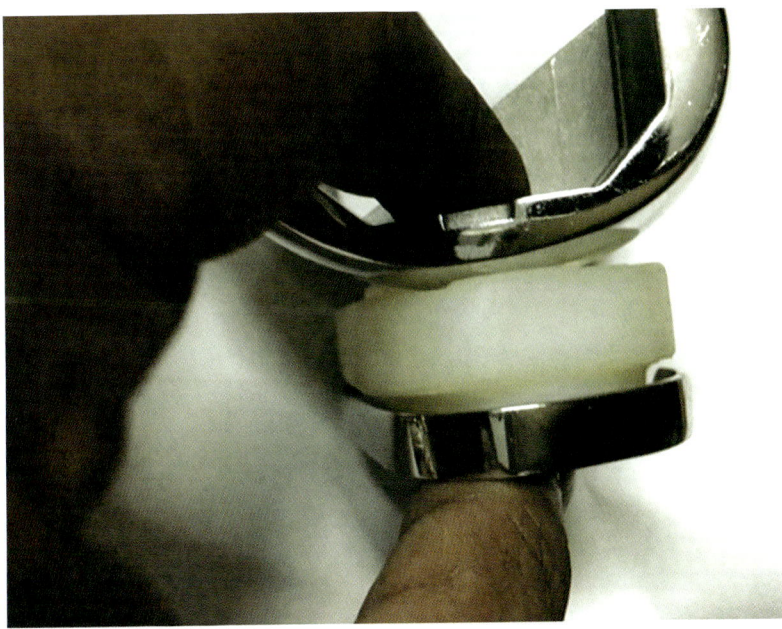

This is a limited contact implant. See areas of point contact stresses.

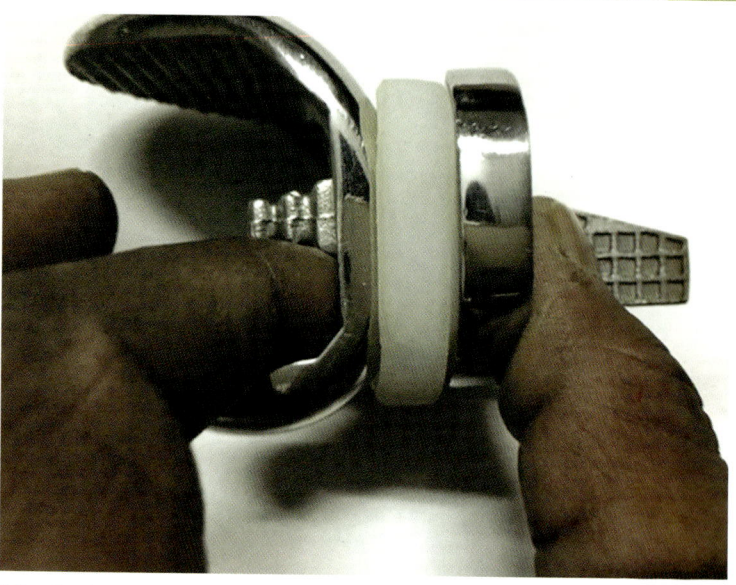

In this design of implant, the contact is more uniform and a larger surface area articulates.

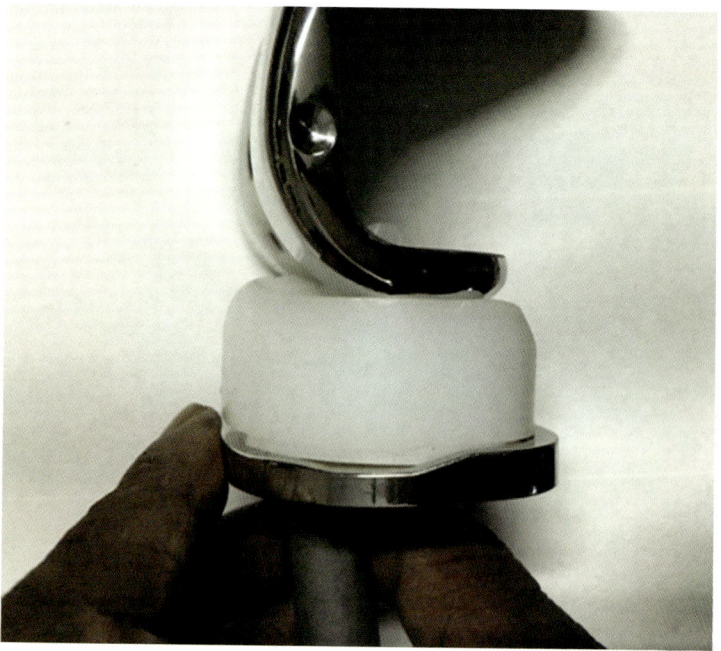

A newer design knee allowing limited contact in full flexion, but rather full contact in extension.

Limited areas of contact causes point loading and rapid boring sort of wear at areas of high stresses. Thus designs should avoid small areas of intense contact. If both the components are spheroidal in shape, it would increase conformity and constraint. An increase in constraint will cause increased stresses at the implant bone interface, leading to early loosening.

Another important point is that a normal physiological knee has femoral condyles articulating with a rather flat tibial surface, with its contour enhanced by the presence of menisci. In a normal knee, the area of contract in flexion is lesser than that in extension. So the design of knee should also take this factor into consideration.

Thus the optimal knee design should allow for a large area of contact between the femoral and tibial components, but the two surfaces should only roughly match in profile and not be very congruent. Moreover, the areas of contact should be shaped so as to allow a slight glide and roll as the knee moves from extension to flexion.

Inbuilt implant constraints: Unlike a hip joint (which is a simple ball and socket joint), a normal knee has cruciates, which are strong structures that keep the knee stable. The collaterals too play an important part in the stability of the knee. If any of these

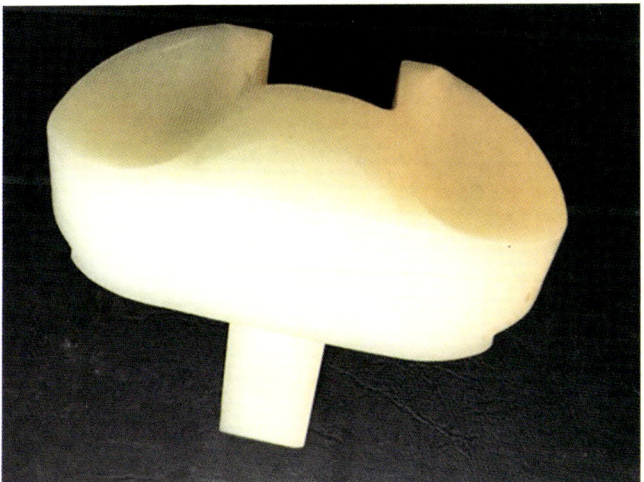

The PCL retaining designs have a central projection to compensate for ACL that has been removed.

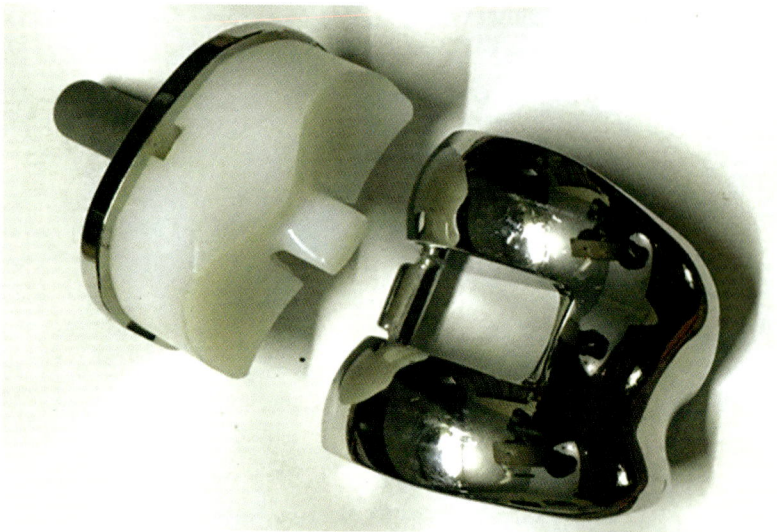

A knee design in which both cruciates are removed should have a projecting cam from the middle of tibia to provide an inbuilt constraint for the joint.

stabilizing factors are missing, the design of the implant should build in a constraint to overcome the deficiency.

Thus with an absent posterior cruciate, the tibial and femoral surfaces should have a posterior stabilizer. Most designs achieve this by sacrificing the anterior cruciate and having a central bridge on the tibial surface.

With collateral laxity, the lax side has to be fine tuned by stretching that side, either by using bone or wedges incorporated into the prosthesis. And if all stabilizing structures are deficient, a hinge joint may be needed, especially in salvage procedures and after resections. However, one has to remember that the more one depends on the implant to provide constraints, greater will be the loosening and wear.

Soft tissue balance: As discussed previously, the restoration of alignment prior to the bony resections is the key to long-lasting results of replacement. If an arthroplasty is performed where the limb looks aligned but the straightness of the limb is achieved by obliquity of bone cuts rather than release of tight structures, the joint will invariably fail due to the unbalanced loading of the surfaces.

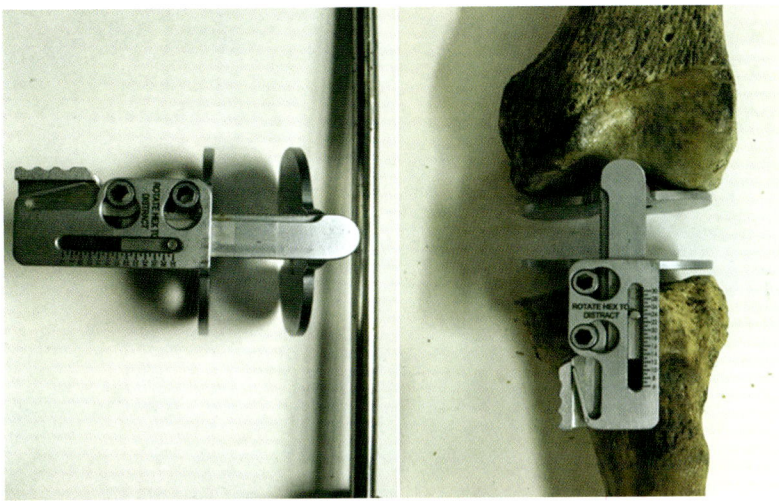

The author's design of a soft tissue balancer and flexion extension gap measurement device.

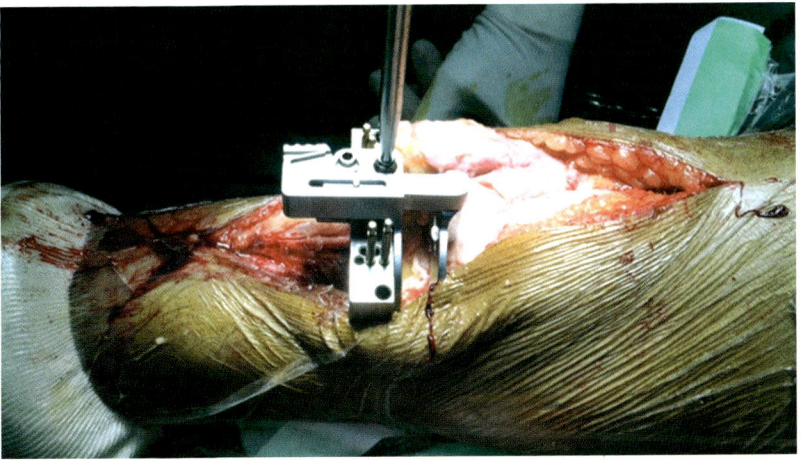

This instrument measures and balances the flexion and extension gap, a step very important for the long-term survive of an implanted knee prosthesis.

To achieve long-lasting results, all deformities should be corrected by correct soft tissue release procedures prior to bone cuts. Despite earlier observations to the contrary, it is now well-established that knees with perfect alignment, adequate soft tissue balance and precise bone cuts will be the only ones that succeed in the long run!

Knee Design Considerations and Types of Knee Replacements

Introduction: Till date, well over 1000 designs of total knee replacements have been described. With continuous additions of newer models and more recent Mark XXXs, telling us that (a) the ideal knee is still under development and (b) we as surgeons lack the patience to wait long enough to know if a particular design works well. Based on theoretical studies, an ideal knee should perform the following functions:

1. It should allow motion as near to the normal knee as possible in all three planes.
2. The joint surfaces should contribute to an excellent stability in extension and reasonable stability in flexion.
3. The artificial articular surface should provide a constantly changing centre of rotation like the normal knee.
4. The design should allow for maximum preservation of available ligaments and supporting structures in the knee that is being replaced.
5. By its shape and structure, the design should compensate ligaments and structures that are deficient.
6. The shape should lend itself to an equal transmission of load through its entire surface to minimize wear and assure a long-lasting joint.

As discussed in the previous chapter, a greater congruency of the tibial and femoral surfaces leads to a fairly uniform distribution of stresses, which will lower the wear. However, a greater congruency will definitely increase the constraint and thus contribute to greater stresses at the implant cement interface, which will lead to loosening. The converse is also true:

A very limited contact will have a minimal constraint and hence no implant bone stresses; however, the very minimal articulating surfaces will be subject to tremendous point contact loads and thus lead to disproportionate wear and failure. The compromise will be a joint in which the surfaces roughly match but are NOT an exact fit.

Types of Knee Designs

Over the years, the various knee joints that have made their appearance can be classified into the following designs based on the shape of the articular surface:
1. Spherocentric designs
2. Roller trough designs
3. Condylar designs
4. Anatomic designs
5. Single radius medial contact designs
6. Meniscal designs

Based on the implant criteria and instrumentation, the designs can be classified as:
1. Universal designs (left and right interchangeable)
2. Anatomic femoral only (left and right femoral components)
3. Anatomic femoral and tibial
4. Gender specific knees.
5. Patient specific implants
6. Modular designs

Regarding metal-backing of the plastic and patellar shapes, the following designs are available:
1. Non metal-backed tibial component
2. Metal-backed fixed HDPE tibial component.
3. Metal-backed detachable HDPE tibial component
4. Non metal-backed patellar component
5. Metal-backed patellar component.

As we move from the minimally constrained towards the more constrained implants, the use gets restricted to grossly unstable knees, revision cases, bone loss, and resection in tumours. These hinged or constrained devices are of the following types:
1. Fixed hinge joints

2. Axial hinge joints

3. Rotating hinge joints

In so far as the method of fixation is concerned, the following types of fixation are available:

1. Fixation with bone cement

2. Fixation with porous coating for bone ingrowth

3. Fixation with hydroxyapatite (HA) coated implants

It follows that each type of knee design will incorporate features from all the above criteria. Some of the above criteria have distinct proven advantages over the other. I shall now give a brief description of the parameters and also list their advantages and disadvantages. This would help you to choose the ideal design that incorporates all the desirable features and avoids features proved to be undesirable.

Spherocentric surface design: These were the very early shapes that came in immediately after the fixed hinge joints failed. The femoral component is a section of a large sphere and the tibial component is a mirror image of the same. These early designs have now been more or less given up. They are mentioned just for the sake of completeness. Examples of this design are the now obsolete. Spherocentric knee and Stabilocondylar prosthesis.

Roller trough design: Here the femoral component is a part of a cylinder rather than a sphere. It is relatively flat at the distal end. The tibial surface roughly matches the femoral condyle but is not an exact fit. Its advantages are:

1. Low constraint, hence less stresses at the implant bone interface.

2. Differential contact in flexion and extension, with an increased contact in full extension providing inherent stability.

3. Range of motion up to 130° possible in a properly implanted knee.

Its disadvantages are:

1. There is no constant changing centre of rotation.

2. The stability in flexion is less.

3. There is a definite constraint in extension that may theoretically lead to implant bone interface loading.

Examples of this design are Freeman-Samuelson Mark II knee, Whiteside knee, etc.

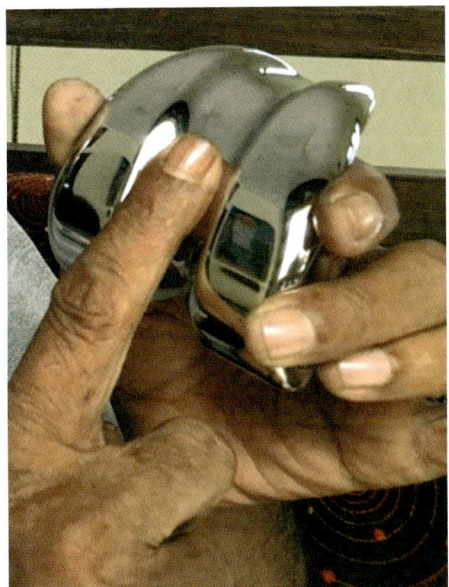

Freeman-Samuelson Mark II knee.

Condylar Designs: Possibly the most implanted knee design in existence, it also has the longest follow-up amongst all knees that have been replaced to date. The shape is a mix between the above two with rather spherocondylar femora and somewhat flat tibial bearings. The edge between the two tibial compartments is raised and may provide an additional constraint by locking with the femur in cruciate deficient knees. The surfaces give a fairly uniform and wide area of contact in extension, good contact in flexion, and over 100° of motion. Its advantages are:

1. The design is a compromise between total contact and extreme low contact designs.
2. Instrumentation is easy and implantation is more or less automatic.
3. About 110° or more of motion is achieved.
4. Wide dissipation of forces allow for reduced wear.

Its disadvantages are:

1. The increased conformity increases the cement-bone interface stresses, with a theoretical chance of increasing failure.
2. The flexion achieved is less than the more anatomic or meniscal designs.

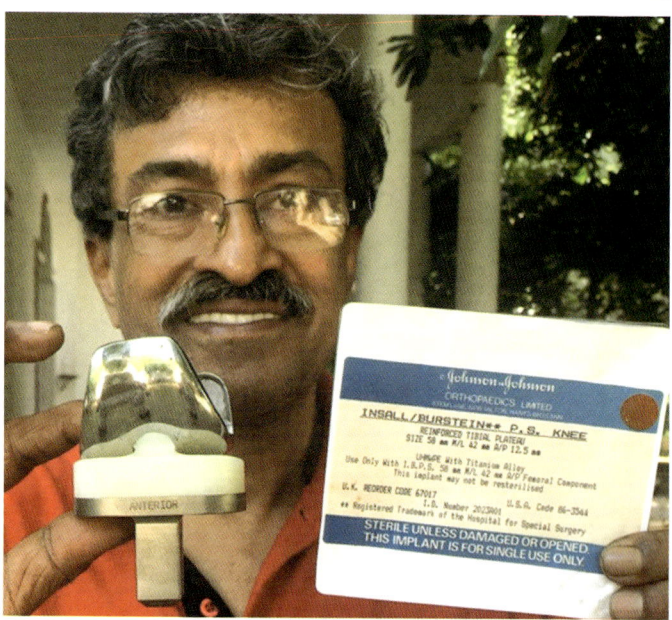

The original total condylar knee.

The most popular examples of this design are the Insall Burnstien II, Total Condylar II, Ranawat Total Condylar, etc.

Anatomic Designs: These copy the normal anatomy of the human knee. The femoral condyles are reasonably flat distally and well cylindrical posteriorly. The medial and lateral femoral condyles are shaped differently to match the anatomic model of the knee. The tibial surface is flattish and approximates a bony tibia with the meniscus. The contact areas in flexion and extension are different. Its advantages are:

1. Good range of motion, which may exceed 120°.
2. Excellent total contact in extension, leading to good contact and low wear.
3. Roller glide from extension to flexion, allowing a constant changing centre of rotation as in a normal knee.
4. Low contact in flexion allowing diminution of implant bone stress and hence lowering chances of failure.

Its disadvantages are:

1. Point contact in flexion may lead to increased wear.
2. The roll on glide increases the laxity of the knee.

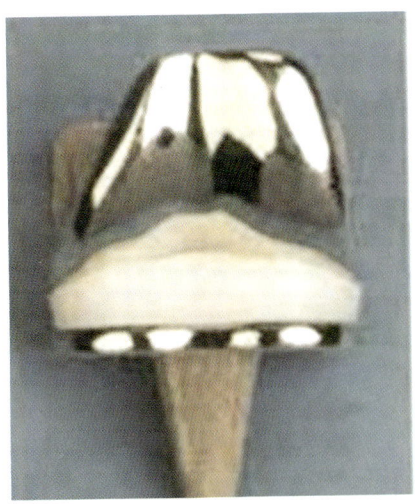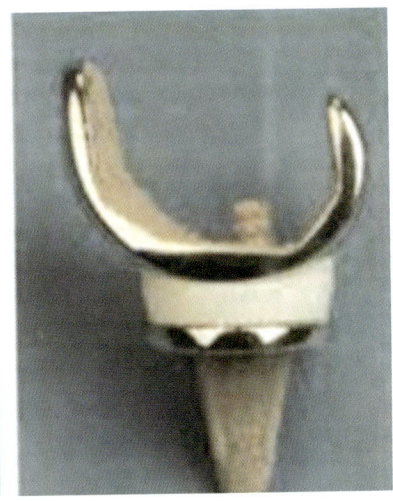

The porous coated anatomic PCA knee.

3. Because of the precise shape of the components, the implantation has to be perfect; even a little mal-alignment will result in tremendous loads across the joint and lead to early failure.

The common examples of this type are the PCA, Kienamatic, Genesis II, Miller Galante, etc.

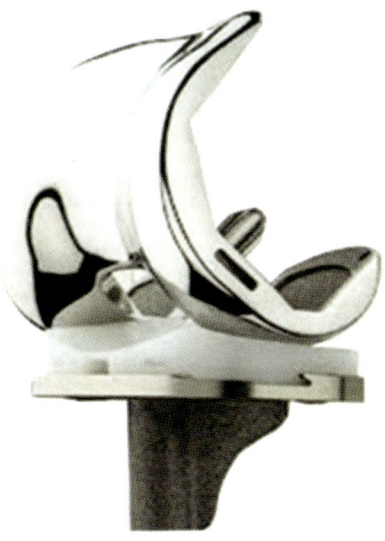

Genesis II knee.

Meniscal Designs: These are new generation knees designed to overcome the problems faced by anatomic designs. The tibial plastic acts as a bipolar bearing and articulates with polished femoral as well as tibial surfaces. This design has a good total contact with both surfaces, yet avoids increased contact stresses. Its advantages are:

1. Bipolar movement and thus less wear.
2. Good contact between the metal and HDPE in almost all phases of movements, which will lead to a very uniform stress distribution.
3. Glide roll more than other designs; hence possibly a few more degrees of flexion.

Its disadvantages are:

1. New design, hence sufficient follow-up is not available.
2. An additional moving part is introduced.
3. Wear on both surfaces of tibia rather than one.
4. Possibility of dislocation of the meniscus.
5. The implant relies very heavily on the precision of ligamentous balance and perfection of the bone cuts. Thus the procedure has a long learning curve and mistakes are not forgiven.

The common examples are the New Jersey LCS, Oxford, etc.

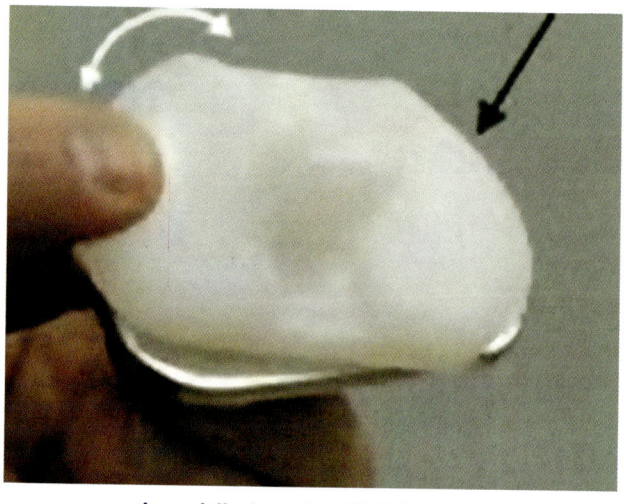

A mobile bearing tibial insert.

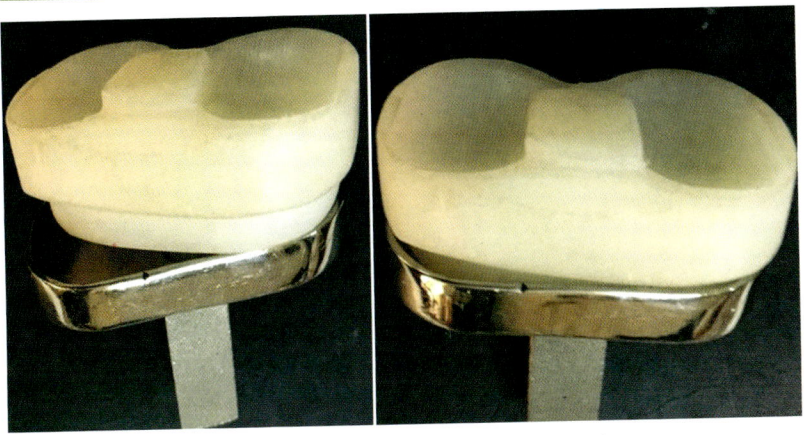

The author's design of a mobile bearing.

The other criteria useful for choosing implants are listed below. One has to take all the points listed into consideration before making an intelligent choice about the right type of implant for a patient.

Universal Designs: Advantages:

1. Simple and easy to use.
2. Less inventory in the operating room leading to lesser patient costs.
3. Simpler and easier instrumentation.

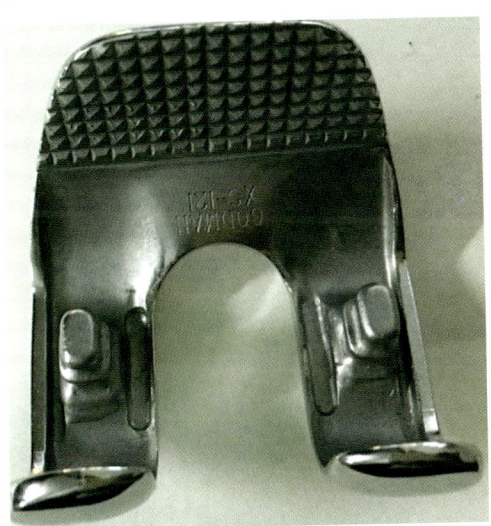

Universal femoral component fits both left and right.

Disadvantages:

1. Need for greater surgical skill for precise alignments.
2. Patellar tracking is not as good as anatomic knees.
3. Prosthesis cannot have inbuilt features for left and right. Consequently bone cuts should differ on left and right side to allow for a valgus positioning of the prosthesis.

Anatomic femoral components: Advantages:

1. Better patellar tracking.
2. Prosthesis insertion is easy.
3. Instrumentation needs much less eye balling.
4. Designs can have a thicker medial and thinner lateral part of the femoral component, needing a much lesser amount of bone to be removed.

Disadvantages:

1. Increased inventory and costs.
2. More (number) and more complicated instrumentation.

Anatomic Tibial Components

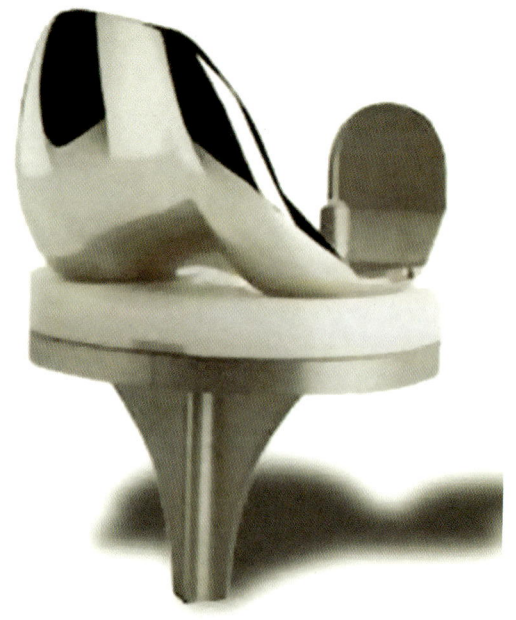

The anatomic femoral component.

These are very recent designs in which the medial and lateral tibial articulations differ in shape and size. The medial aspect is larger and slightly deeper compared to the lateral side. It has a lot of theoretical advantages, but the follow-up is short and it is much more expensive.

Nonmetal-backed tibial component: Studies have shown that a metal-back in tibia dissipates forces much better, leading to much lesser stresses and lesser plastic deformation. However, the thickness of the plastic should be a minimum of 5 mm in the thinnest part. Otherwise if the plastic wears out over the years, there will be a severe metallosis by the grinding between the femoral component and the tibial metal base plate.

There is an increasing interest and resurgence of studies towards nonmetal-backed tibial components now. All poly tibias have now made a comeback and still have a place in the very elderly low demand knee.

Metal-backed fixed and modular tibial components: Most tibial components presently available are metal-backed. More recent ones are all modular. However, there are a few designs that still have a fixed metal-back. The modular design has an advantage of greater control, especially in the final stages of surgery. Here

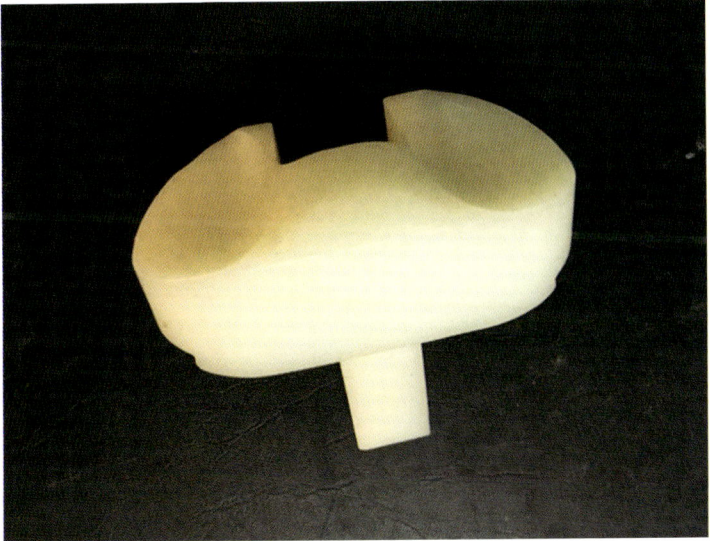

An all poly tibial component, which is now making a comeback.

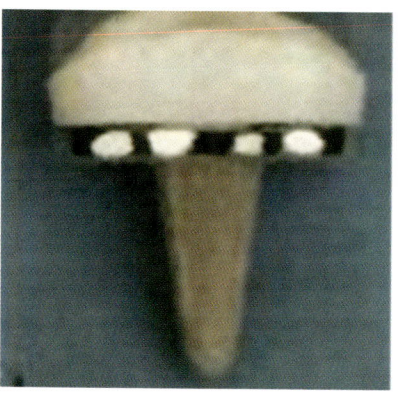
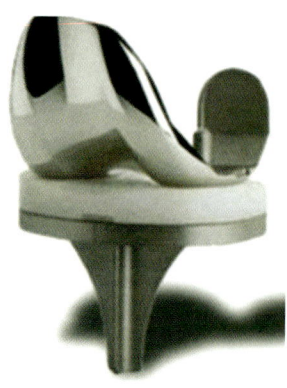

Fixed and mobile tibial bearings.

if one finds that after cementation, the knee is a bit tight or loose, one can just change the polyethylene liner to get a better fit.

Modular designs: Here the modularity pertains to the interchangeability between the tibial and femoral components. In the first generation knees, one could use only the same-sized femur with the same-sized tibia. Later designs became compatible one size up or down. The present generation modular knees are practically universal, where one can allow articulation with any femur and tibia.

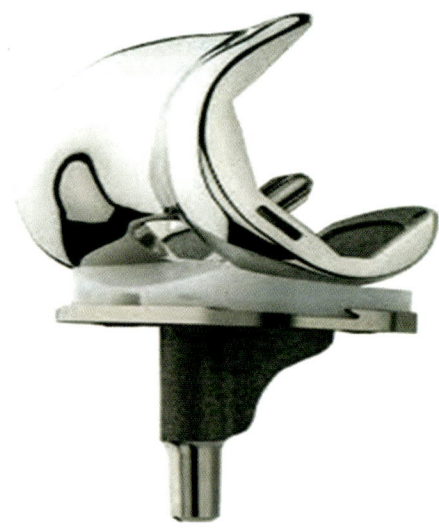

A current modular knee.

For example, if a patient takes a medium or large femoral component, and the tibia is cut a bit too low because of bony defects, leading to the use of a much smaller tibia, the components will still match and articulate perfectly.

Patellar components metal-backed and nonmetal-backed: Though there was an initial surge of interest in metal-backed patellar components, these are seldom used now. The reason is that the thickness of the patellar button even normally is lesser than 4 mm. To accommodate the metal-back, one will have to make a thinner button. This will wear off pretty soon and result in a knee where the femoral component rubs directly against the patella, leading to severe wear debris and associated problems.

Status of hinge designs: Hinge designs are no longer used as primary replacements. However, there are specific indications for their use, mainly in the following conditions:

1. After resection in bone tumours.
2. As a last stage for revisions with severe bone loss and complete ligamentous instability.

However, one must understand that a hinge only offers a temporary solution and the patient must be informed that it will definitely fail over a period of time.

Fixation of the implants: Of the various modalities available, fixation by bone cement has the longest and most successful outcome. However, the difficulties in revision and bone loss associated with loose cemented components has made some surgeons consider alternative methods of fixation, especially in younger patients. The Freeman HDPE serrated pegs, which snap fit without cement for both femur and tibial components, have a reasonable amount of success in the medium to long term. Recent results of the cementless porous coated and hydroxyapatite coated implants too are fairly impressive.

For a beginner, the following points should act as a reasonable guideline:

Elderly, low demand patients and rheumatoid knees at any age should have a cemented knee.

Relatively younger patients and those with good bone stock should have a cementless implant.

Indications and Contraindications of Total Knee Replacement

Indications: Pain, stiffness and deformity are usually co-existent in most patients and together form a triad of symptoms for which knee arthroplasty is indicated. Of the three symptoms, pain is the primary and main indication. Pain interfering with normal daily activities, pain at rest and pain not relieved by nonsurgical methods—all account for a reasonable indication for a knee replacement. The common conditions where this amount of pain is present and where the procedure is indicated are:

1. Osteoarthritis: Primary osteoarthritis of the knee is a very common problem, especially in the Asian patient. The social activity of squatting somehow protects the hip against primary osteoarthritis, and this is probably compensated by a much larger incidence of knee arthritis.

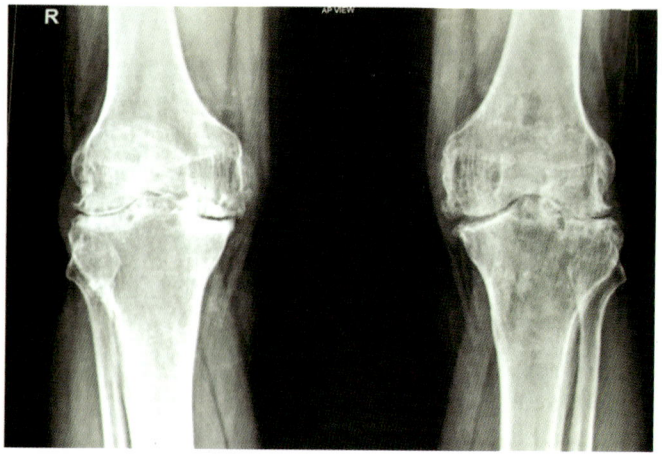

Severe osteoarthritis of the knee.

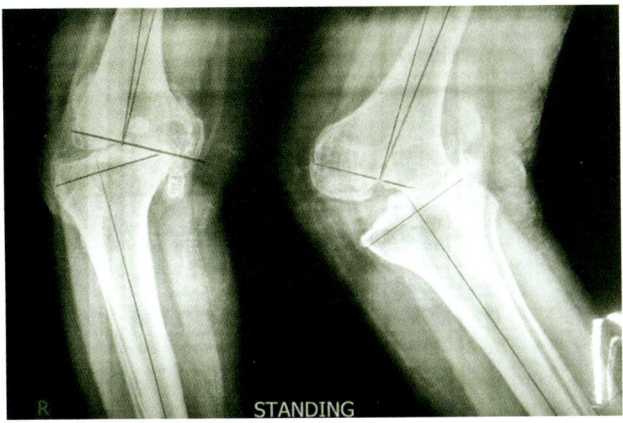

Bilateral OA with wind swept deformities.

2. Rheumatoid arthritis with increasing pain and stiffness.

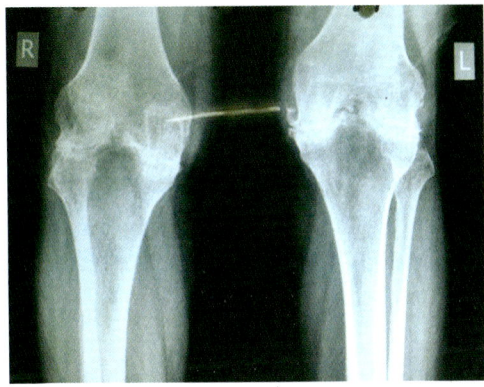

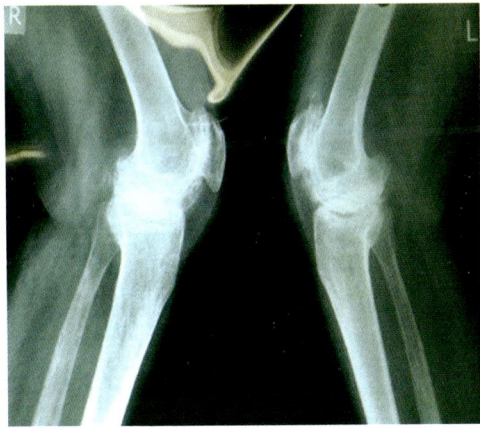

Tri-compartmental rheumatoid arthritis.

3. Other seronegative spondylo-arthropathies like ankylosing spondylosis, psoriatic arthritis, gout, Crohn's disease, etc. (provided the first criteria of pain is met).

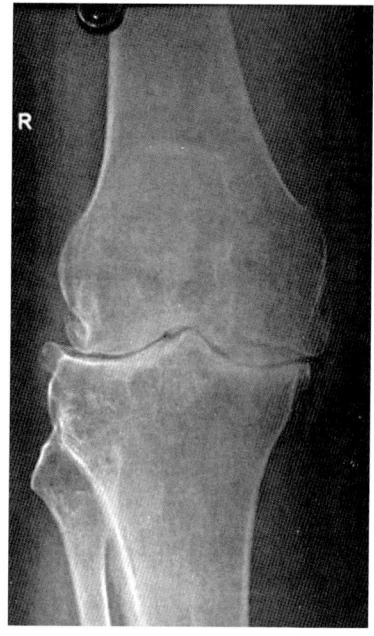

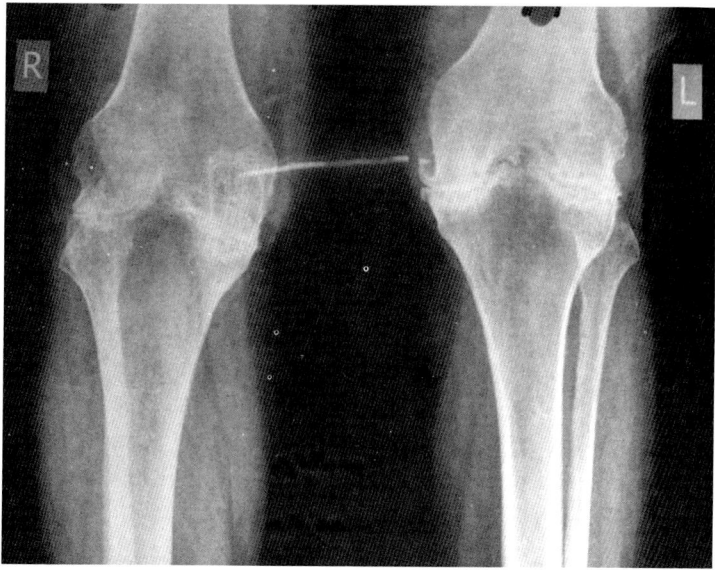

Seronegative knee arthropathy.

4. Post-traumatic arthritis, secondary to trauma, or intra-articular fractures. One must ensure that the knee is sufficiently painful before contemplating an arthroplasty.
5. Arthritis that has started to become painful after a high tibial osteotomy.
6. Haemophiliac arthritis with severe joint destruction. Due care should be taken to manage the haemophilia and sufficient factor replacement should be available prior to contemplating surgery.
7. Post-tubercular degenerated knee, provided the disease process is quiescent. A prophylactic course of anti-tubercular treatment is mandatory prior to taking up surgery.
8. Painfully stiff knee ankylosis, with an incomplete arthrodesis.
9. Old septic arthritis with painfully degenerated or ankylosed knee in which the infection has been eradicated and the knee is quiescent.

Contraindications

Absolute Contraindications

1. Active sepsis, either in the knee or elsewhere in the body. However an old septic arthritis is not a contraindication as mentioned above, so long as the infection has been eradicated.
2. Charcot's disease with absent joint proprioceptive function is doomed for failure because of abnormal and un-mechanical loading of the joint.
3. Absent quadriceps mechanism likewise is an absolute contraindication.
4. A painless arthrodesis in a good functional position.

Relative Contraindications

1. Young age is a contraindication, as this is at best a salvage procedure, the reliability and longevity of which are still under investigation. However, even young patients with very severely crippling disability and a low life expectancy can be favourably considered.
2. Obesity is a relative contraindication. Increased body weight puts an increased demand on the replaced joint, thereby reducing the life expectancy of the implants. In my setup,

patients weighing over 110 kg are refused the operation unless they reduce their weight.

3. Level of Activity: Patients with a very high demand may well be treated with other methods as palliative procedures until such time that the demand on their knee reduces and they become fit for surgery.

4. Mechanical problems like malunited fractures in the femoral or tibial shaft, an absent patella, old partial patellectomy, predominant patellofemoral or unicompartmenal disease, etc. form relative contraindications for a beginner who is advised to refer these problems to more experienced colleagues.

Checklist for a Knee Replacement Programme

In my set up, I follow the following checklist and document the answers. I give points for each parameter and only then reach a decision regarding arthroplasty. Surgeons contemplating to start this procedure or use it routinely are advised to check this list and modify it to suit their needs. In these days of increasing litigation and consumer protection, one is better off being cautious in case selection, meticulous in surgical technique, precise in patient monitoring and advice, and critical in follow-up and documentation to avoid problems.

1. Diagnosis
2. Range of motion
3. Walking distance
4. Degree of pain, including night pains. Analgesics taken presently, dosage, frequency
5. Age and gender
6. Body weight
7. Septic focus: Teeth, prostrate, bowels, bladder, others.
8. Associated conditions: Diabetes, hypertension, benign prostatic hyperplasia
9. Anaesthetic fitness.
10. Chest expansion, cervical spine and lumbar spine in rheumatoid arthritis and ankylosing spondylosis.
11. X-ray findings, involvement of all three compartments, stress and weight bearing films.
12. Occupation and lifestyle. Demands on the replaced knee.

13. Social background. Rural or urban. Religion. Squatting. Namaz.
14. Psychological profile. Motivation. Demands and expectations.
15. Financial status. Affordability of hospitalization, implants, western toilet facilities, etc.

In my clinic I have a model of the implant on a plastic bone. In addition, I also have a short video clip of the operation and a few pictures of the pre-operative and post-operative activities of some patients. Detailed counselling is done and all the pros and cons of the operation are explained fully.

In addition, a specific day of each month is the *long-term follow-up day*. All old patients are asked to report on this day for clinical and radiographic evaluation. New patients on the waiting list for this procedure are called on the same day and invited to interact with old patients to get first-hand "user feedback" about the operation, its advantages and limitations.

General Principles of the Surgical Technique

Total knee replacement is a surgical procedure that is an *epitome of perfection in component placement.* For good long term results, it is imperative that all the components are placed precisely and all the soft tissues surrounding the implants perfectly balanced to allow for a uniform stress and load distribution over the components and consequently produce a longer life of the implant and a pain- and complication-free functioning knee joint to that patient.

It is not an exaggeration to state that the procedure *is more of a soft tissue surgery rather than a bony surgery.* One must desist from making even the first bone cut unless a perfect soft tissue balancing has been achieved. Attempts to correct deformities by obliquity of bone cuts will surely lead to disastrous results!

On a review of the literature, the fact that emerges very clearly is that long-term success of knee replacement is dependent upon precise bone cuts and perfect component placement. Irrespective of the knee design used, it is imperative that the following critical steps be followed:

1. The distal femoral cut should be in *5° to 7° of valgus.*
2. The upper tibia should be in neutral to *2° of varus and a 3° to 5° slope* from anterior to posterior.
3. All ligaments should be *balanced* so that there should neither be *instability* nor *tightness.*
4. After bone cuts, the gap between the femur and tibia *should be the same in flexion and extension.*
5. The instrumentation should allow an *exact fit* of the component used.

Most designs of total knee replacement have their own instrumentation to achieve the above goals. These instrumentation vary from very simple limited instrument sets that rely heavily on "eye balling", to the very recent highly complex ten tray instrumentation sets that are a pain to learn and far too complex for the theatre sister.

I am now describing the essentials of the procedure irrespective of the instrumentation used.

Preoperative evaluation: We are treating the patient as a whole, not just replacing a knee. Thus a preoperative planning and evaluation schedule is very important and should be strictly followed. My personal schedule that has stood me well is to check and document:

1. History of past and present problems, special mention of diabetes mellitus, hypertension, bleeding and coagulation disorders. History of infections or sepsis anywhere in the body. Drug allergies and past medication.
2. Clinical examination of the affected and opposite knee, both hips and spine. Peripheral vascular status of the affected and opposite limb to be examined.
3. General examination to assess heart, lungs, exclude systemic diseases, status of teeth and prostate. On occasions, it may be wise to get a physician's opinion as to the fitness of the patient for such a major surgical procedure.
4. Blood and urine examination and chest radiograph are mandatory, both from the surgical and anaesthetic point of view. Specific compulsory investigations include bleeding and clotting times, blood urea and creatinine, haemoglobin , PCV and a urine culture.
5. Average blood replacement needed is about two units of fresh blood; adequate preparation for the same should be made.

Preoperative radiographic planning: A correct preoperative radiographic planning allows us to achieve the following objectives:

1. Choose the correct sized implant.
2. Assess the stage of the disease.
3. Know about the bony defects that need to be filled.
4. The axial alignment of the joint that needs to be restored.

5. The status of bone density.

6. Old fractures or malunions above or below the joint line.

It is not enough to just have a small film with the anterio-posterior and lateral radiographs of the knee joint. A lot of information is missed and one may get into serious trouble at the operation by not having anticipated the unexpected!

In our set up we take the following X-rays:

A. Standing AP and lateral views of the affected and opposite knees.

B. Varus/valgus stress X-rays.

C. Full length ortho roentgenogram with the hip, knee and ankle in a weight bearing, standing stance to assess the true axial alignment.

D. Cervical and lumbar spine X-rays to assess the possibility of intubation or spinal anaesthetic. This is especially important in rheumatoids and ankylosing spondylosis.

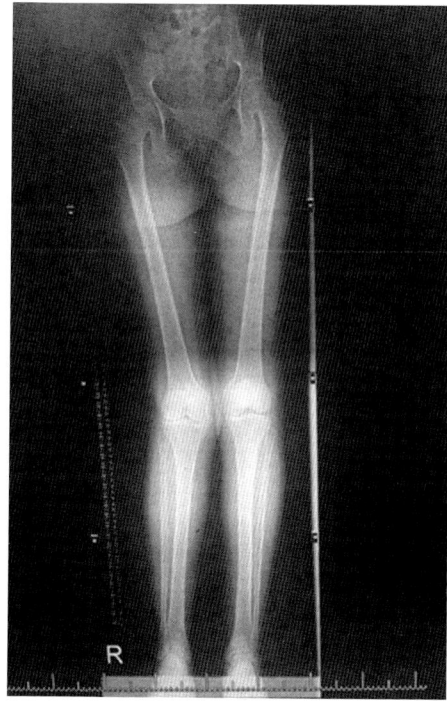

A full length X-ray with hips, knees and ankles in a single frame helps to plan the surgery properly.

Preoperative surgical planning: A complete range of instrumentation is a must for a proper job. Different implants need different instrumentation sets and are supplied by the manufacturers. A full set of retractors, all the cutting blocks and a saw system are mandatory. Full sets of femoral and tibial trials are essential and it would be unwise to embark upon the surgical procedure without them.

If there is a preexisting internal fixation device or prosthesis, instrumentation needed for its removal is also necessary. For revision knees, one must have the special cement removal chisels. Bone cement of the appropriate type and in sufficient quantity is mandatory. Adequate range and sizes of the prosthesis, including one size above and below, and all thicknesses of tibial components must also be kept ready and handy. Though the preoperative evaluation would have indicated the approximate size and removed much of the guesswork, a cautious surgeon is always prepared for the unexpected.

Preoperative anaesthetic planning: An anaesthetist reviews the patient a few days before the operation and does all the

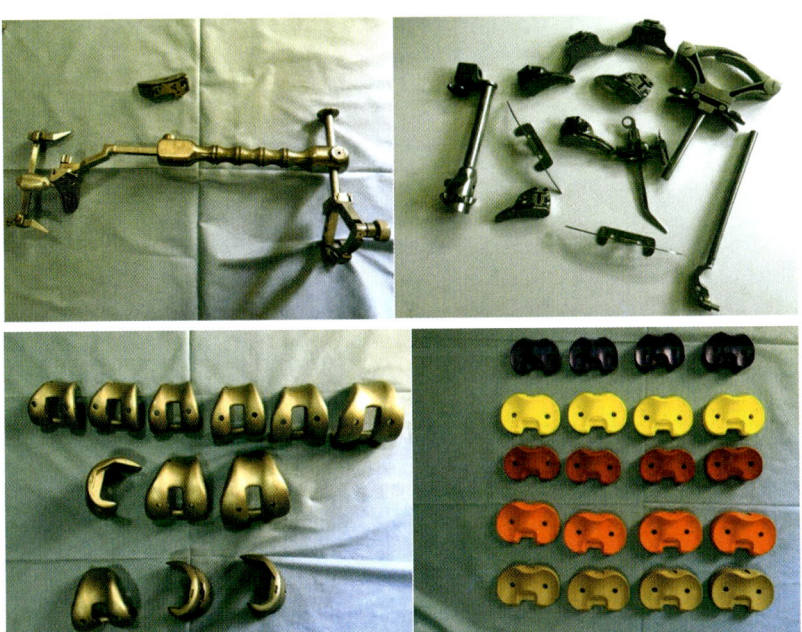

Each instrumentation set comes with its own trials.

assessment needed. He reviews the investigations and plans for the type of anaesthesia depending upon the patient's condition. A regional anaesthesia is always preferred; over 97% of our knees are done this way. In simple uncomplicated cases, a Sensorcaine spinal anaesthesia is used. If the surgery might take longer, a continuous epidural anaesthesia administered with a plastic catheter is used. General anaesthesia is rarely used in our set up. The final choice of the anaesthetic agents and mode of administration is left entirely to the anaesthesist. An anaesthetic chart is maintained in which preoperative, intraoperative and postoperative parameters are recorded.

Preoperative theatre requisites: Much has been written about the operation theatre conditions needed for arthroplasty. A lot has been said about the unsuitability of average operating rooms for a knee replacement. A laminar flow with space suits, though ideal, is a very expensive proposition for most average operating rooms. Bio-occlusive clothing too is not easily available in our country as it is all imported. If one looks into the literature, the original Charnley series of total hip replacements had an incidence of about 8% infection. He opined that airborne microbes were the cause and set about to remedy it. Whilst working on this problem, he took the help of persons maintaining clean air in breweries and distilleries, where a strict abacterial status is essential for proper fermentation. He postulated that the air in the operating room must be changed many times and the fresh air blown into the theatre should be ultra filtered, abacterial and aparticulate. Further, he postulated that the surgeon emits bacteria from his skin and breath. So if the surgeon is encompassed in a space suit-like contraption with hoods and if all the air expired by the surgeon is let out through a separate outlet, infection must be reduced. He was correct!

Using these methods, he managed to reduce his infection rate from 8% to less than 1%. Simultaneously, surgeons found that prophylactic antibiotics also reduce the infection rate despite the surgery being performed in a conventional operation theatre. Nelson and Phillips reported a reduction of infection in a conventional theatre from 5.8% to just 1.3% with the use of antibiotics. It has been postulated that clean air, prophylactic antibiotics and clothing all act complementary to each other and their use together reduces the infection rate to less than 0.5%.

In our circumstances, not all hospitals are equipped with a laminar air flow, though most modern orthopaedic operating rooms have them. Proper clothing and prophylactic antibiotics are easier to achieve. As far as the cost effectiveness goes, prophylactic antibiotics are the cheapest, followed by clothing, then air delivery systems.

It is the personal experience of the author that the infection rate has been acceptably low just by meticulous observation of detail and prophylactic antibiotics. With just 3 infections in the first consecutive 300 knees done, of which about 250 were performed in our set up and the others in district hospitals all over the country, a special protocol for the Indian circumstances has been devised.

The following are the steps to be taken:

1. The operating room must not be used on the previous day and must be cleaned thoroughly. It should be properly fumigated and an ultraviolet lamp illuminated all night.
2. One or two air conditioners allow for a flow of clean filtered air into the theatres. This also keeps the temperature of the operating room cool, avoids the surgeon and theatres staff sweating, and allows the cement to set slowly.
3. The Boyle's machine, theatre furniture, and all loose and bulky machinery and objects in the operating room are cleaned and wiped with lysol the evening before surgery.
4. The patient is prepared in a side room; all ward clothing is discarded and the patient re-gowned prior to entering the operation theatre.
5. The operating team's outer garments are all autoclaved. Two caps and masks are worn; in the case of female personnel, the hair should be completely covered.
6. The procedure proceeds with proper planning, minimum time is wasted, and a quick, precise job is done with a minimum of the wound being exposed to the outside.
7. In the initial stages, entry of too many personnel into the operating room was not allowed. But subsequently, as the

number of visitors from outside the city rose, the rule was relaxed. So as many as six observers were inside the theatre on many occasions without any problems, so long as all personnel followed the theatre protocol.

8. Special drapes are used. Made of thick cotton, very large in size, they completely drape the patient and isolate the operating field from the anaesthesist's end. Further details of the type of drapes used and the method of draping is described in the section on operating technique. The currently available disposable paper drapes are also good, so long as one uses large drapes that stretch from floor to floor on both sides.

It has been found that it is easy to enforce this sort of a discipline in operation theatres where only orthopaedic operations are routinely performed. In general nursing homes, and those with a great turnover, it might be sometimes difficult to enforce all the above conditions. However, it must be emphasized that each of the above needs to be followed religiously to avoid any complications. An infection in an arthroplasty is a disaster. Sir John spent all his life working towards 0% infection. We all must treat an infection as our own personal responsibility, taking all precautions and making all efforts to minimize it.

Antibiotic prophylaxis: The current pharmacological literature tells us that airborne bacteria are prone to cause infection only during the actual surgical period. Sufficient concentrations of antibiotics present at and immediately after the operation are sufficient to avoid infection. Prolonged administration of antibiotics will only encourage resistant strains to grow and cause problems. Any of the newer wide spectrum antibiotics can be used. A good rule of thumb is to avoid popular antibiotics commonly used by general practitioners as rarer the antibiotic, lesser the chances of resistant strains. Presently we use Cefuroxime sodium 1.5 gm in 6 doses every 12 hours beginning from just before anaesthetic induction.

An intravenous administration assures peak serum concentrations, especially when the joint is open. I do not use antibiotics in the cement (except in revision cases and tubercular hips where I add streptomycin to the cement).

The Scrub and Drape Routine

I shall now describe my own personal theatre scrub and drape routine. There are no very hard and fast rules so long as one pays meticulous attention to the principles of asepsis. Most surgeons start off with a routine; over a period of time, they add append and modify the same until the system and routine gives optimum results. Once the standards have been set, it usually remains a fixed routine unless there is overwhelming evidence that modifications in the routine can result in a better outcome, or fewer complications. The following points will be described in the same order as it is performed!

1. Initial cleaning and ward preparation.
2. Scrub routine for surgeons, assistants and nurses.
3. Role of tourniquet in knee replacement surgery.
4. Cleaning and draping of the operative part.
5. Special tips and tricks.

Initial cleaning and ward preparation: The patient preparation starts a day before the surgery. A shampoo bath and thorough cleaning of head and hair is done. All nails are cleaned and clipped, and the limb is thoroughly cleaned from the toes to the groin. Special care is taken to clean the inter-digital area between the toes. No shaving is done. In the case of a hairy individual, it is a standard practice to shave just a small strip of skin especially in the operative area inside the theatre just before the surgery.

Studies have shown that small cuts occurring during shaving tend to become infected. Also, shaving performed in the 12 hours before surgery actually increases the chances of infection. That is why *no shaving is done in the ward*. From umbilicus down to all toes (including the inter-digital area), povidine iodine scrub solution is applied with a cotton gauze, thoroughly scrubbed and wiped with water. No brush is used, as this may cause deeper layers of skin to scale and bring out *Staphylococcus epidermidis*.

The night before the surgery, the patient has a mild laxative like paraffin or Cremaffin gel, and takes a liquid diet. Fasting is started from appropriate intervals.

On the morning of surgery, the operative side is again cleaned with povidine iodine solution. A glycerine enema is given. The patient then wears a sterile theatre gown and is shifted into the operating room after administration of the appropriate premedication. In our set up, we have two stretcher trolleys and stretchers: (a) a "clean set", which does not leave the operating room complex, and (b) another set, which goes between ward and OT entrance. Once the patient reaches the theatre, he is shifted to the theatre trolley and stretcher, and re-dressed in another sterile theatre dress. All ward clothing goes back with the ward stretcher.

The surgeon and other theatre personnel: Enforcing strict discipline and a strict protocol are mandatory in each case. There are no relaxations to any of the rules. Bio-occlusive clothing and paper gowns were not easily available in our country when I began this, hence I used specially tailored garments: Standard theatre uniform (pyjamas and tops made of fine cloth with very small pores) for all theatre staff (anaesthesist, nurses, radiographers and theatre boys). The groin and chest areas had double layers of cloth. These dresses were autoclaved.

Now of course if the patient can afford it, I do not hesitate to use disposable bio-occlusive clothing.

Disposable theatre caps and masks are used. I routinely use two caps and two masks. All theatre staff is instructed to have a bath on the morning of the surgery. All theatre personnel wash their feet and wear rubber slippers. No panty hose or stockings allowed for nursing staff. Each item of apparel worn is autoclaved prior to use. A separate set of linen is kept exclusively for joint replacements and is not used for other routine orthopaedic cases.

The Scrubbing Routine

This again is the standard practice with minor modifications. With a povidine iodine scrub solution the hands, and forearms down to the elbows are thoroughly washed. A nail brush may be used, but is optional. We do not advocate the practice of rubbing a thick bristled brush on the entire forearm and causing the deeper layers of staphylococci to rise up.

A thorough wash continuously under clean running water is done for the whole duration of the scrub. Then the hands and forearms are doused in povidine iodine solution which is allowed to stay on for about 30 seconds, then washed off with boiled water. A handful of sterilium or spirit is then rubbed up to the wrist and the personnel enter the operation theatre.

In the theatre, each person first dons a glove of the appropriate size. The sterile gown is picked with the gloved hand; once it has been tied, the second glove is worn. This is because even after a good surgical scrubbing routine, the hands are just clean, not sterile. By picking the gown with bare hands, one tends to unsterilize it. Once a sterile glove is worn, the gown can be handled.

On occasions, the surgeon uses a third pair of gloves. All this may seem too exacting, but a recent study did show that over 26% of gloves developed holes after surgical procedures and two or three gloves considerably minimize the risk of contamination by hand.

The Theatre Infrastructure

A special set of linen, maintained exclusively for arthroplasties, consists of eight large sheets 275 cm by 366 cm. Each sheet has 2 layers of thick green cloth stitched together at the edges, also stitched across the surface to keep the layers aligned uniformly. In addition, about 6 smaller sheets (183 cm by 122 cm) are needed. A large sheet (about 183 cm by 305 cm) with centre hole is also needed. A big stockinet at least 92 cm long is stitched at one end and rolled (for the foot). Bio-occlusive plastic adhesive (transparent, adhesive polyurethane film which allows the skin to breathe) for opposites are an optional extra and are indeed useful if available.

A closed suction drain system is essential and should be kept ready. Appropriate suture material as described later must also be within reach. All the requisite implants and the cement are prominently placed on a trolley for easy retrieval.

The geography of the actual operation theatre is very important. We prefer to avoid shelves, racks and unnecessary equipment, all of which tend to gather dust and glove powder, and require extensive effort to keep clean. Four stainless steel trolleys are routinely used. One is for linen placement, later used as a cement mixing area and also to place the actual implants before final cementation.

The second keeps all the general surgical instruments and is set in the standard manner of keeping all tips and clean ends towards the centre and all handles towards the periphery. The assisting nurse makes it a point to only handle the 'dirty' end of each instrument; the ends of the instruments entering the wound are scrupulously kept untouched.

The third trolley contains the knee instrumentation and cement bowls. The latter are transferred to the linen trolley once the draping has been completed. The last trolley contains power instruments on fully charged batteries.

It is our standard practice that the nurse only handles instruments from the linen and basic trolley. The first assistant can on occasion help to pick up instruments from the instrument trolley. The power instrument trolley is handled by the surgeon alone. All these trolleys are placed on the side from which the surgeon is operating.

I do not encourage the scrubbing up of company personnel, because I find that most possess no medical qualification.

The suction and diathermy machines are placed on the opposite side. As the regularity of these operations increases, a specific protocol evolves and each member of the team exactly fits into his or her role.

The Role of Tourniquet in Knee Replacement Surgery

Tourniquet application does make the surgery elegant and the bloodless field makes the life of the operating surgeon very easy. Furthermore, the bloodless cancellous cut surfaces allow for a proper cement application. In my early practice, it was a matter of routine to use a tourniquet in all cases. However, with the passage of time, based on the available data in literature, the frequency of tourniquet application became lesser.

The editorial by Klenerman in JBJS questioned the need for a routine tourniquet application in all knee replacement surgeries and also listed the complications of the same in elderly rheumatoids with a poor skin condition.

At about the same time, I started a small study to assess whether the benefits of a tourniquet outweigh the resulting complications. In this simple study, all patients undergoing bilateral simultaneous knee replacements had a tourniquet applied for one side but not on the other side during surgery. If one knee was more severely damaged, surgery without a tourniquet was done on this knee. This study is still continuing; its conclusion and results shall be published at a later stage. However, the preliminary findings of this study reveal that:

1. The average time taken for operation with tourniquet was 55 minutes (63 minutes without tourniquet).
2. Immediate postoperative pain was significantly less on the side without the tourniquet.
3. Total blood loss was more or less the same with or without a tourniquet.
4. Intra-operative bleeding was higher without a tourniquet.
5. But drainage was significantly higher when a tourniquet was used.
6. The sum total of both was more or less the same.
7. Skin problems and delayed healing were significantly lower in the group without the tourniquet, rather than the tourniquet group.

Hence I have presently stopped using tourniquet in almost all cases. However for a beginner, I still recommend the use of a tourniquet, except in cases of rheumatoids with a very soft and papery skin.

Operative Scrub and Drape Routine

Once anaesthetized, the patient is laid supine on the table. I do not use any sand bag or other aids. With the theatre assistant holding the foot, the whole limb is painted with povidine iodine based surgical scrub solution. The upper level is the groin and buttock and the lowest level is the heel. The same area then is painted with povidine iodine solution, followed by an alcohol-based sterilizing solution. Now the scrubbed and gowned operating assistant holds the calf using a thick multi-layered sterile towel and the foot is prepared.

The operating table is covered with a rubber sheet or a plastic sheet, with three large sheets over it, covering the table from all three sides. The fourth large towel is put across the patient above the limb, brought down and clipped with a towel clip. Three more large sheets are used on the upper half of the patient. The last of these is drawn up like a curtain and clipped to two saline stands to isolate the anaesthesist from the operating area.

A small towel is used for covering the foot, as the toes should be identifiable under the drapes. Stockinet is now wrapped from the foot until mid-thigh and clipped with a towel clip to the upper drape. Suction and diathermy connections are given and these leads and tips are kept in specially tailored pouches clipped to the drapes on the table.

Special Tricks and Tips

1. Wear the first glove before wearing the gown.
2. Wear two gloves and keep changing the outer glove every 30 to 40 minutes.
3. Use large drapes which provide adequate cover.
4. Do not use a bulky drape for the foot lest it camouflages the toes and make toe identification difficult at the operation.
5. Do not shave the operative part.
6. Follow strict theatre discipline!

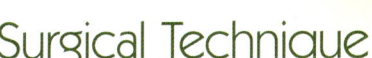

Surgical Technique

The basics of the surgical technique for all knee arthroplasties remain the same, irrespective of the knee design used, or whether the implant is cemented or not. This chapter will cover the basics of the procedure independent of the knee design.

The Skin Exposure

Of the various exposures available for knee arthroplasty, the most favoured is the straight midline anterior approach. A straight incision starts about 6 cm above the patella, extends down over the centre of patella and stops just below the tibial tubercle. Using a soft pad, the skin is gently teased from the incision, making sure that a generous amount of underlying soft tissue is retained along with the skin.

Using a deep knife, the quadriceps tendon is cut in the middle, with this incision extending up to the upper surface of the patella. Another incision is made from the lower border of patella till the tibial tuberosity. The two incisions are joined on the medial side skirting along the medial border of patella leaving enough soft tissue attachment for subsequent reattachment. Using a big gauze, the patella is held between the operating surgeon's thumb and index finger and everted out laterally as the knee is flexed. This will deflect the patella laterally and afford a clear view of the interior of the knee. We have to be very careful in this step and ensure that we have given enough clearance above and below the patella. Unless this has been done, there is a likelihood of avulsing the patella at the patellar tendon.

Soft Tissue Techniques

Once the interior of the knee is visualized, we proceed with soft tissue methods to achieve the following:

1. Thorough visualization of the interior of the knee.
2. Release of contracted structures and achieving soft tissue balance.
3. A thorough pericapsular release of the distal femoral and upper tibial surfaces to allow for an adequate anteroposterior translation of the femur over the tibia and vice versa.
4. An adequate clearance of the osteophytes for full visualization of the articular surfaces.
5. Soft tissue releases to allow for accommodation of all the jigs and instrumentation.

These are achieved in the following manner:

All bleeders are caught and coagulated. Using a cutting diathermy, a portion of the patellar fat pad is excised for better visualization. The anterior cruciate is excised to allow for an anterior translation of the tibia over the femur. Both the menisci are removed. Using a nibbler, all osteophytes are removed from the circumferences of the distal femur, proximal tibia and patella. The knee is straightened and inspected to see if there is any fixed varus, valgus flexion or recurvatum deformities. If the same are present, then further releases are performed to get a balanced and straight knee in 5° to 7° of valgus.

The Distal Femoral Cut

Using an 8 mm drill bit, a hole is made just anterior to the insertion of the anterior cruciate ligament. Through this, an intramedullary rod is inserted and the distal femoral cutting guide attached to it. The guide and its operation depend upon the type of instrumentation being used.

Some recent guides allow for a choice of the valgus cut from rectus to 9° in 2° or 3° increments. Other systems may have a fixed jig that allows only one angle. Irrespective of the system employed, one must ensure that the distal femoral cut is exactly parallel to the floor in the front-to-back axis and is in some degree of valgus from side to side.

The Upper Tibial Cut

Various jigs are available for this, intramedullary as well as extramedullary. Unlike the femur, which is enveloped in bulky thigh muscles, the medial aspect of tibia is more or less subcutaneous and palpable throughout its length. Thus it does not matter whether one uses an intra- or extramedullary guide. Most guides have a provision for a few degrees posterior slope. The upper tibial cut should be exactly parallel to the floor in the side-to-side axis and tilted posteriorly in the front-to-back axis. Once this cut is made, the knee is straightened and checked for a complete correction of all deformities.

Soft Tissue Balancing and Additional Releases

The original Kenna instrumentation had an instrument called the graduated tensioner. Mike Freeman and John Goodfellow too had their own designs of tensioners. These were devices which would stretch the medial and lateral gaps first in extension, then in 90° flexion and later in mid-flexion.

I too have designed a tensioner which I use at this stage. Unless the medial and lateral structures are in equal tension and when the jaws of the tensioner are opened to achieve this, and the knee is in 5° of valgus at this stage, I do not proceed further. Any ligamentous imbalance is corrected at this stage. This problem is particularly irksome in varus knees, and the following additional steps are performed:

1. Externally rotating the tibia and using a periosteal elevator, the medial structures are stripped further back.
2. This would uncover posterior osteophytes of medial tibial condyle which are nibbled.
3. The tibia is fully anteriorly translated and osteophytes in the intercondylar area, if any, are nibbled away.
4. Now the soft tissue balancer is introduced again and the tissue tension is evaluated.
5. Additional releases are performed, if needed.
6. Unless the knee is dead straight in AP axis and in a good valgus in ML axis, do not proceed to bone cuts.

The anterior and posterior femoral cuts and chamfers: Using an appropriate cutting guide of the correct size, the anterior and posterior femoral cuts are made. These should be parallel to each other and the two surfaces should be parallel in a slight external rotation. This will allow for a better patellar tracking. A cut of these surfaces that positions the femoral component in internal rotation is a disaster and should be scrupulously avoided.

The patellar cut and preparation: Using an appropriate device or instrument, the patella is cut across half of its. It is essential that enough bone should be cut so that after insertion of the patellar prosthesis, the thickness of the remaining patella plus the prosthesis should be equal to the thickness of the patella before the cut!

Trial components and trial reduction: Now appropriate holes, slots and marks are made over the cut surfaces of the femur, tibia and patella. The exact method and system is instrumentation dependant, and varies from design to design. The trial components are inserted and the knee is put through full range of movements checking for laxities, deformities and patellar tracking. The following tips are useful irrespective of the system employed:

1. If the knee is fully extendable and is wobbly in the side-to-side movement, it means that one has to use a thicker tibial component. Try the next bigger size until the knee is stable in side-to-side axis in full extension.
2. If the knee is not fully extendable, either the posterior releases have not been performed or the tibial thickness is too much; a tibia of one size smaller thickness is used.
3. If the tibial base plate does not rest circumferentially over the cortical bone of the upper cut surface of the tibia, or if there is an overhang with the tibial component protruding beyond the bone, an appropriate resizing of the tibial size is done.
4. If the patella does not track into the femoral groove on its own from flexion and extension, or if it is necessary to use a thumb to keep the patellar tracking ("Variance from the no thumb rule"), then lateral release of the patella is mandatory.

The final prosthesis and fixation: After a perfect trial reduction, the actual implants of the correct sizes are removed from their sterile wrappings and inserted without cement. A trial reduction is again performed and due attention is paid towards deformities, laxities, and patellar tracking. Once everything is confirmed to be satisfactory, the implants are fixed with or without cement depending on implant design and method of fixation.

Drainage and closure: The wound is washed and inspected for any bleeders that might be present. All bleeding points are caught and ligated. Check that the implants are in the correct position. The patellar tendon is deflected back medially.

Two drain tubes are connected to a closed suction system. Using thick synthetic suture (like Daxone or Vicryl number one), the patellar tendon is repaired. Subcutaneous sutures are put using a one zero vicryl. Skin is sutured using a one nylon or prolene. We routinely use a continuous suture. I do not use staples and my idea has been vindicated by current studies, which have categorically proved that metal staplers are inferior to nylon.

PREPARATION DRAPING AND SKIN INCISION

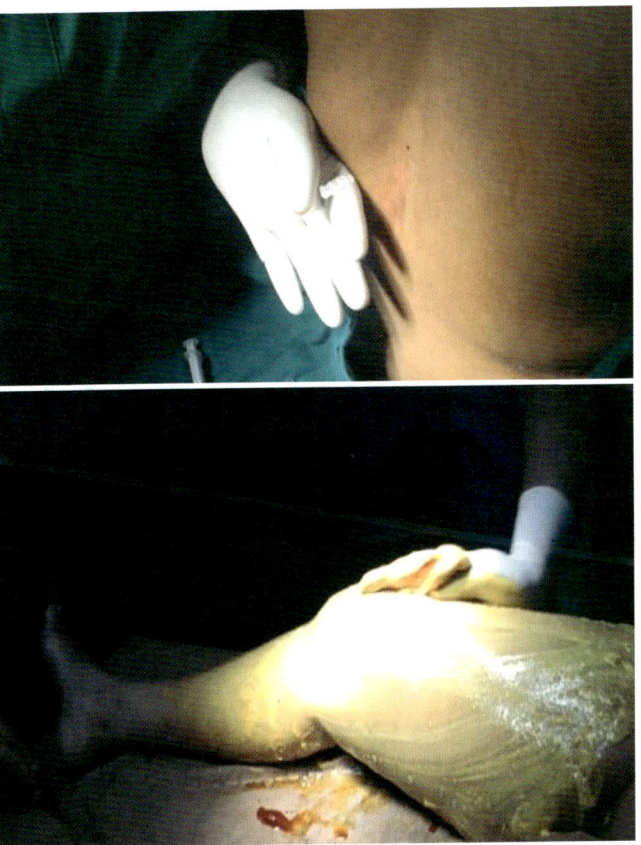

The surgery is performed under general or regional anaesthesia. The limb is prepared from groin to toe.

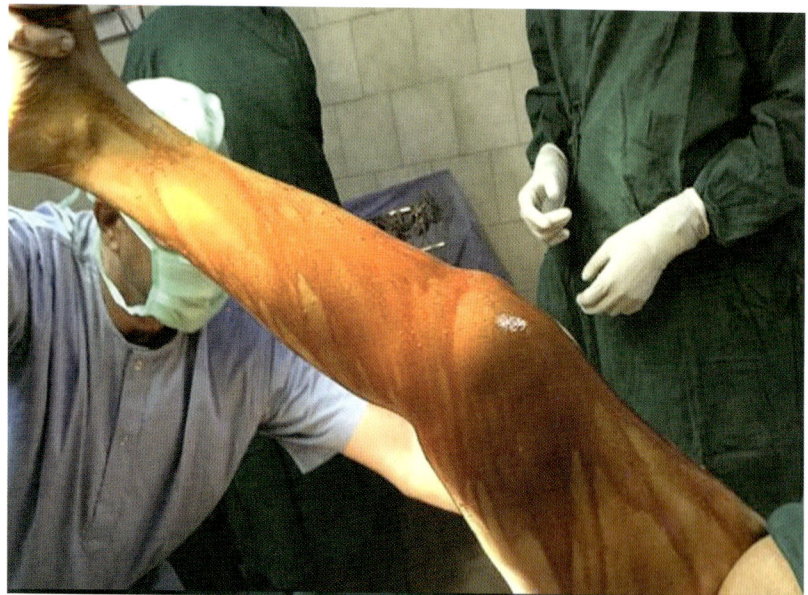

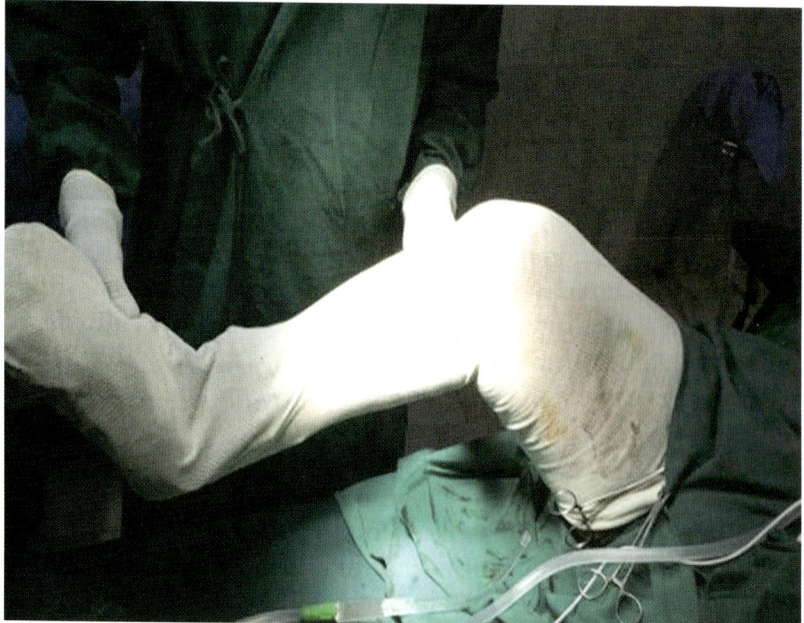

Painting and draping of the limb. Bulky towels should be avoided over foot, as we need to check toe orientation during surgery.

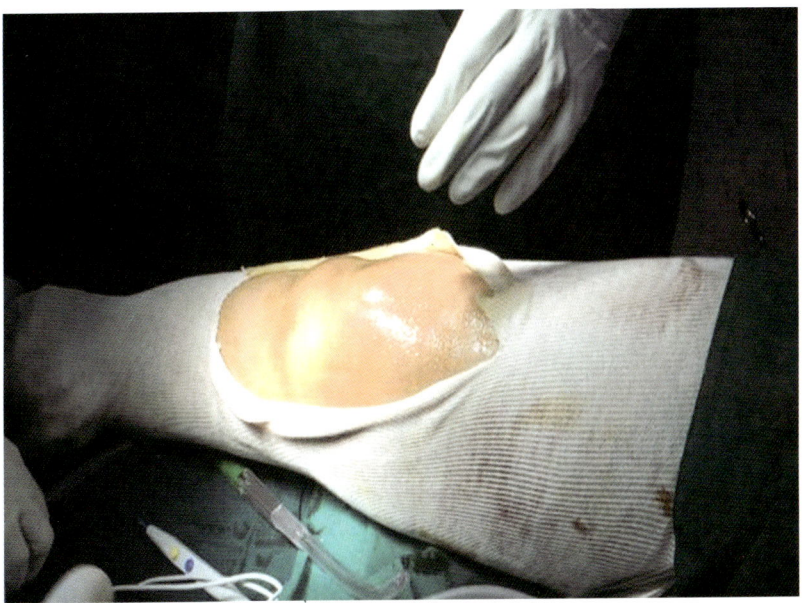

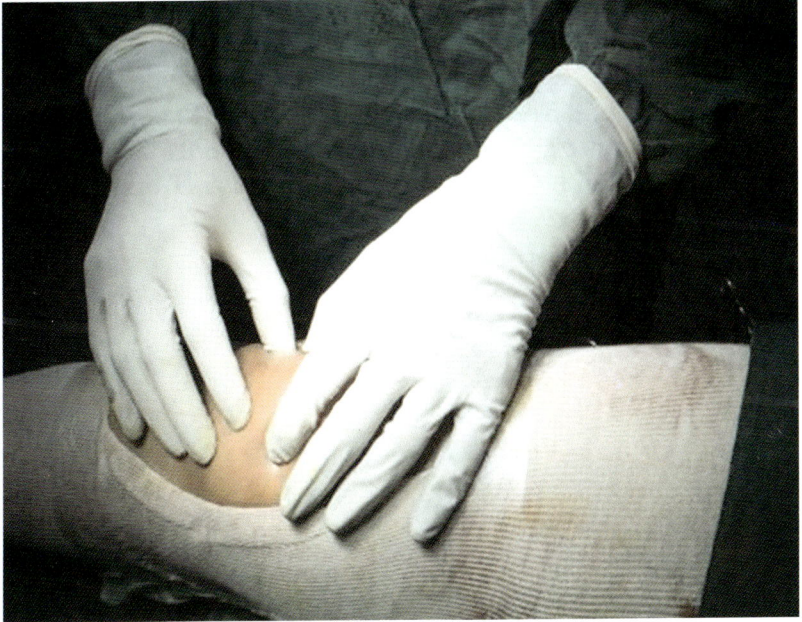

Patella is the landmark over which the incision is centred.

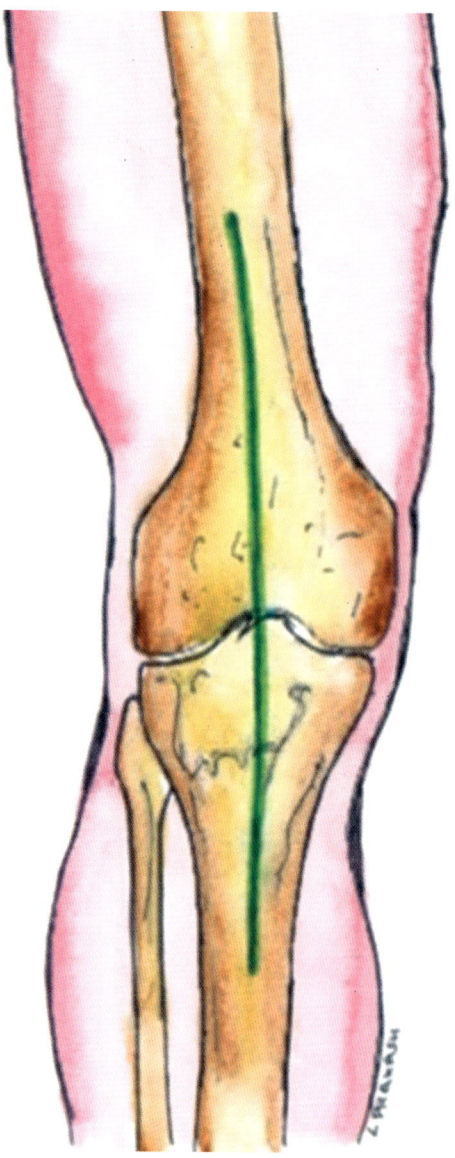

Straight midline skin incision over patella up to the tibial tuberosity.

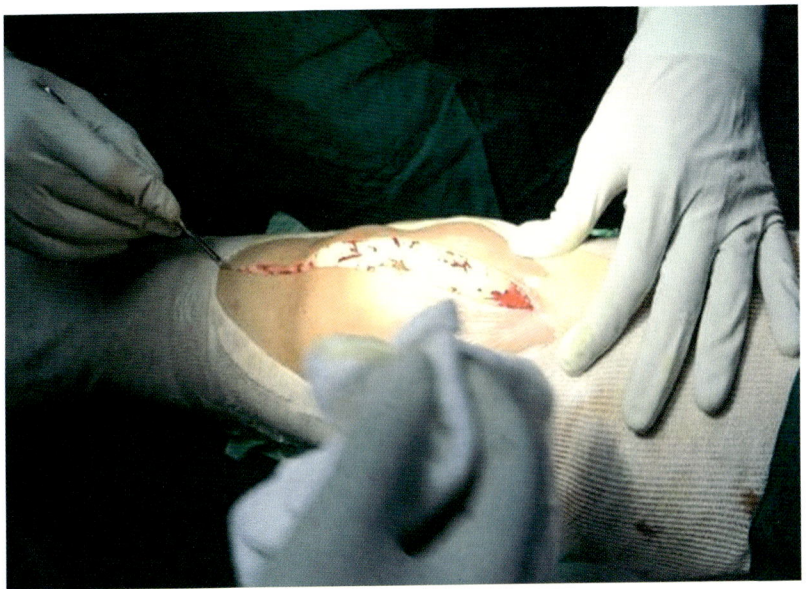

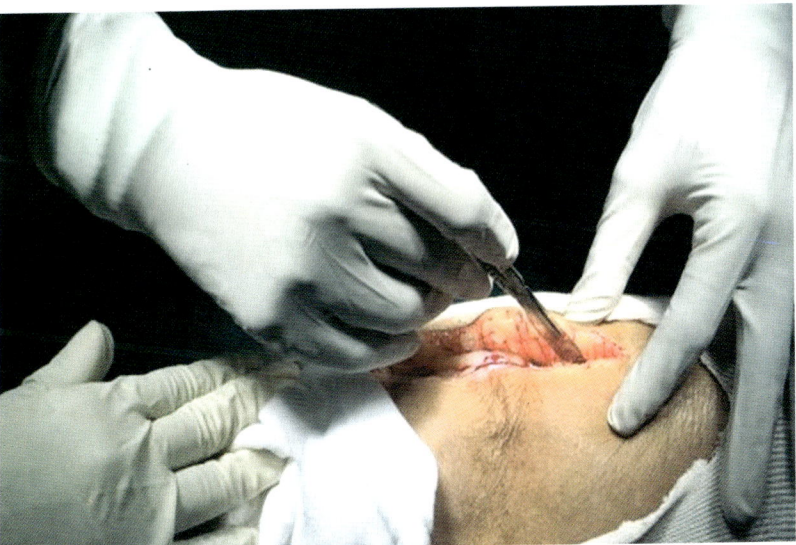

The incision can be extended superiorly or inferiorly as needed in each case.

DEEP INCISION AND EXPOSURE OF THE JOINT

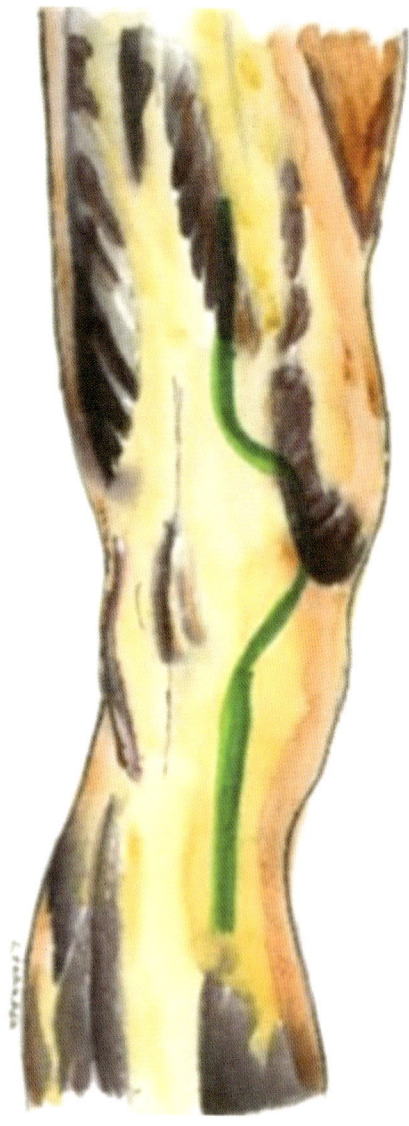

Quadriceps tendon is incised in the line of its fibres, and the deep incision skirts around the medial patellar border straightening down below it, up to the tibial tuberosity.

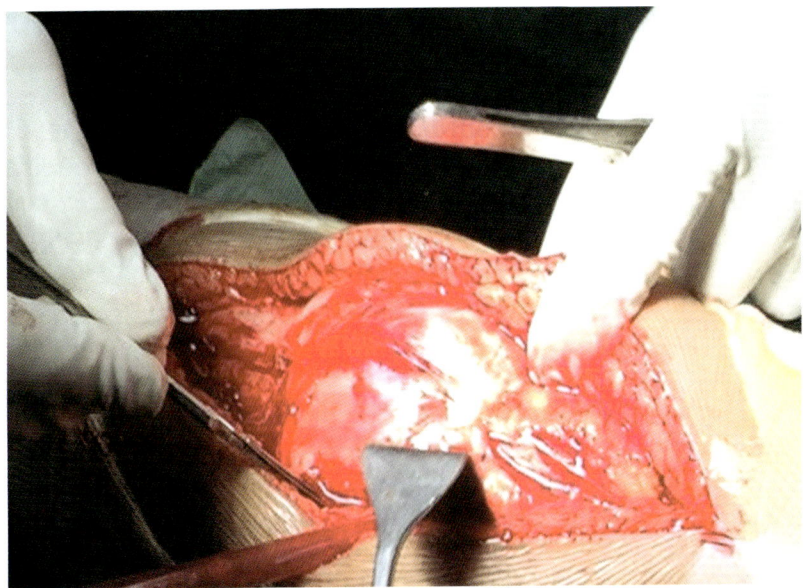

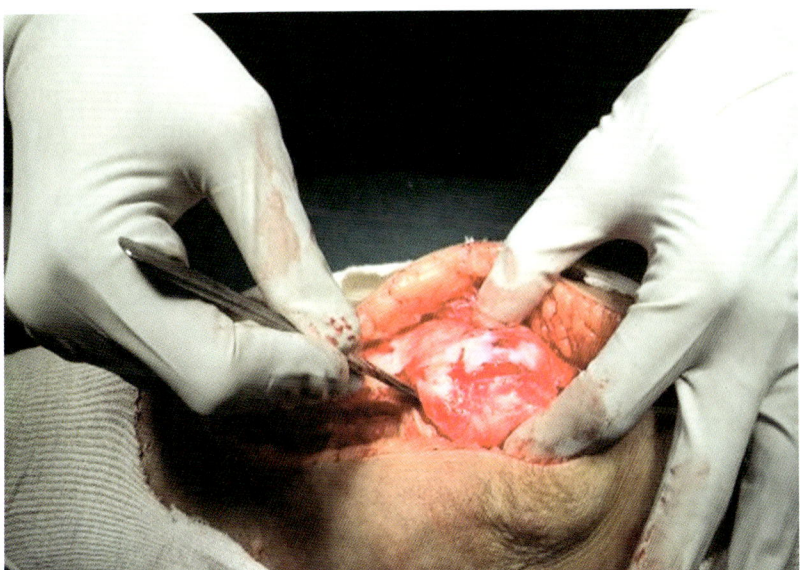

It is usual to make two deep linear incisions, one above and one below the patella and then curve it around the medial patellar border, retaining enough soft tissue for subsequent suturing.

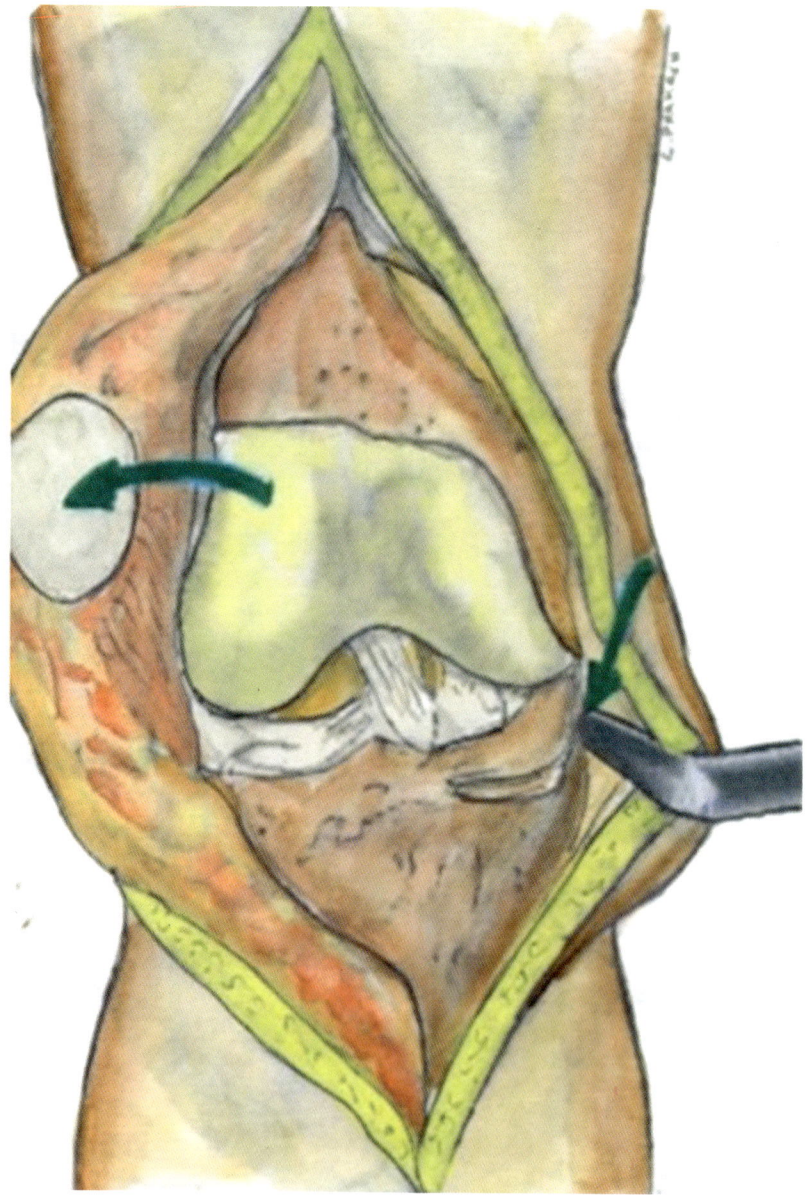

The patella is deflected laterally, exposing the knee.

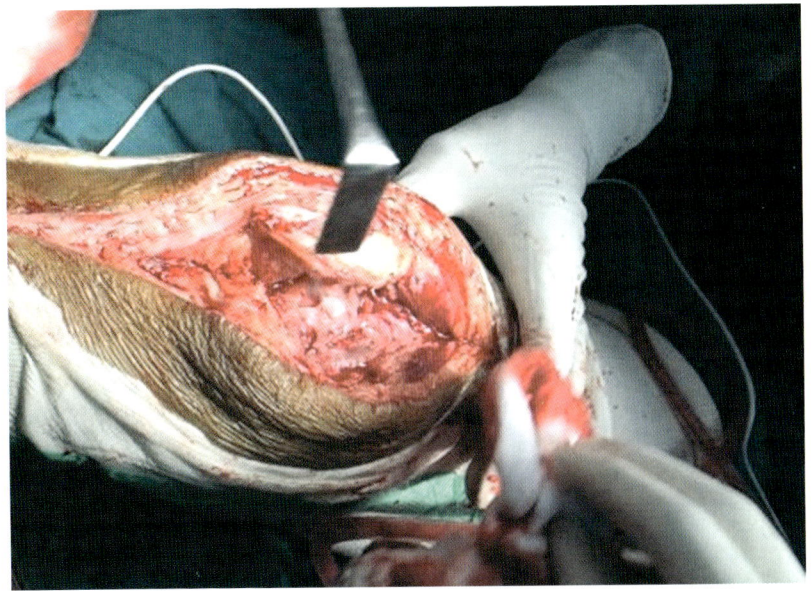

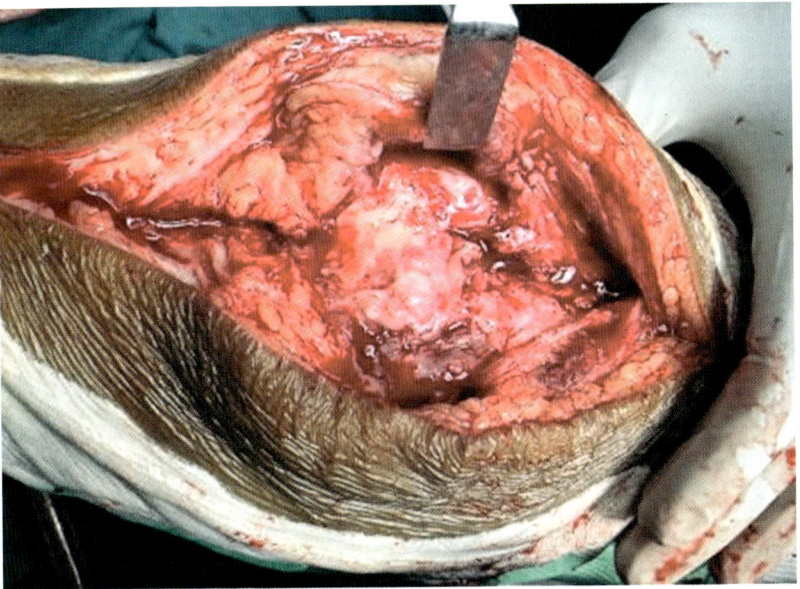

The interior of the knee is now visualized.

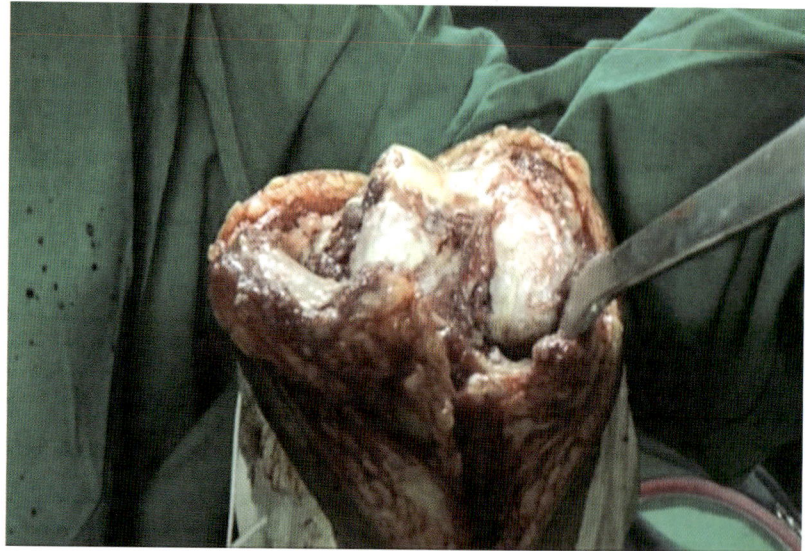

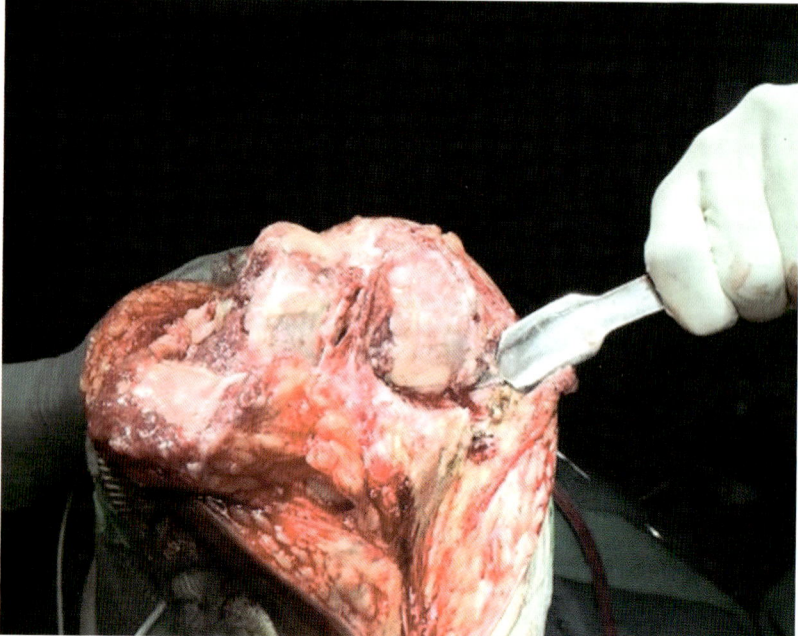

Flexion of the knee shifts the patella further laterally and gives a decent exposure.

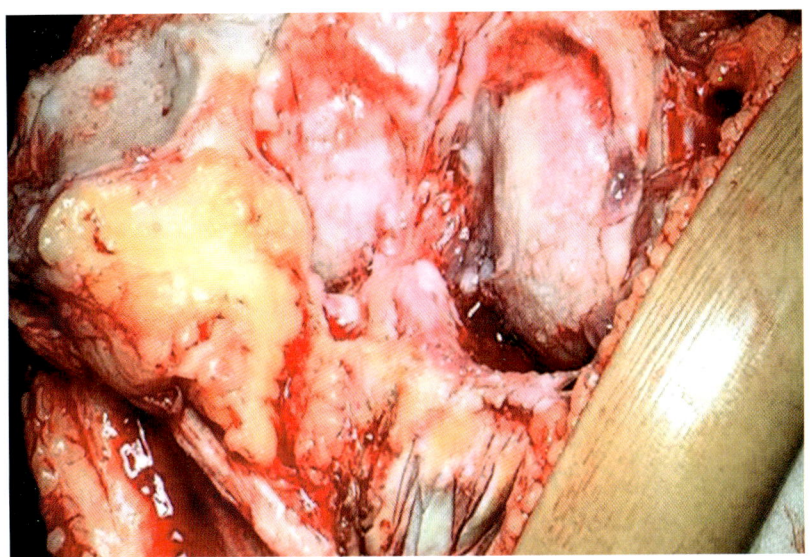

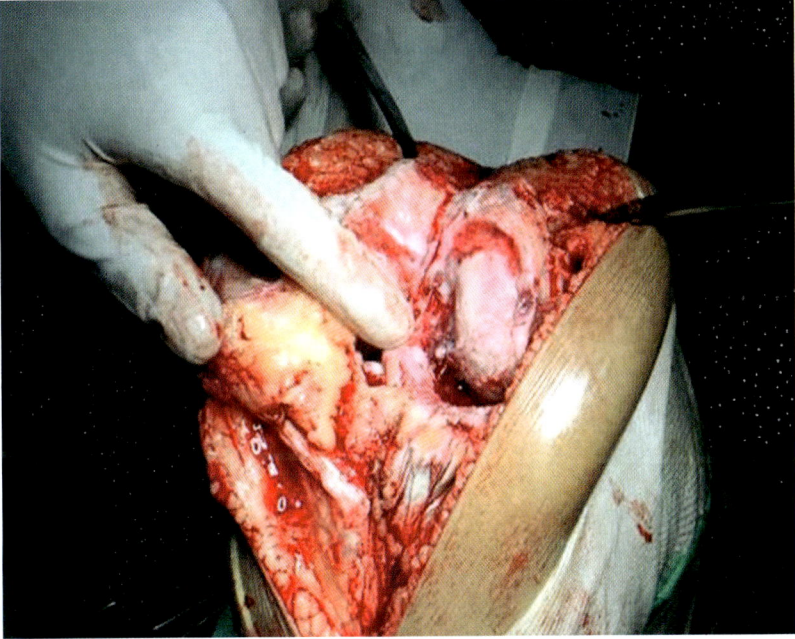

Anterior cruciates are invariably present even in the most damaged osteoarthritic knees, while they are damaged and frayed in rheumatoids.

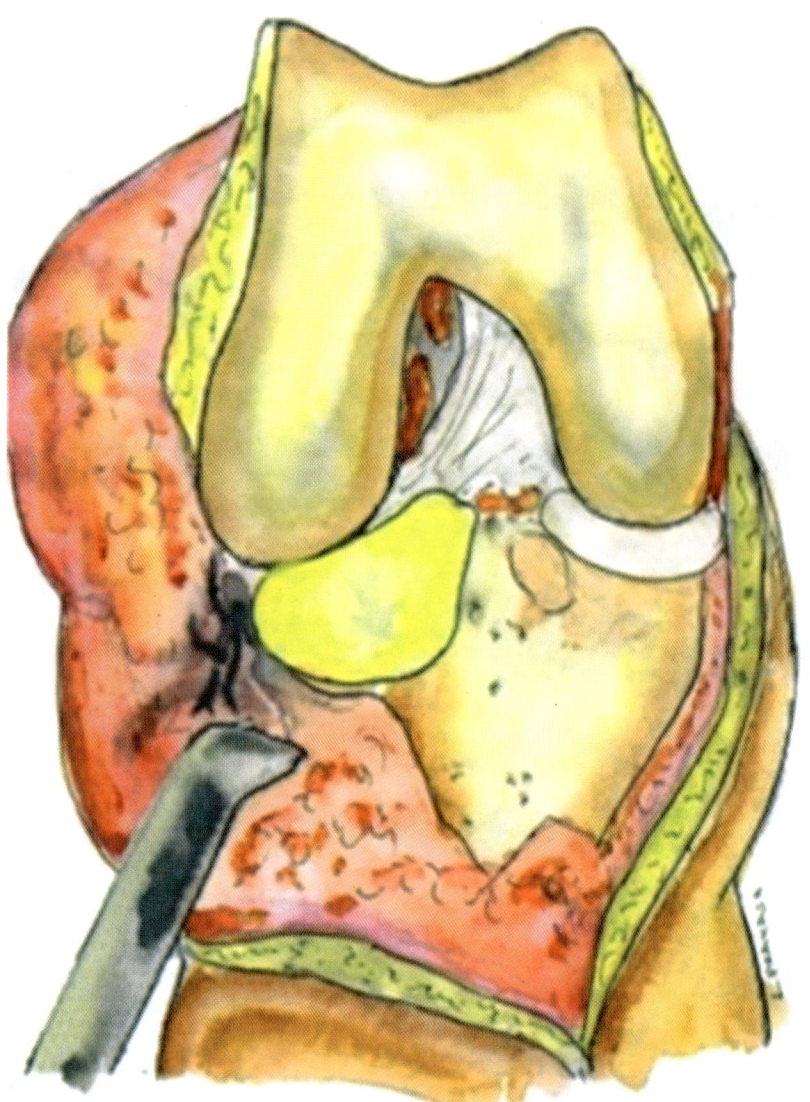

Anterior translation of tibia stretches the ACL.

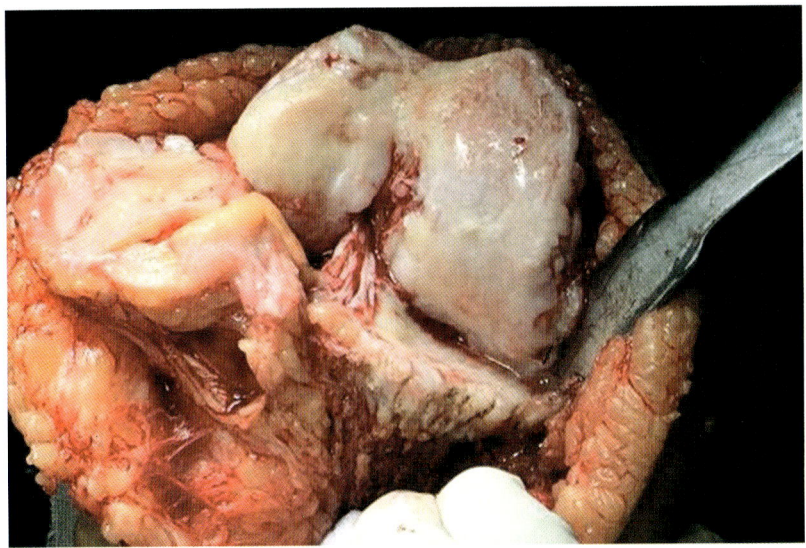

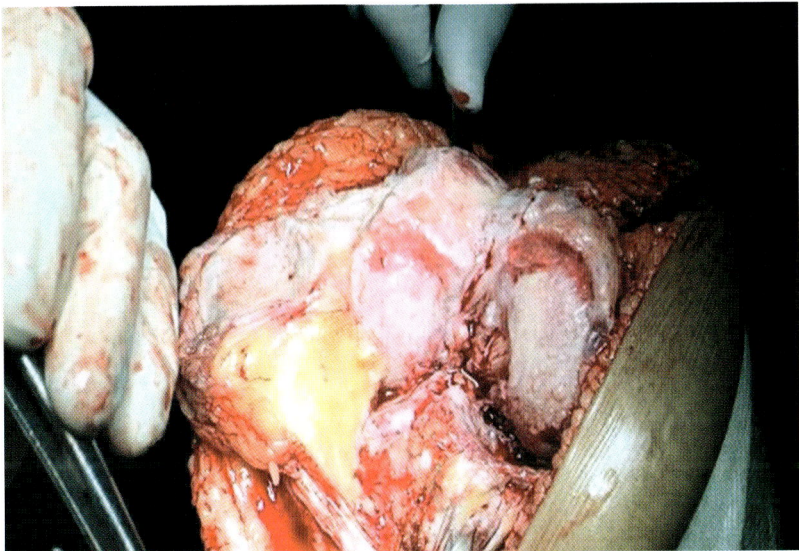

Judicious placement of Homman retractors allows good visualization of knee interior.

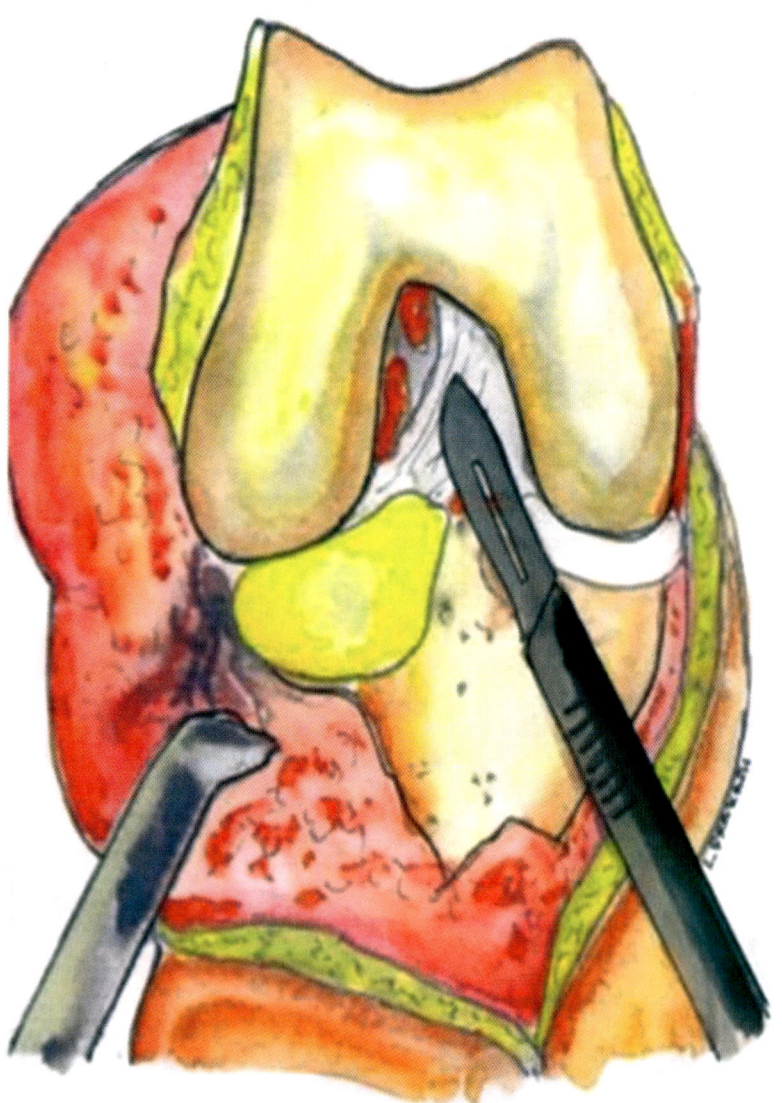

The anterior cruciate is excised.

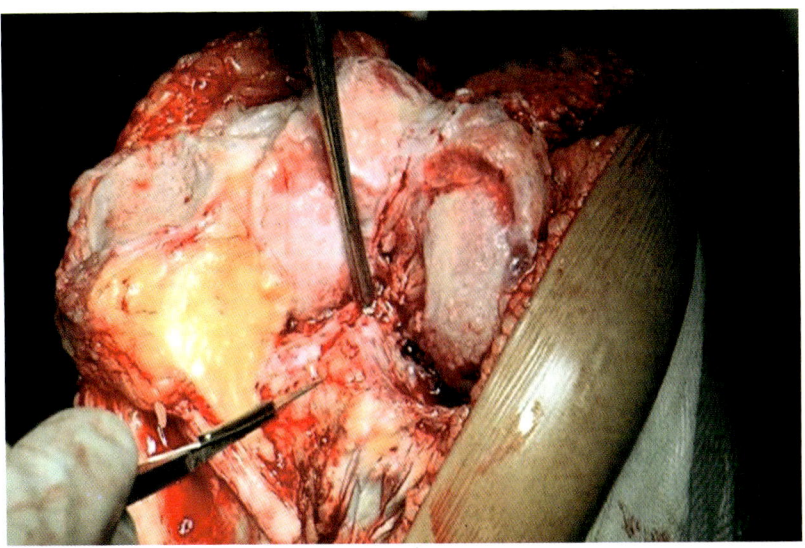

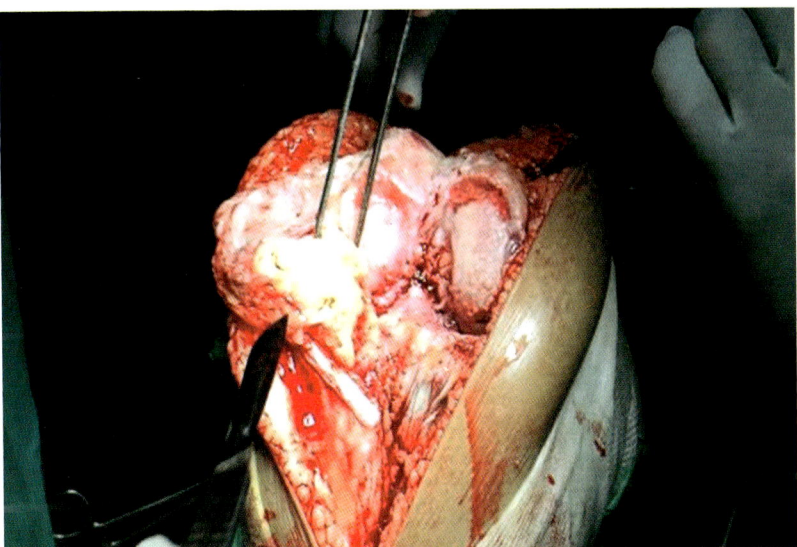

Excision of anterior cruciate and infrapatellar fat pad facilitates full anterior translation of tibia, essential for proper instrumentation.

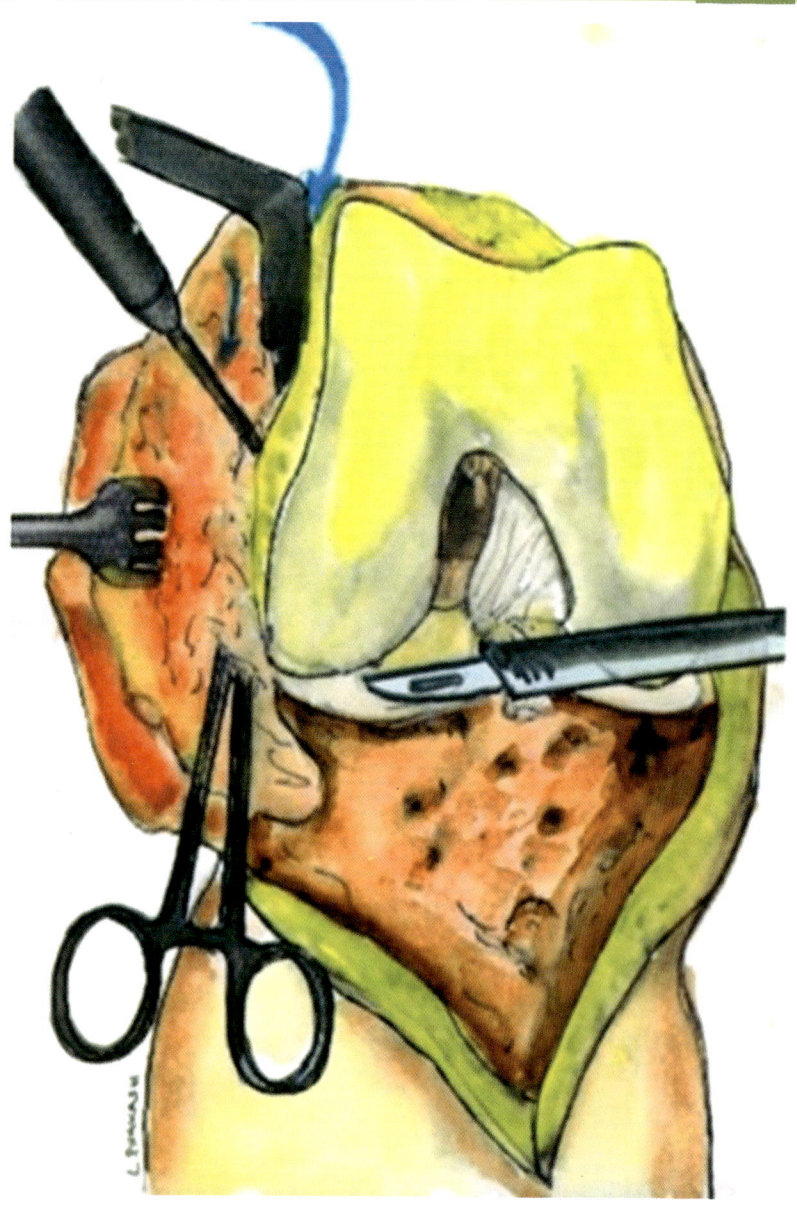

Both menisci are excised.

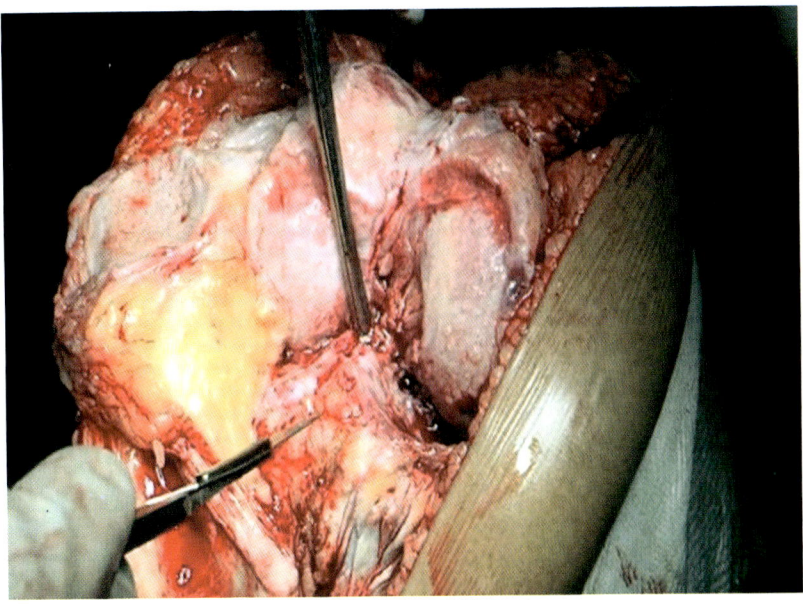

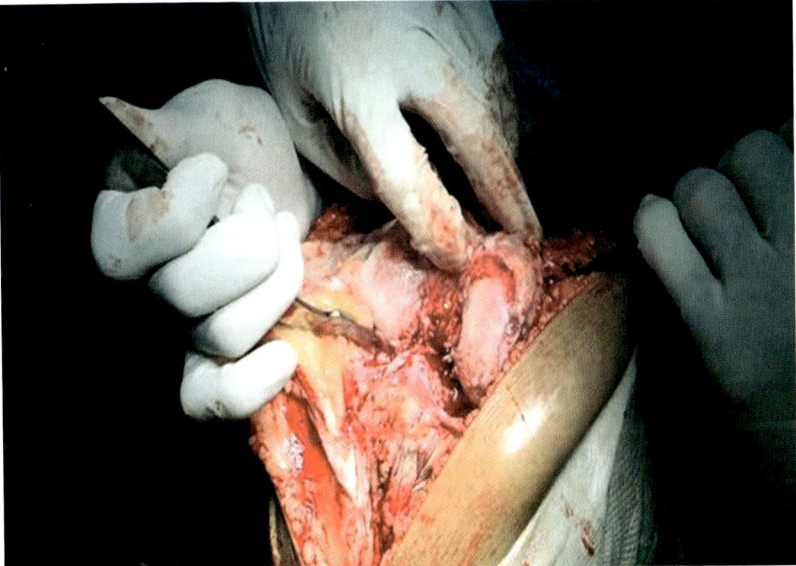

Depending on the compartment involved, meniscus on one side is usually more damaged than the other.

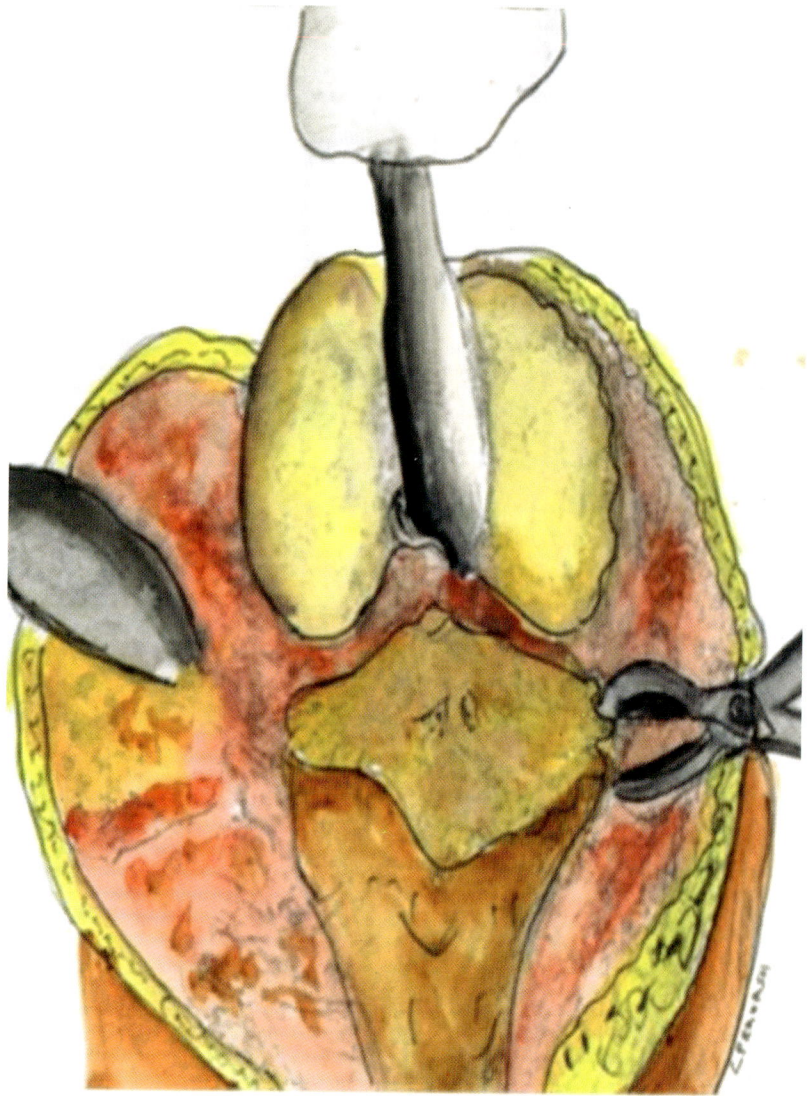

A Homman retractor in the intercondylar area pulls the tibia well forward providing a decent view of the knee interior.

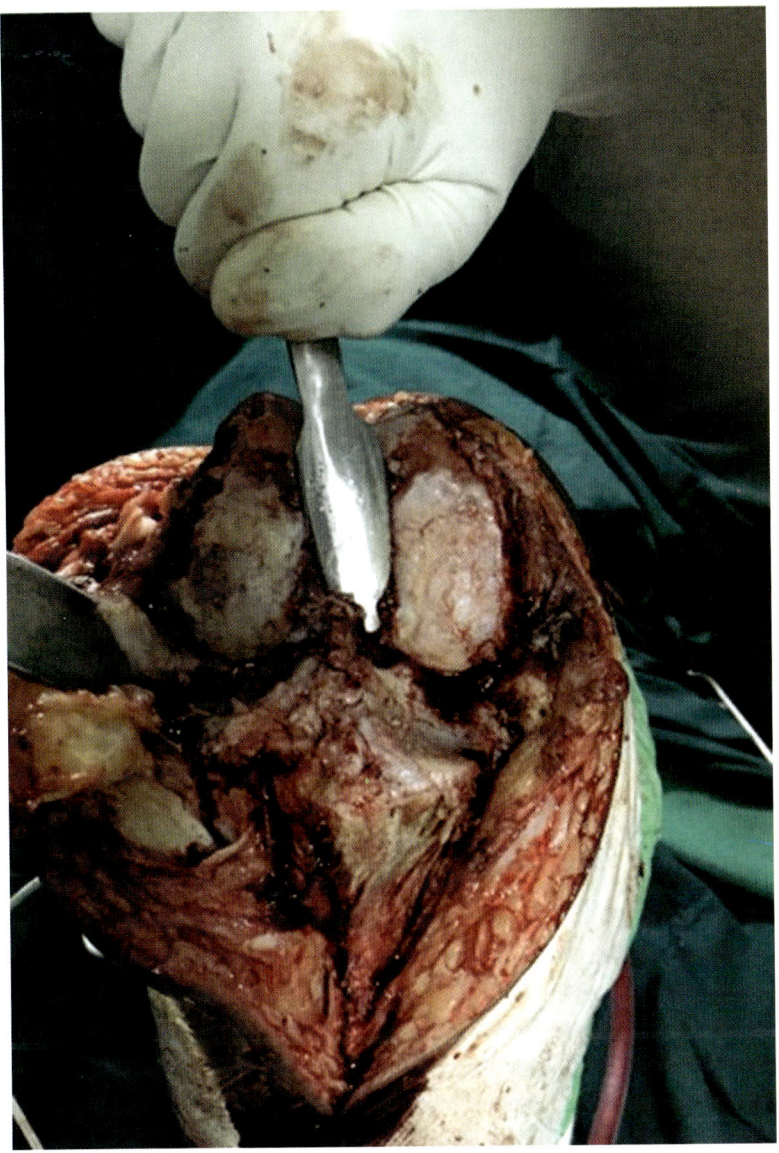

The correct position for Homman retractors.

SOFT TISSUE RELEASES AND DEFORMITY CORRECTION

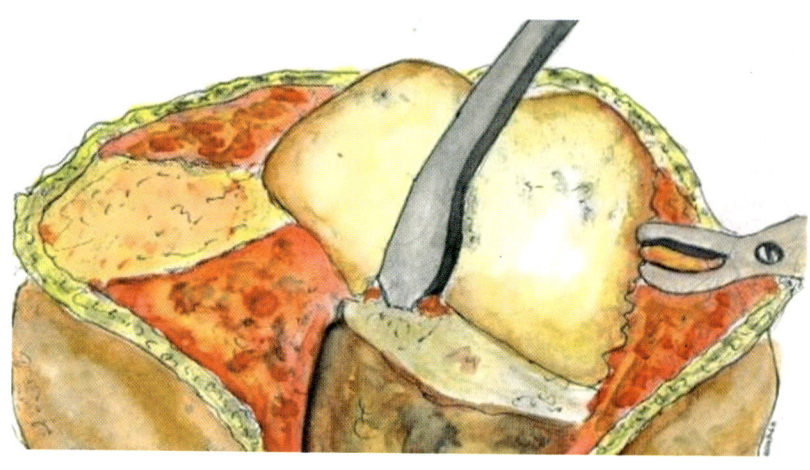

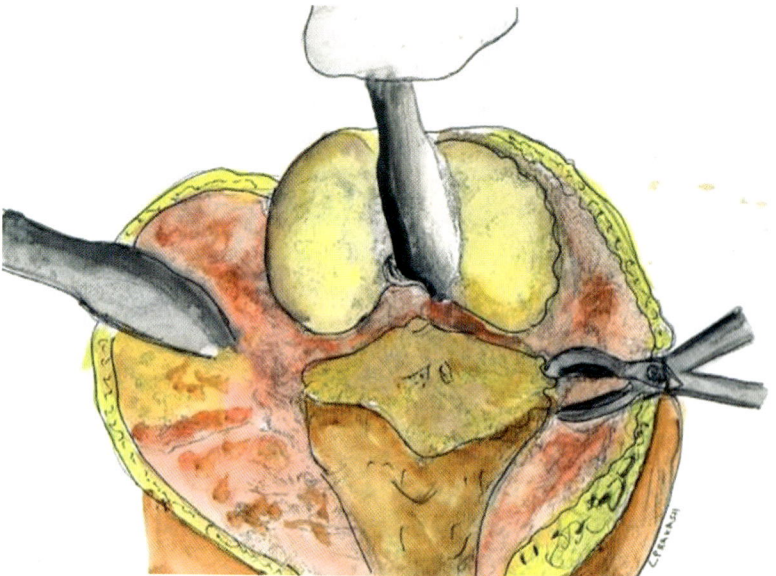

Osteophytes on both femoral and tibial side are removed with a nibbler.

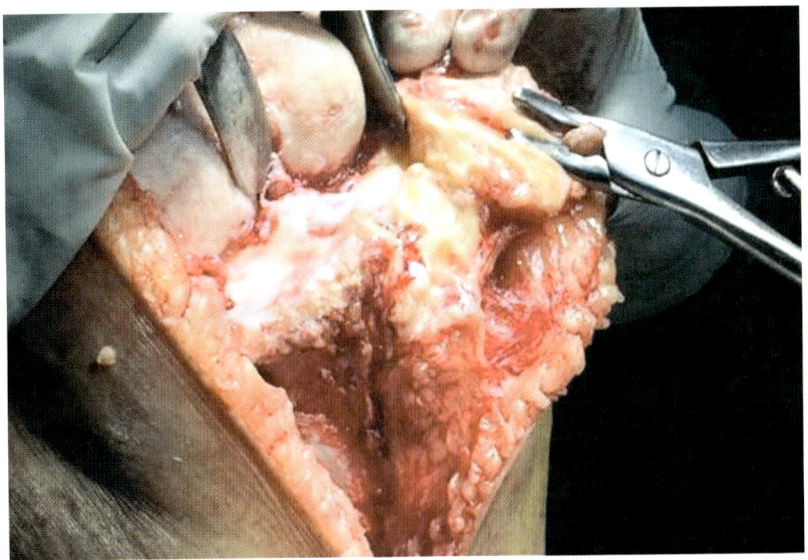

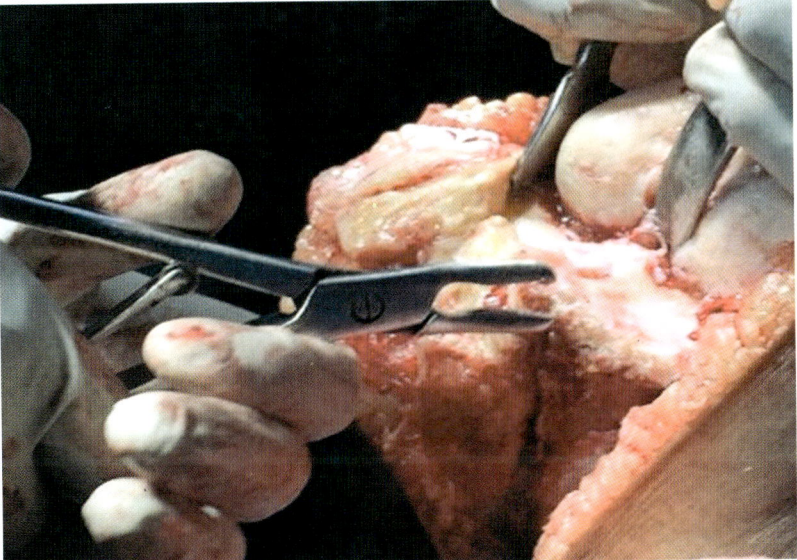

In most cases, removal of overhanging osteophytes corrects a significant amount of deformity.

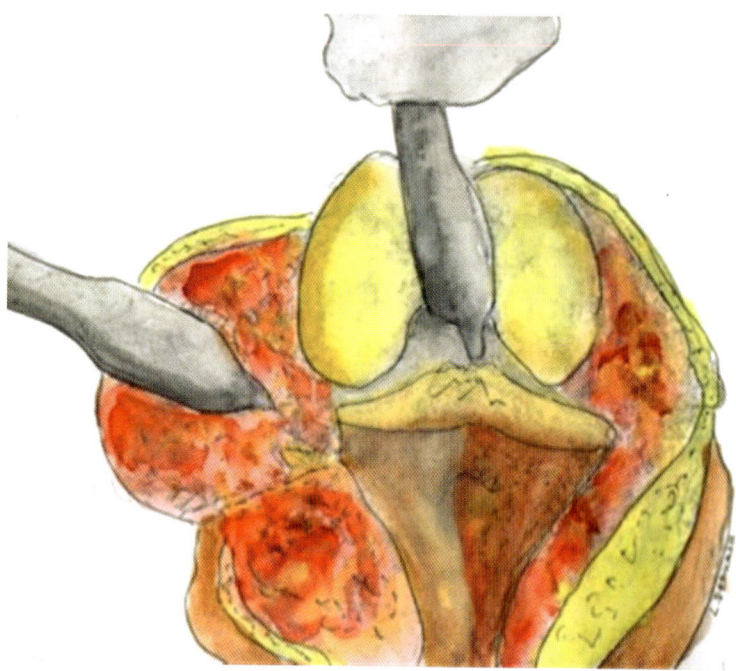

Additional medial or lateral soft tissue releases are done to correct residual deformities.

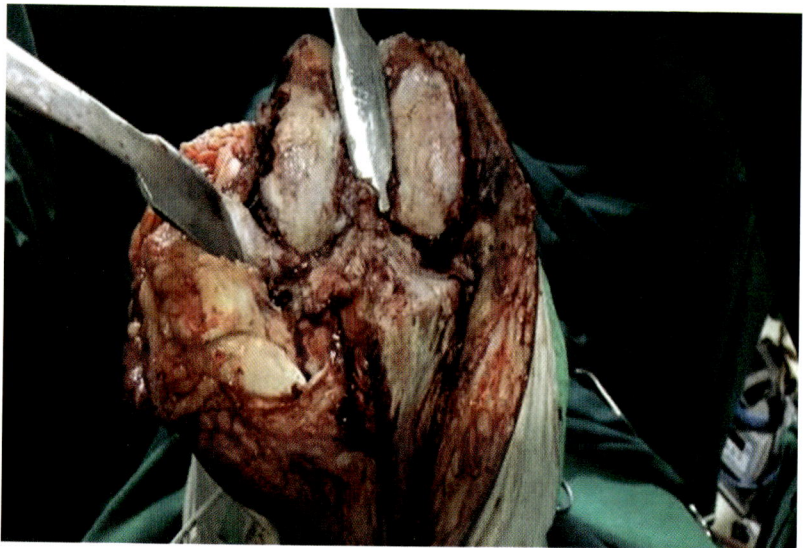

By external rotation and stripping the periosteum with medial collateral structures, a proper medial release is performed.

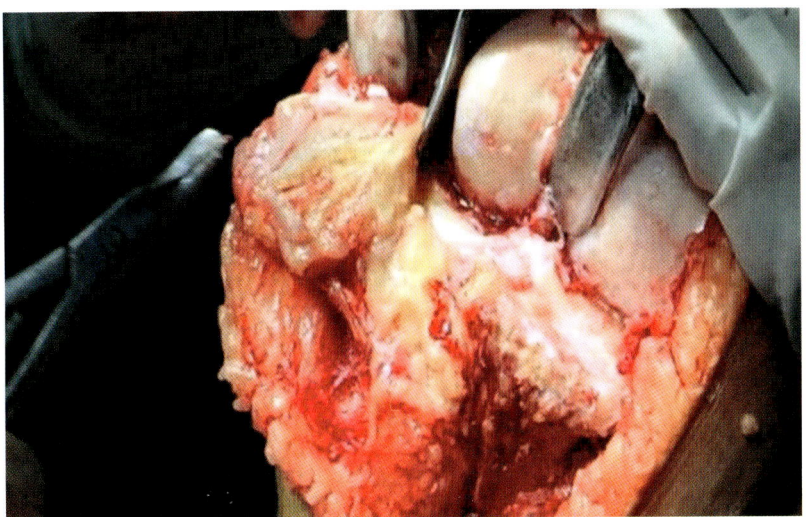

Internal rotation allows for release of tight structures on the lateral side.

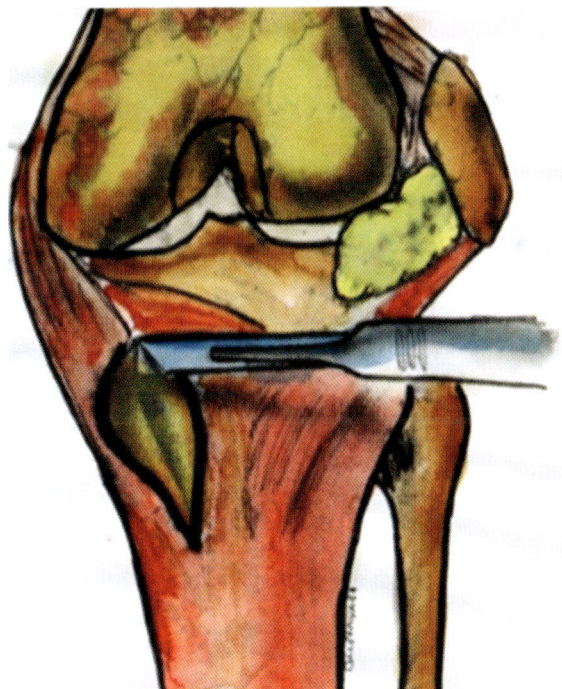

A good method of medial release is to make an incision bone deep and lift a periosteal flap, including all the medial collateral structures.

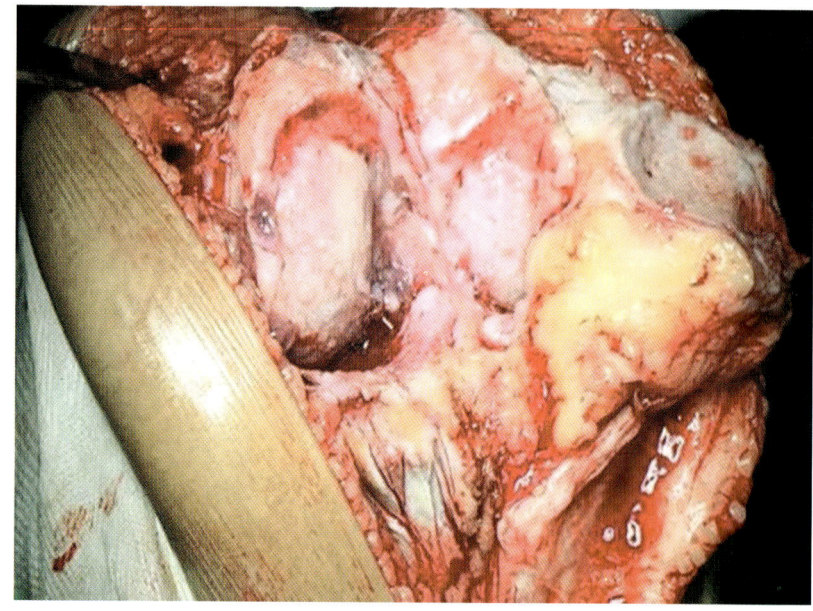

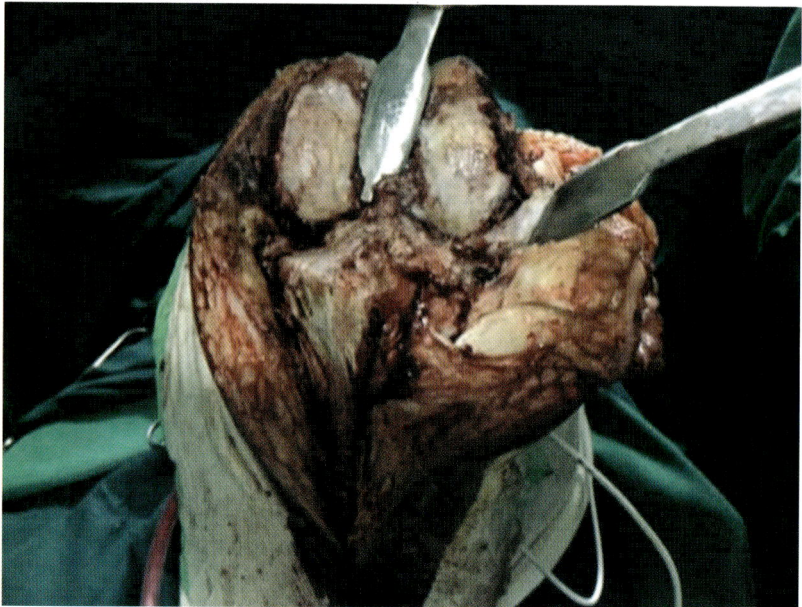

Most stubborn varus deformities can be corrected to a great extent by this method. This is a very important step.

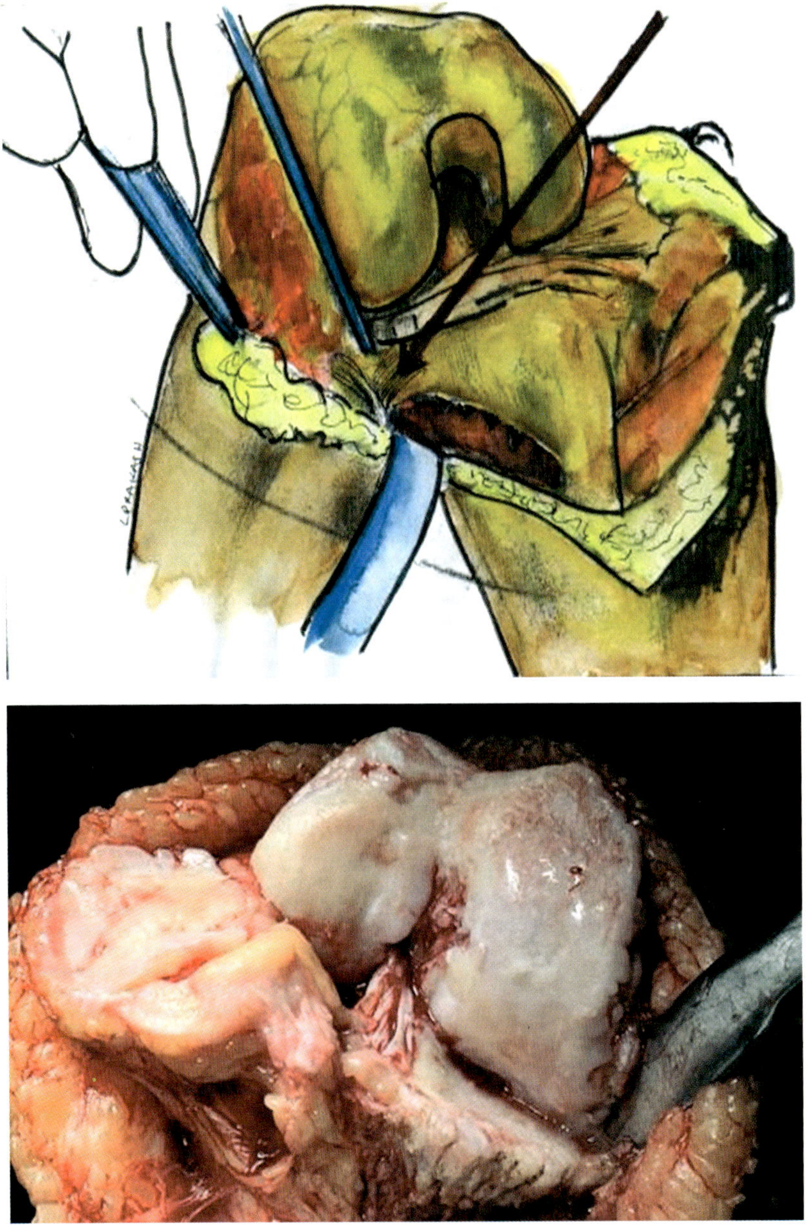

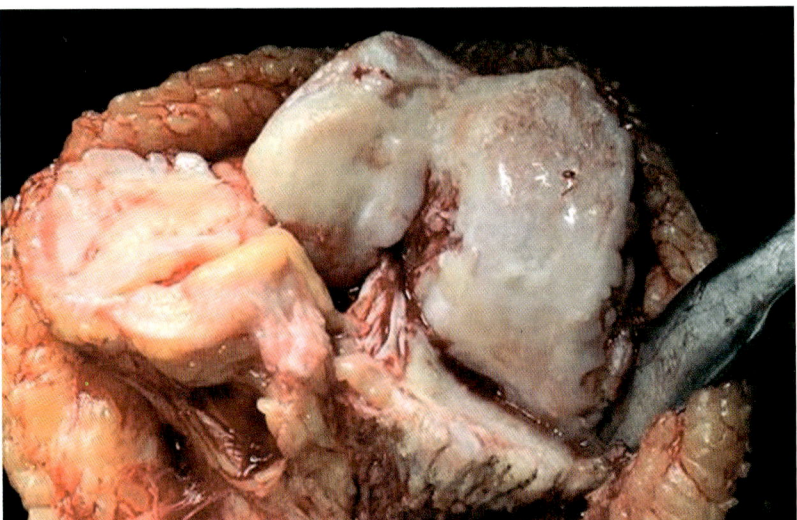

In extreme varus, release up to the semimembranosus tendon may be required.

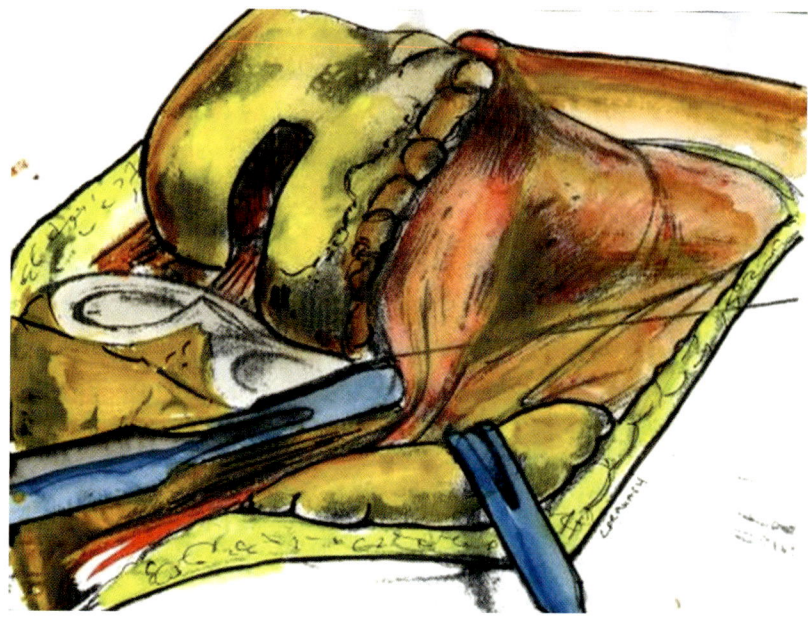

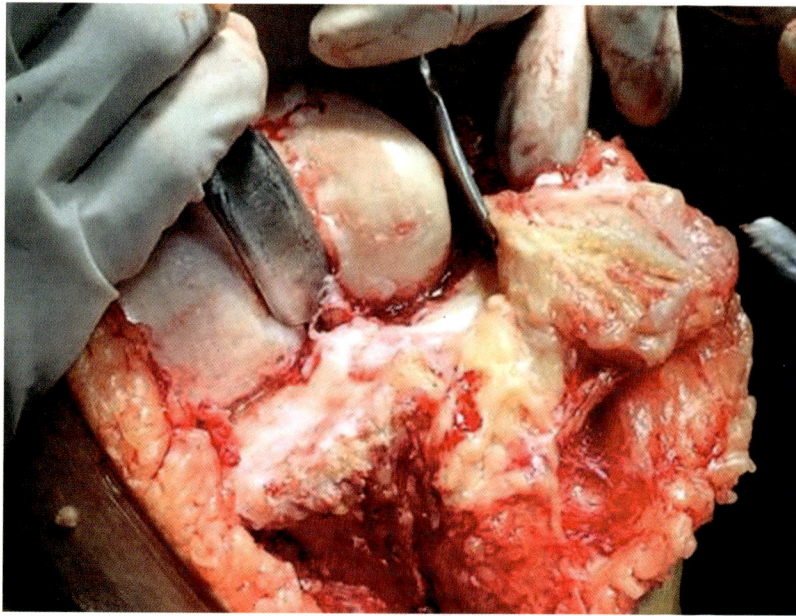

In valgus deformities, an extensive medial release right up to the popliteus tendon is needed. Occasionally, release of the tendon may be required.

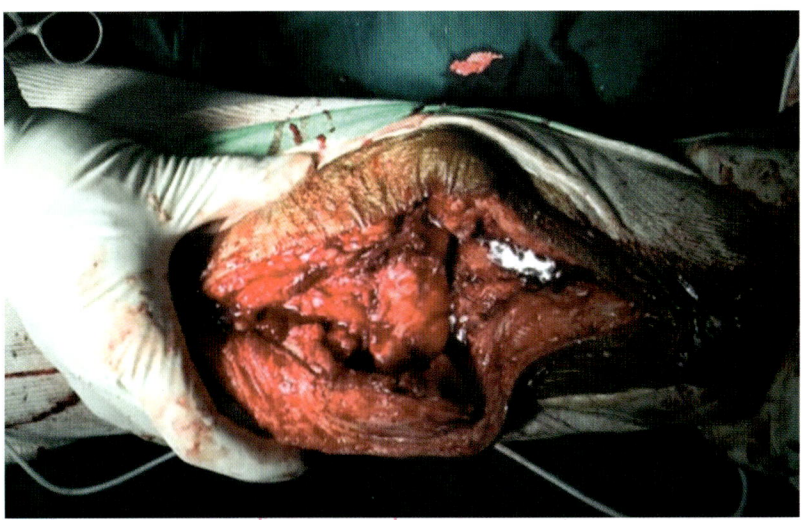

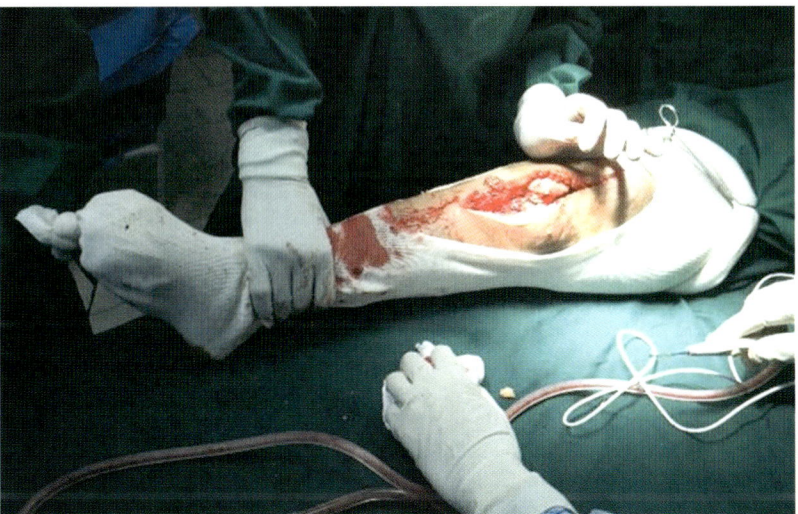

After soft tissue releases, ensure that all deformities are corrected before beginning the first bone cut.

Soft tissue releases are the most important part of a knee replacement surgery.

All deformities should be corrected before the first bone cut.

Knee arthroplasty is more like gardening than carpentry.

TKR needs 5 bone cuts to femur and 1 to tibia in a precise position.

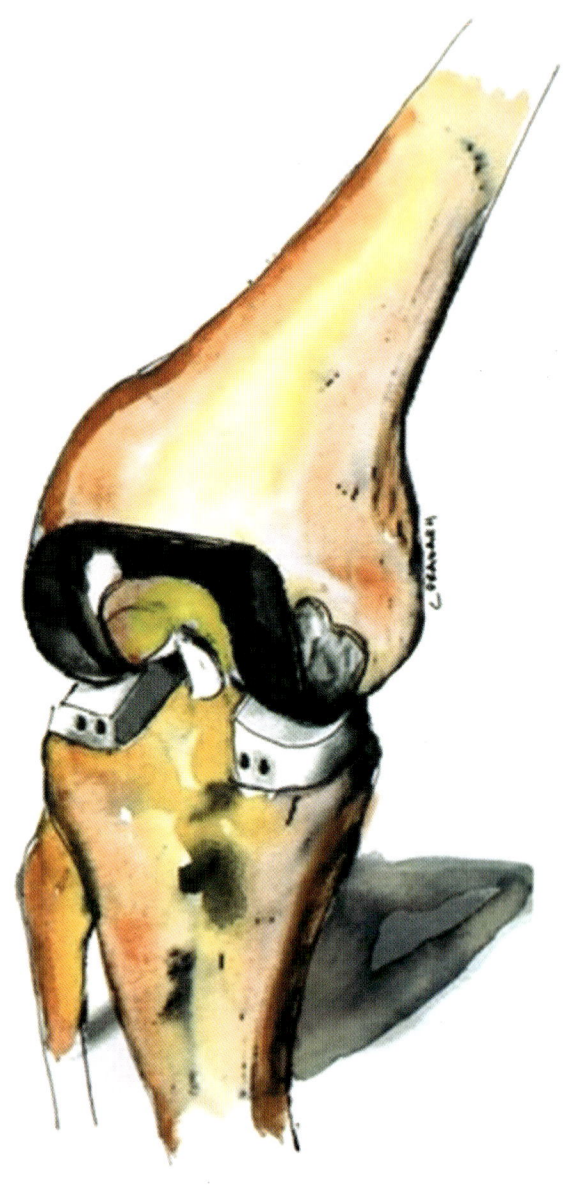

The six bone cuts for every knee arthroplasty independent of the design.

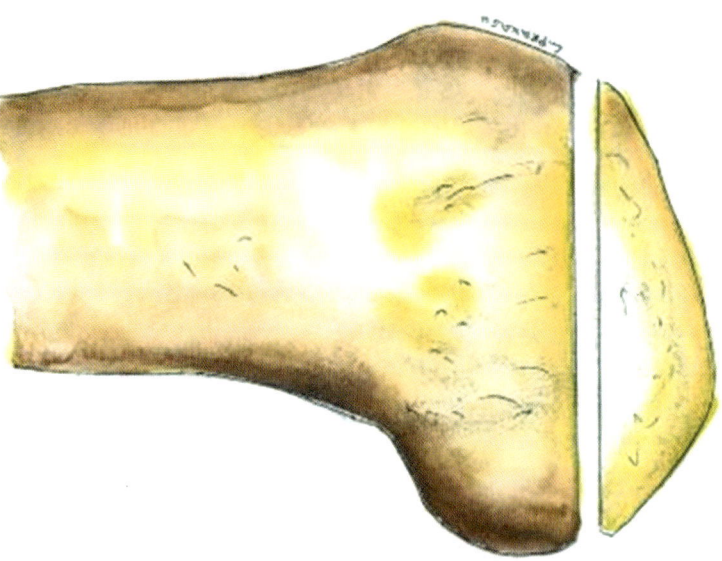

The distal femoral cut should be parallel to the ground in AP axis and in 3° to 5° valgus in ML axis.

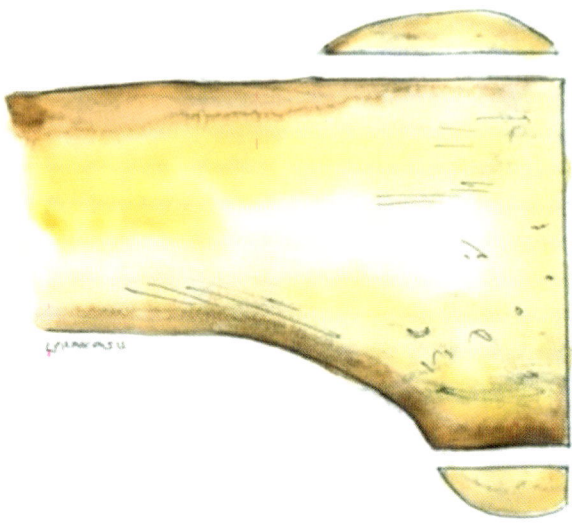

The anterior and posterior femoral cuts should exactly match the inner dimensions of the prosthesis to be used.

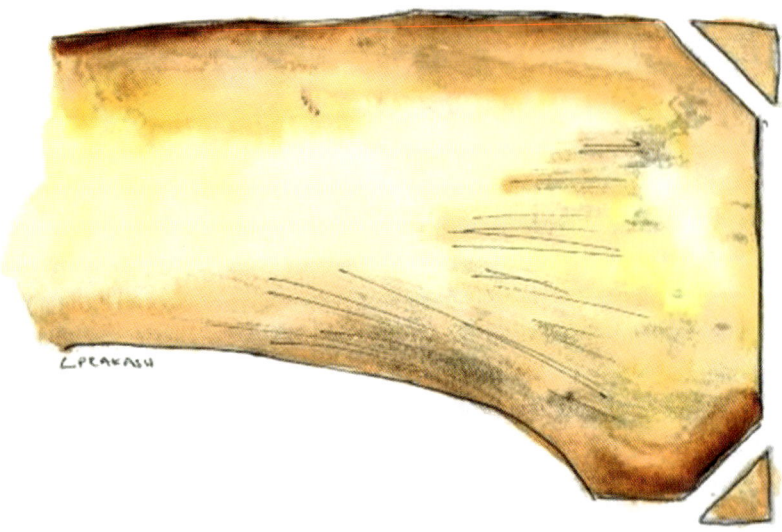

Anterior and posterior chamfer cuts again mirror the implant.

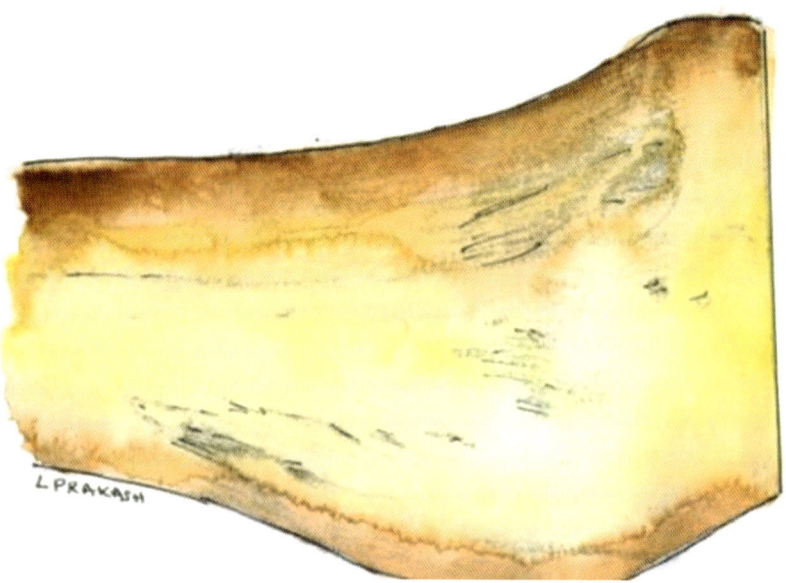

The upper tibial cut should be parallel to the floor front side-to-side and in a 3° to 5° posterior slope in the anterioposterior axis.

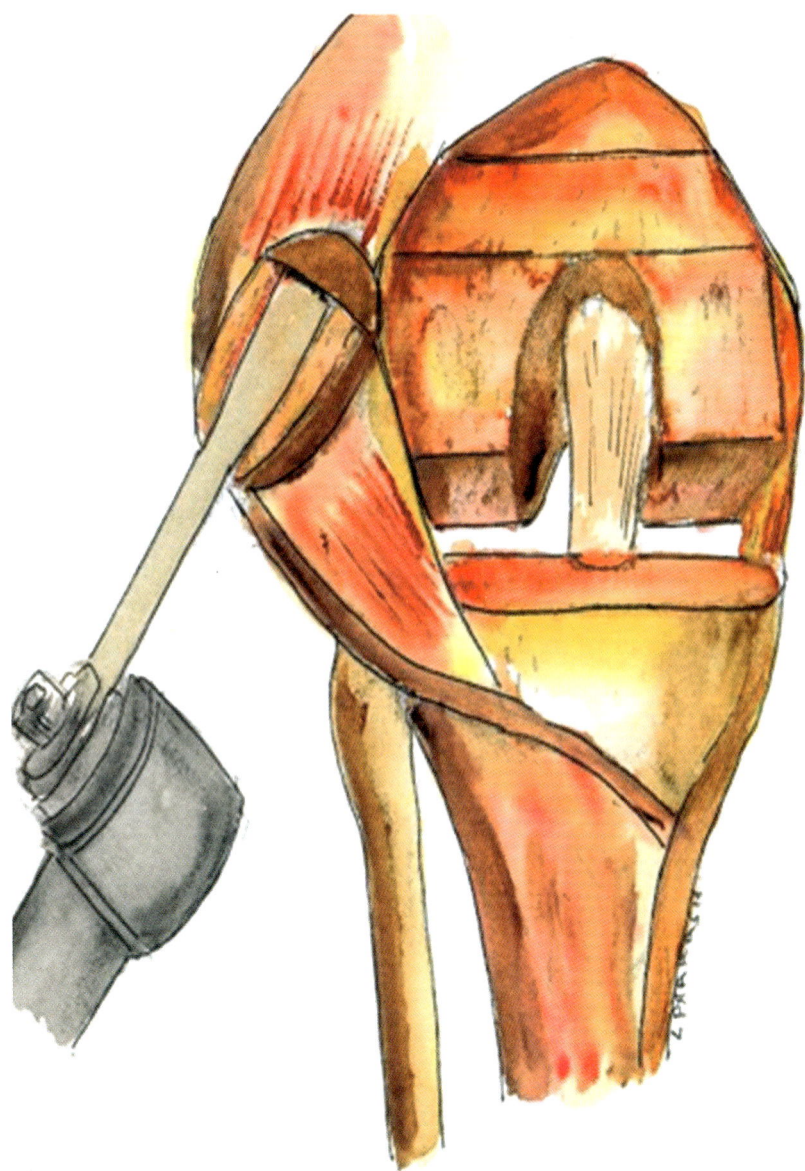

The patellar cut can either be for a replacement or patelloplasty/ debulking.

THE DISTAL FEMORAL CUTS AND PREPARATION

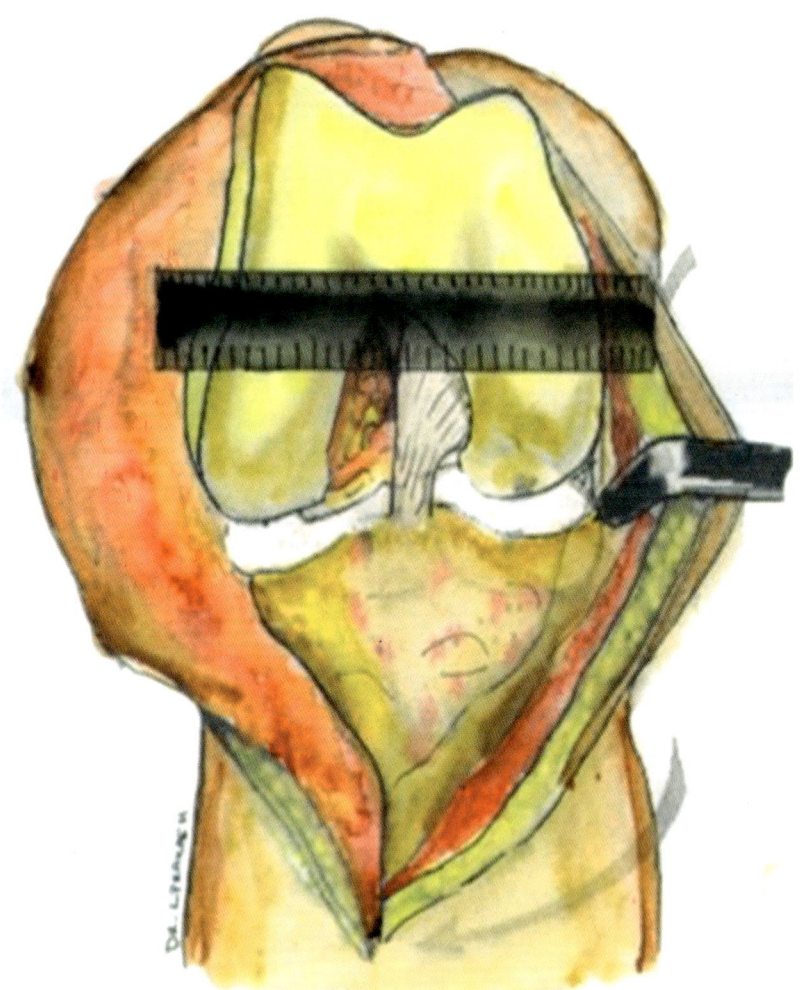

Measurement of the distal femur in AP and side-to-side axes is the first step after soft tissue releases. This tells us about the size of the implant to be used.

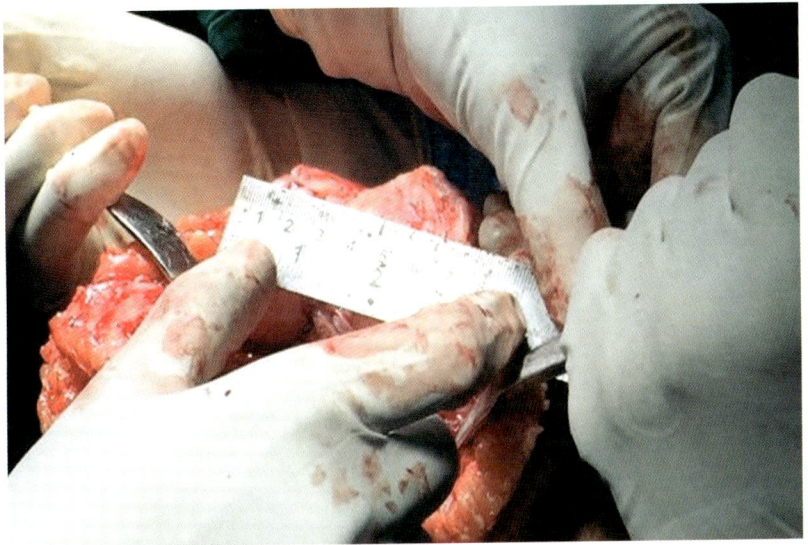

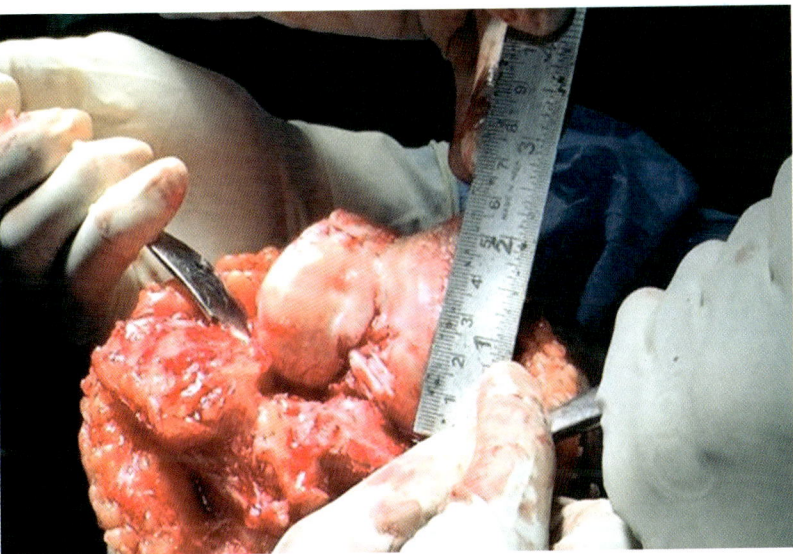

Actual measurement helps us to narrow down on the prosthesis size to be used.

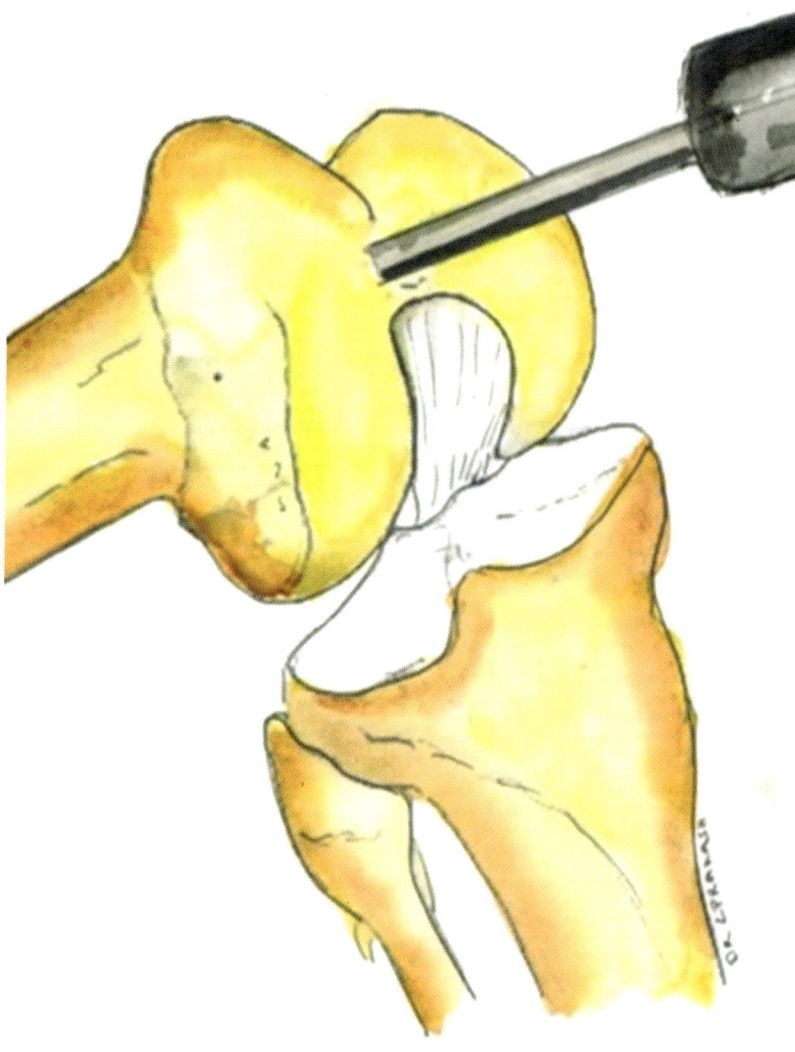

With a chisel, an opening is made in the intercondylar notch above the insertion of ACL.

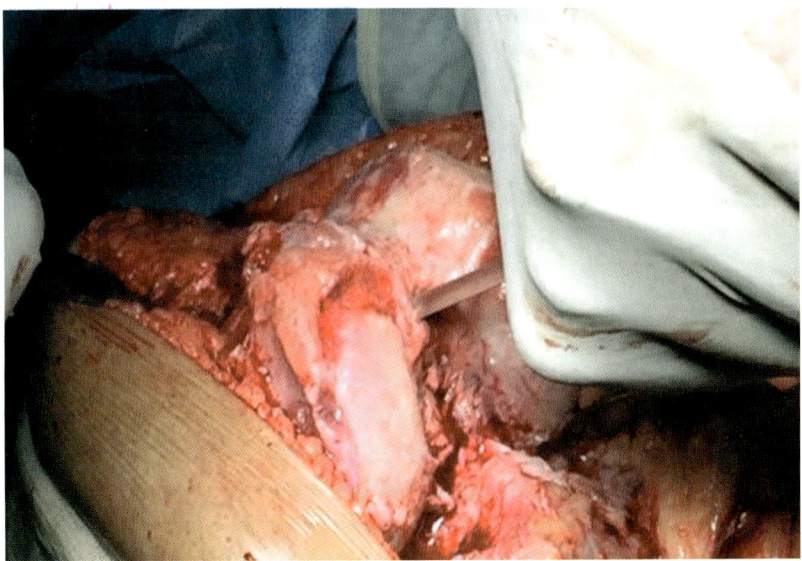

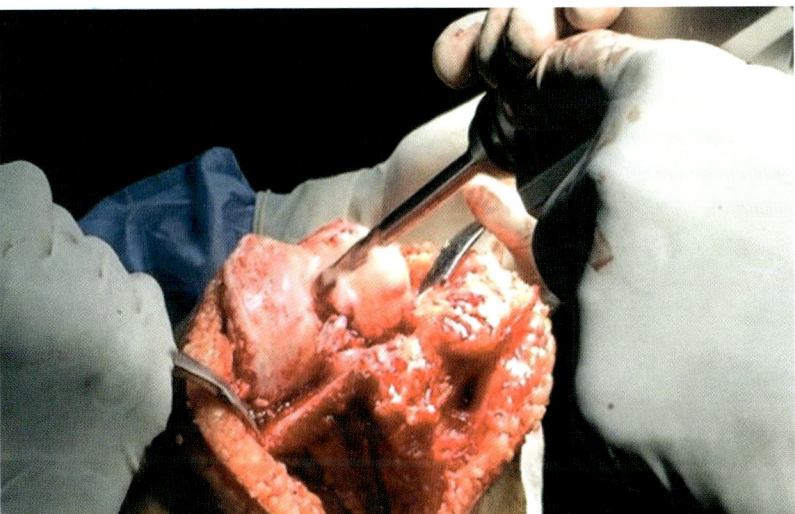

The chisel hole opening will guide the drill bit for intramedullary instrumentation.

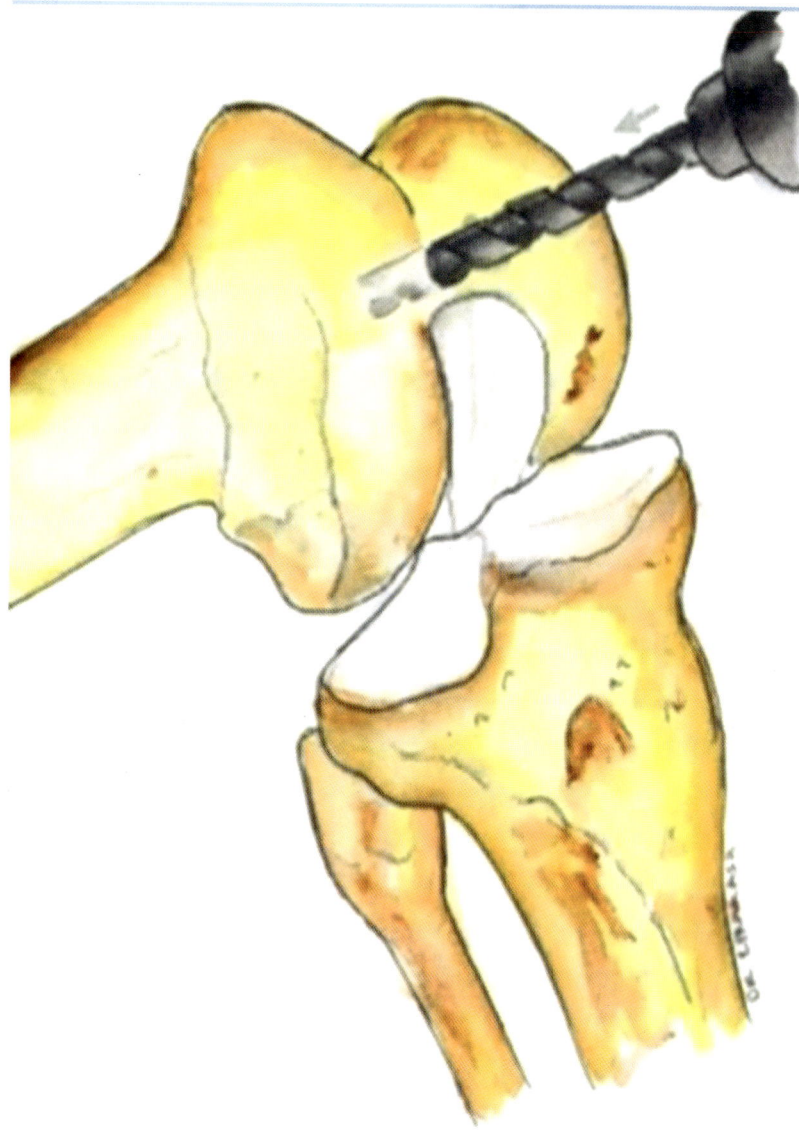

The hole is enlarged with an appropriate drill bit.

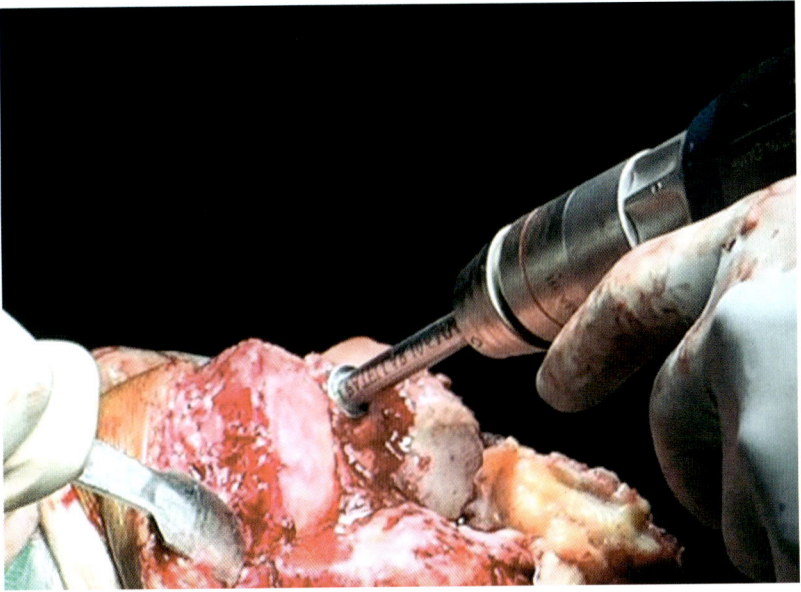

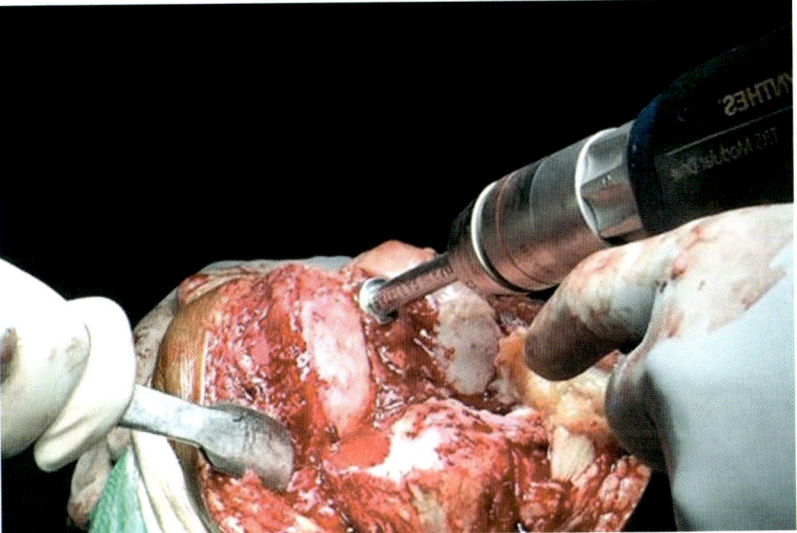

This hole will be used for the intramedullary alignment rod.

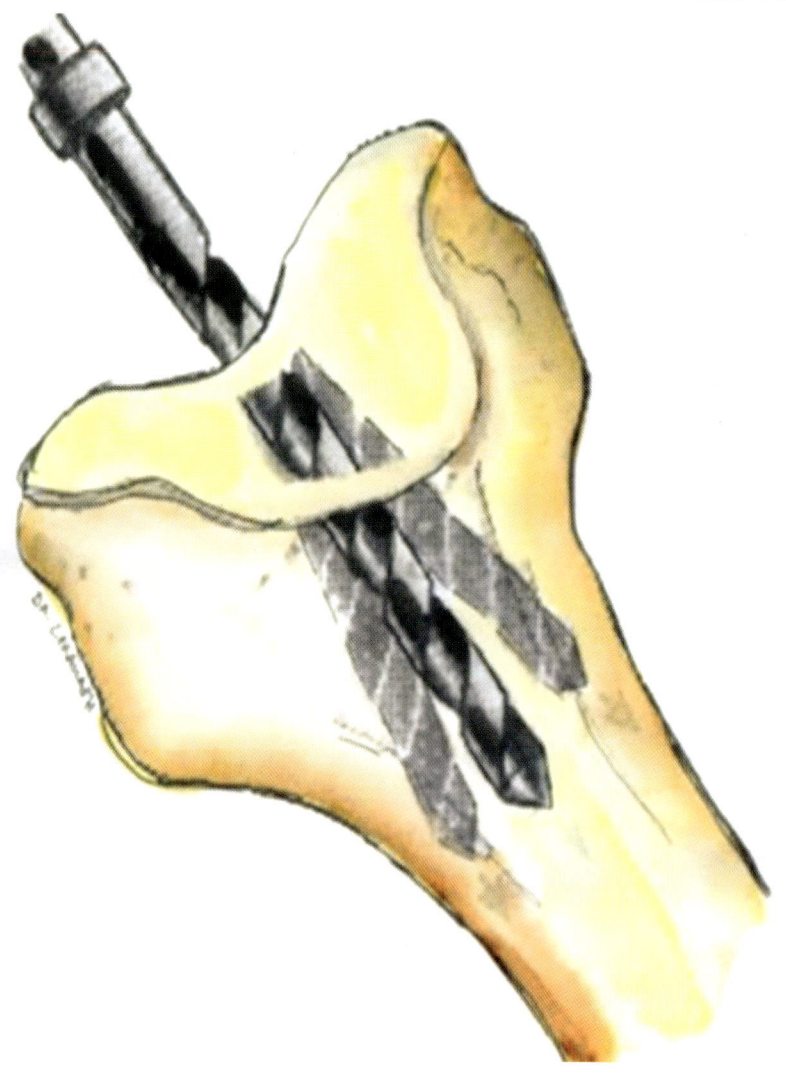

The drill bit is see-sawed to locate central medulla.

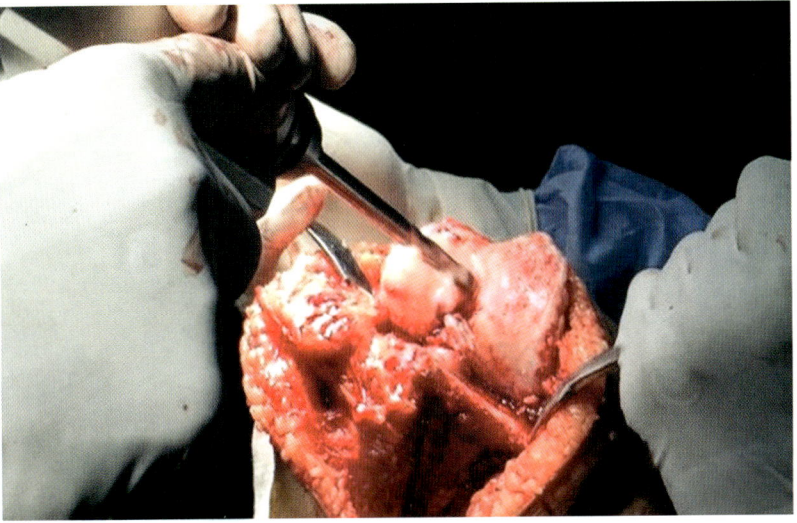

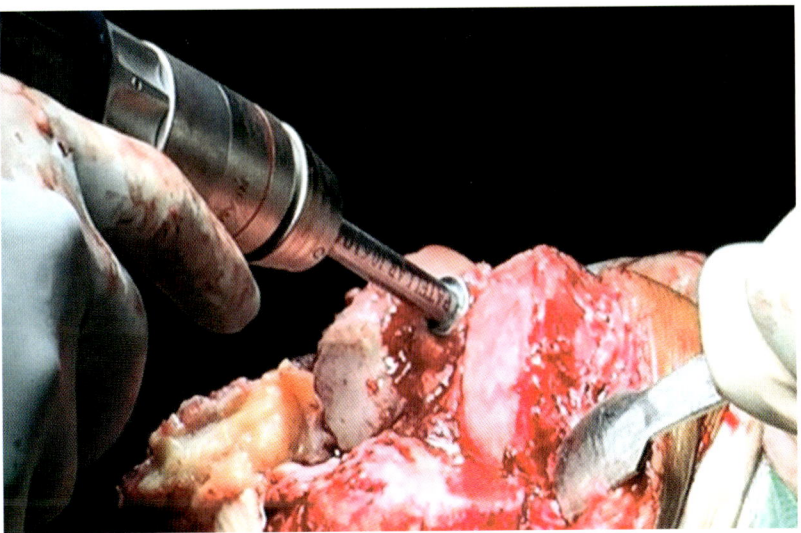

The distal femur is now ready to take the intramedullary broach.

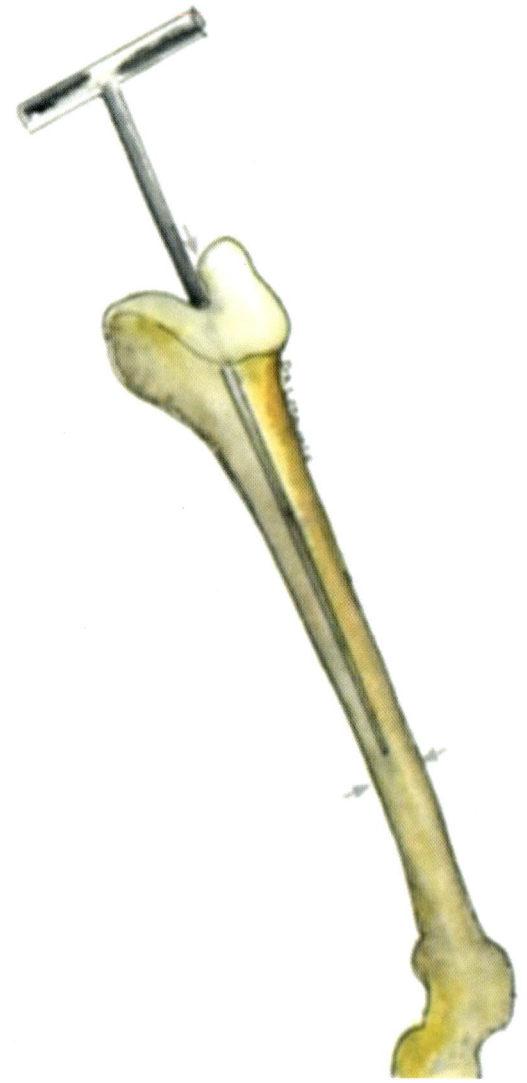

The long broach is pushed right up to the isthumus. This is essential to ensure that the distal jigs are in a precisely defined alignment to the long axis of the femoral shaft.

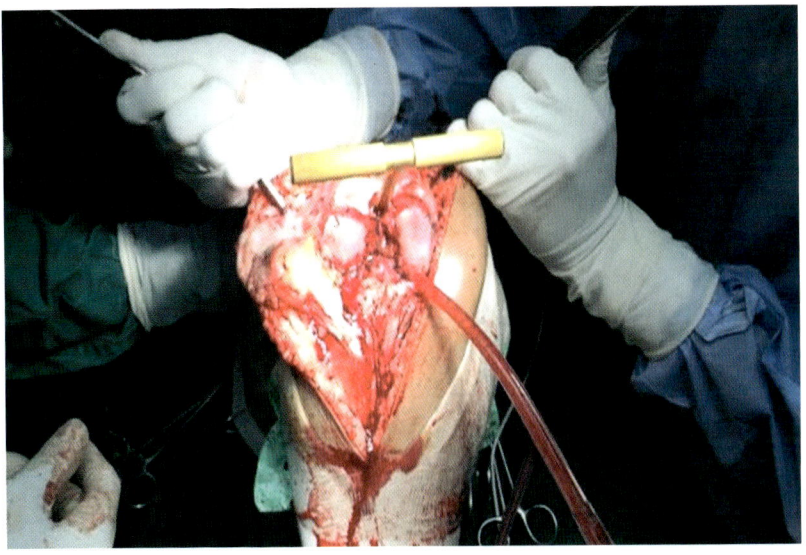

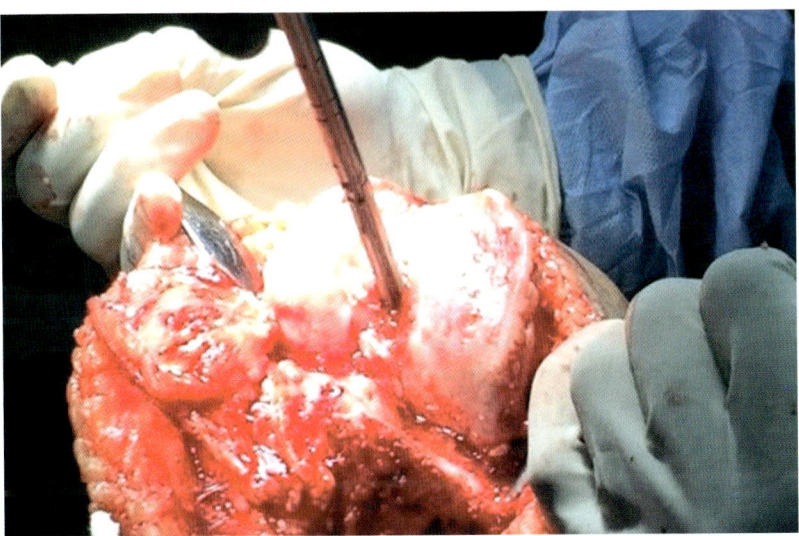

The intramedullary rod thus lies in the long axis of femur.

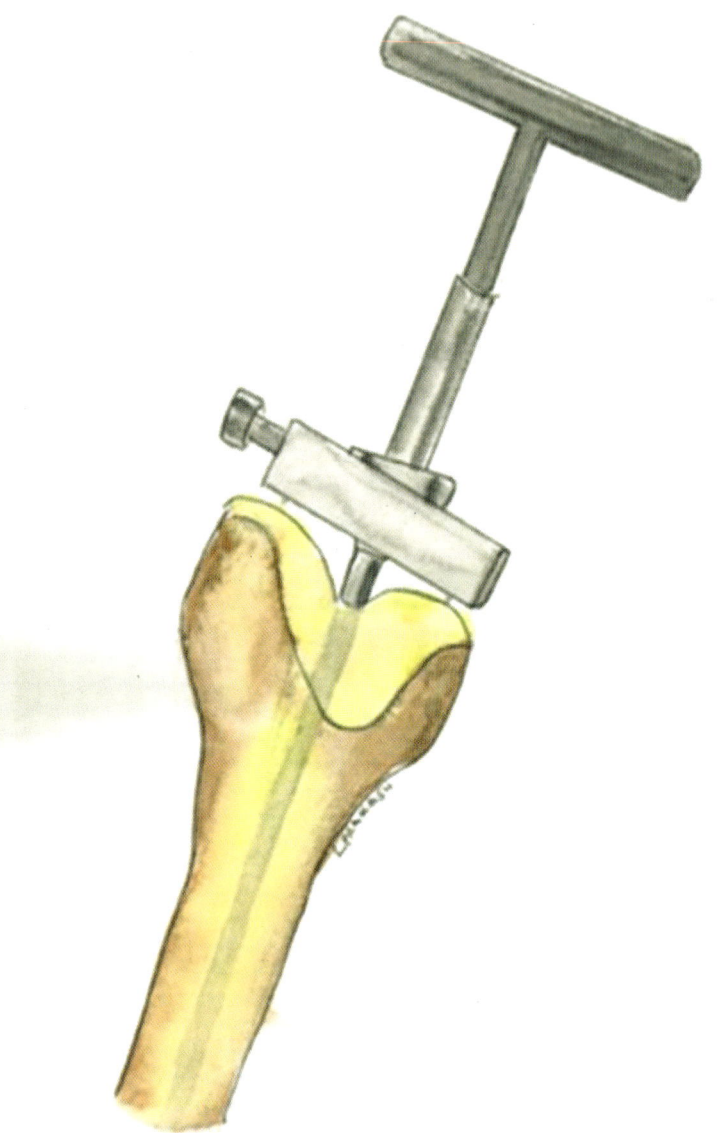

The distal cutting guide is slid over the intramedullary rod.

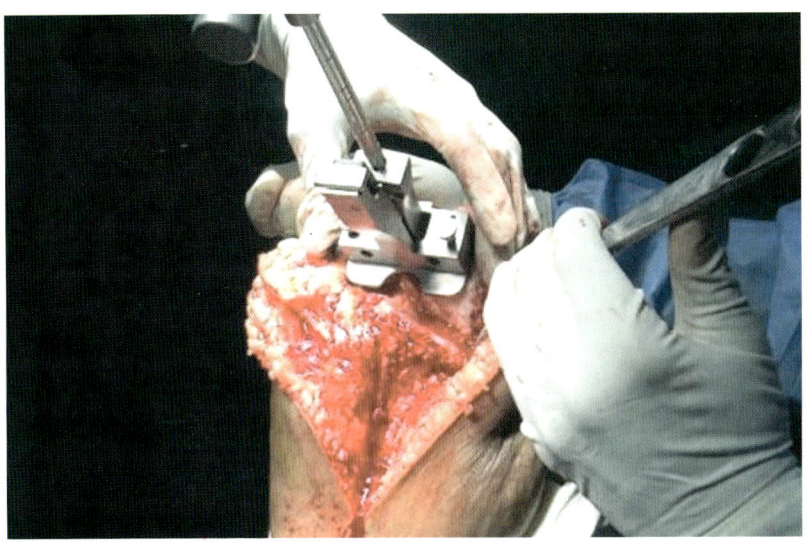

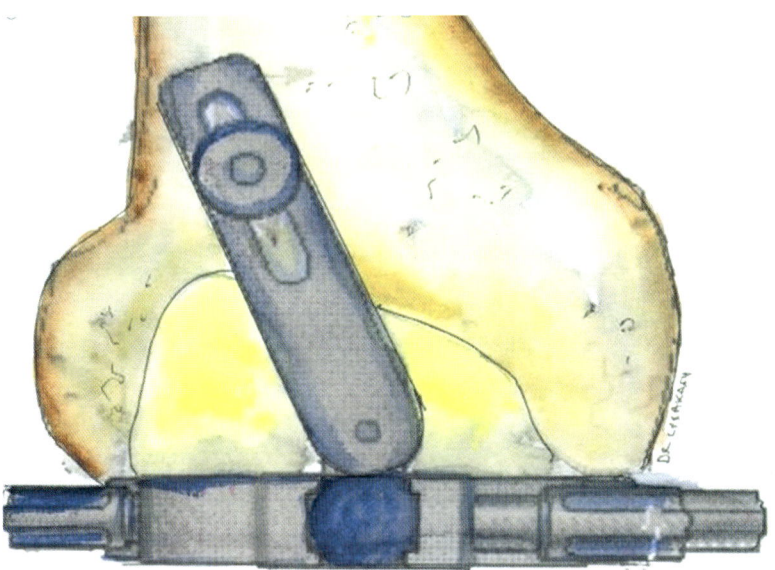

Different designs have their own methods to provide the desired valgus to the femoral cut. However, most systems are based on Kenna's patented universal knee instrumentation system with a few minor modifications.

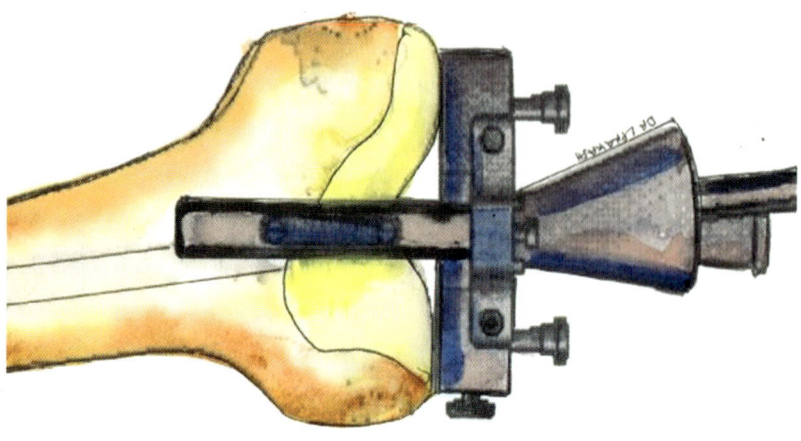

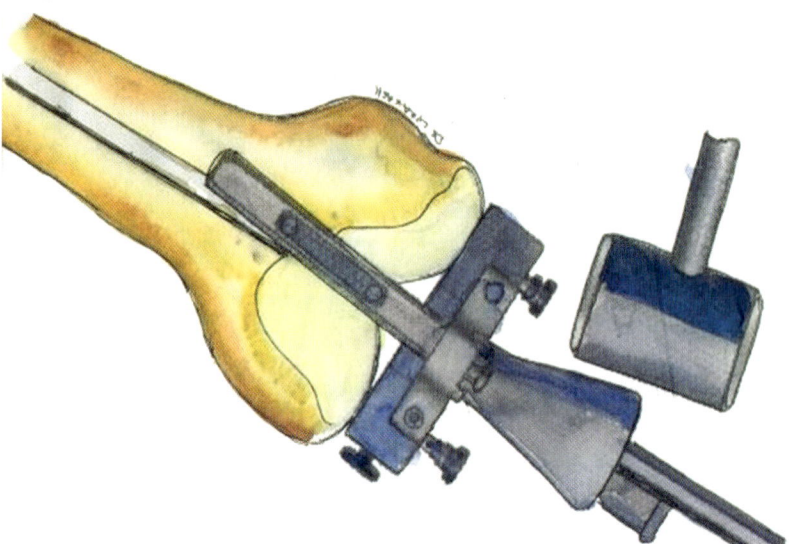

The jigs ensure that the distal femoral cut is parallel to the floor in AP axis, and in 3° to 6° of valgus in the ML direction.

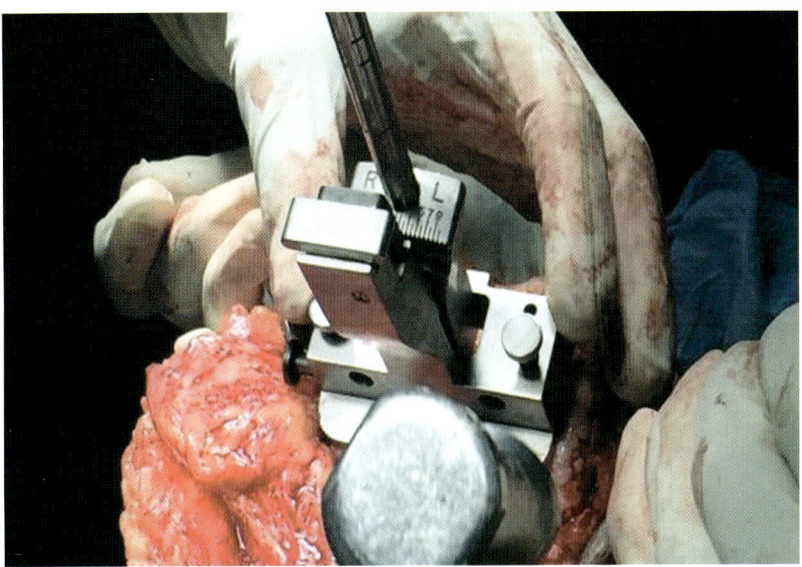

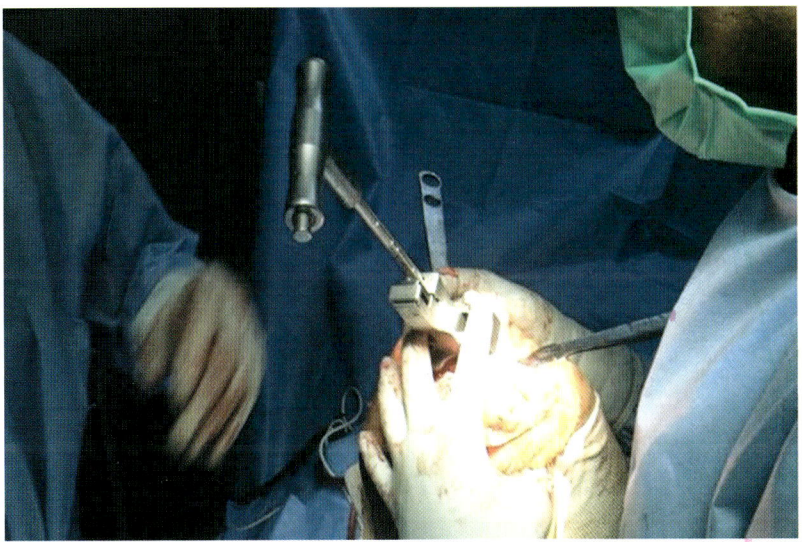

The rotational alignment is then checked.

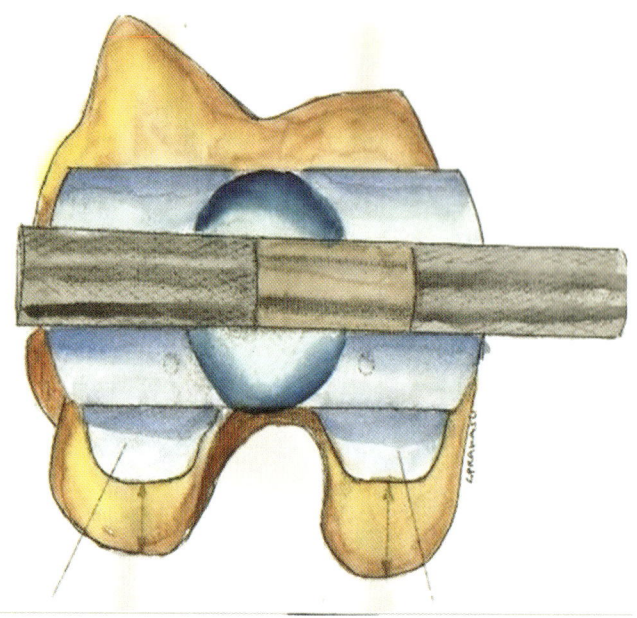

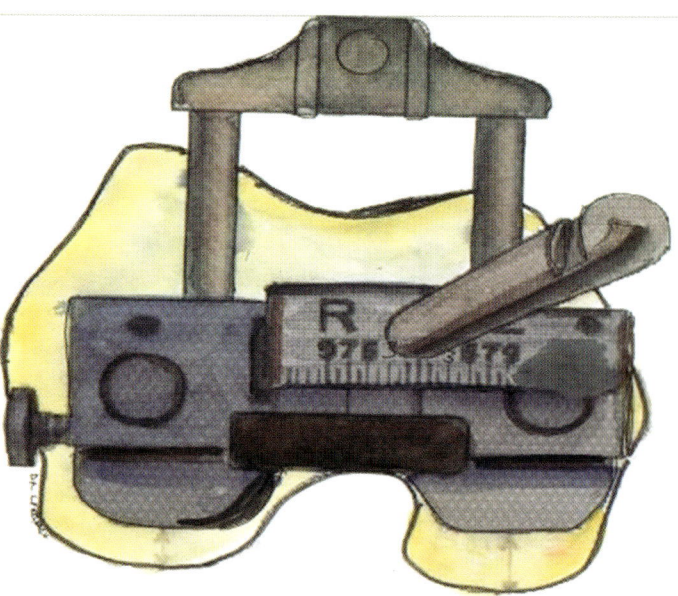

Different designs of instrumentation have their own valgus and rotation evaluation markings.

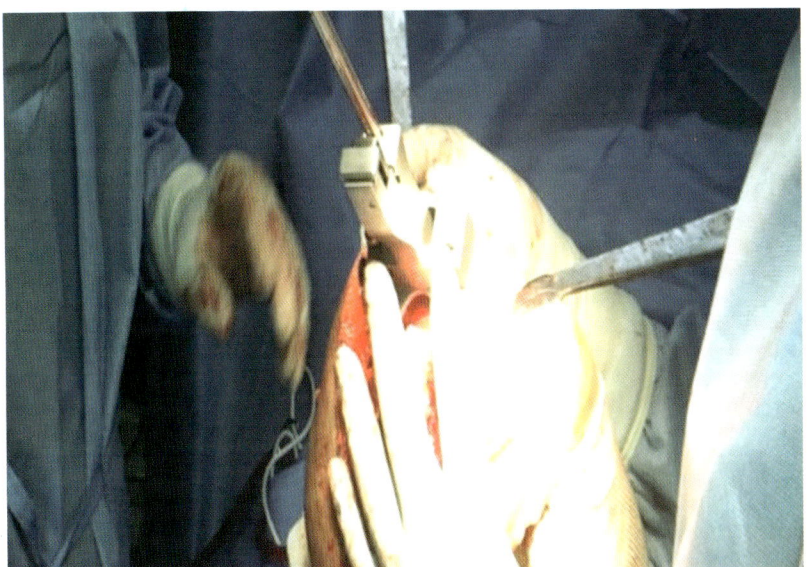

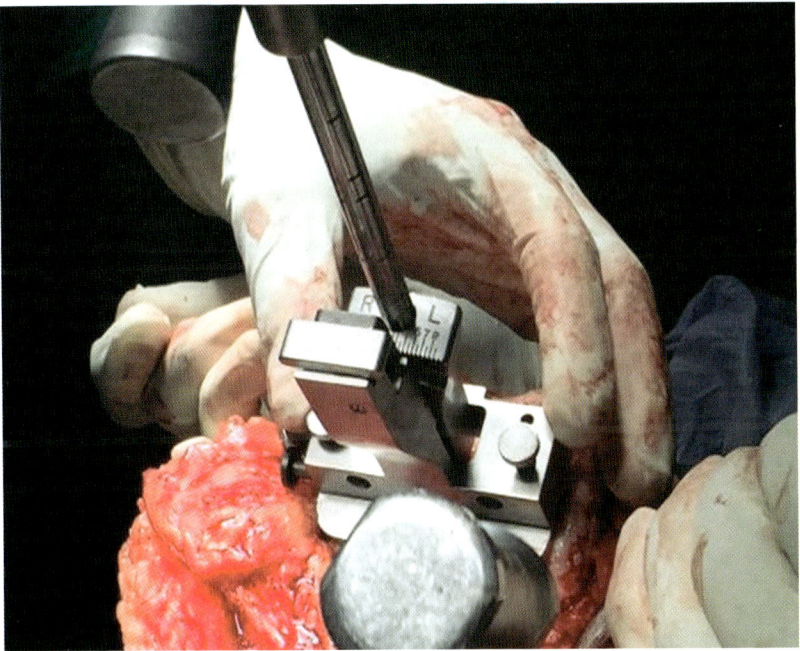

The distal cutting guide is pinned in the correct position.

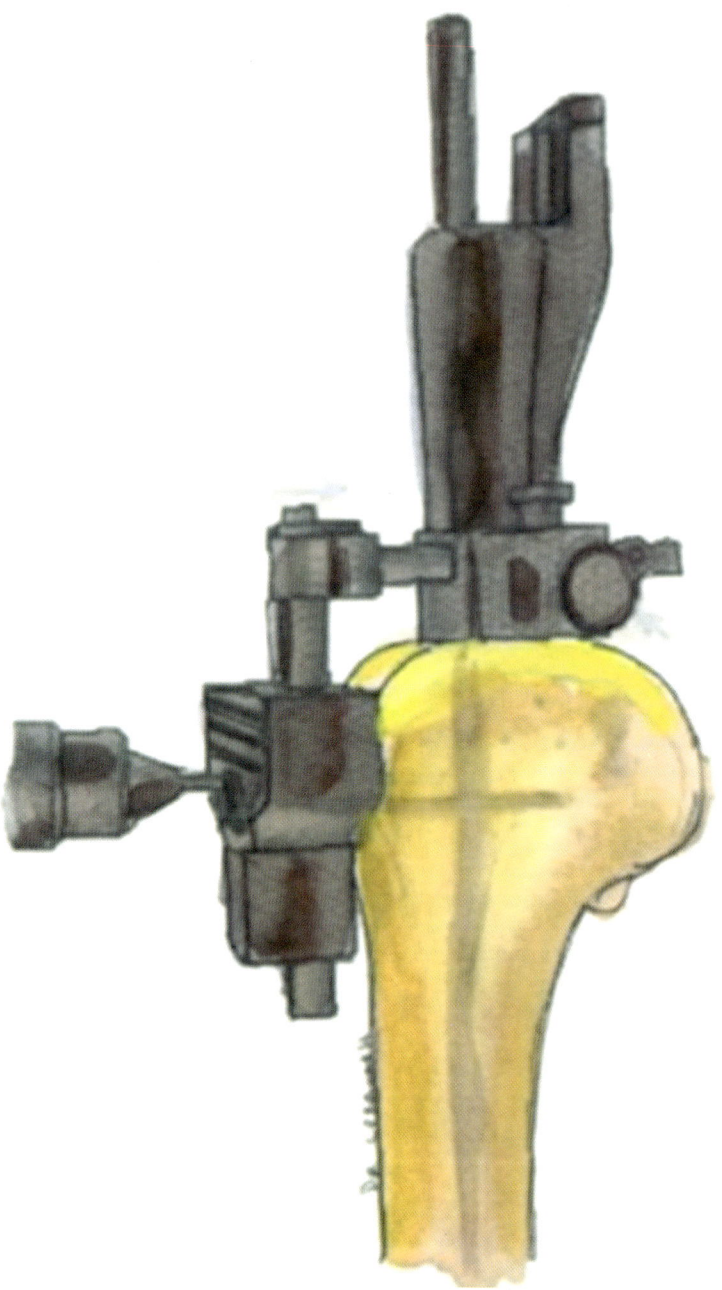

The distal femoral cutting block is now pinned to the anterior aspect of distal femur.

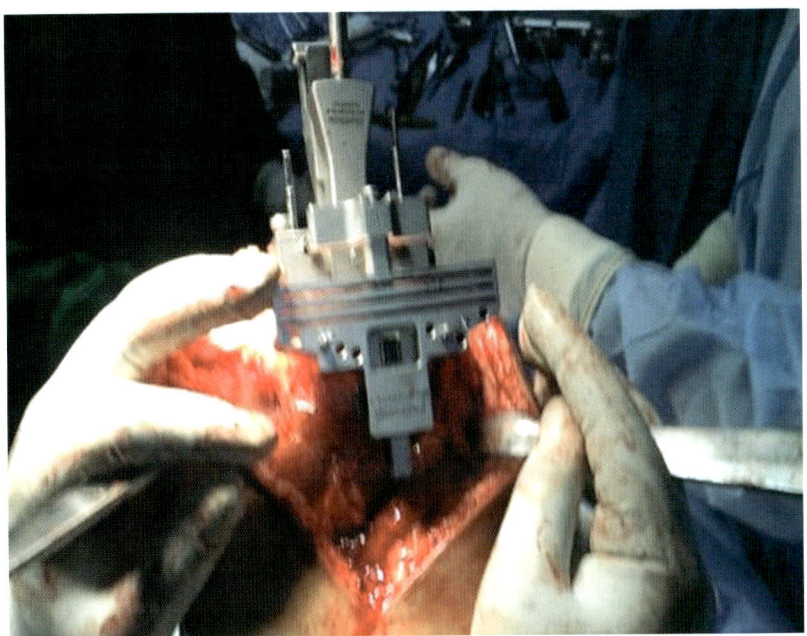

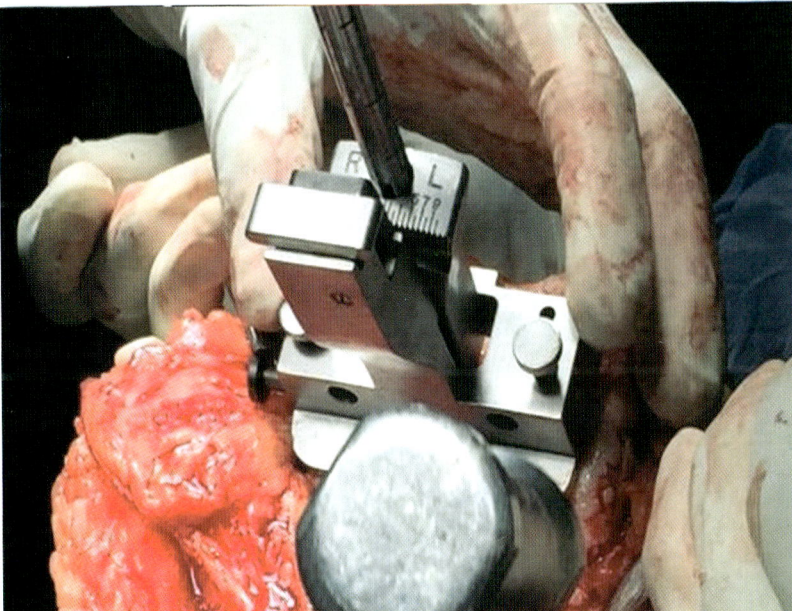

The cutting slot in this block will be in correct relation to the long axis of femur because of the intramedullary guide.

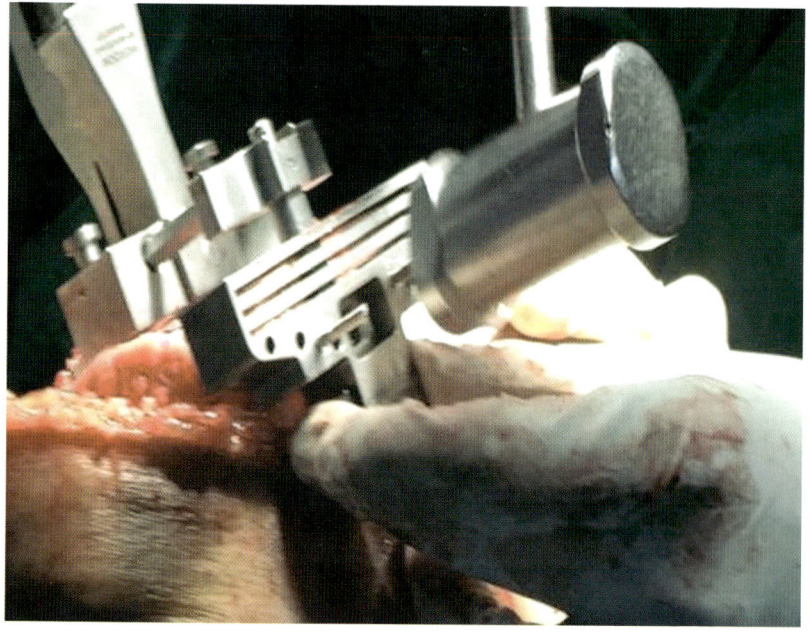

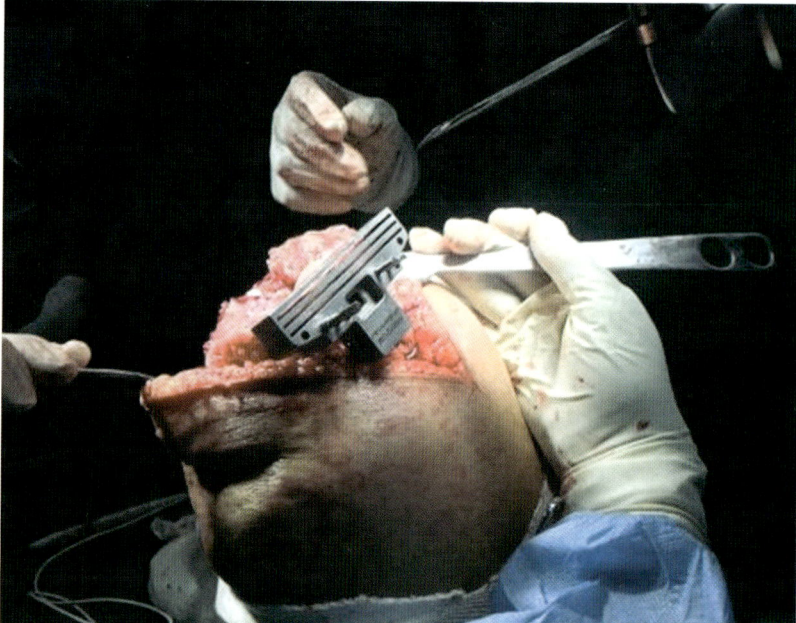

The thickness of bone removed depends on the implant type and the knee condition.

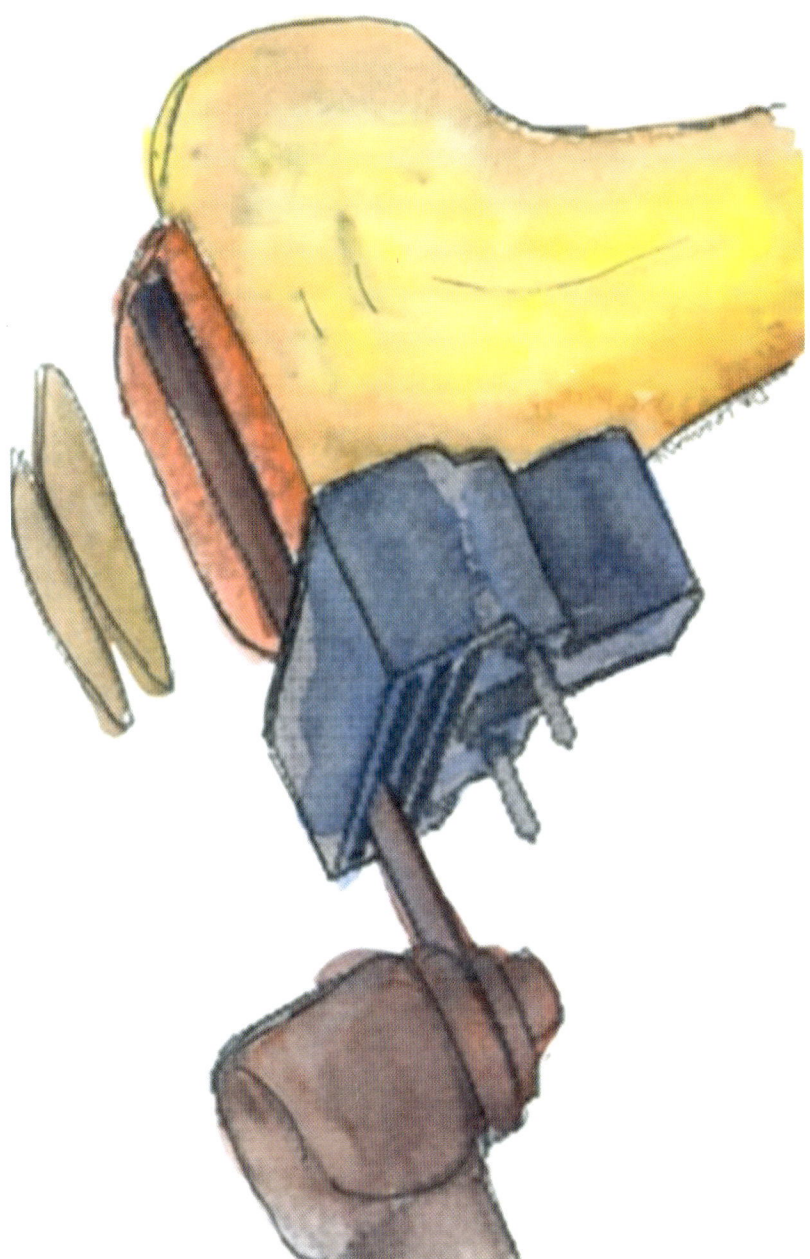

An attempt must be made to cut wafer thin slivers of bone.

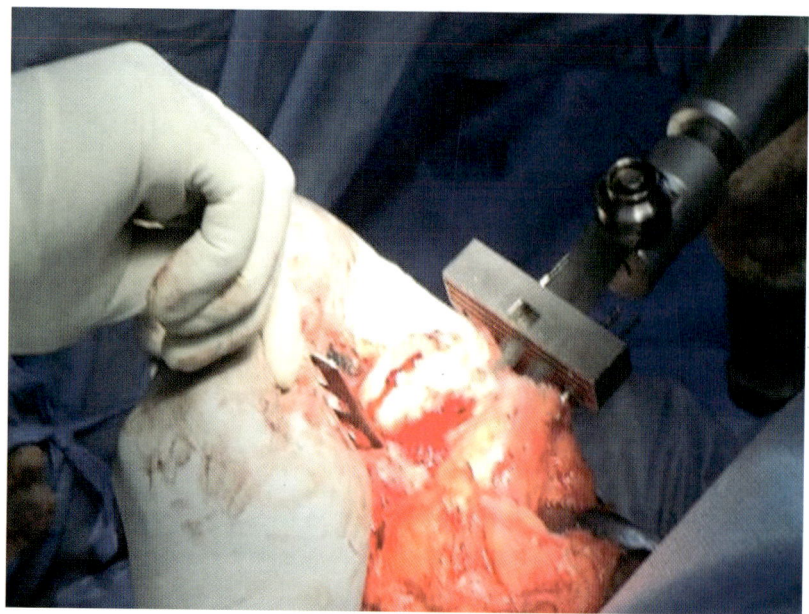

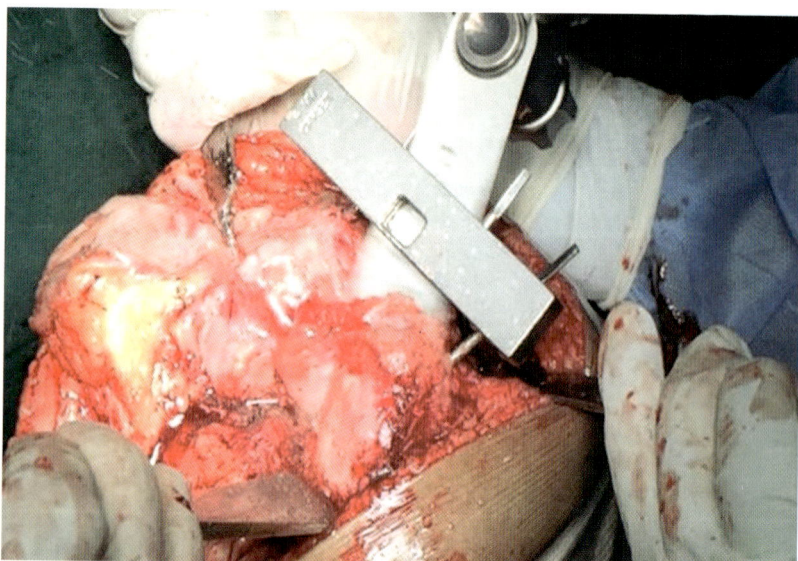

It is better to err on the side of thinner cuts initially, which can be subsequently refined.

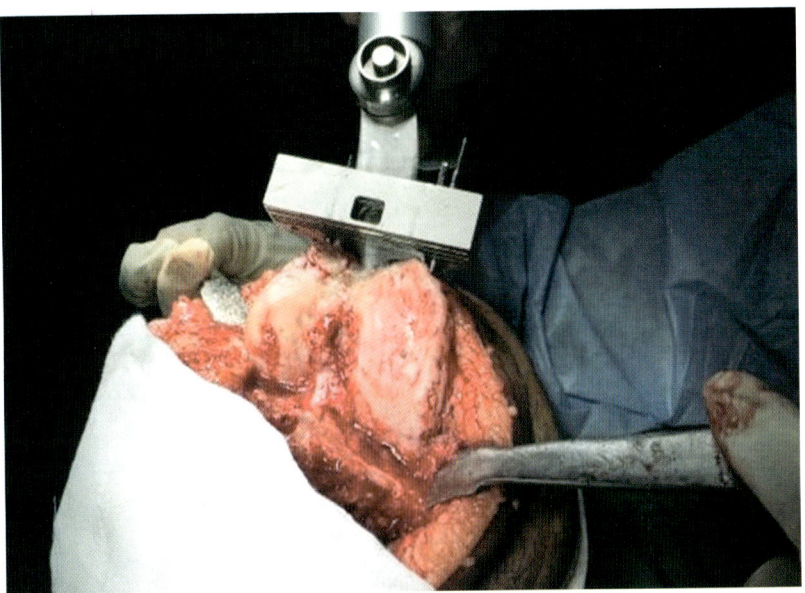

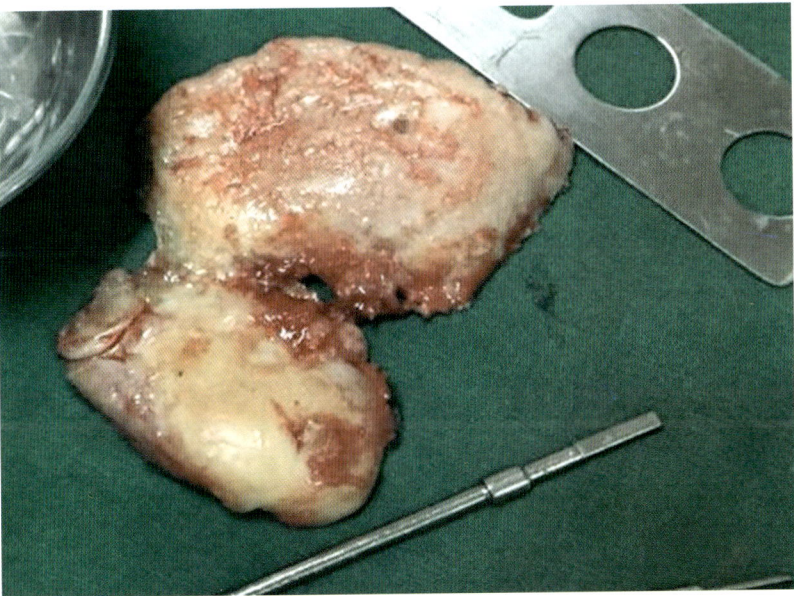

The bone removed should be more or less equal to the thickness of the femoral component.

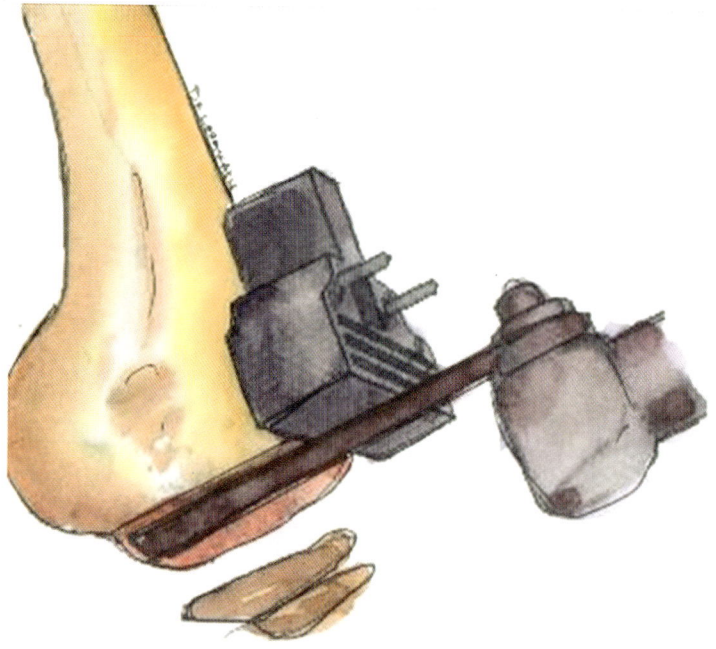

Different instrumentations have different designs of this block.

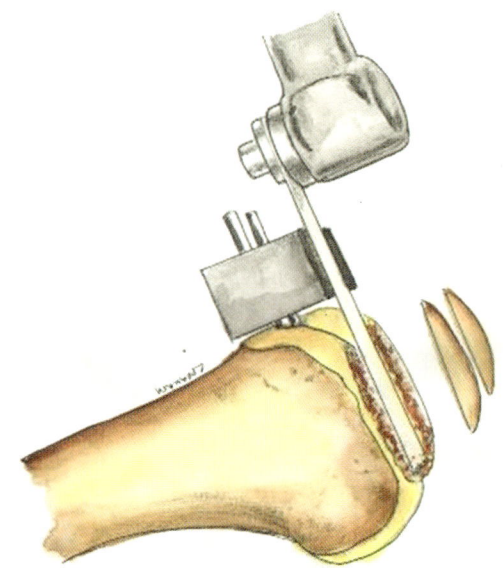

In case a non-slotted block is used, the saw blade should remain flush to the block.

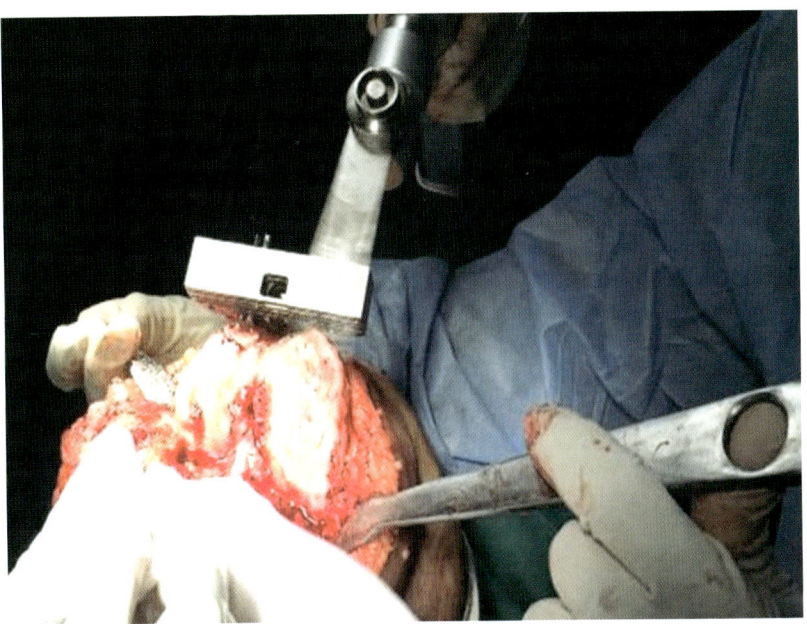

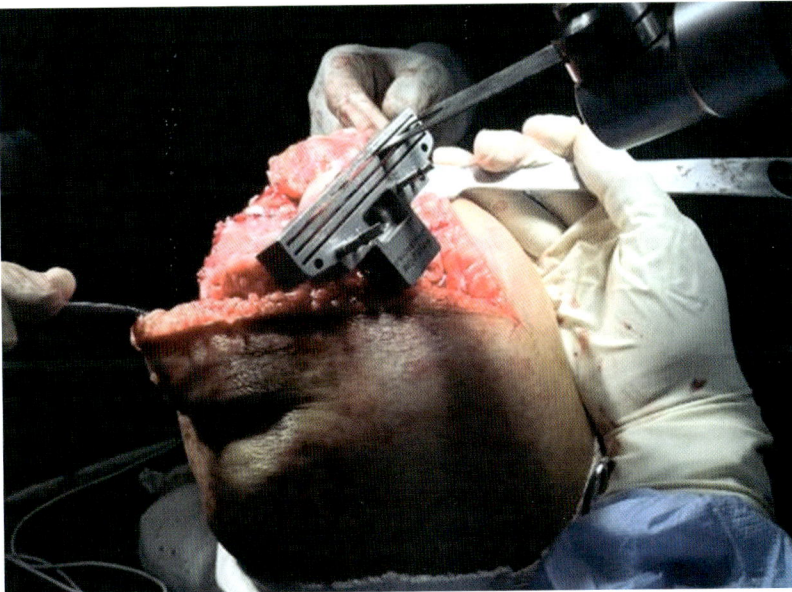

The block pins should be retained in place because after the tibial cut, if an additional femoral cut is needed, the distal cutting block can be reinserted over the same pins.

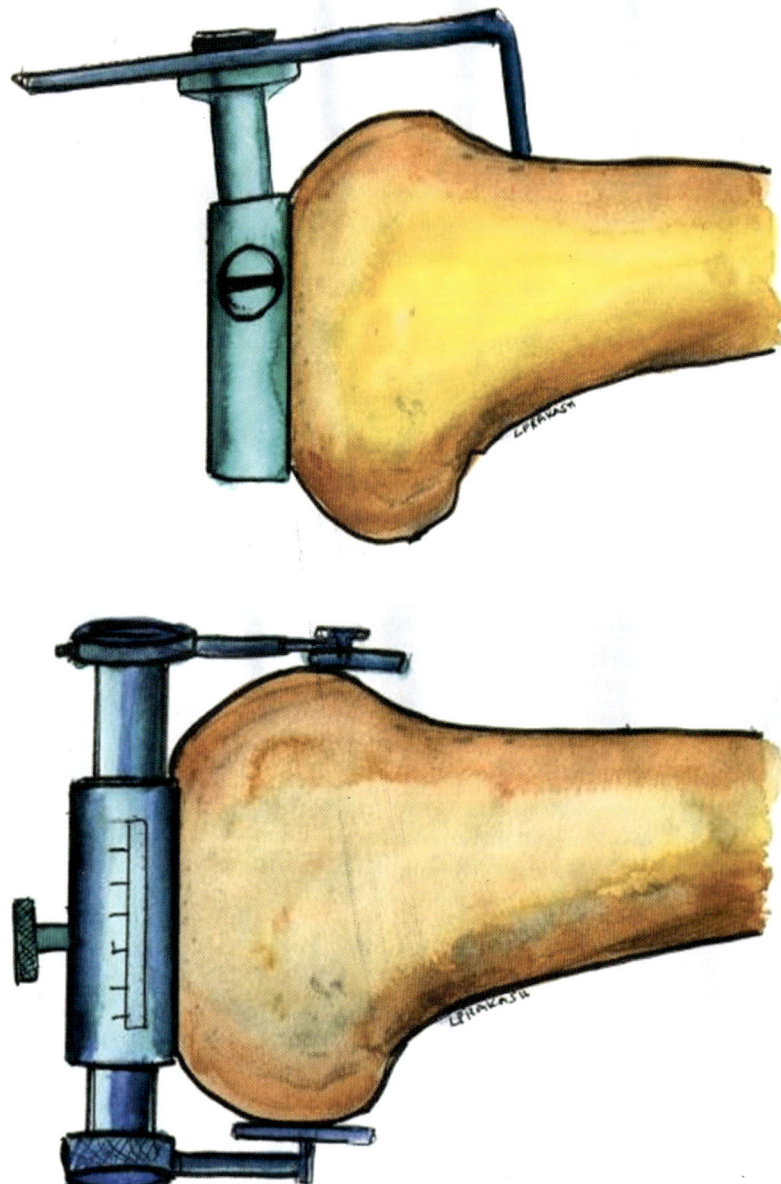

Each prosthesis design has its own femoral measuring gauges.

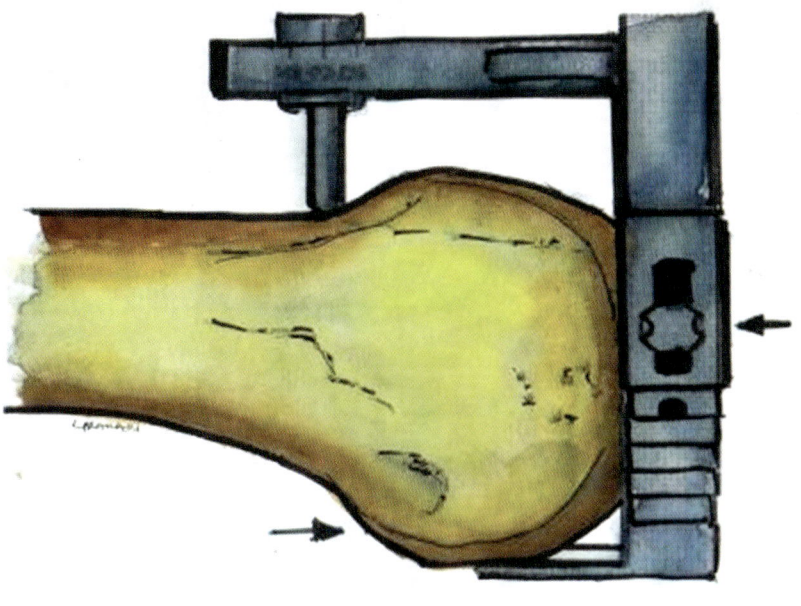

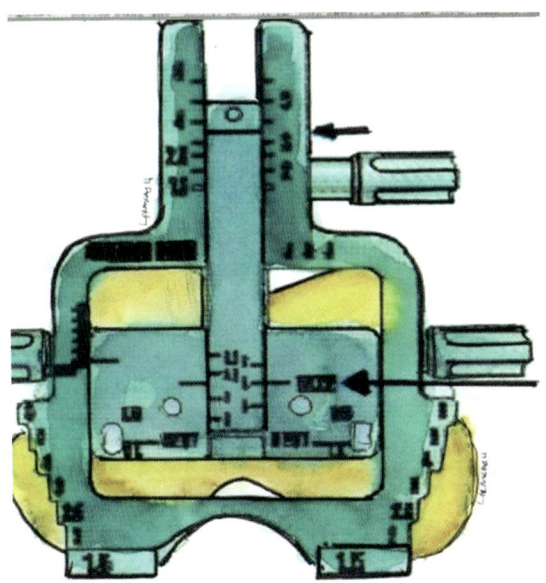

Some devices are simple while others are complicated. This step tells us the correct size of the femoral component that will eventually be used.

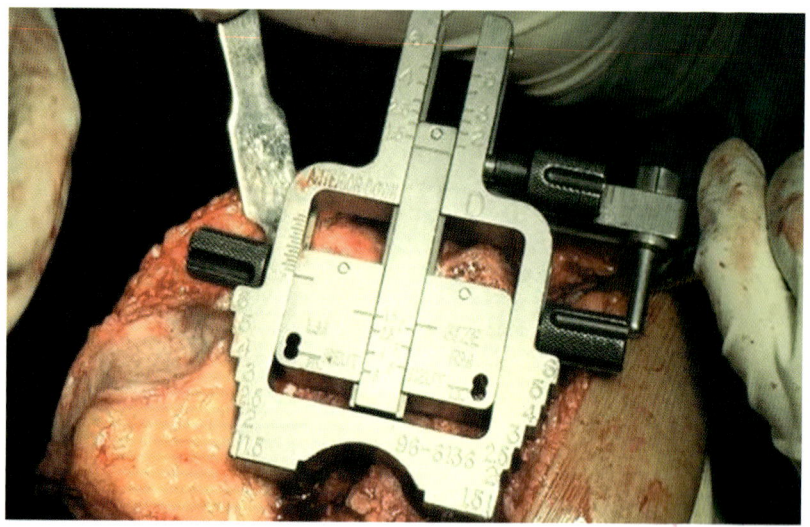

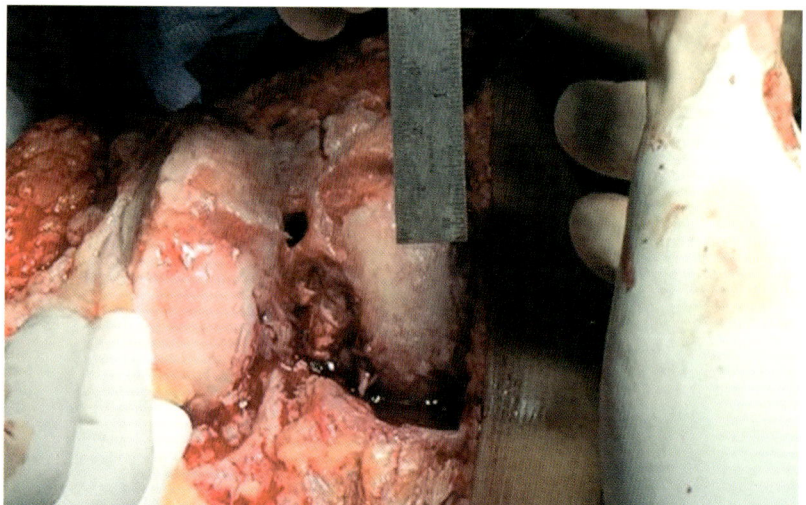

Even a simple stainless steel measuring scale can be used to determine the size of the femoral component.

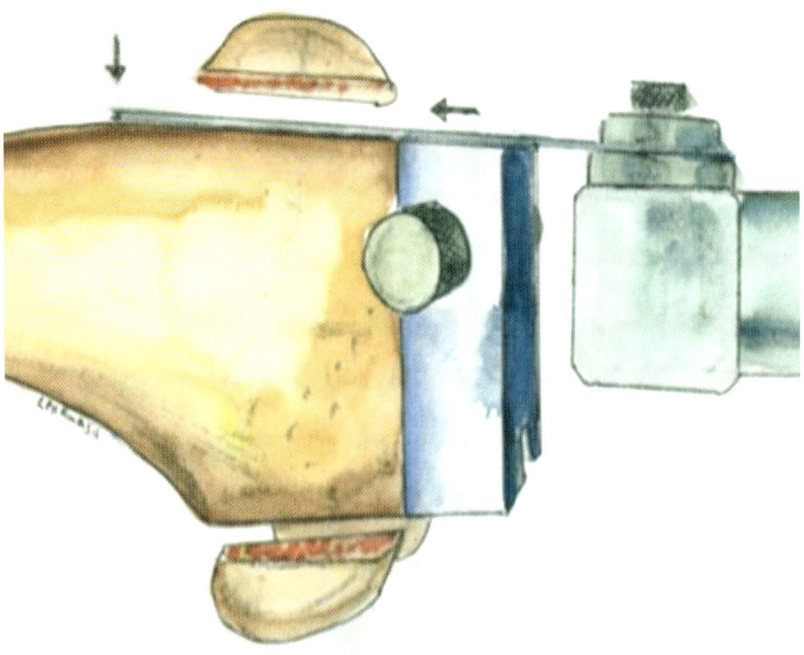

After the correct sized block is pinned, the anterior and posterior distal femoral cuts are made. Thin slivers should be removed, especially anteriorly, to avoid femoral notching.

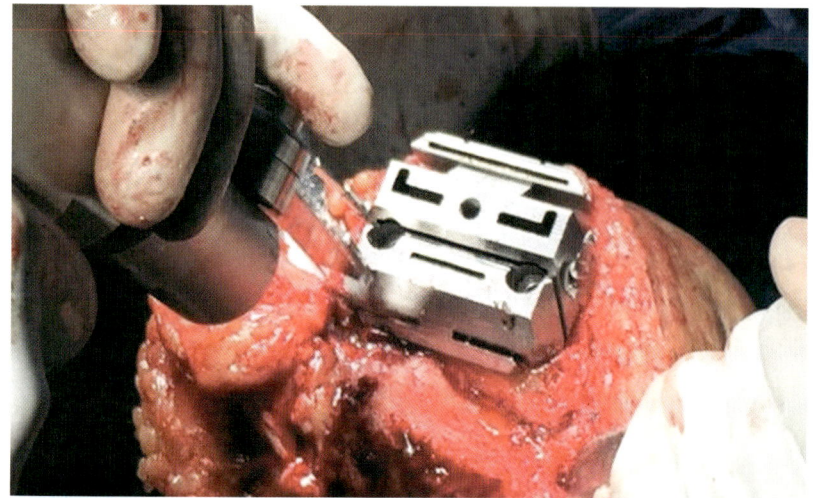

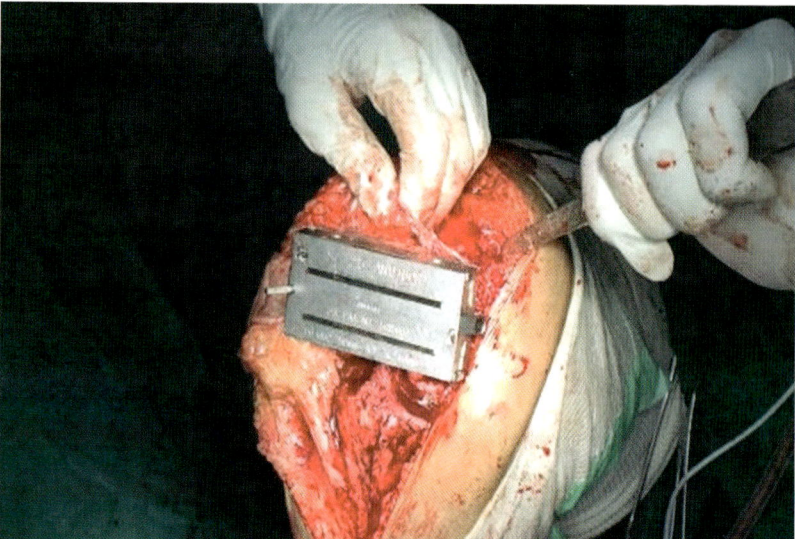

Each company has its own design for the block. If the saw blade is not passing through the slot, one should keep it flush with the block to ensure the correct axis of the cut.

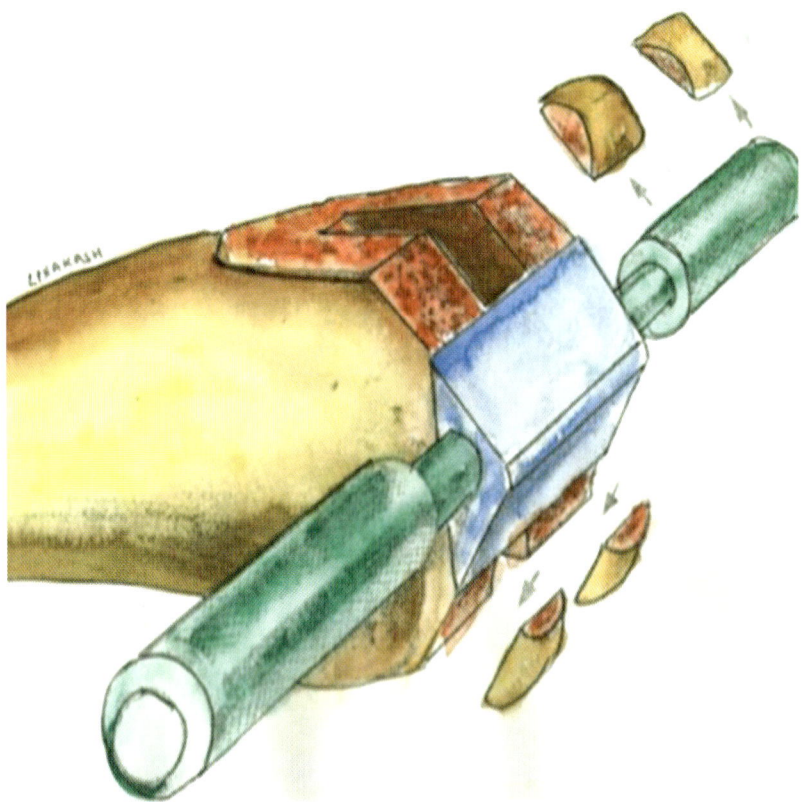

The next step is chamfer cutting. This block can either be a prismatic wedge or a solid block with beveled slots.

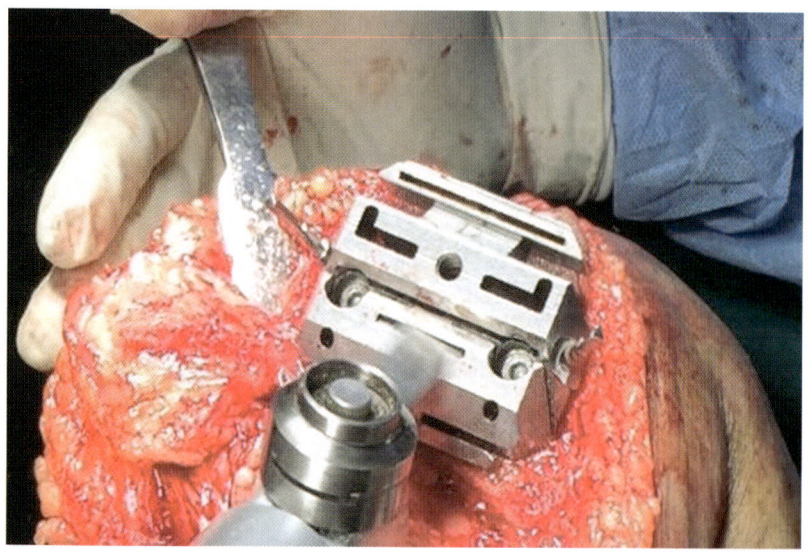

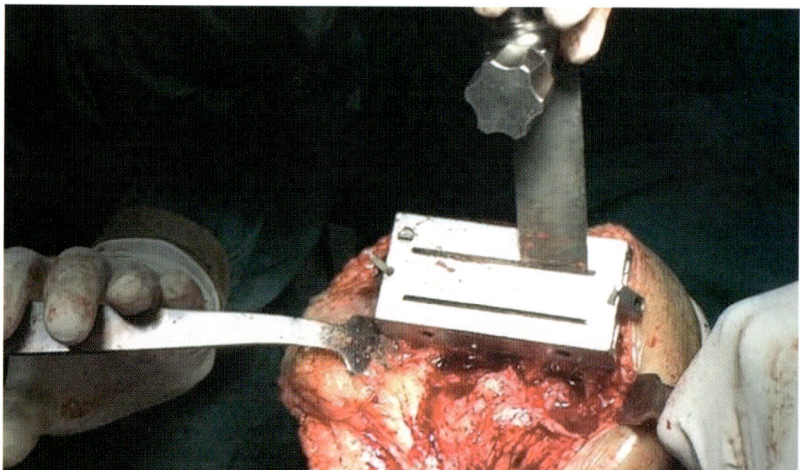

These cuts are in the precise angle to match the interior of the femoral component and will ensure a perfect fit, especially in a cementless implant.

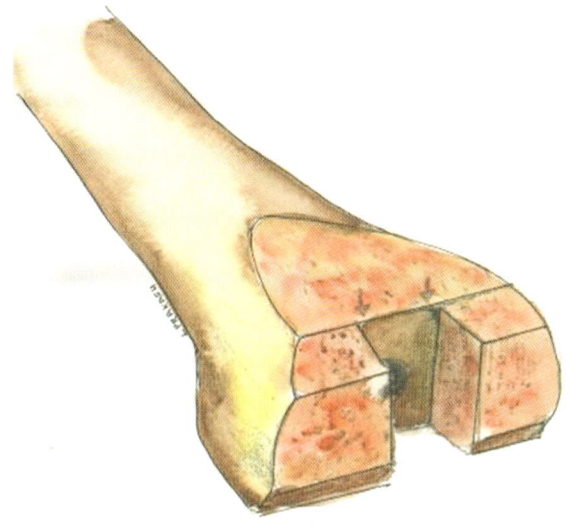

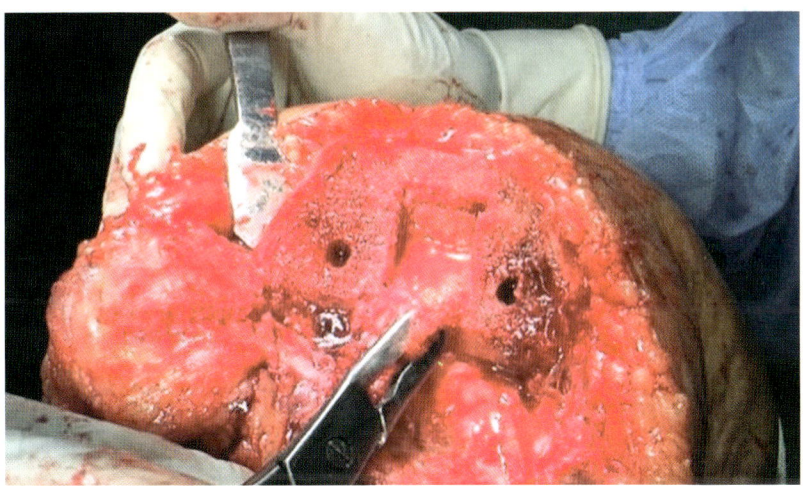

After the distal bone cuts, the femoral surface should match the interior of the prosthesis perfectly.

THE PROXIMAL TIBIAL CUT AND PREPARATION

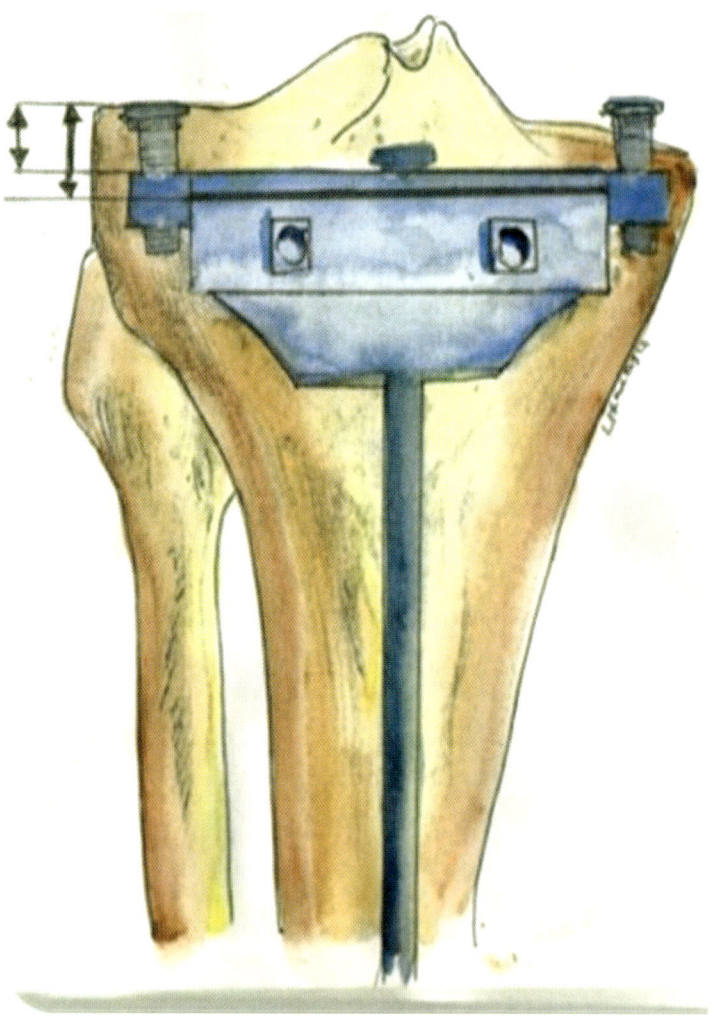

Tibial referencing is usually done by an extramedullary guide, which is a straight rod extending from tibial tuberosity to the centre of the ankle.

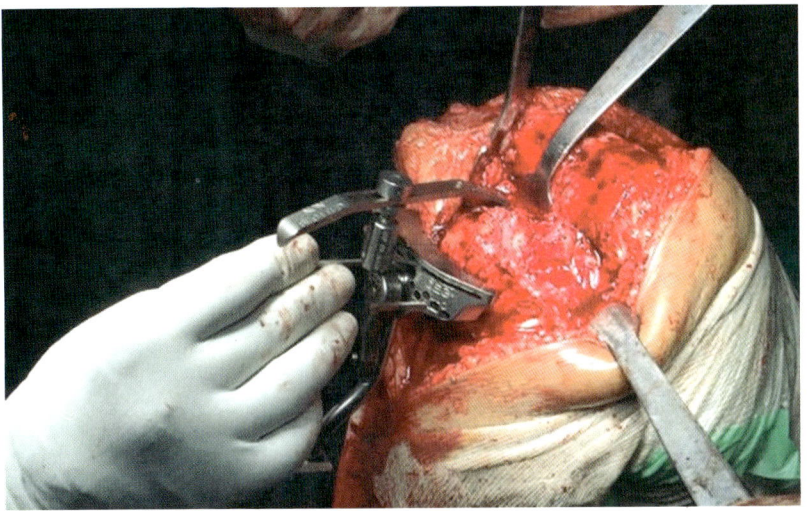

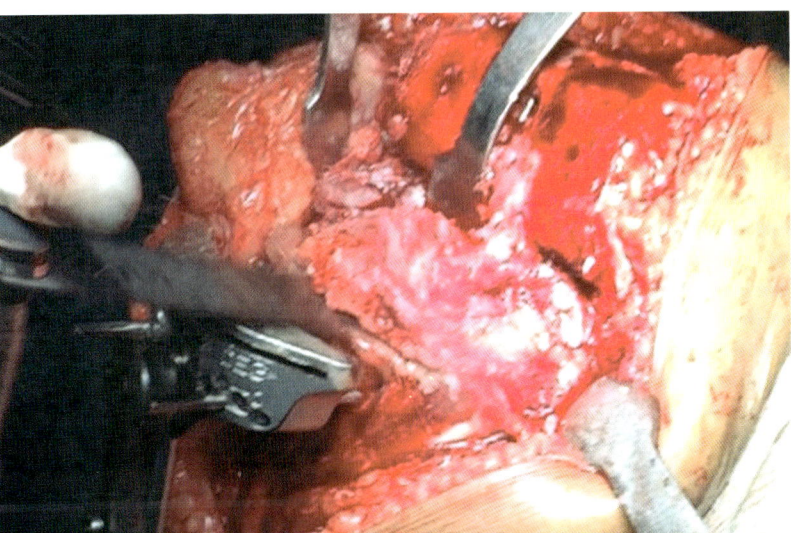

The slot in the jig ensures that the upper tibia is in 3° to 5° of posterior slope.

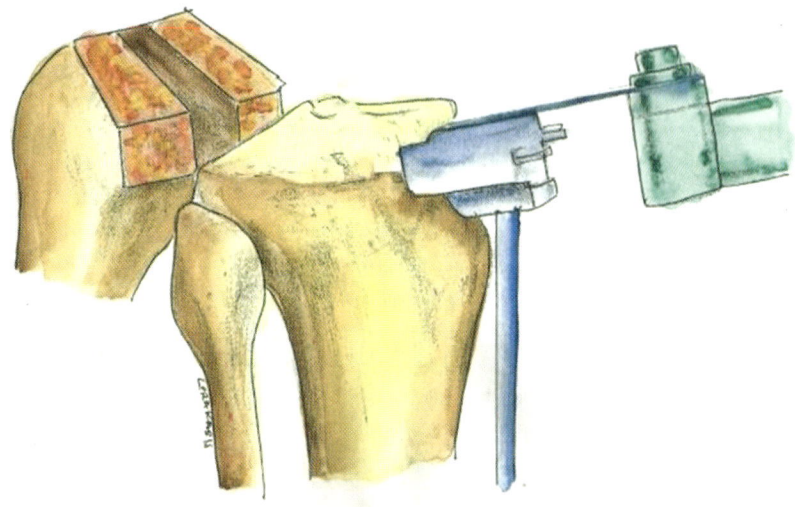

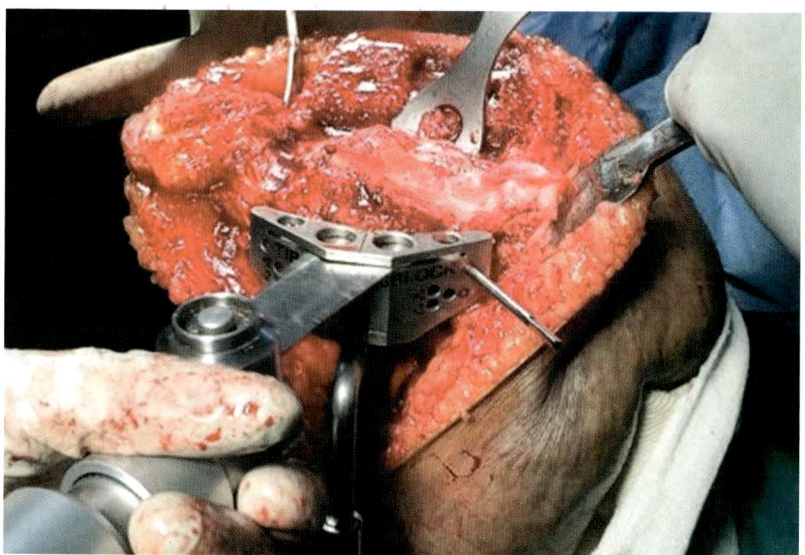

One should attempt to take the thinnest possible wafer thin cuts. It is always safer to err on the side of thinner cuts, which can later be improved upon if needed.

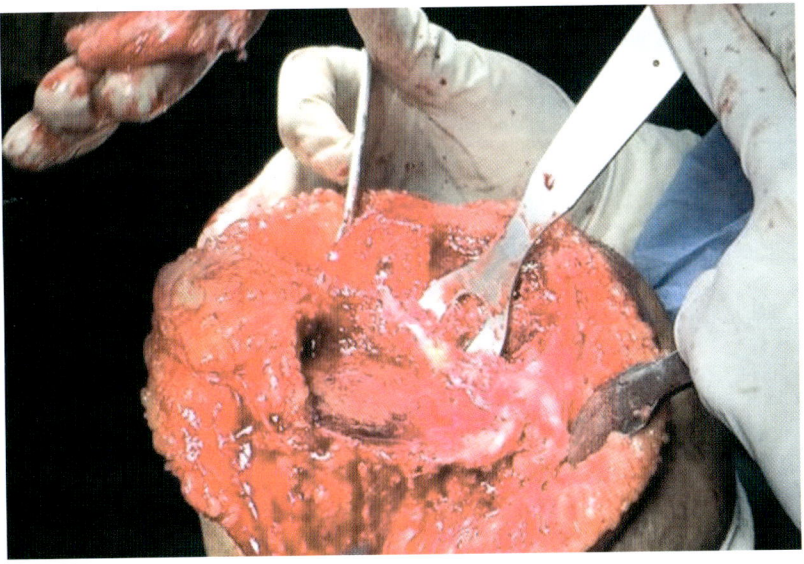

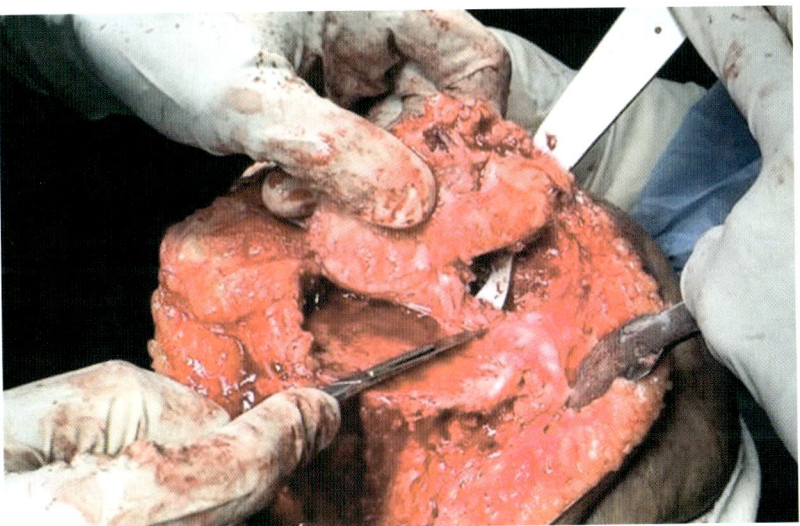

The combined thickness of the femoral and tibial cuts should match the thickness of the two components combined.

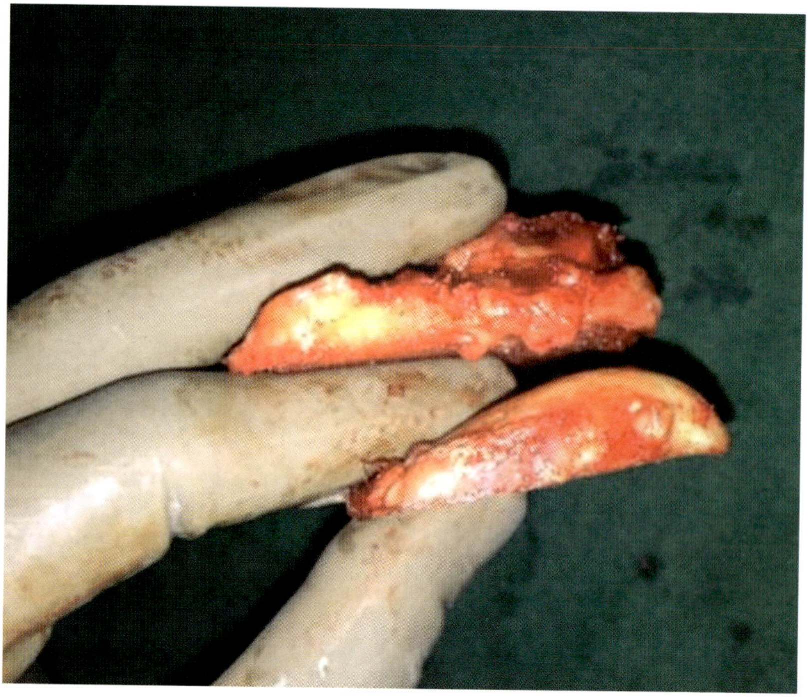

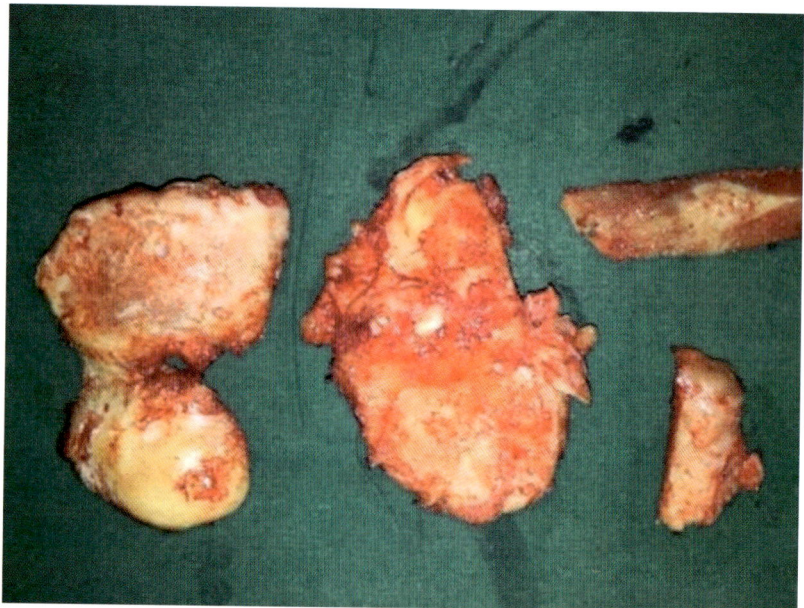

The average bone cuts in a typical knee replacement.

BALANCING THE FLEXION AND EXTENSION GAPS

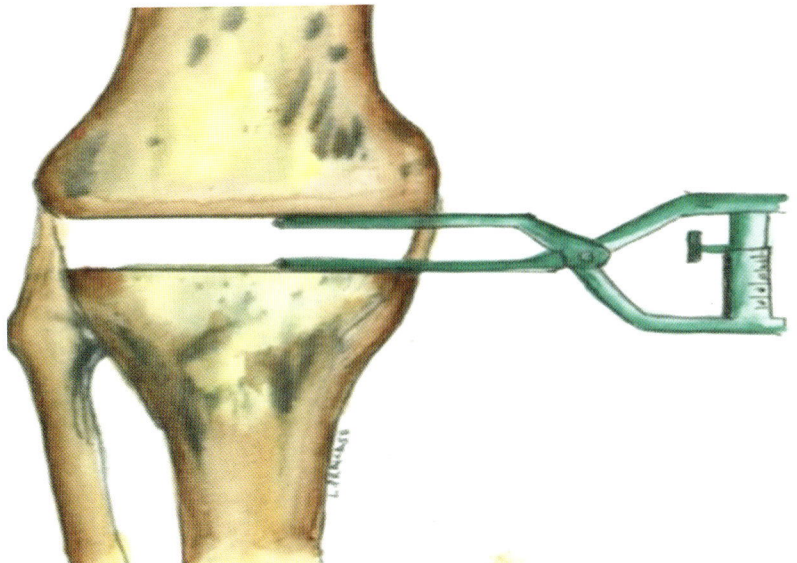

The earlier soft tissue releases will ensure that the gaps in flexion and extension are equal. This is the most important step in a knee replacement.

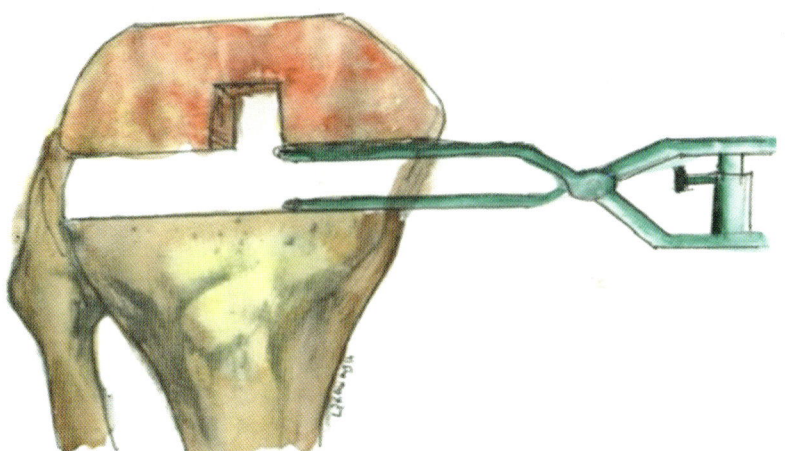

Most gap balancers also measure the gap to indicate the correct size of HDPE insert thickness.

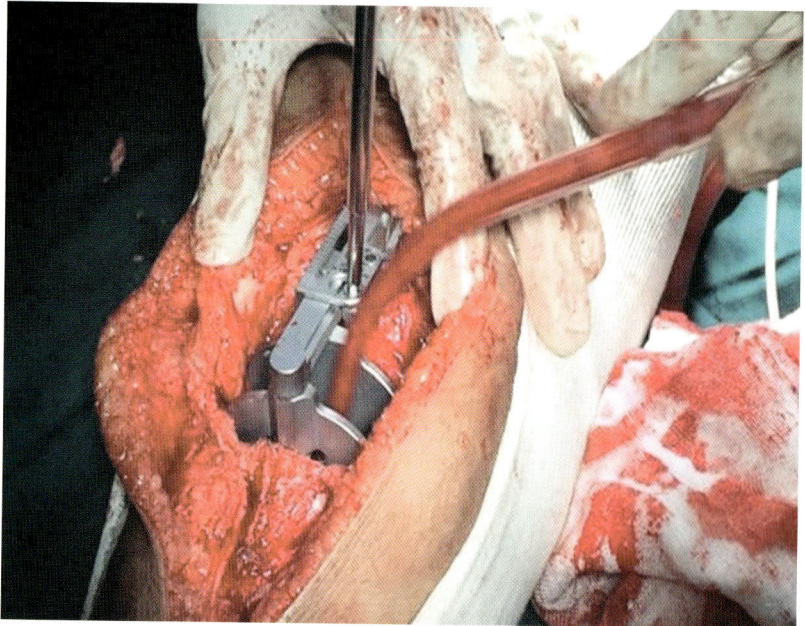

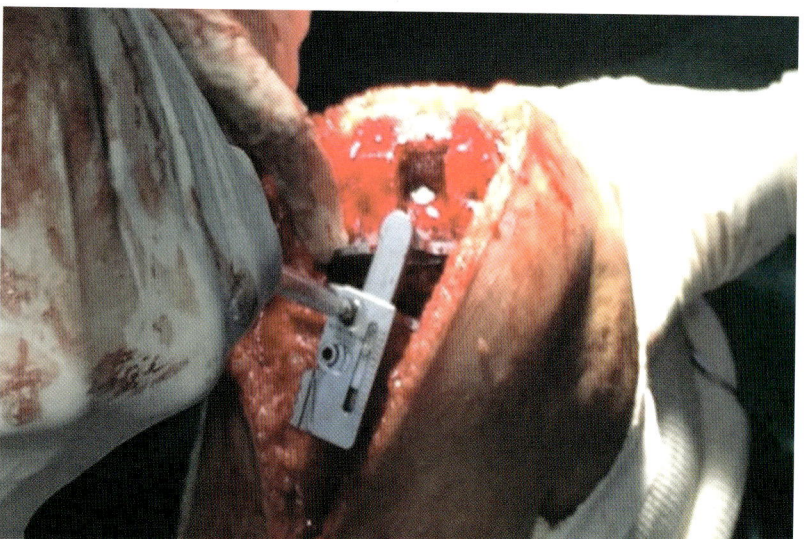

Different instrumentation deigns come with different gap balancers.

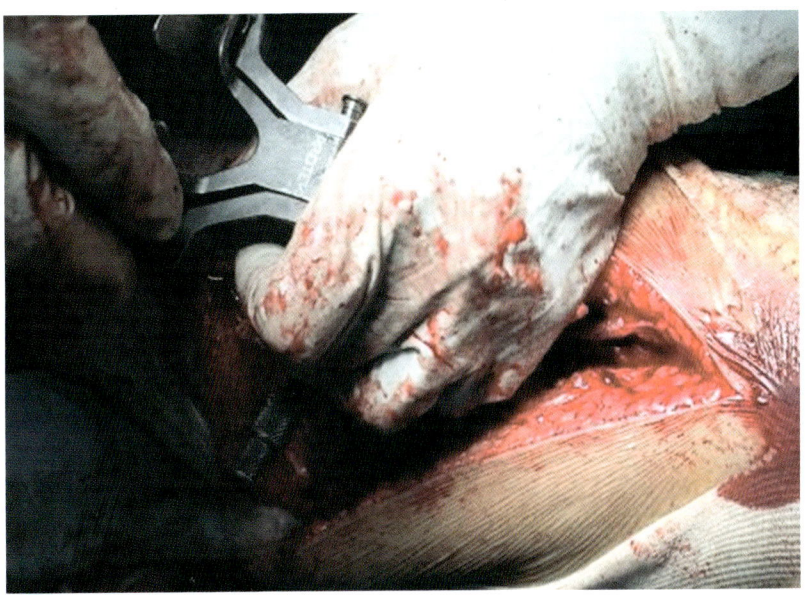

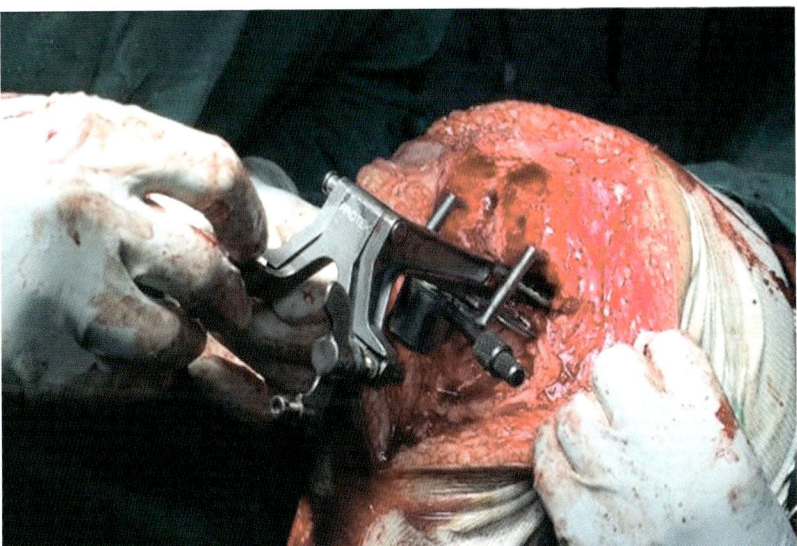

The basic design invented by MAR Freeman is an easy and precise instrument for this purpose.

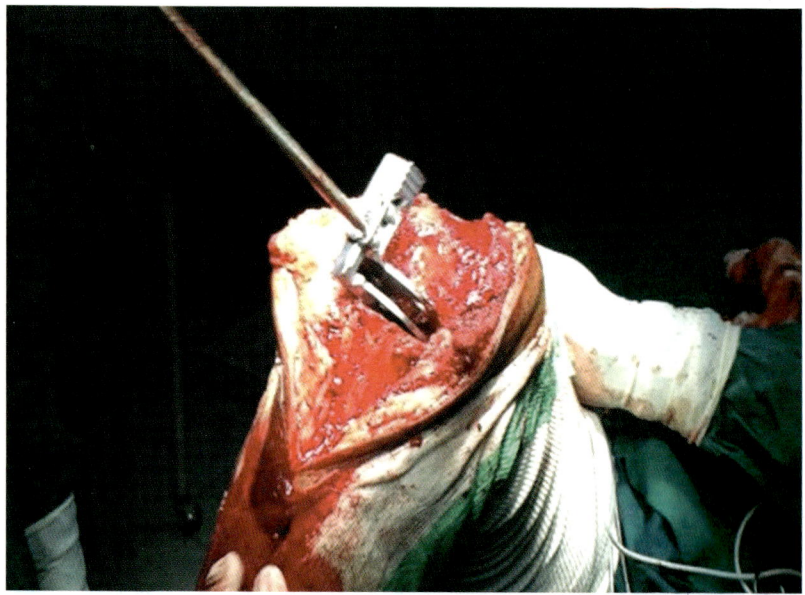

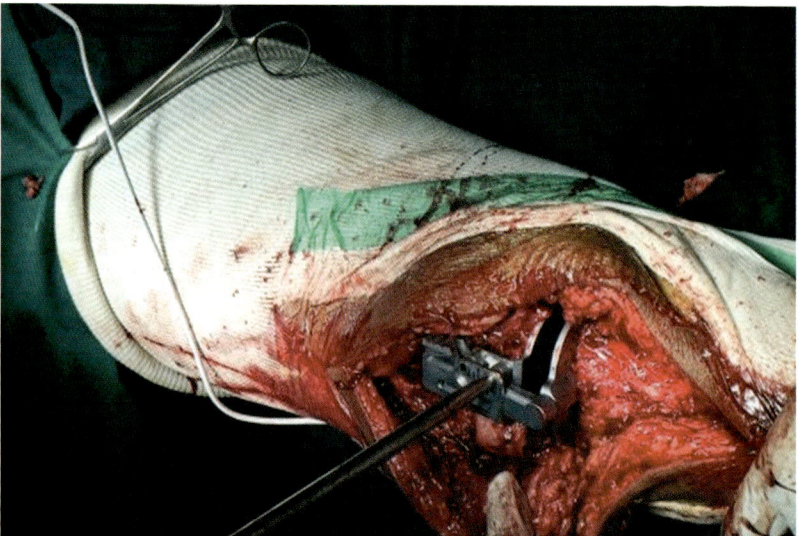

My design of the gap balancer. I consider this the most important instrument for the long term success of a TKR.

TRIAL COMPONENTS, TRIAL REDUCTION, AND PRE CEMENTATION PROCEDURES

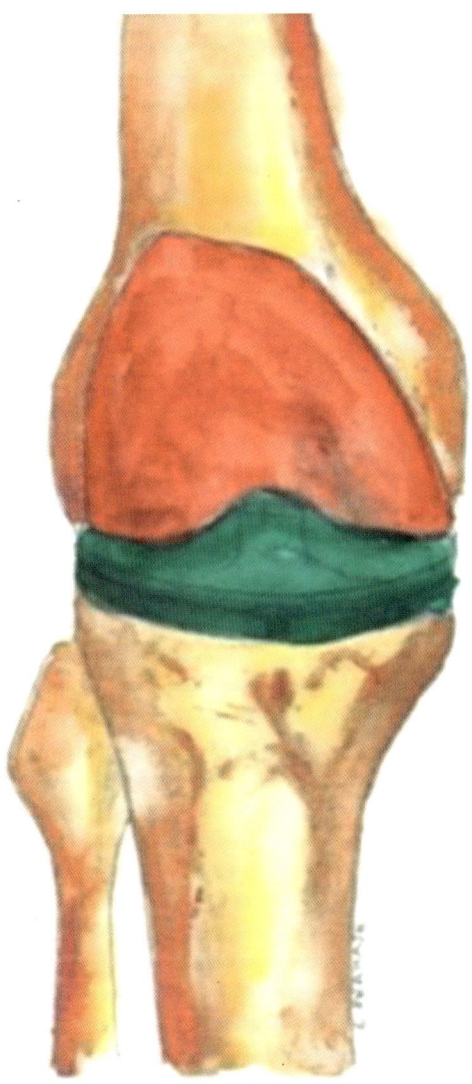

The next step is insertion of the trial implants and a trial reduction.

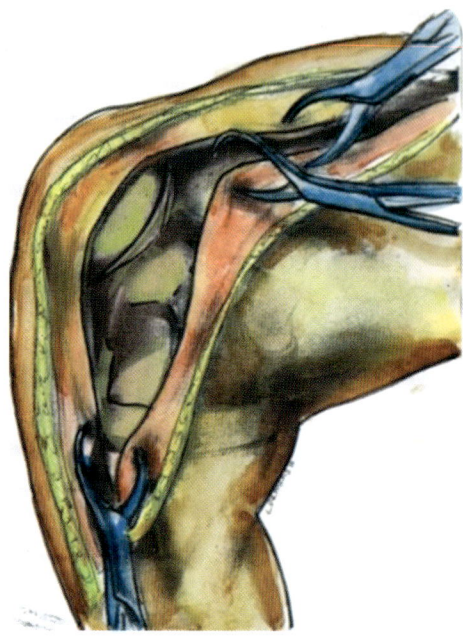

Towel clips to deep medial structures ensure correctness of patellar tracking.

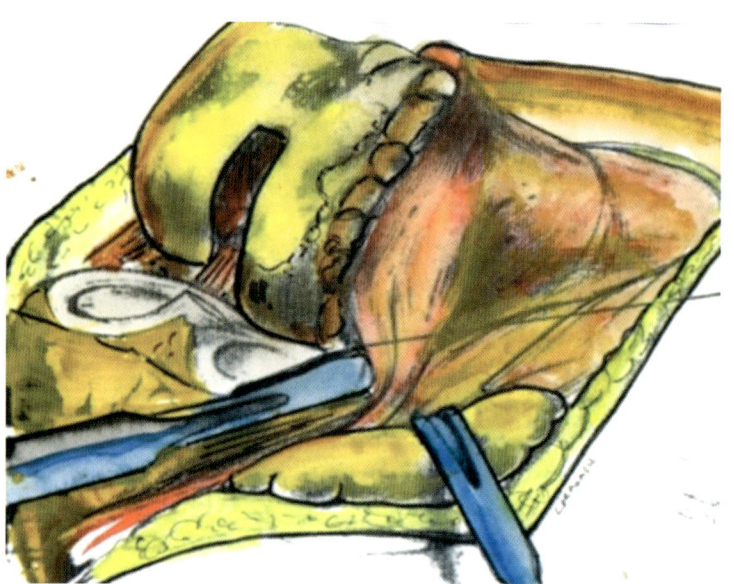

The clips will indicate the state of tension in the quadriceps mechanism.

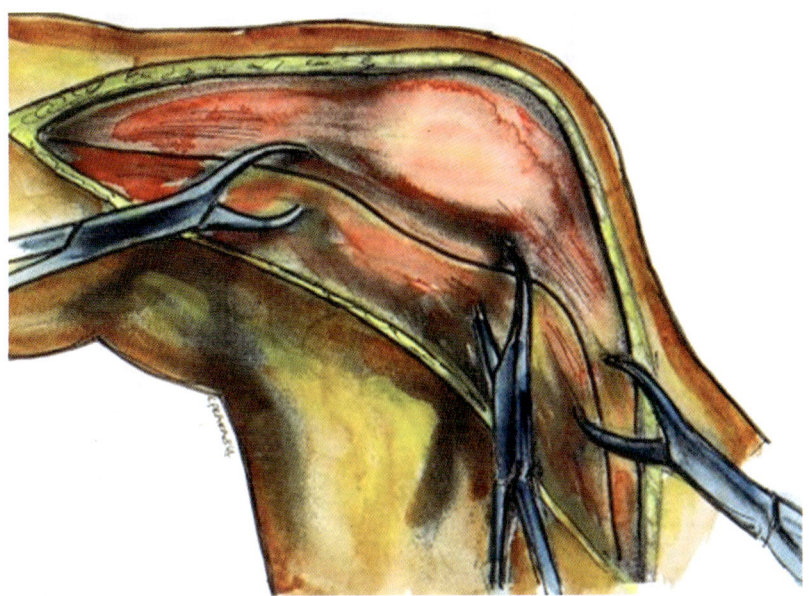

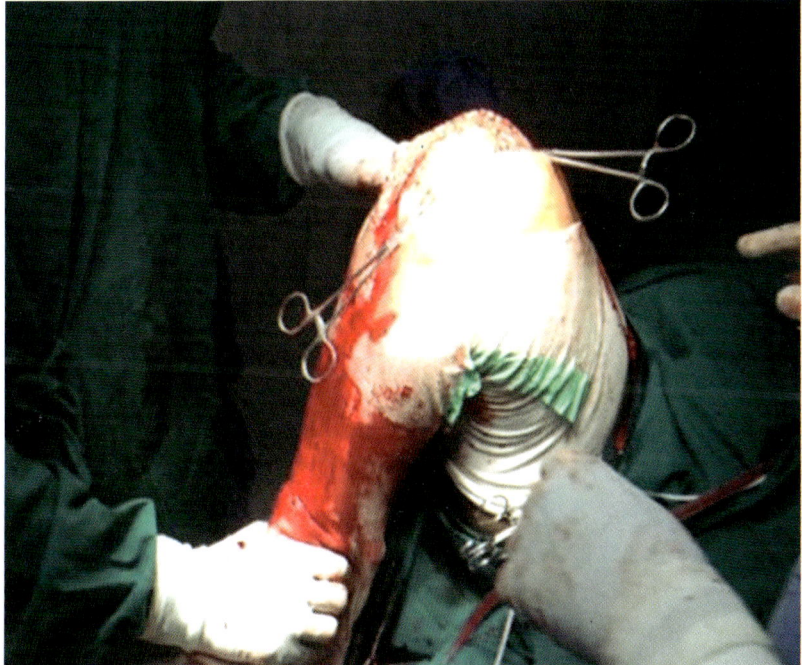

Extremes of flexion should not open the clips. If they do, additional soft tissue releases may be required.

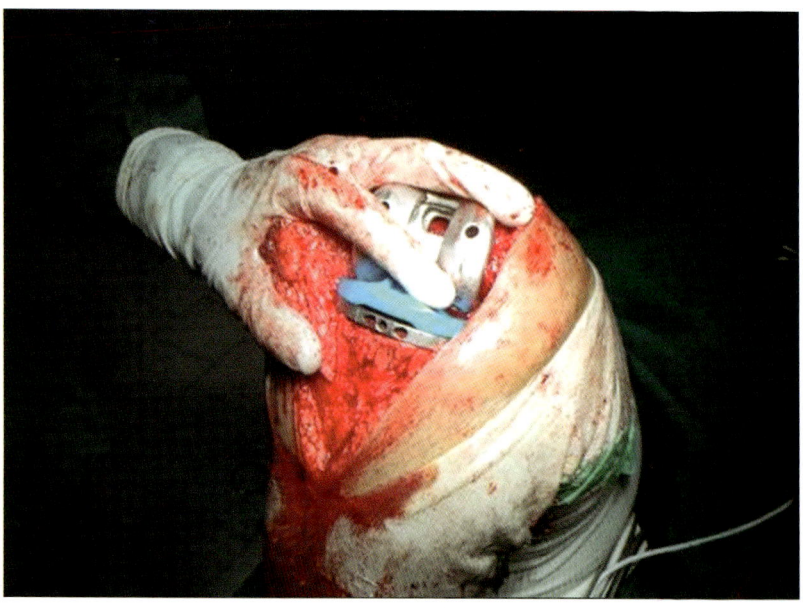

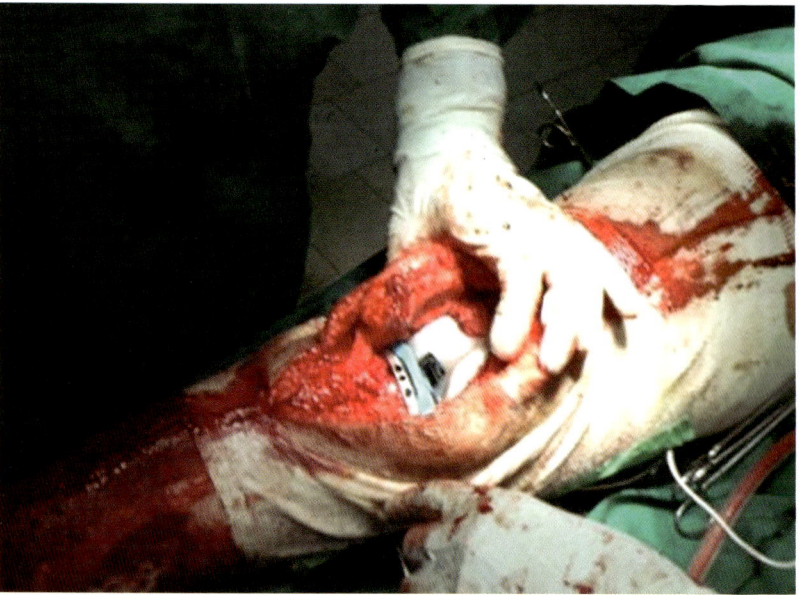

Insertion of trial components.

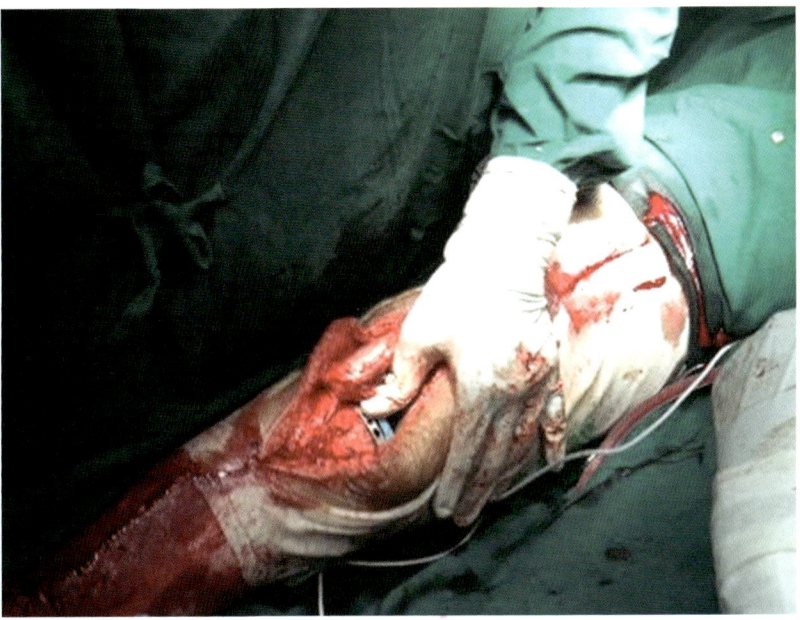

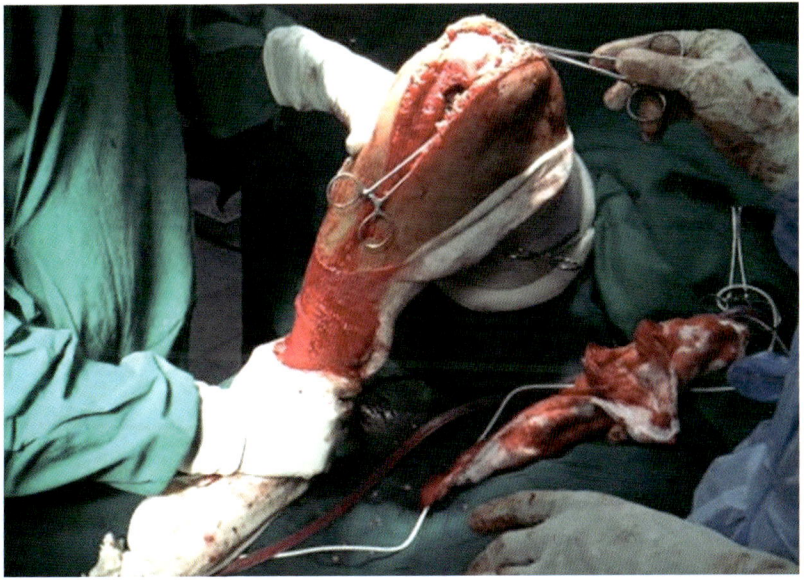

Towel clips and checking of stability in flexion and extension.

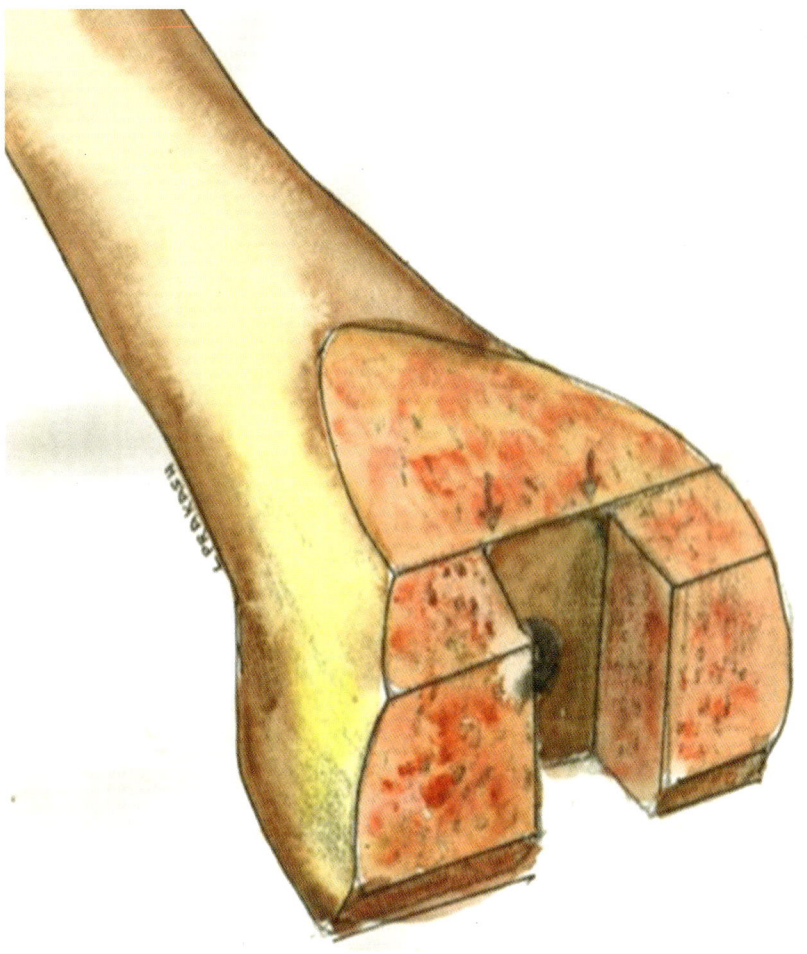

If a posterior stabilized implant is used, this is the time to make the notch cuts.

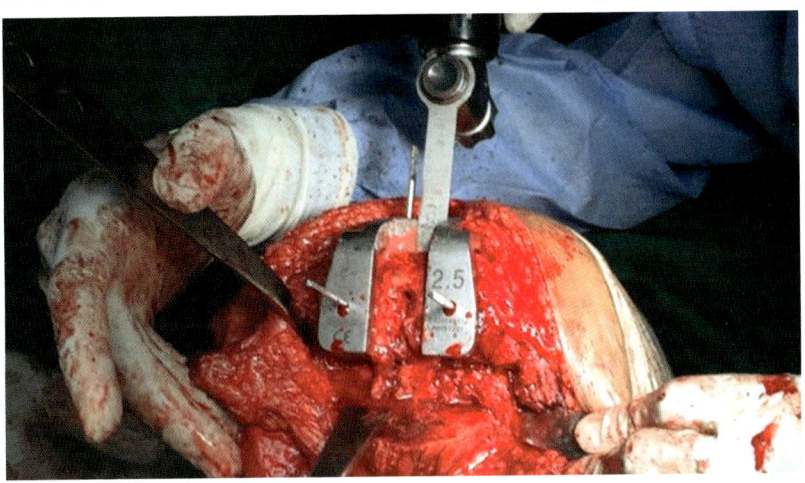

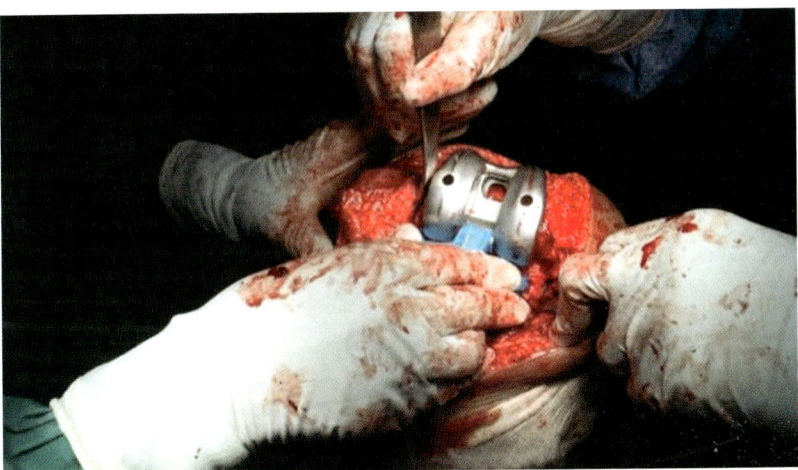

After the notch cut, a posterior stabilized implant is put through the same range of motions.

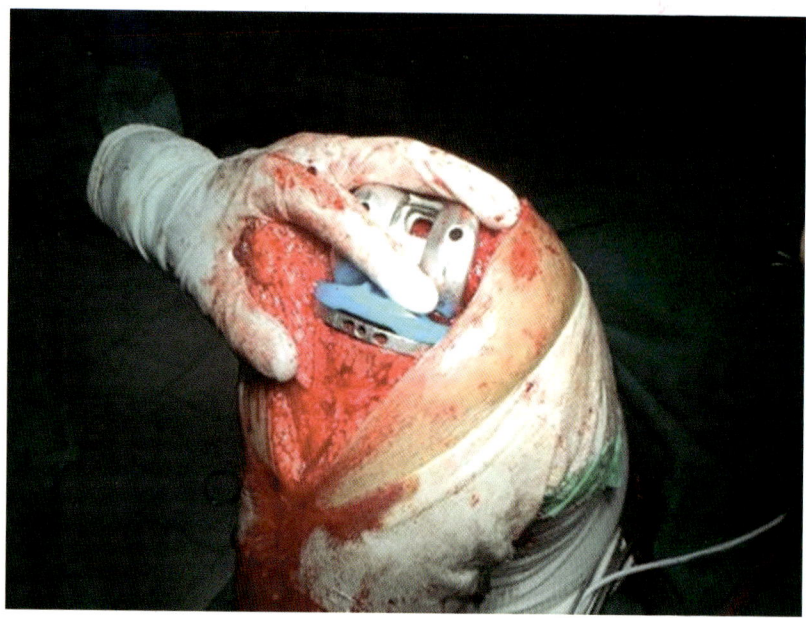

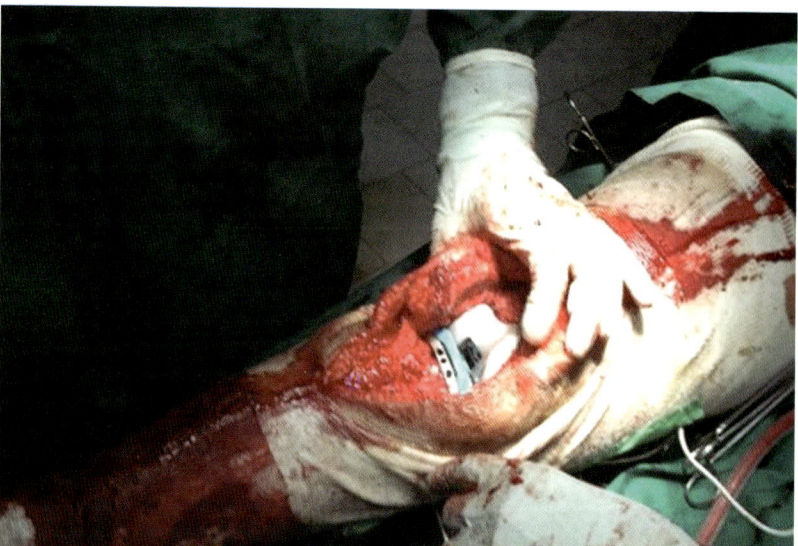

There should be no deformities in full extension and the knee should flex up to 110°.

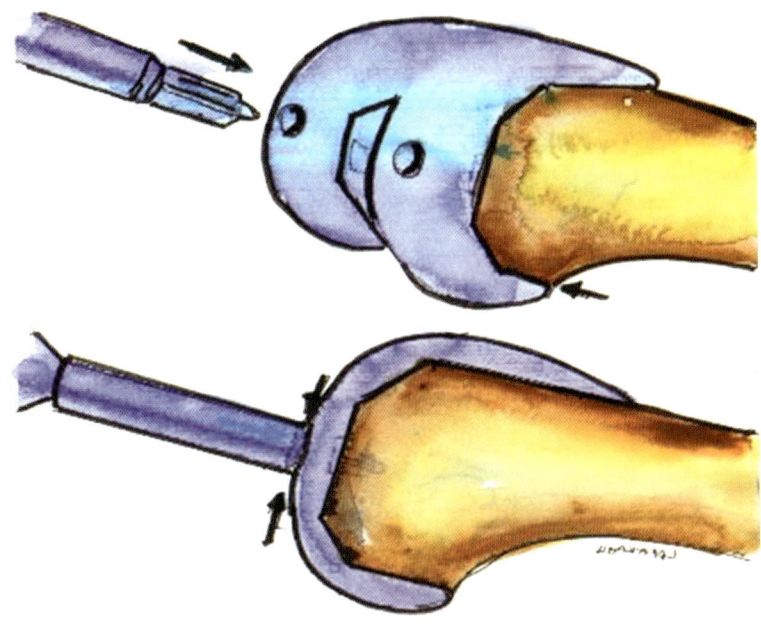

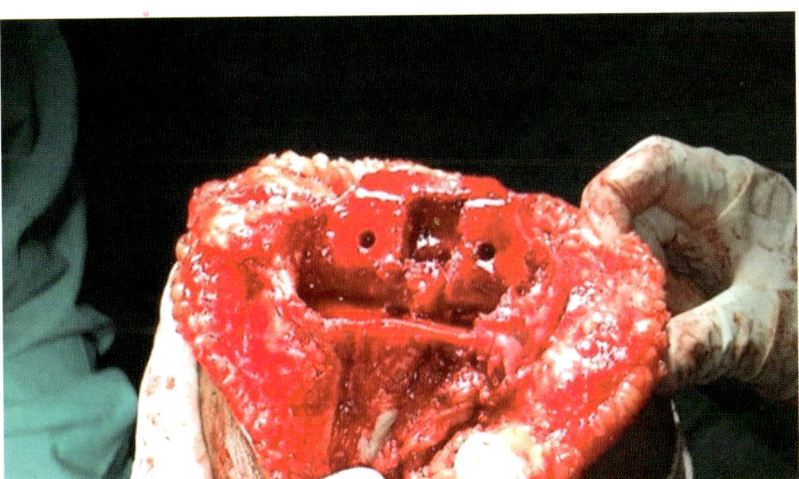

If the design of femoral components has pegs, now is the time to make peg holes.

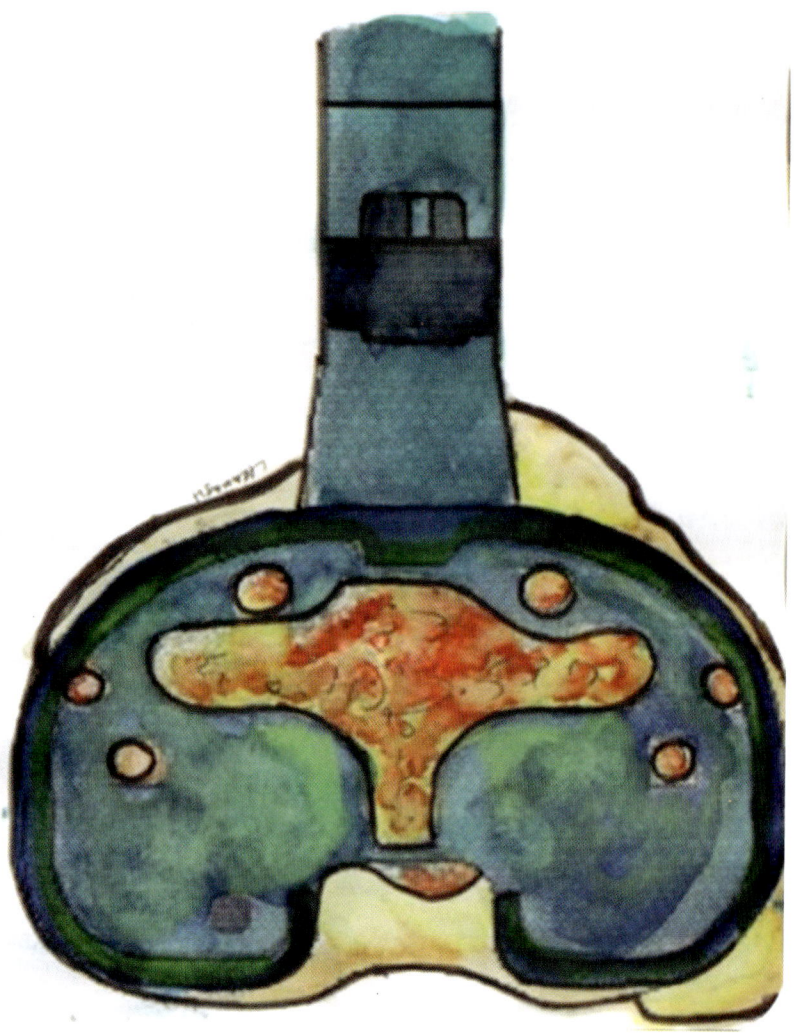

The tibial size is next measured.

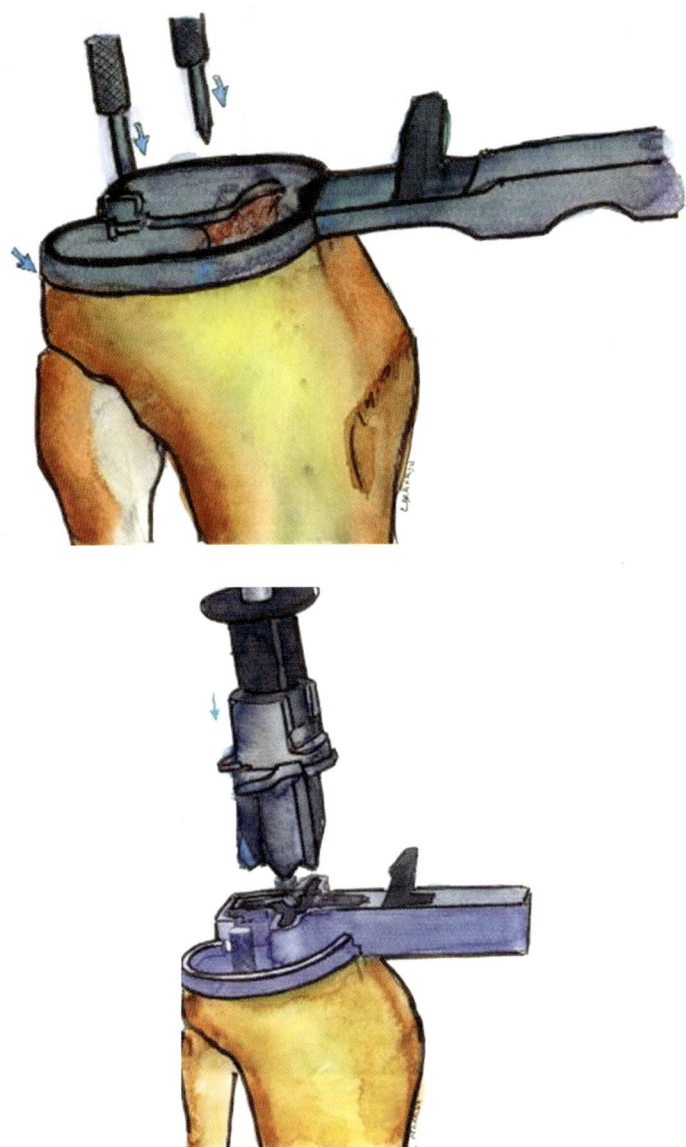

There should be no medial or lateral overhang. The seating should be uniform over the upper tibial surface.

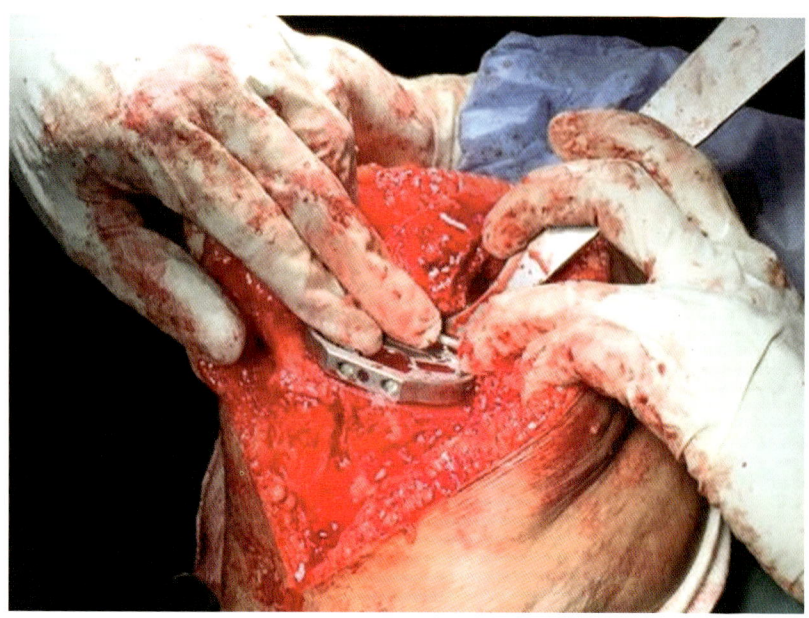

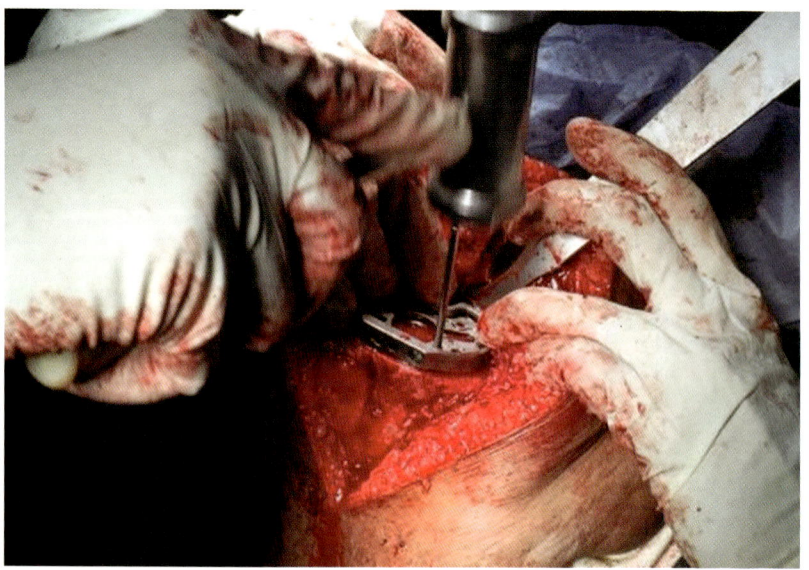

Pinning of the correct sized tibial guide.

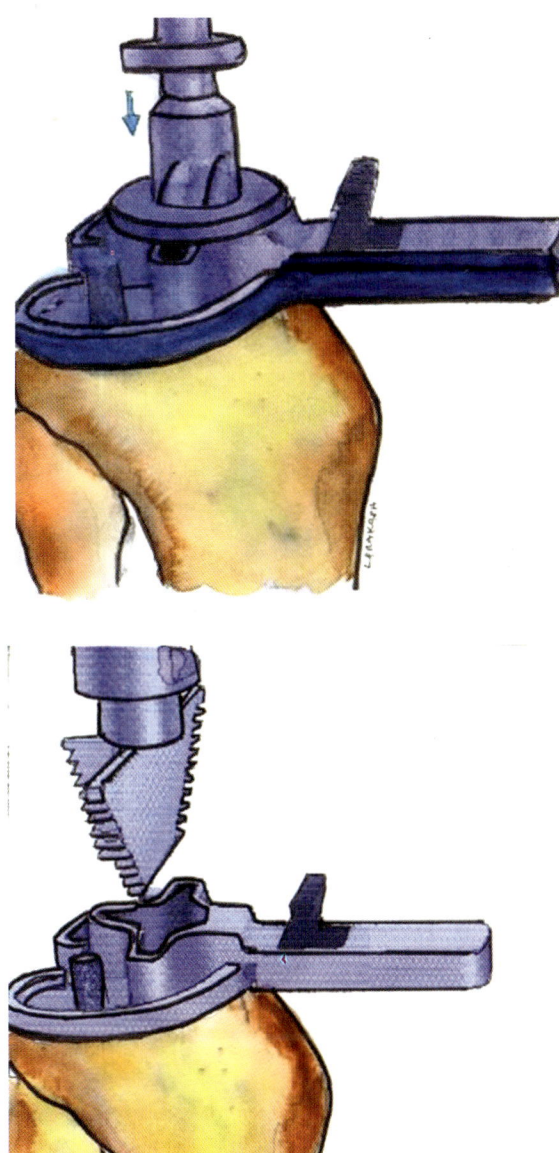

Depending on the design, the proximal tibial notches are drilled and slotted.

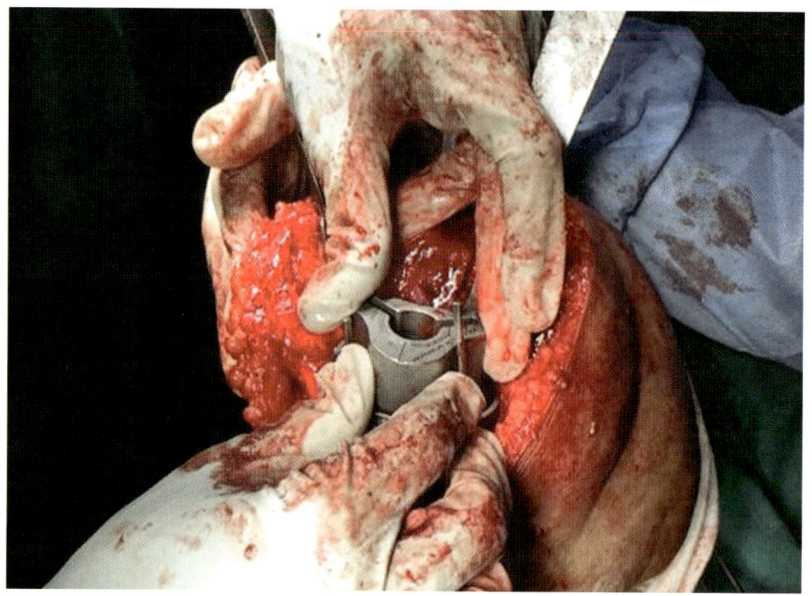

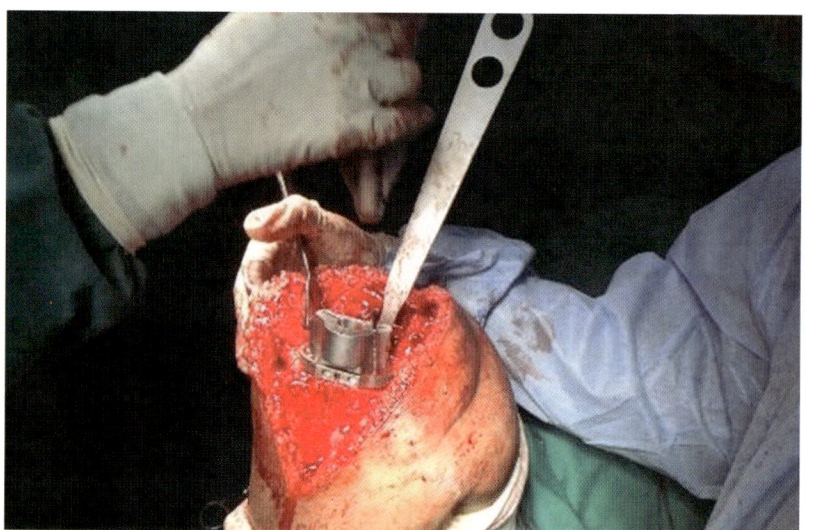

Proximal tibial preparation.

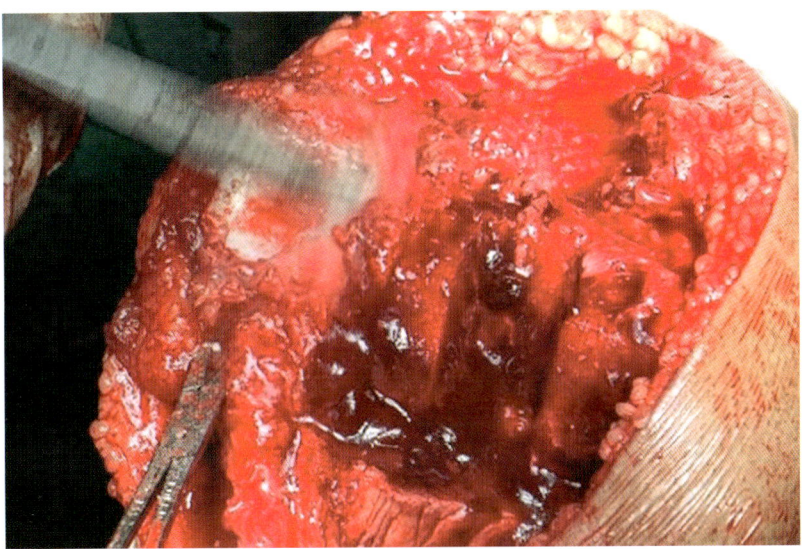

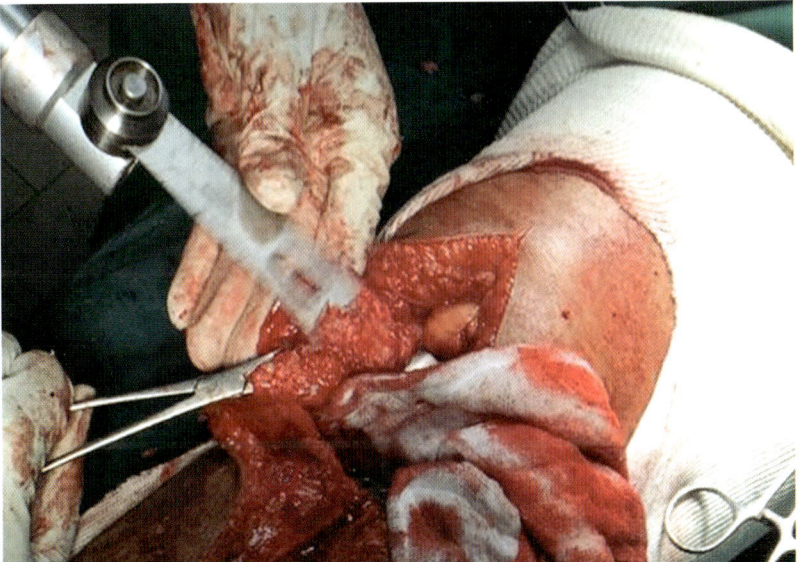

The next step is patellar shaving. One can either replace patella or just resurface and trim the edges.

PRE-CEMENTATION TRIAL WITH ACTUAL PROSTHESIS (ALSO THE STEPS FOR FIXATION OF A CEMENTLESS PROSTHESIS)

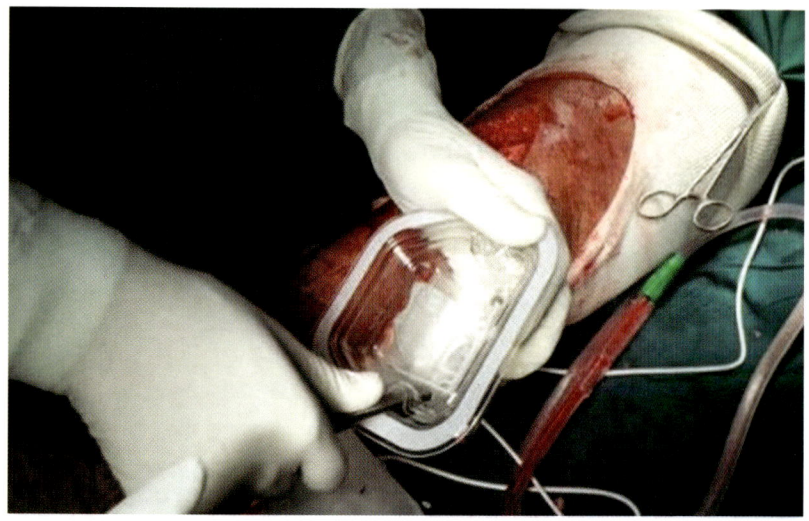

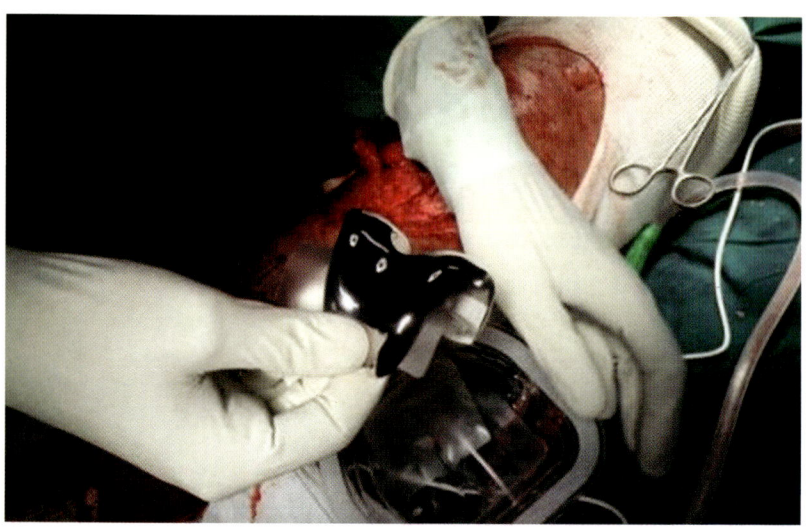

The actual implants are now unpacked.

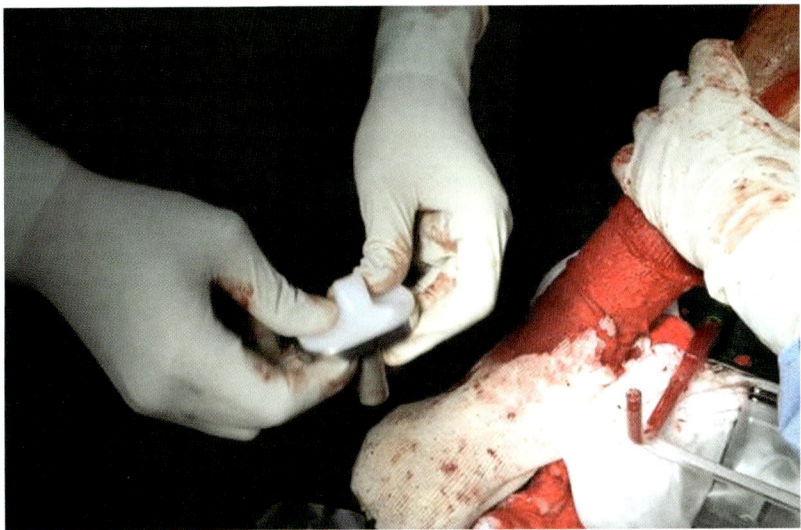

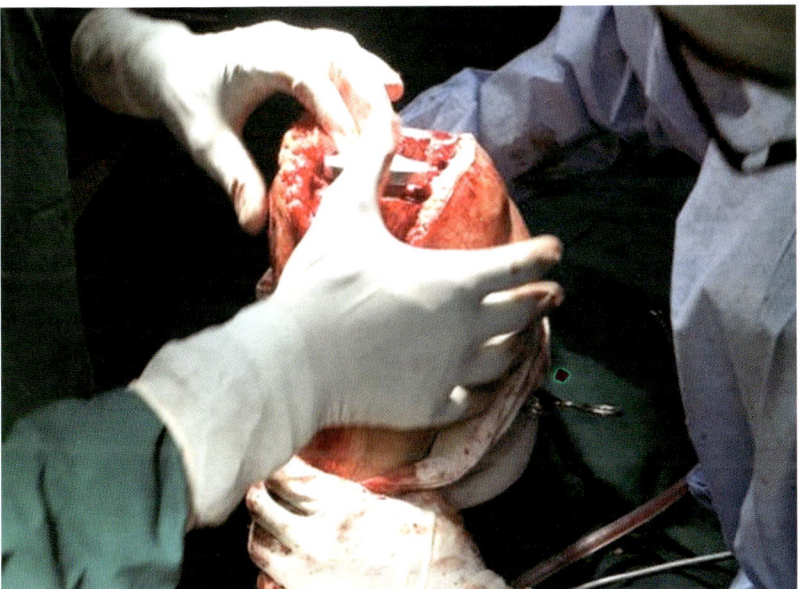

The actual components are inserted without cement and pushed in place. If cementless implants are used, proper impaction of the prosthesis completes this step.

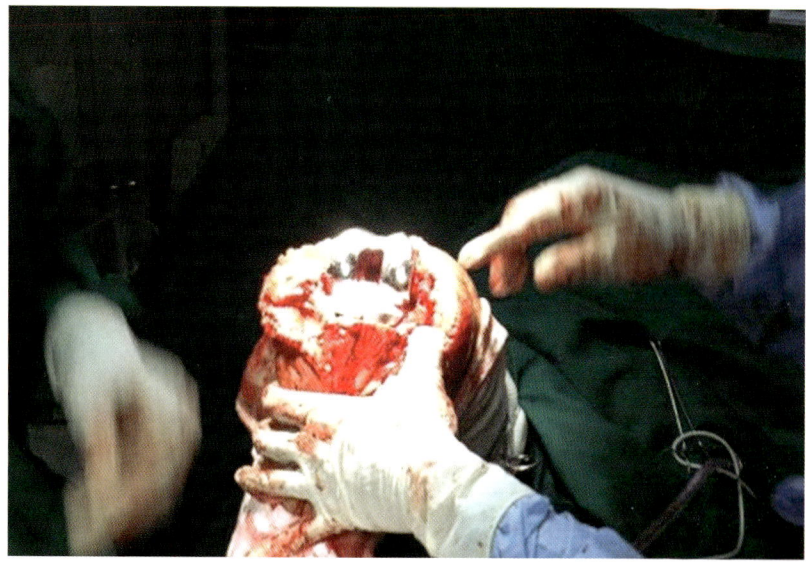

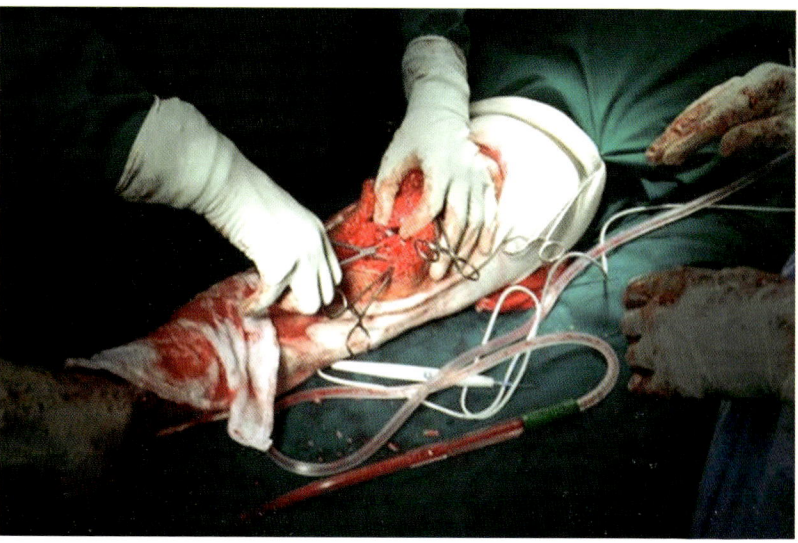

Once again a trial reduction is performed and knee stability is rechecked.

CEMENTATION OF THE COMPONENTS

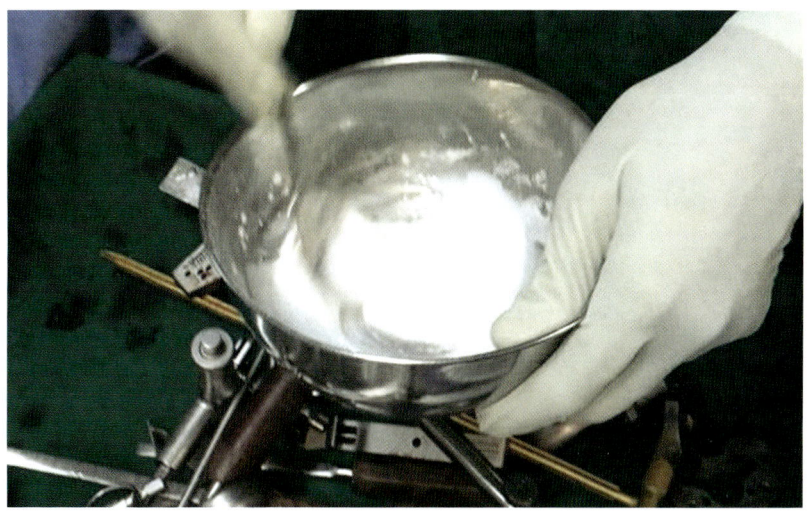

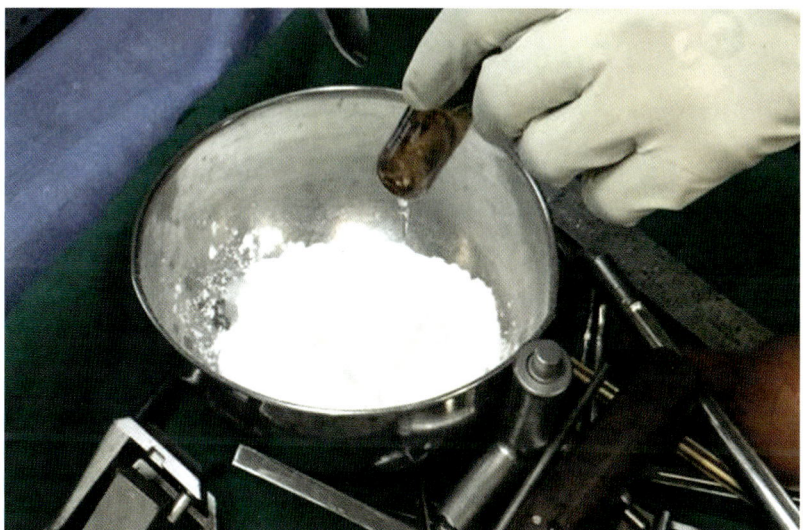

In case of a cemented knee, this is the time to open and mix the cement.

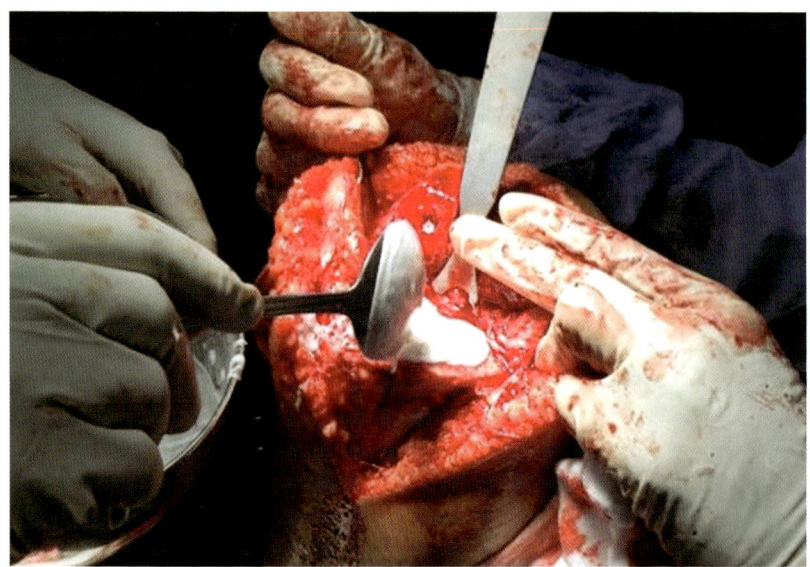

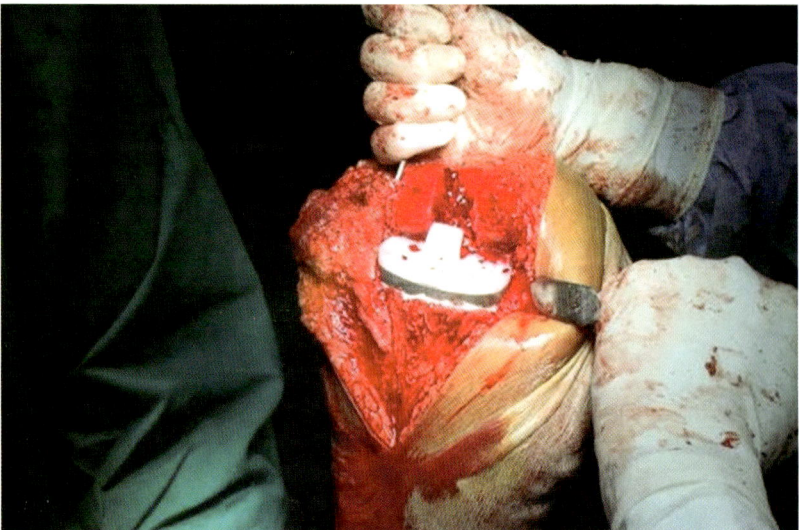

The surfaces should be clean and dry. Liquid cement is poured over the tibial cancellous surface and the component pressed in.

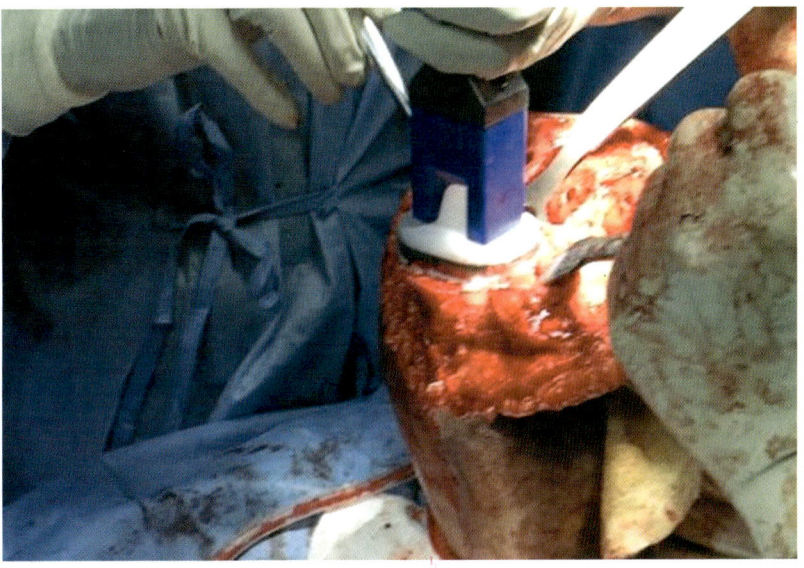

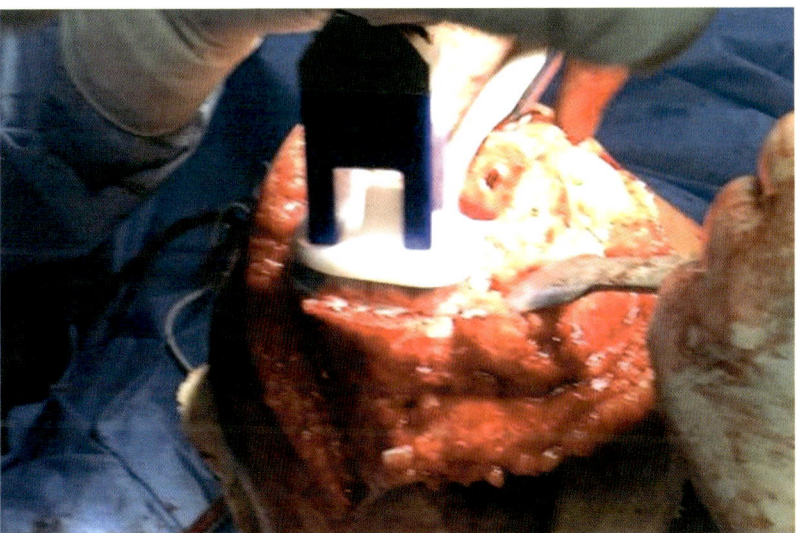

Rather than hammering the tibial component, a sustained pressure is applied until the cement sets.

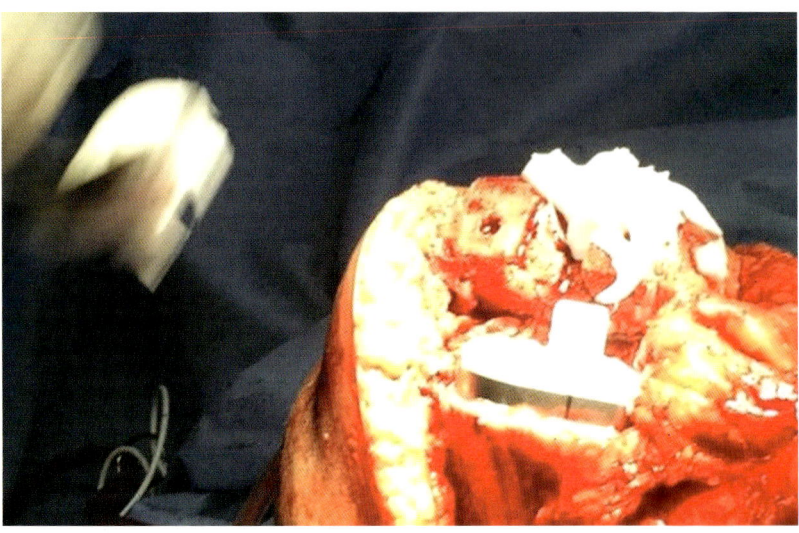

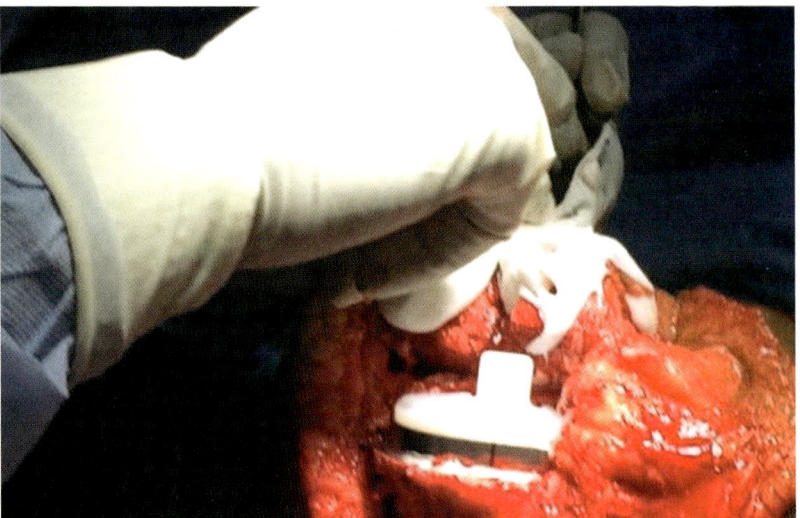

Liquid cement is now poured over the lower femoral cut surfaces. Nonantibiotic loaded cements are more liquid in the initial stages and provide better cancellous integration.

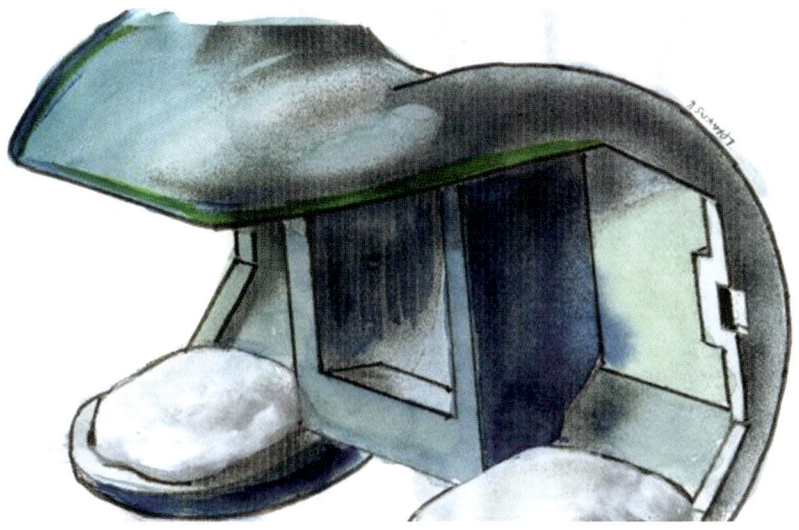

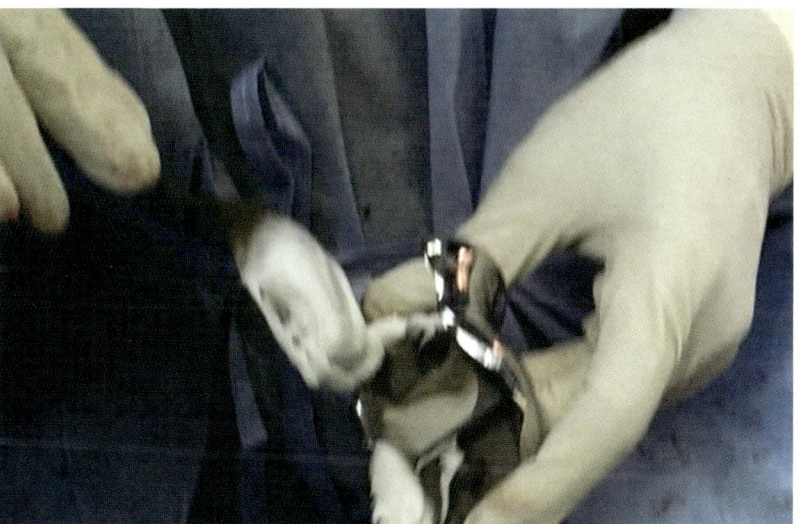

An important step is to put cement in the posterior condylar area in the prosthesis itself.

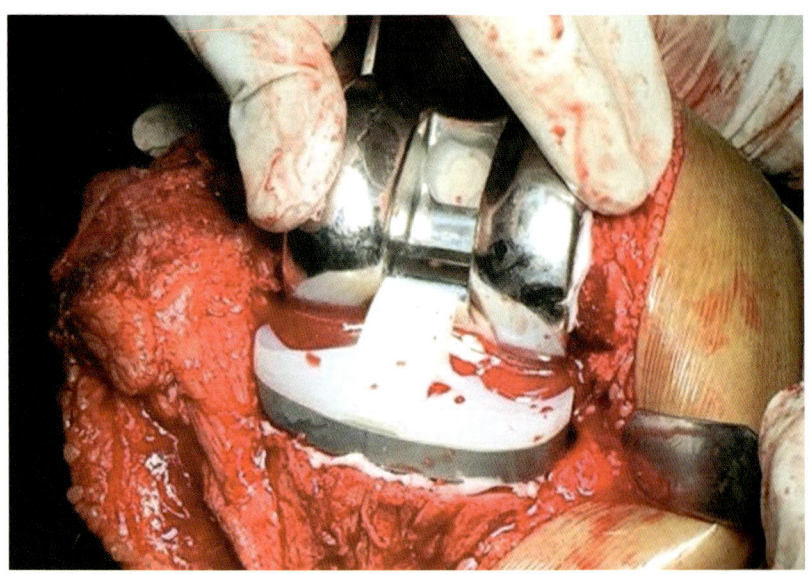

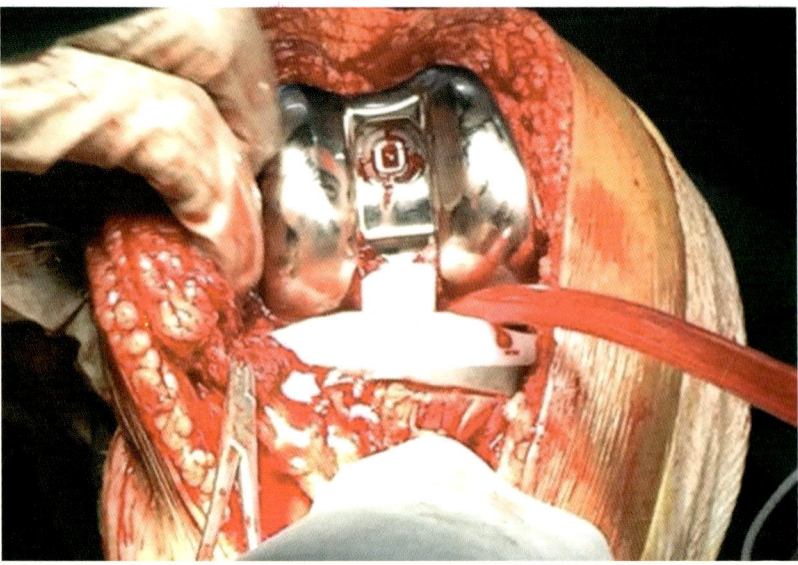

The femoral component is now pushed in place. Again, hammering should be avoided and sustained pressure should be applied.

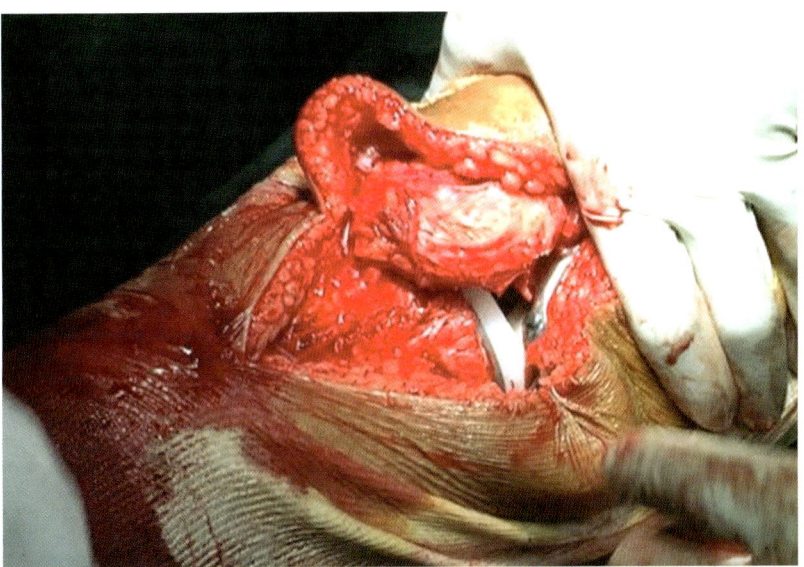

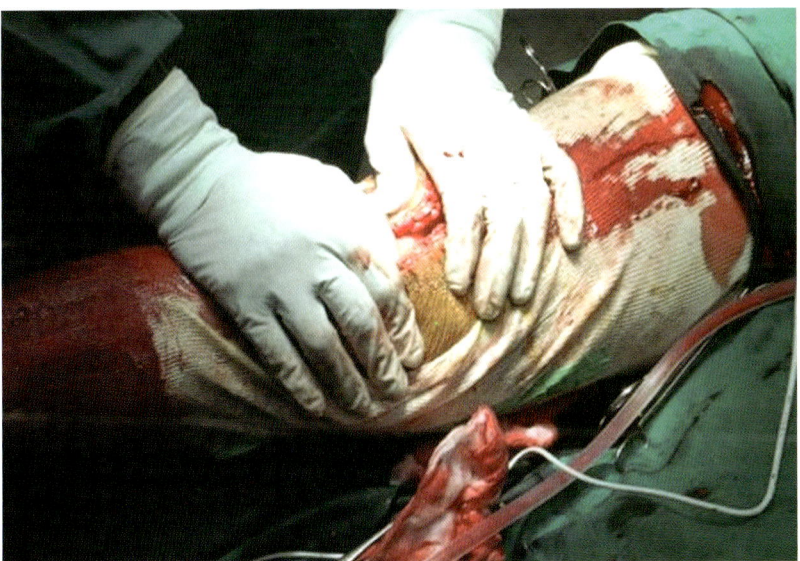

Extending the knee and holding it in hyperextension for 15 minutes will ensure that the cement bonds both components.

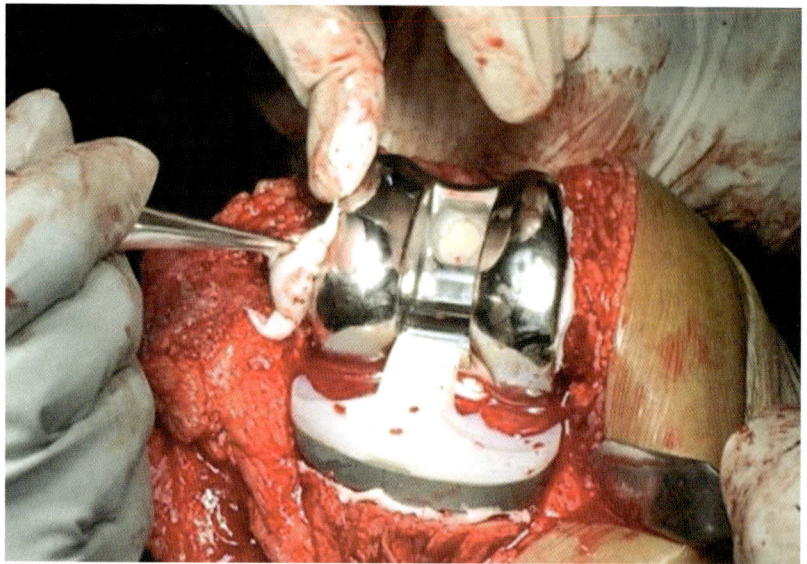

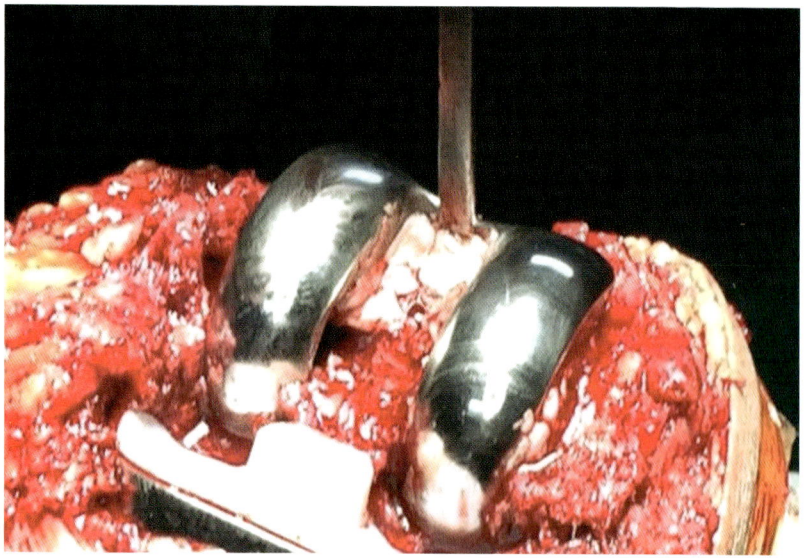

Excess cement is removed either by a chisel or a curette.

The six basic knee arthroplasty cuts:

1. Distal femur
2. Proximal tibia
3. Anterior femoral
4. Posterior femoral
5. Anterior chamfer
6. Posterior chamfer

THESE ARE THE SAME IN BOTH CEMENTED AND CEMENTLESS TKR.

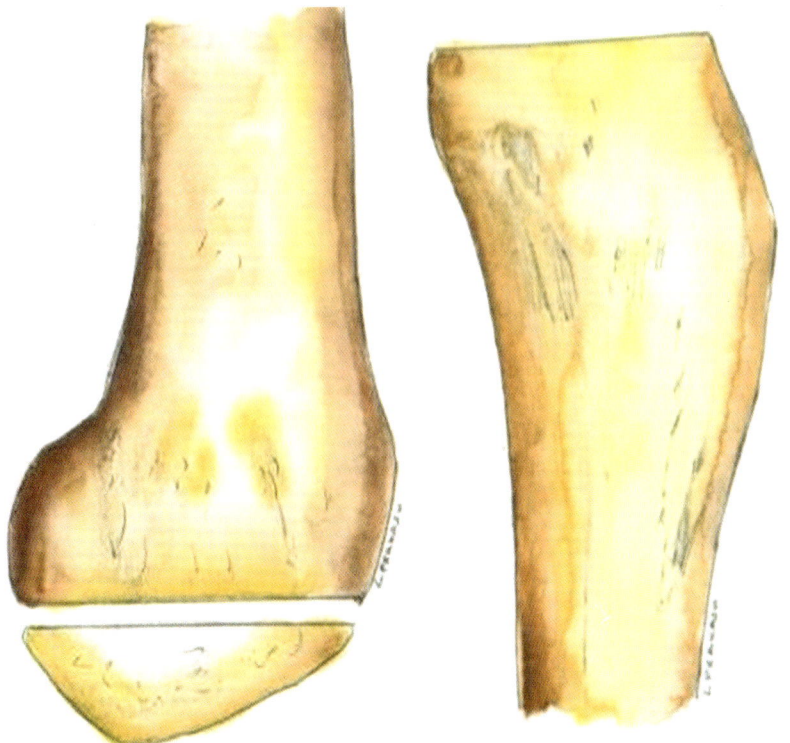

The lower tibial and upper femoral cuts.

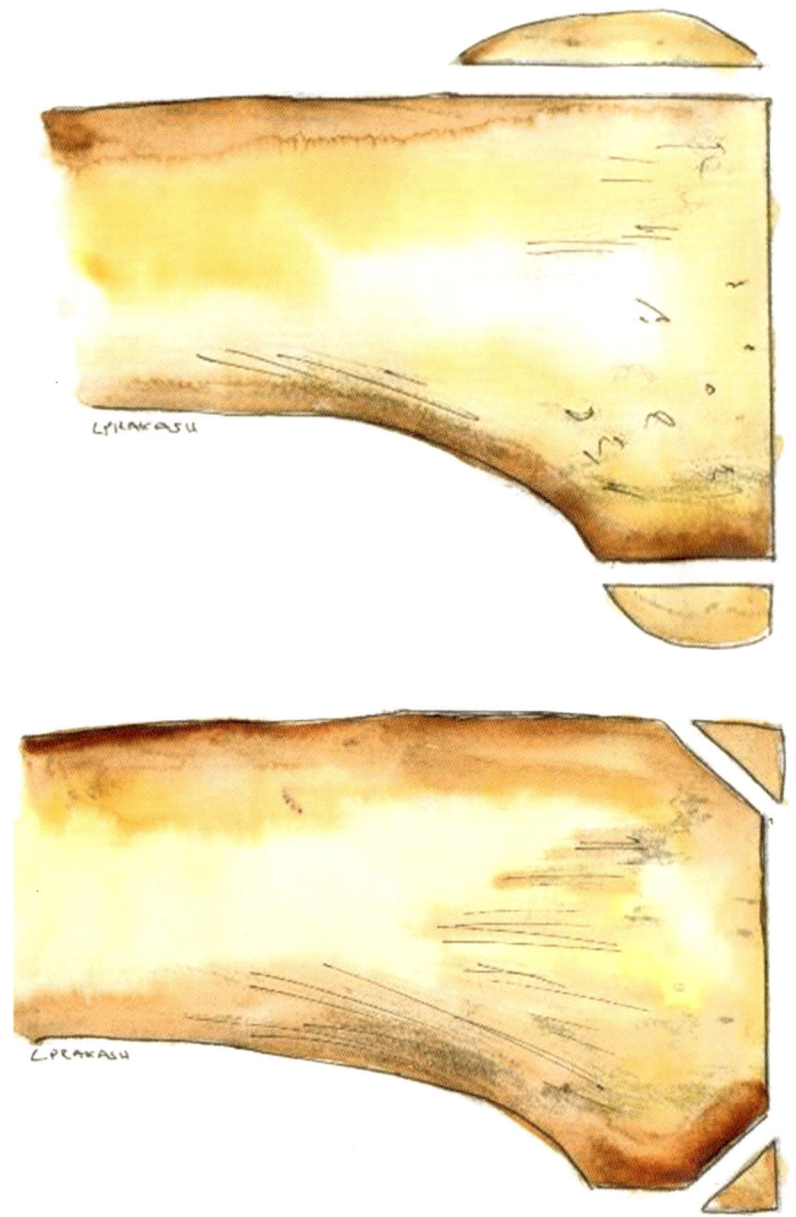

The anterior posterior and chamfer cuts.

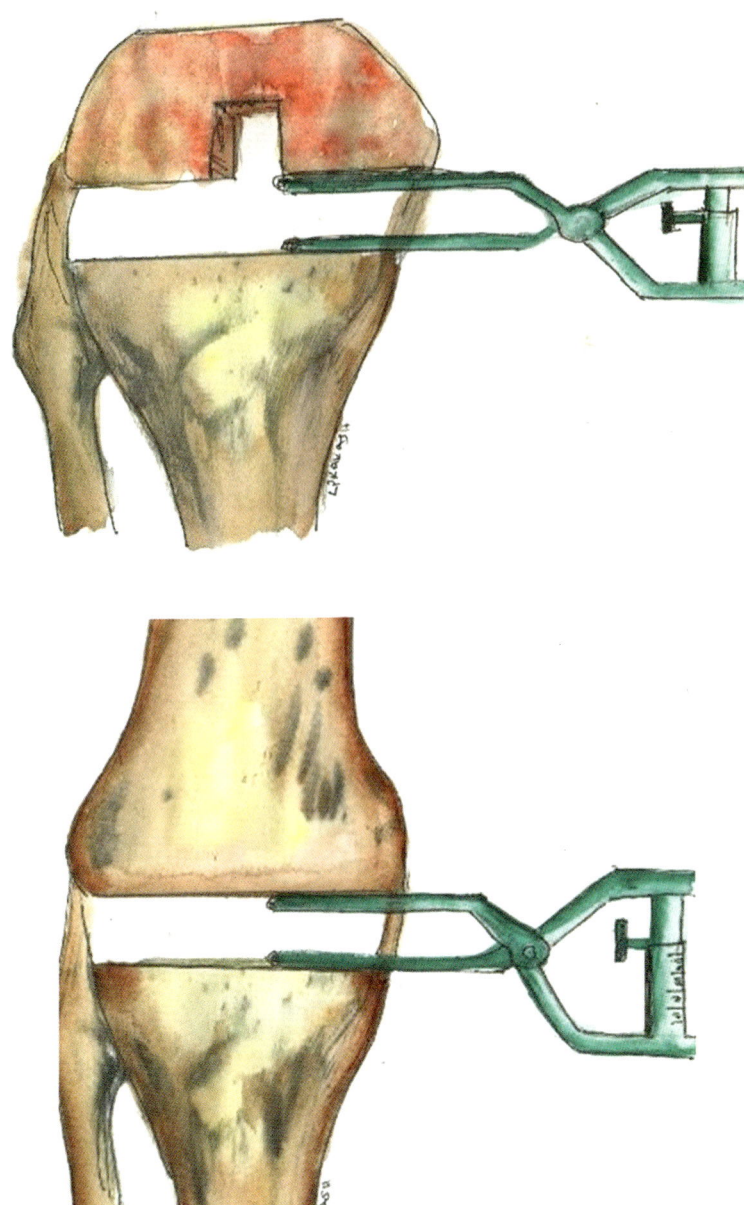

Flexion and extension gap balance is the most important step of total knee replacement.

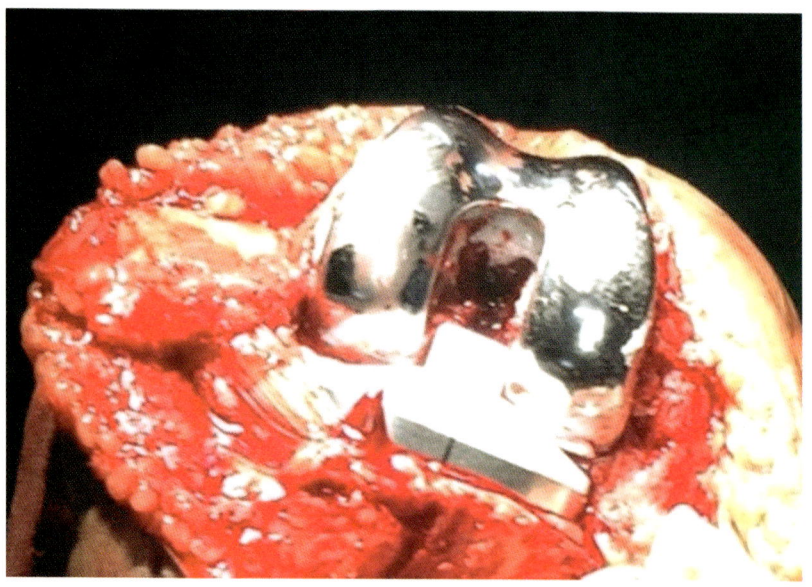

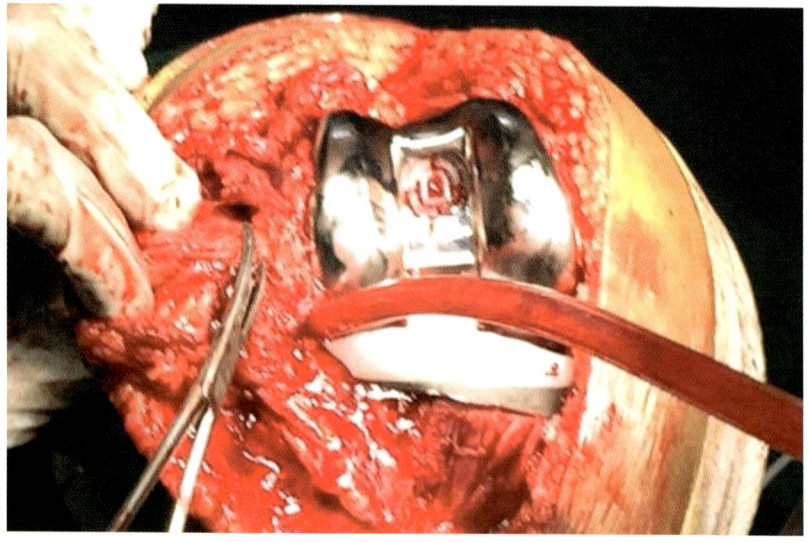

After removal of excess cement, the joint is thoroughly washed.

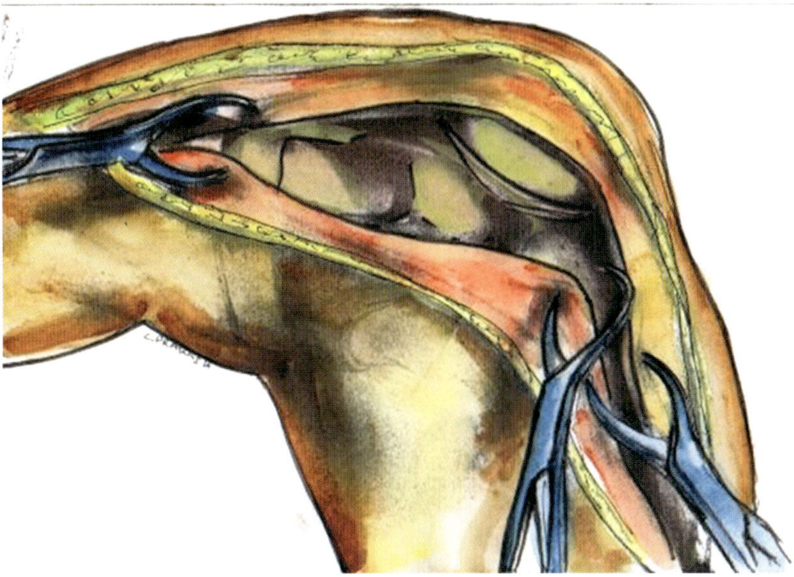

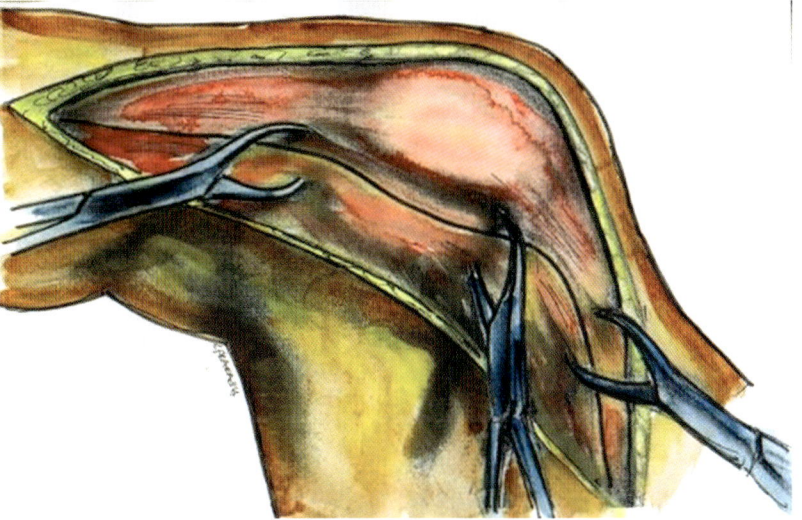

Towel clips will confirm that the patella does not tend to snap out during flexion.

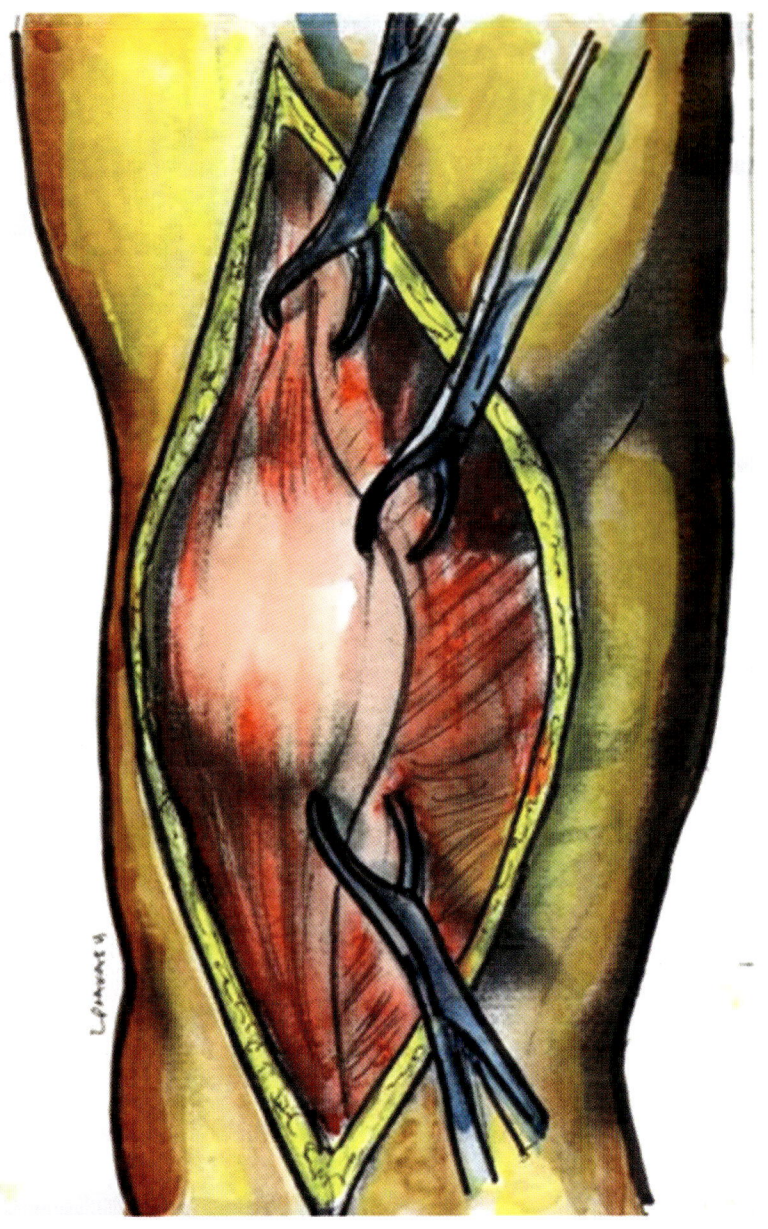

The knee can be put through a full range of motion at this stage.

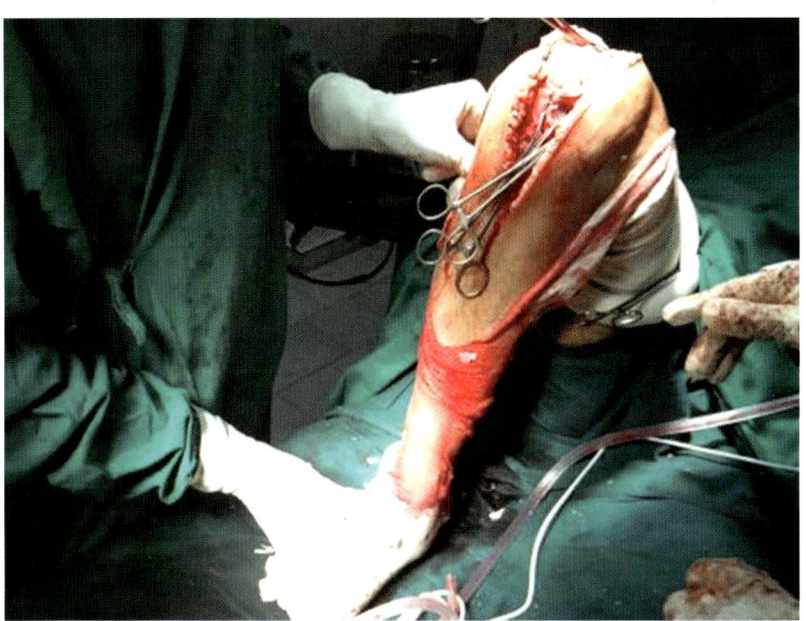

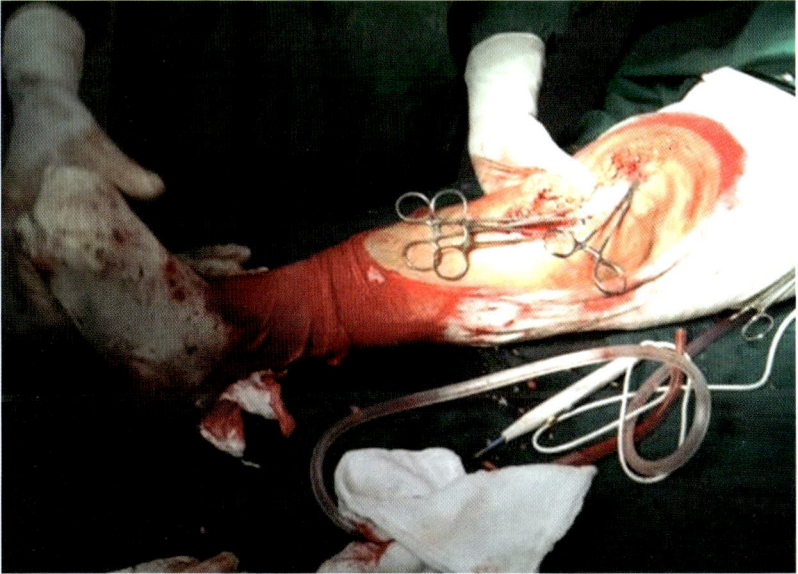

No deformities should be present now. The knee should be extendable fully, be in slight valgus and lock steady in mediolateral axis.

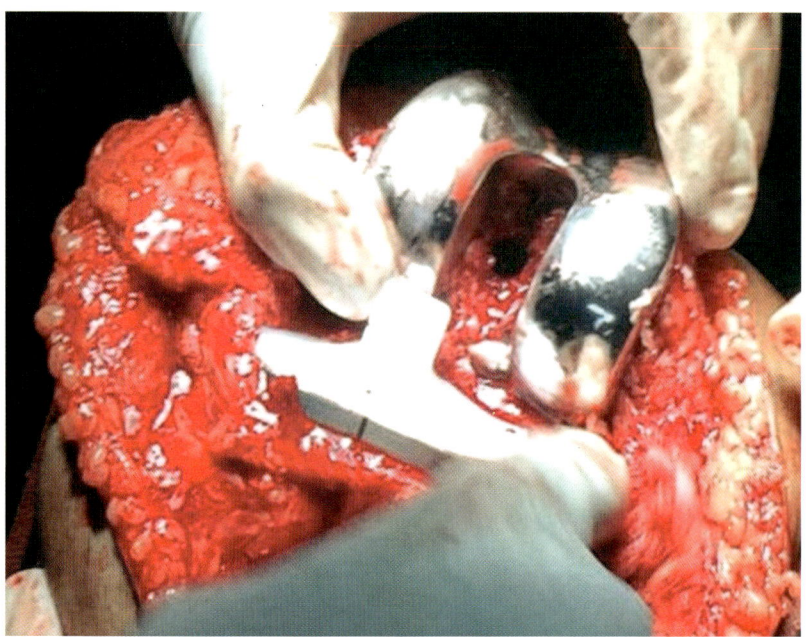

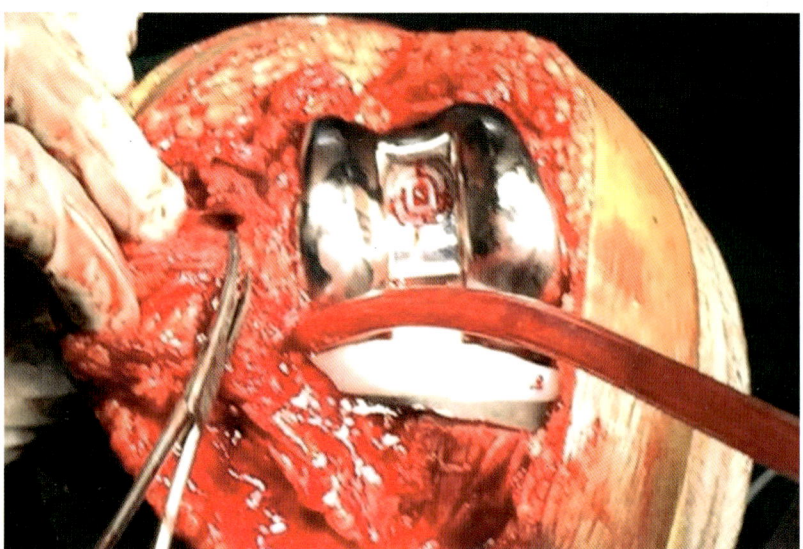

The knee is now inspected carefully, washed thoroughly and all loose cement bits removed patiently.

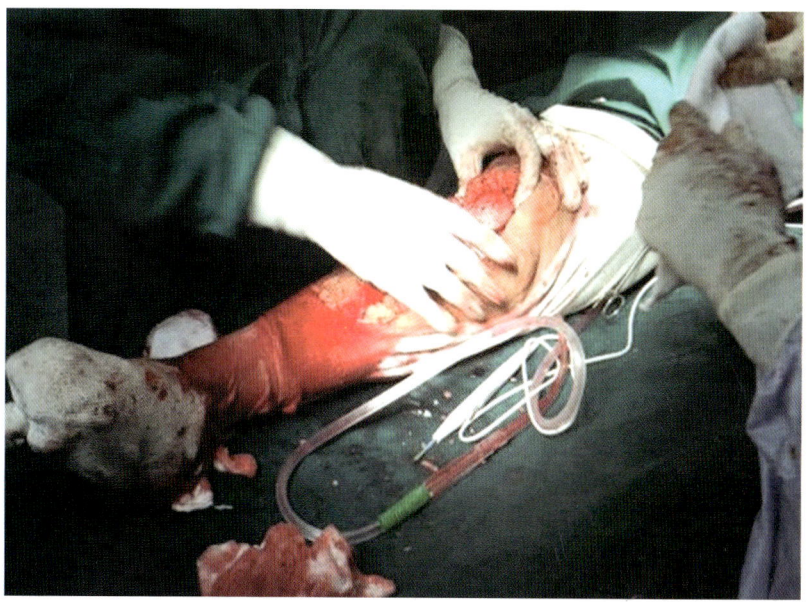

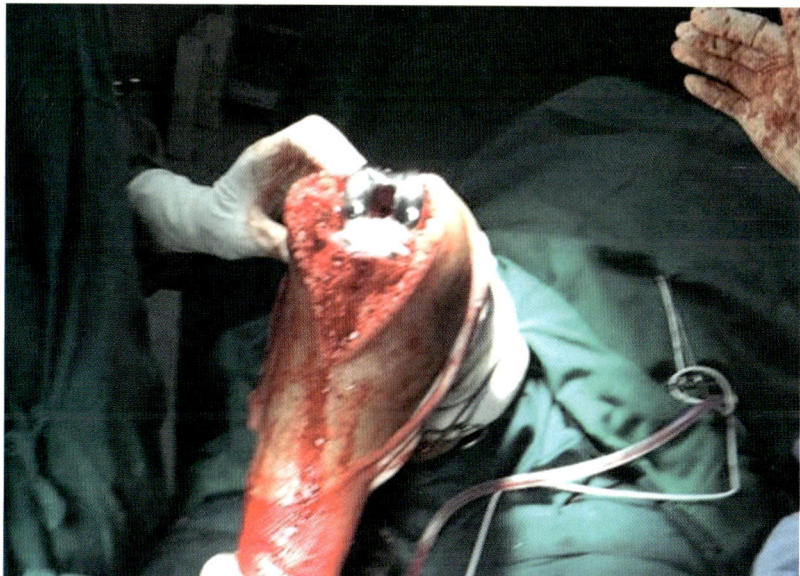

The joint is again put through full range of movements with and without the towel clips.

REDUCTION, DRAIN, SUTURE AND BANDAGES

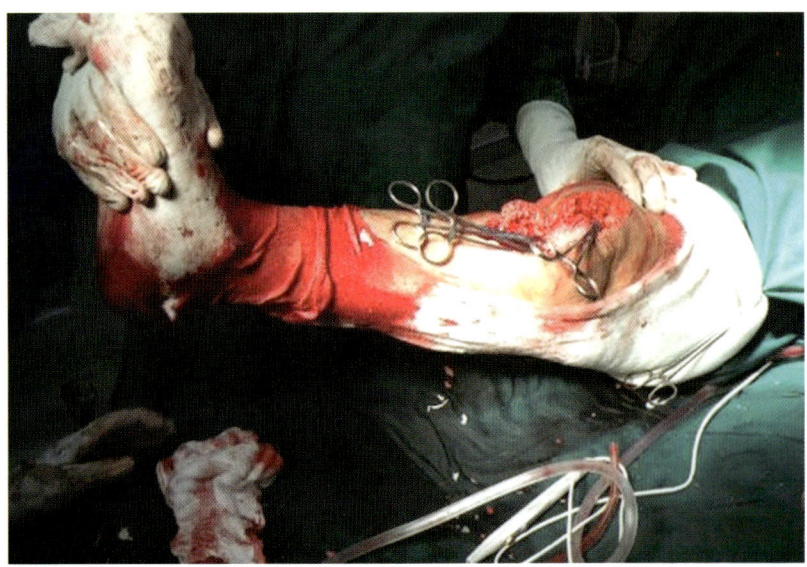

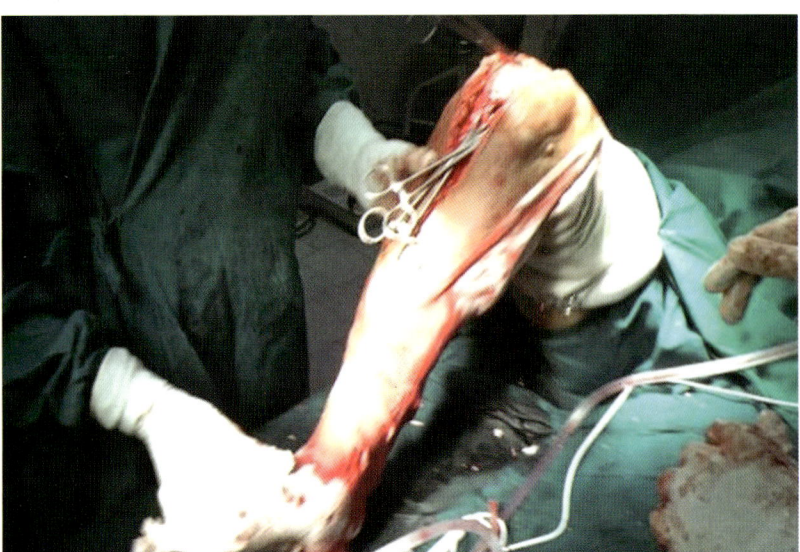

The joint is again put through full range of movements with and without the towel clips.

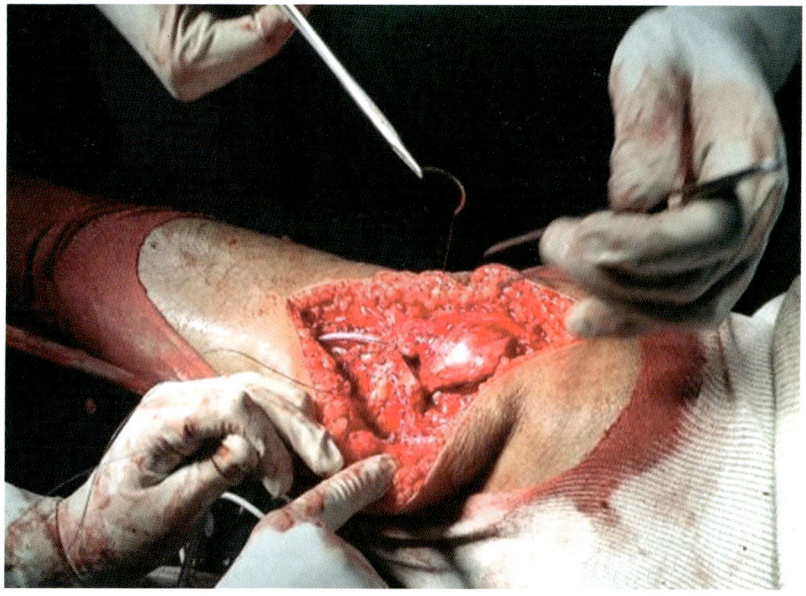

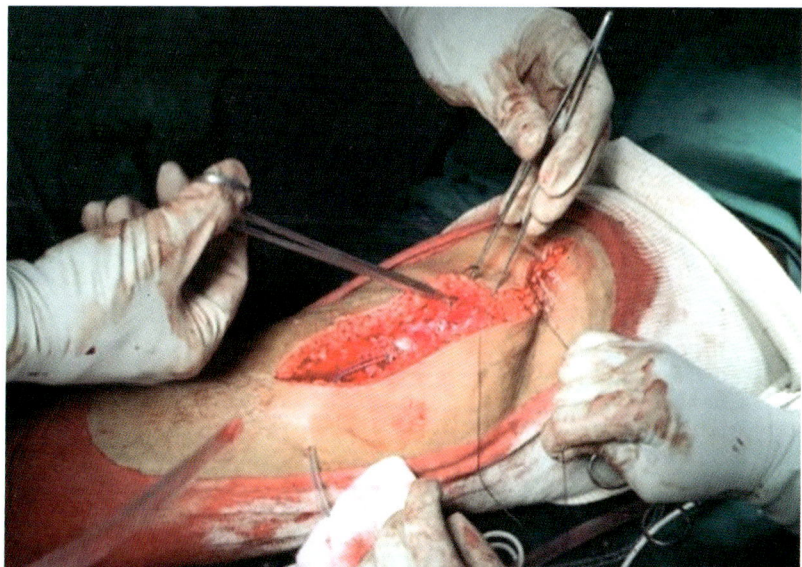

The quadriceps mechanism is sutured by strong absorbable sutures. A suction vacuum drain is inserted deep into the knee.

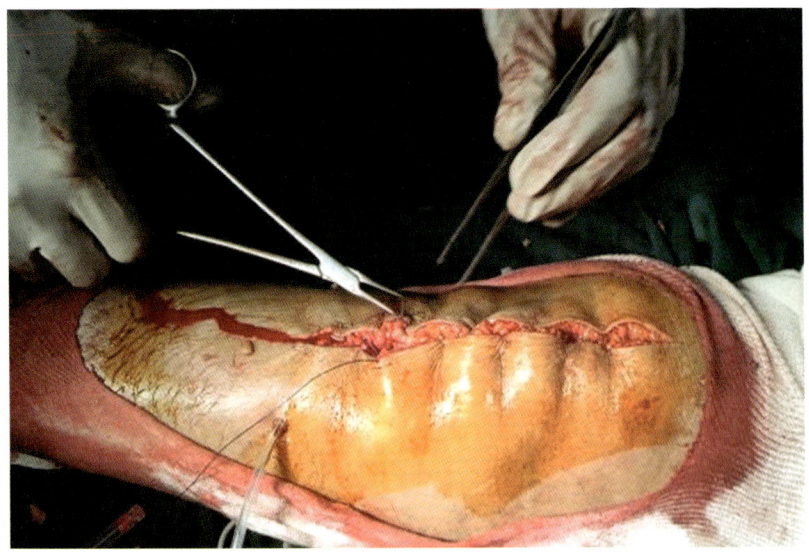

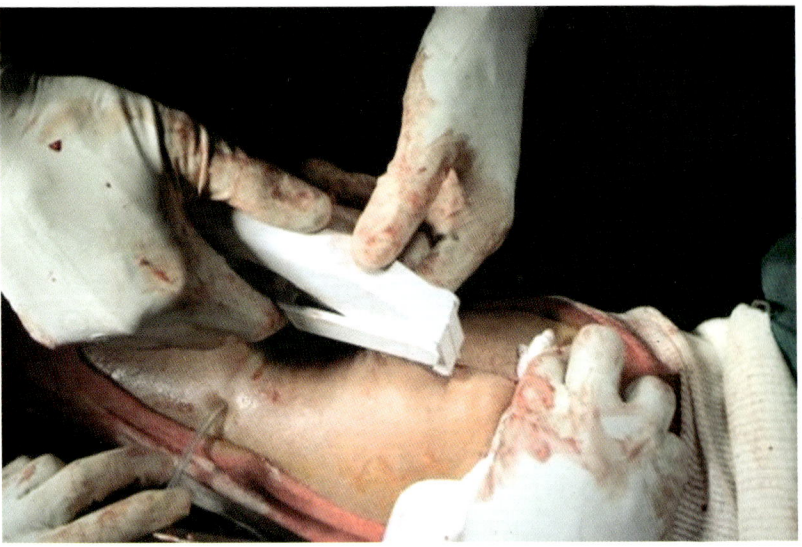

Subcutaneous absorbable sutures approximate the skin, which is closed by stapler application.

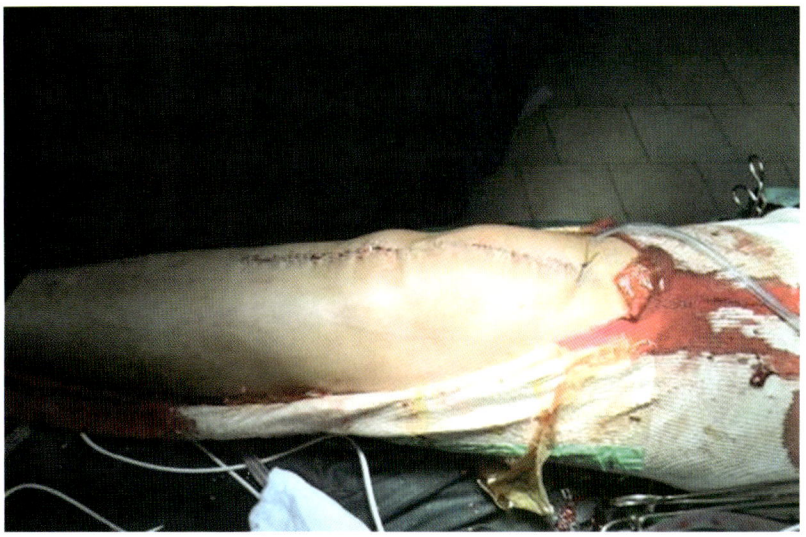

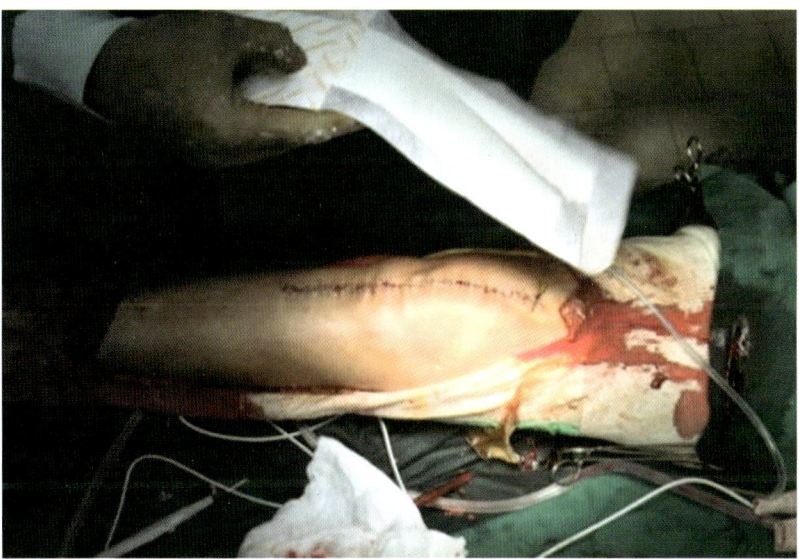

A sterile adhesive bandage is now pasted over the incision.

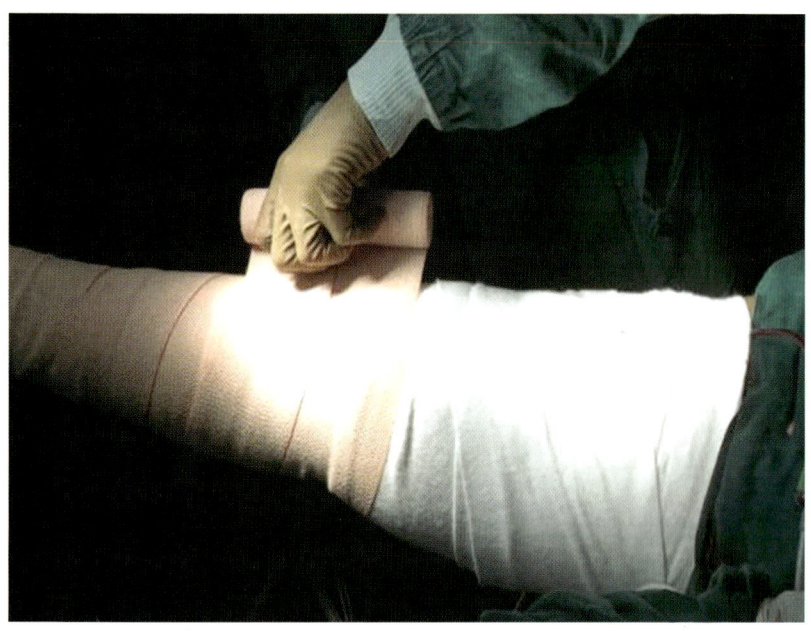

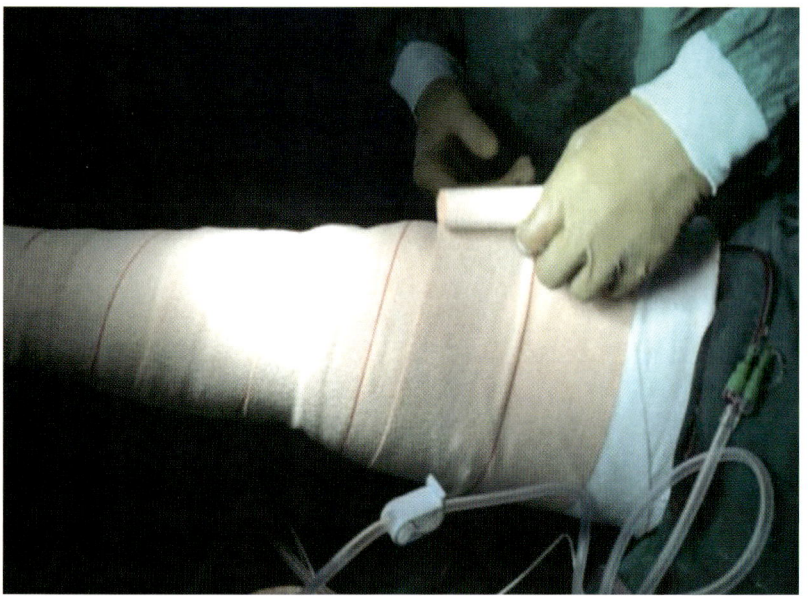

Cast padding and crepe bandage provide compression.

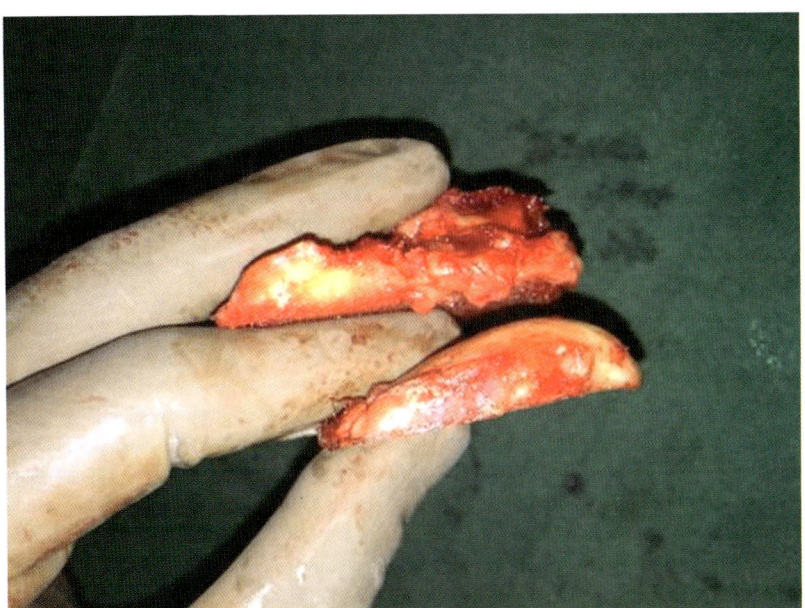

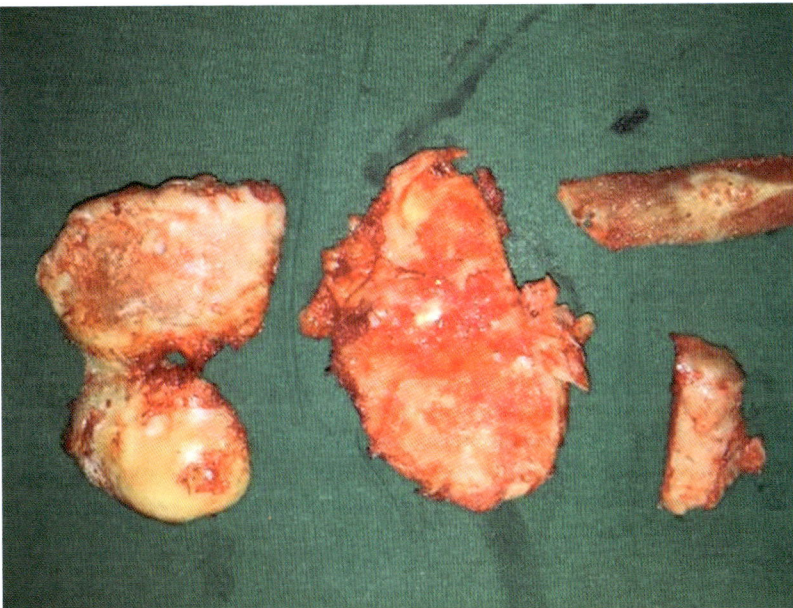

As mentioned previously, the total bone removed should not be more than the thickness of the two components.

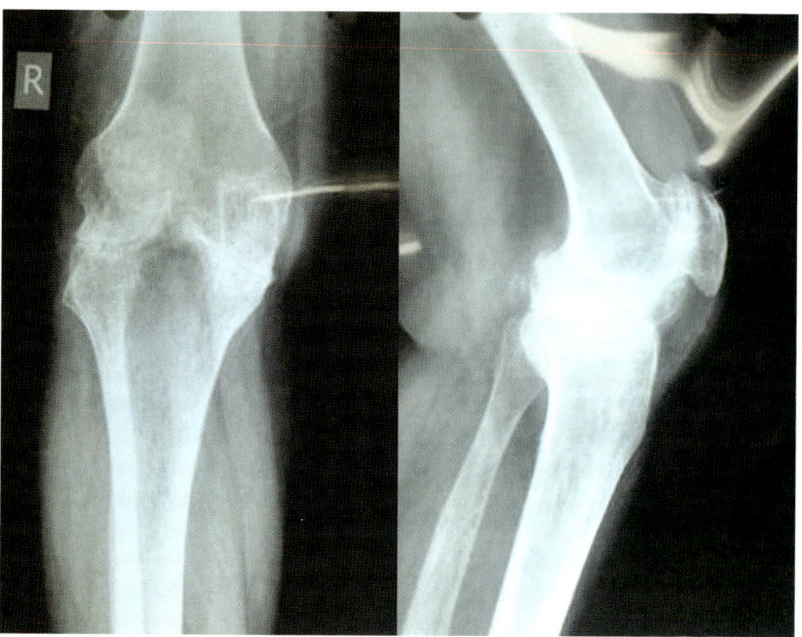

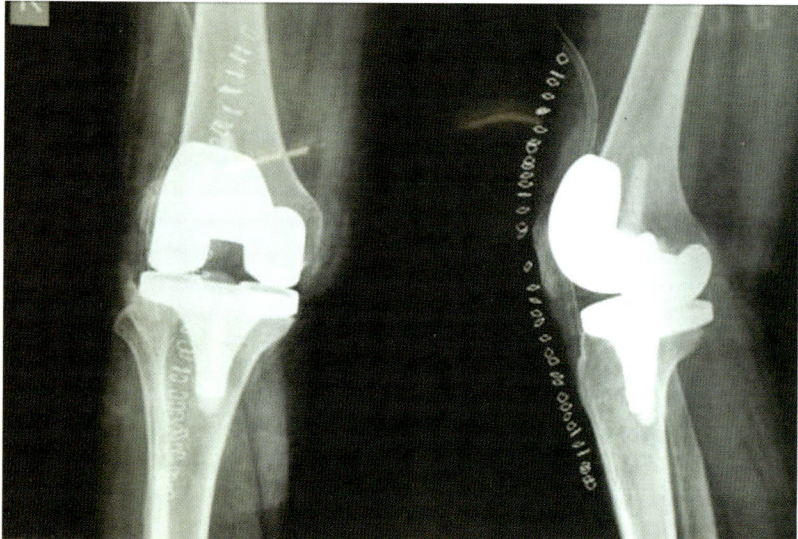

A postoperative radiograph is taken for evaluation of component position.

Instruments for Primary
Total Knee Replacement

Irrespective of the implant design or brand, the instruments achieve exactly the same goals, namely:

1. Cutting the lower femur in a few degrees valgus and parallel to the floor.
2. Cutting the upper tibia neutral to floor mediolaterally but with a slight posterior slope.
3. Ensuring a proper rotational alignment during anterior, posterior and chamfer cuts of distal femur.
4. The surface and taper cuts of distal femur should exactly match the undersurface of the femoral component.
5. Adequate trials for checking all cuts and releases before implantation.
6. Instrumentation to ensure that gaps in flexion and extension are equal.

CHARNLEY FEMORAL BROACH

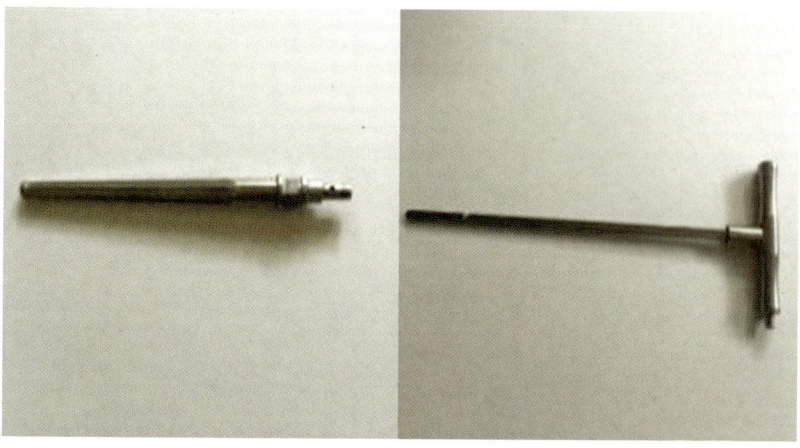

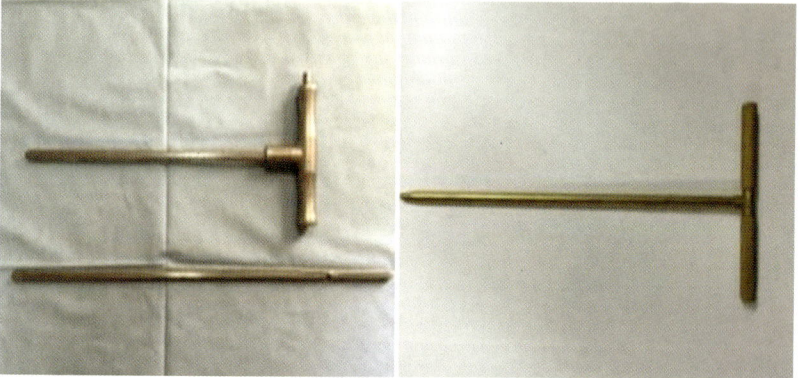

The intramedullary broach and alignment rod is available in different combinations from the simplest to the most complicated. This is the first instrument used and locates the long axis of the femur. The rod should be inserted deep enough into the medulla to catch the isthmus to ensure that a wrong axial identification is avoided. The distal femoral cutting guide is attached to this block.

DISTAL FEMORAL CUTTING ASSEMBLY

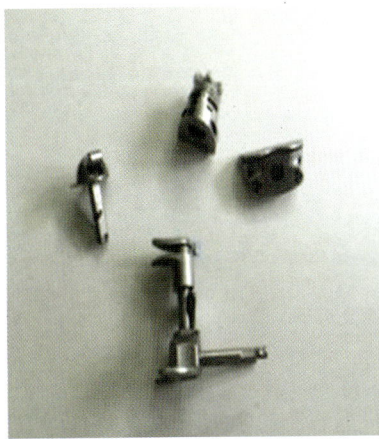 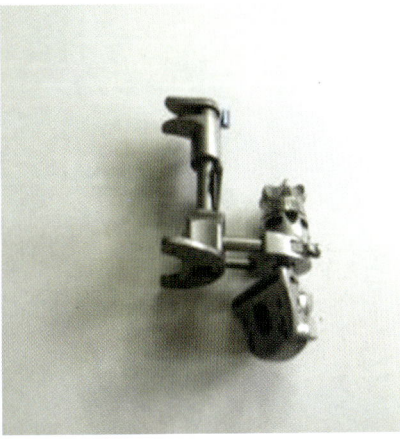

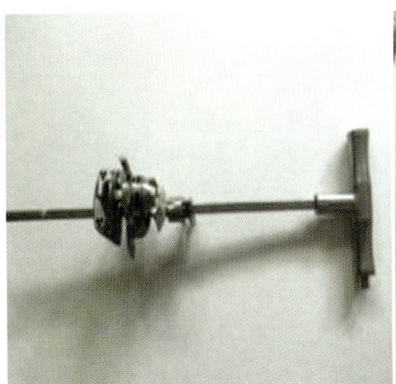 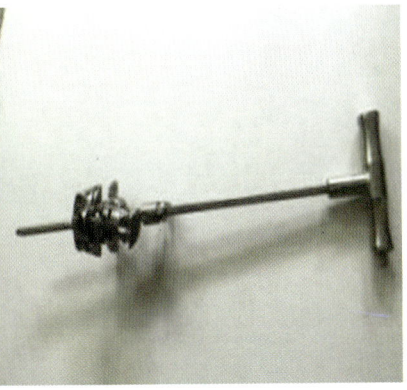

Various designs of distal cutting blocks achieve the same purpose with minor technical variations in the instrumentation.

EACH SYSTEM PROVIDES A VALGUS CUT

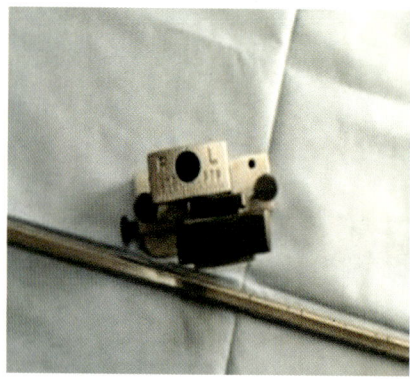 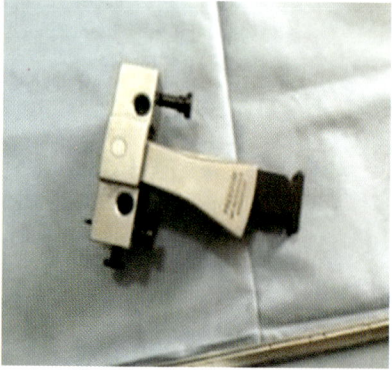

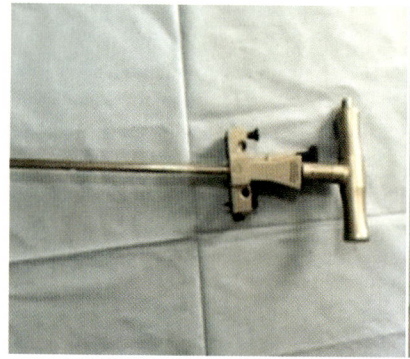 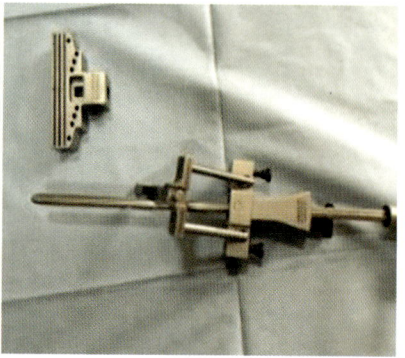

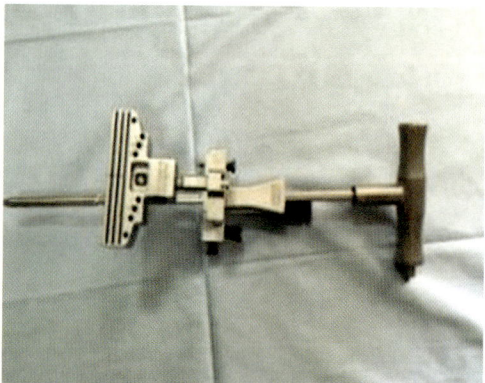

Each instrument can provide valgus cuts from 3° to 7° in small increments to tailor the cut according to the patient.

BLOCK DESIGNS VARY

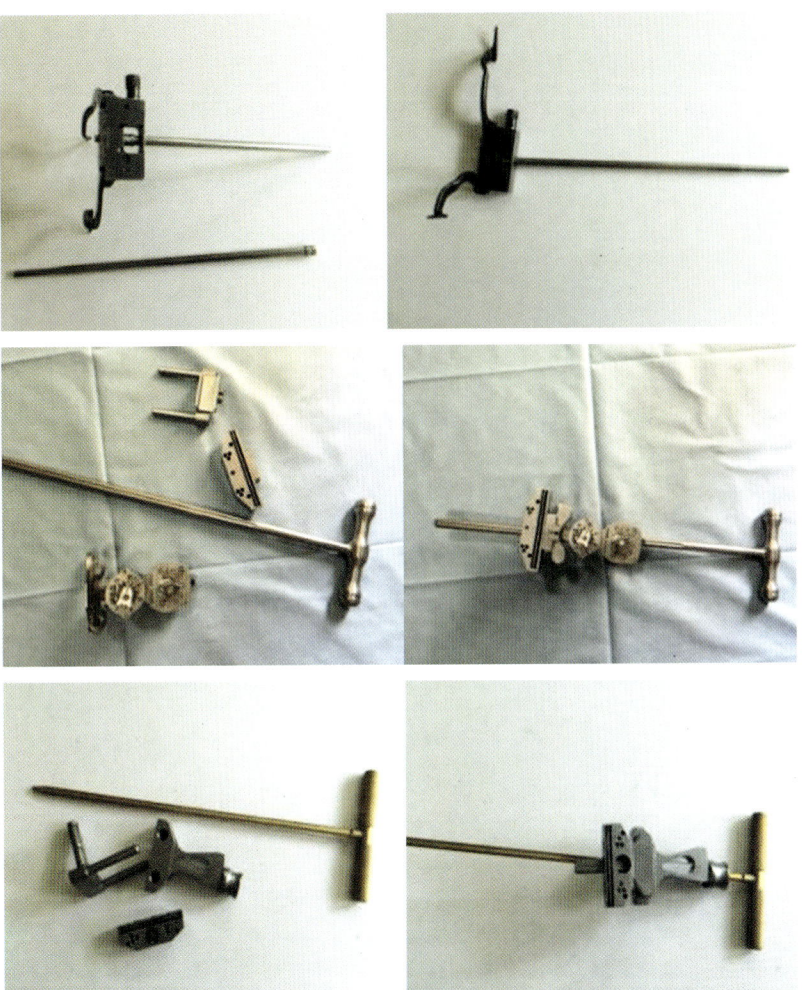

These blocks can vary from simple Freeman and Insall designs (top and bottom) to the complex fourth generation magnetic snap-on jigs.

THE UPPER TIBIAL CUTTING GUIDE

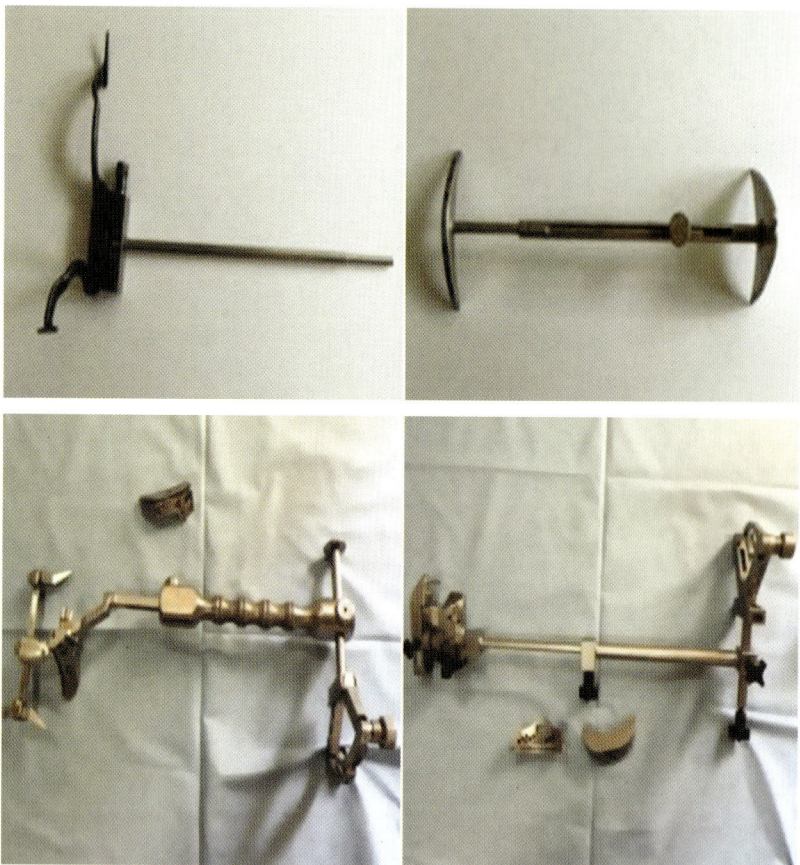

The upper tibial cutting guides too come in various designs. They cut 7 mm of upper tibia with a slight posterior slope.

STATIC GAP EVALUATION DEVICES. THEY CANNOT MEASURE MID-FLEXION GAPS

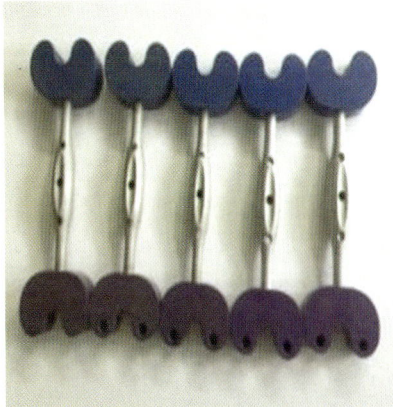
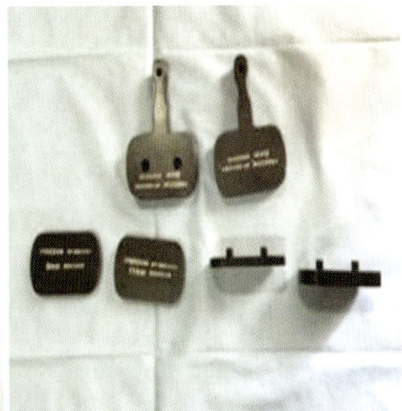
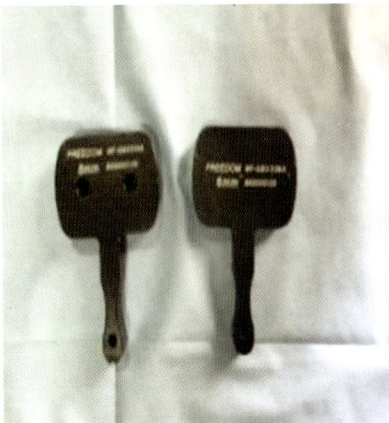
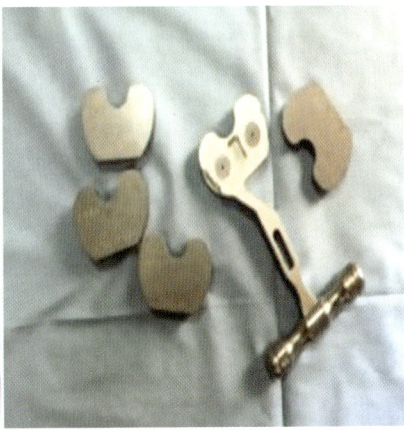

The gap balancing can be either static or dynamic. Static balancers are just spacers of different thicknesses which are tried in flexion and extension to ensure that the knee is neither too tight nor too wobbly.

DYNAMIC GAP BALANCING INSTRUMENTS

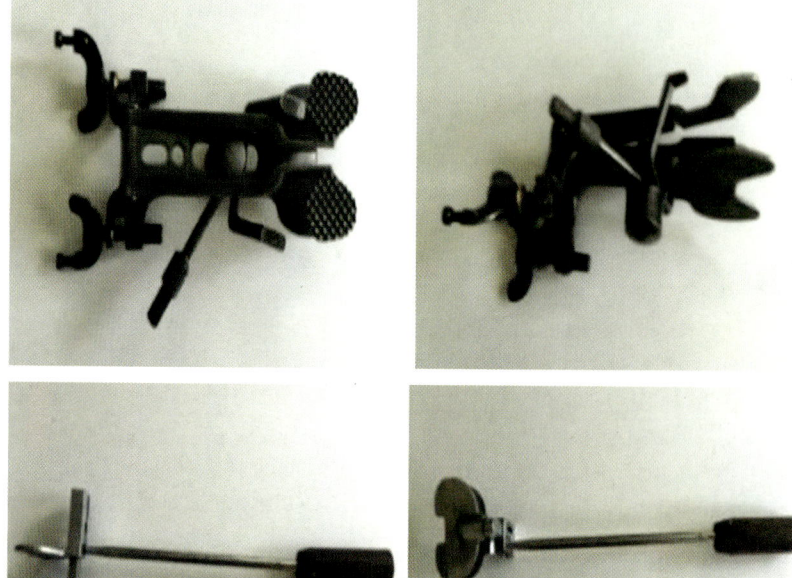

The dynamic gap balancers expand the gap with a turn screw and even mid-range gaps can be measured. Long-term success of a knee depends on proper gap balancing and equalization of tension in all quadrants.

FEMORAL COMPONENT SIZE MEASURING

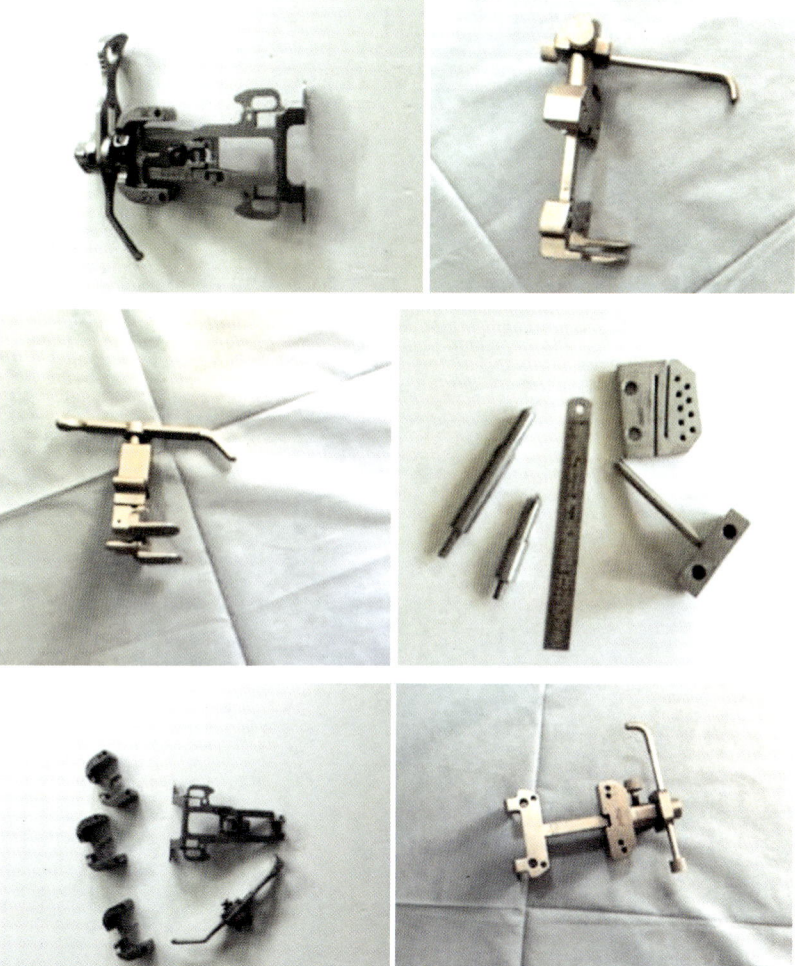

Each implant design has its own femoral size template. It is useful to have a metal scale to correctly measure the cut dimensions and ensure that the right size implant is used.

THE FOUR-IN-ONE CUTTING BLOCK, COMMON TO ALMOST ALL DESIGNS

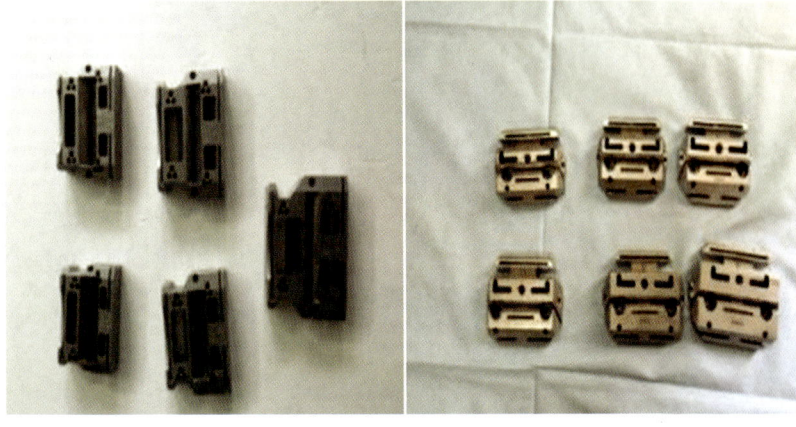

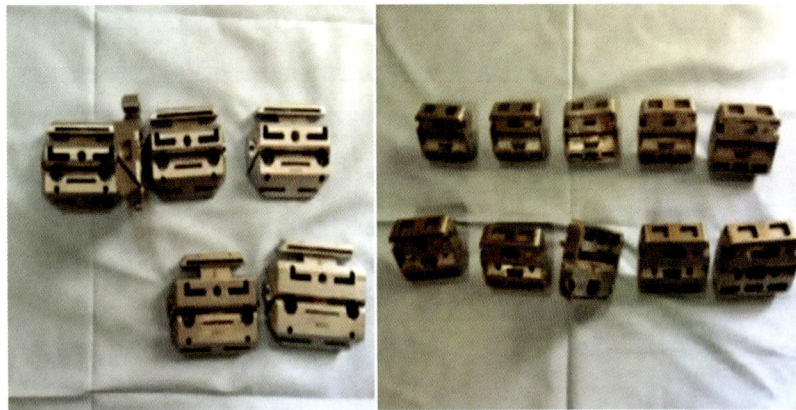

The four-in-one cutting blocks do the anterior, posterior, anterior chamfer and posterior chamfer cuts.

THE FOUR-IN-ONE CUTTING BLOCK, COMMON TO ALMOST ALL DESIGNS

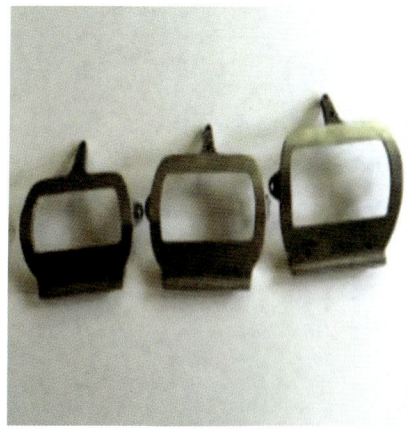
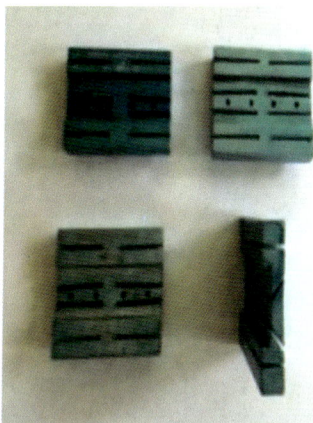
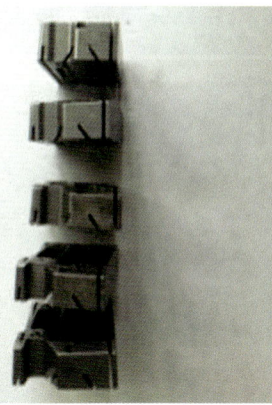
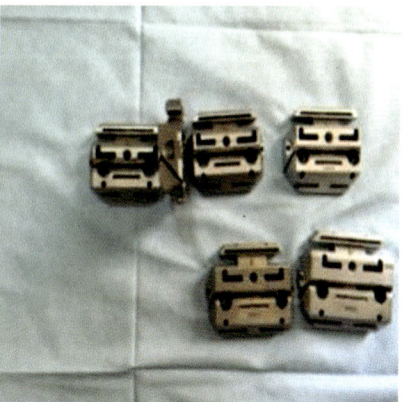

Each design is different, but they are all based on the same scientific principles and produce the same end result. The one in blue is a light titanium cutting block designed by me in 1994.

TIBIAL SIZERS

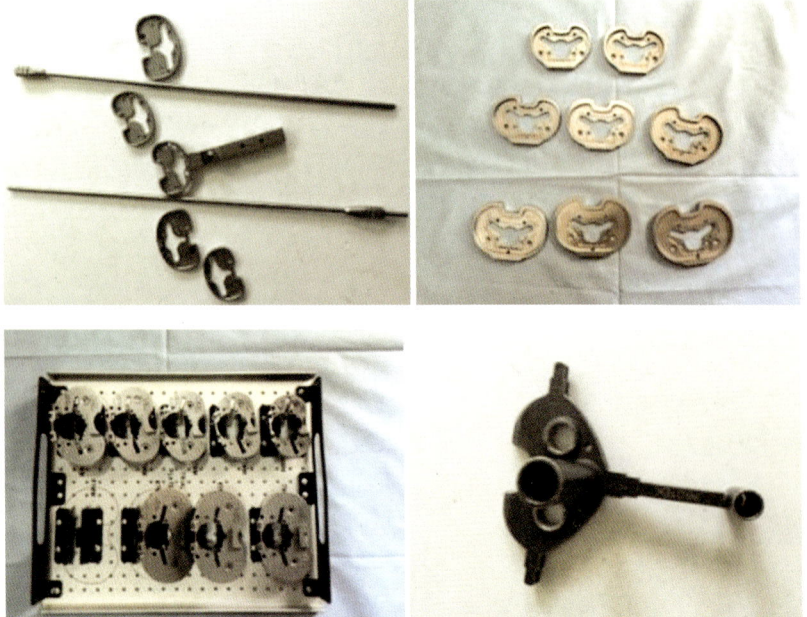

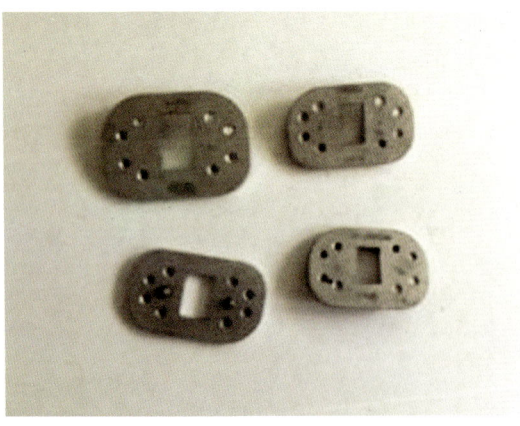

Tibial sizers match the implant and differ from company to company.

BOX CUTTERS ARE NEEDED IF A CRUCIATE SCARIFYING DESIGN IS USED

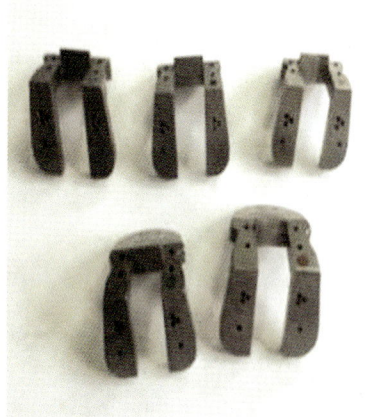
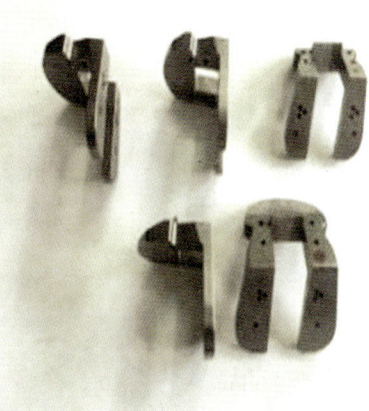

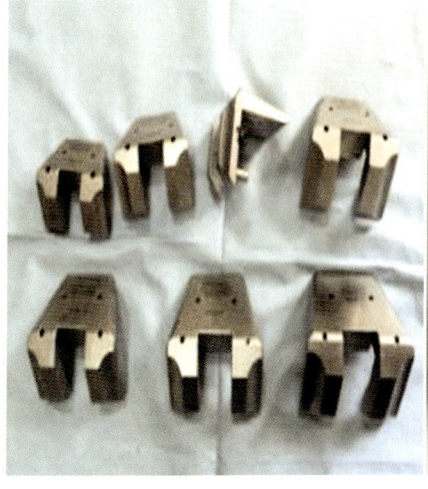
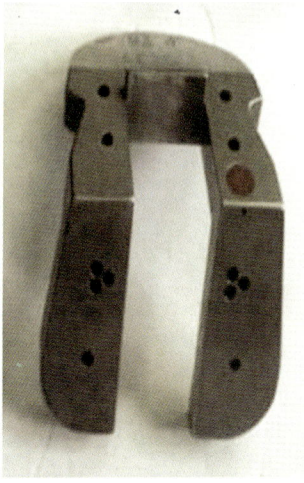

In case a posterior cruciate ligament scarifying design is used, a box cut is needed; each implant design has its own box device.

CS AND CR IMPLANTS HAVE THEIR OWN TRIALS

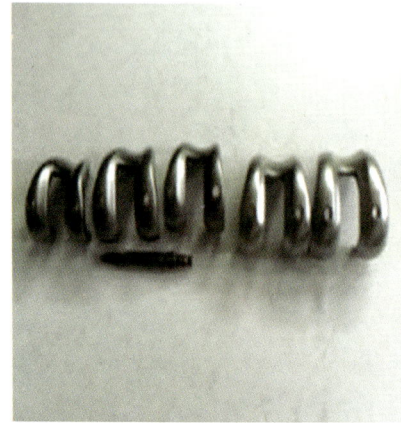 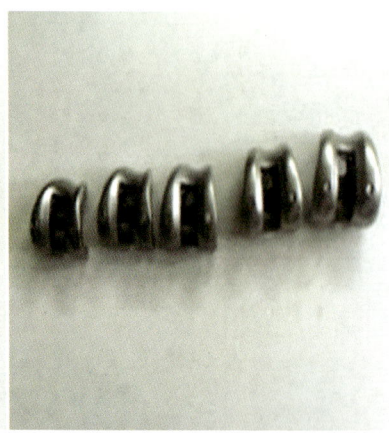

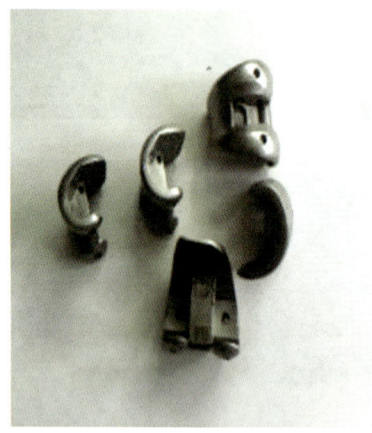 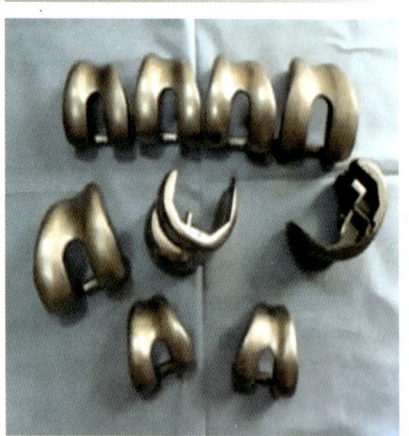

Femoral trials are available in many sizes and designs depending on the manufacturer.

COSTLIER DESIGNS HAVE A LARGER INVENTORY WITH MINIMAL SIZE AND THICKNESS INCREMENTS

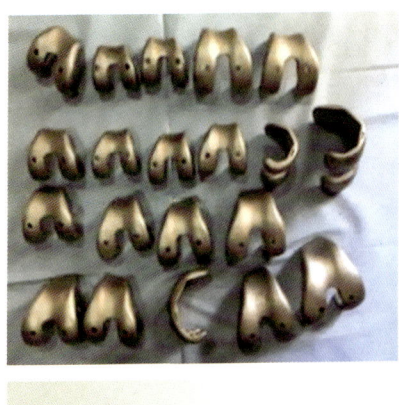
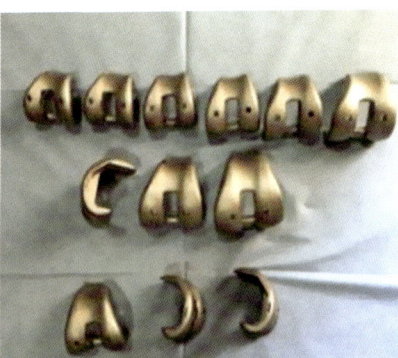
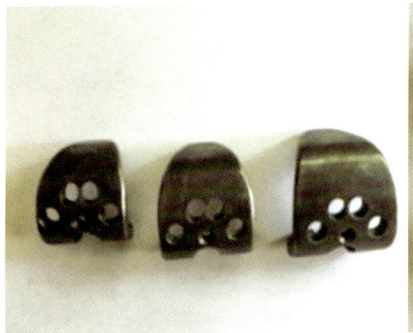
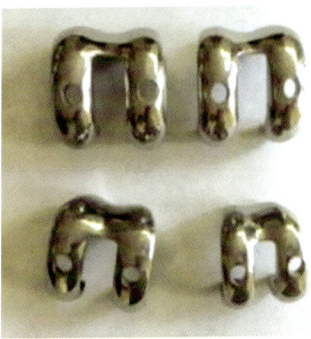

Early generation knees had universal (common left/right) femoral components in 3 or 4 sizes. Modern knees have 10 left and 10 right femoral components each in CR and CS designs.

TIBIAL TRIALS IN VARIOUS SIZES AND THICKNESSES

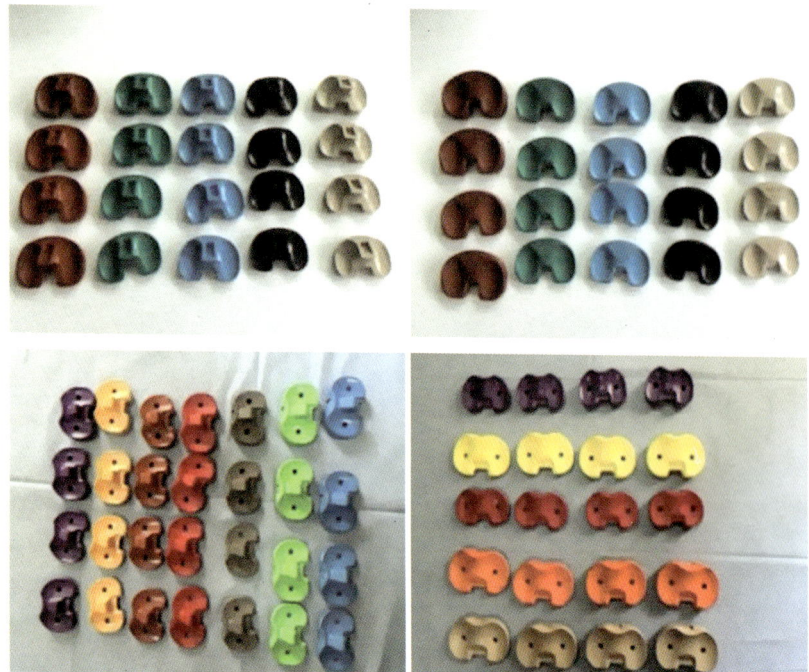

Each set comes with its own tibial trials, some in 1 mm difference, others in 2, 3 and 5 mm differences. Separate trials exist for CS and CR designs.

TIBIAL TRIALS IN VARIOUS SIZES AND THICKNESSES

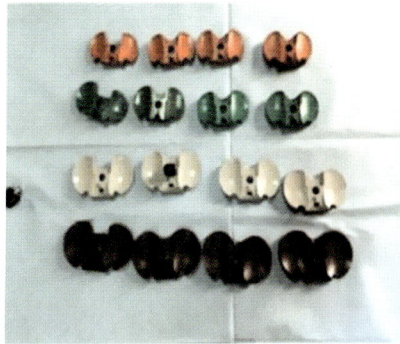
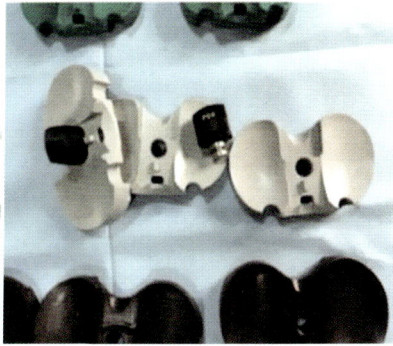
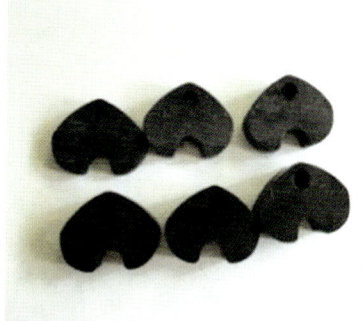
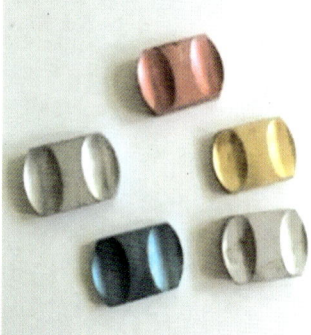

Some designs have pegs to convert CR trials to PS ones. Some have as few as 4 thicknesses, while others have up to 9.

TRIAL REDUCTION

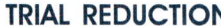

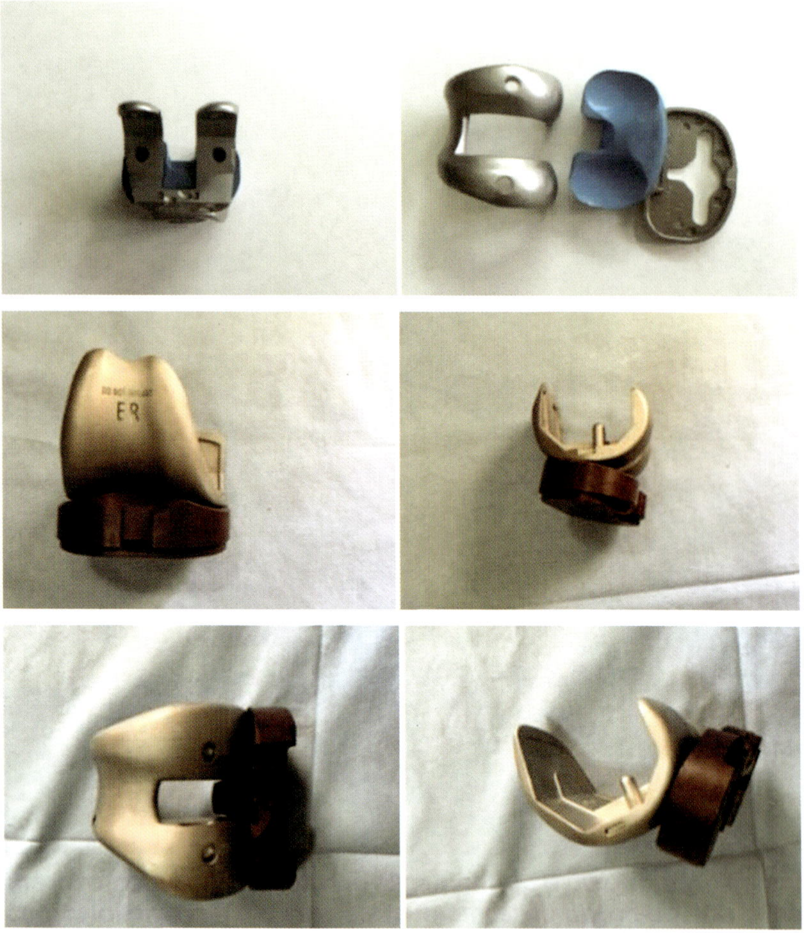

Different designs and their trial reductions.

THE TWO CLASSIC OLD DESIGNS

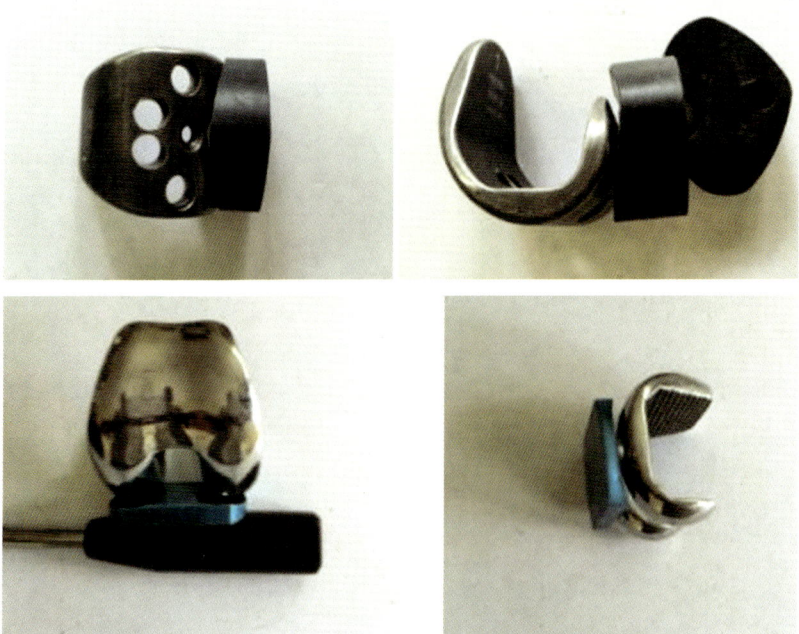

On top is Freeman Mark II and at bottom is IB I, both time-tested classic gold standard designs.

TIBIAL PREPARATION DEPENDS ON THE DESIGN

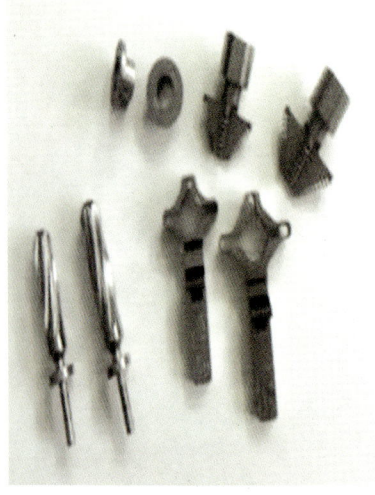 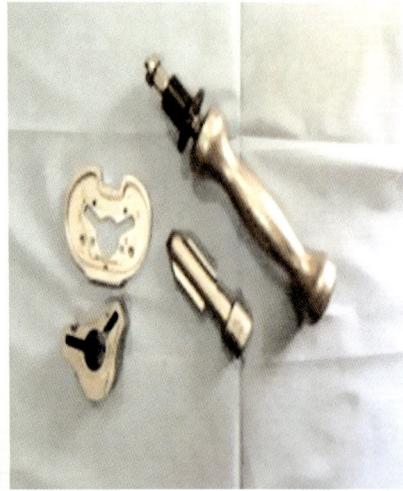

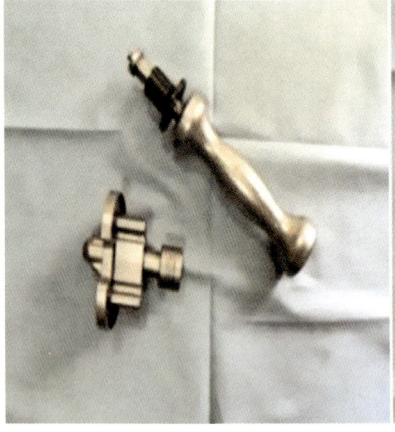 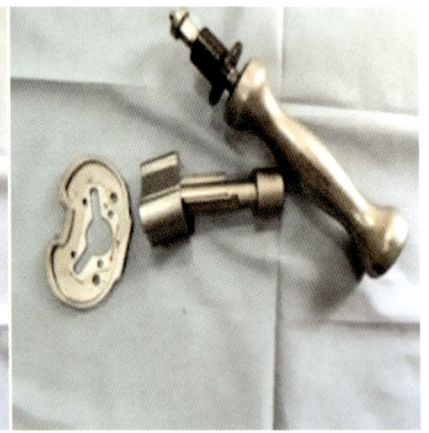

Tibial preparation depends upon type of implant, and includes guides, drills and fin cutters.

TIBIAL PREPARATION DEPENDS ON THE DESIGN

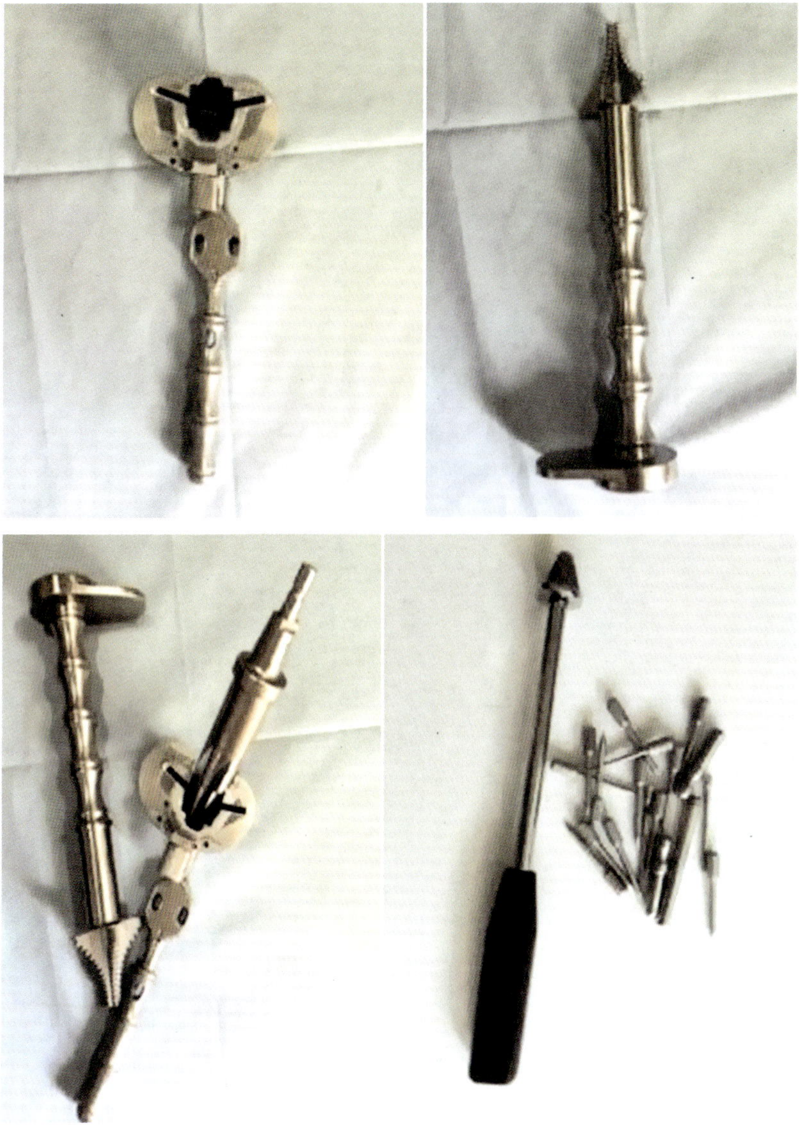

Other designs use box chisels or broaches to match the tibial metal-back.

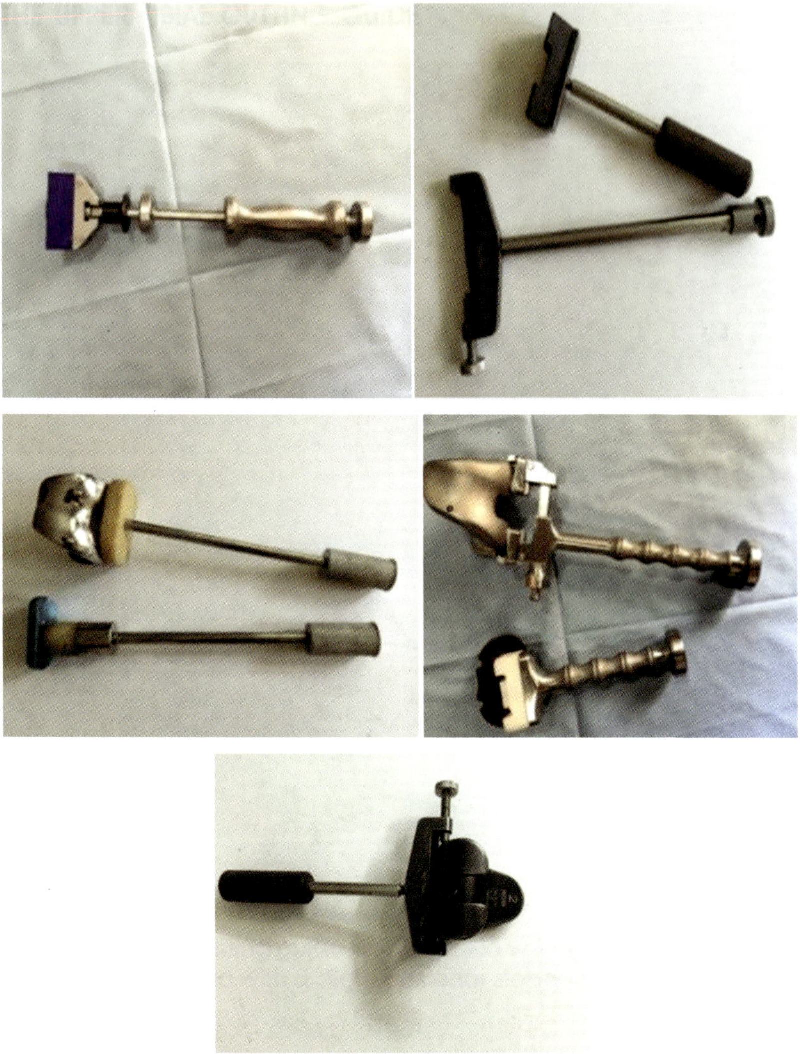

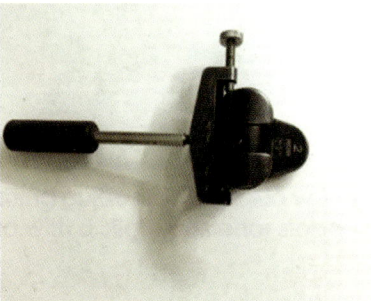

Impactors for femur and tibia.

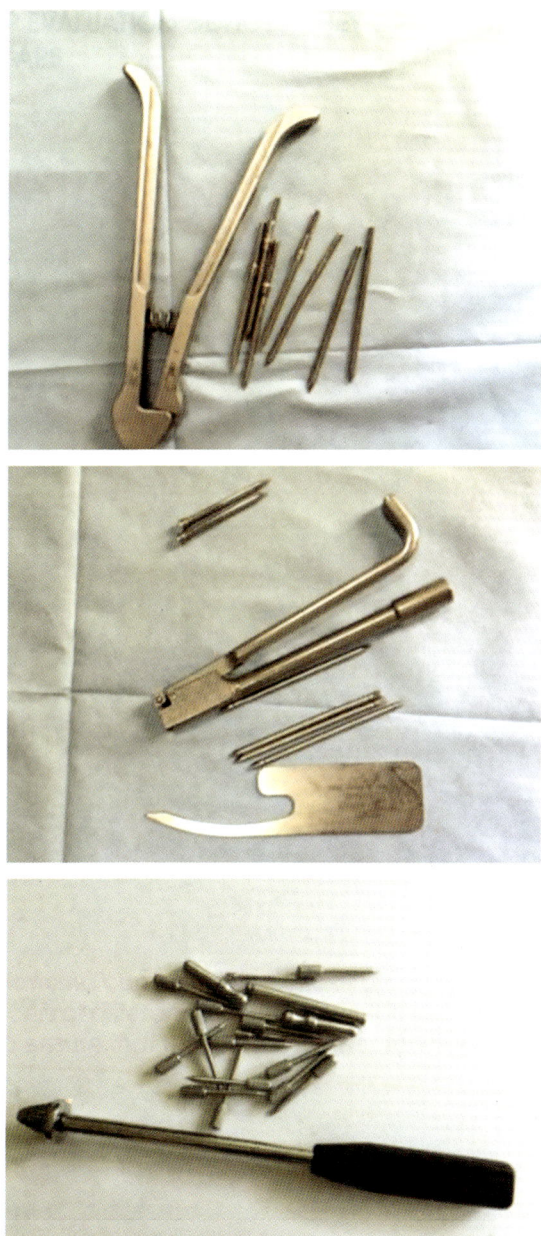

Block pins, extractors, angle strips, and other nuts and bolts.

Postoperative Treatment, Mobilization and Physiotherapy

The patient is shifted to the ward. In case a spinal anaesthetic is used, and for elderly patients with a history of prostatic or urinary symptoms, it is usual to catheterize in the theatre itself.

On the first postoperative day, the catheter is removed. If the patient has a good pain threshold, one can make him stand. Walking with a walking frame is started on day two and weight bearing is allowed up to pain tolerance.

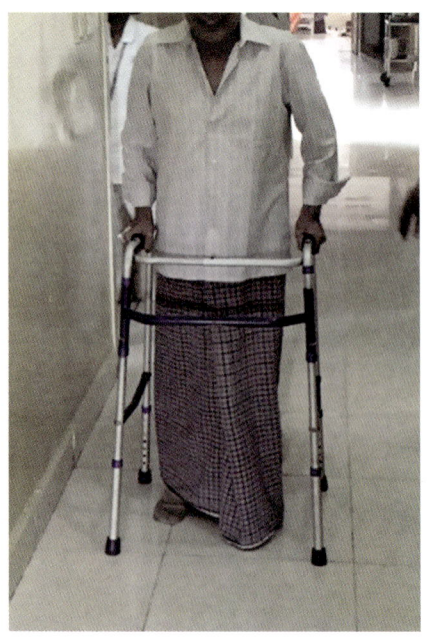

Patient is mobilized with a walker early.

Drain is removed on second or third day after it has stopped collecting.

The bandages are loosened on the fifth day and knee flexion is started. Using a smooth mica board with talcum powder on it, the patient is encouraged to rub the heel on the board allowing gradual flexion.

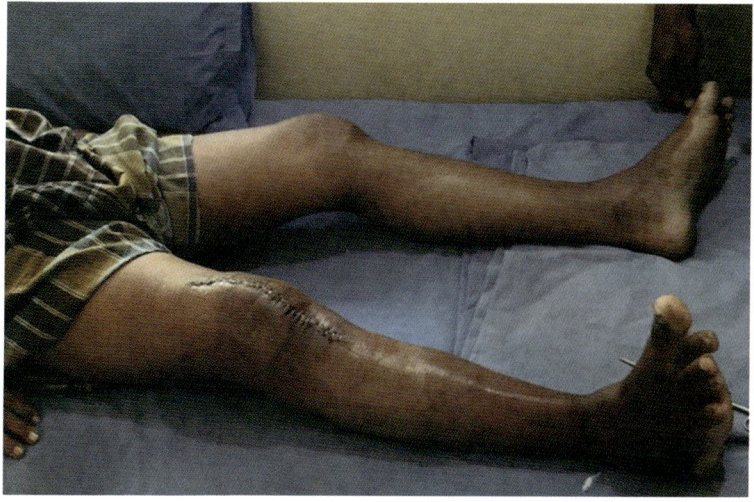

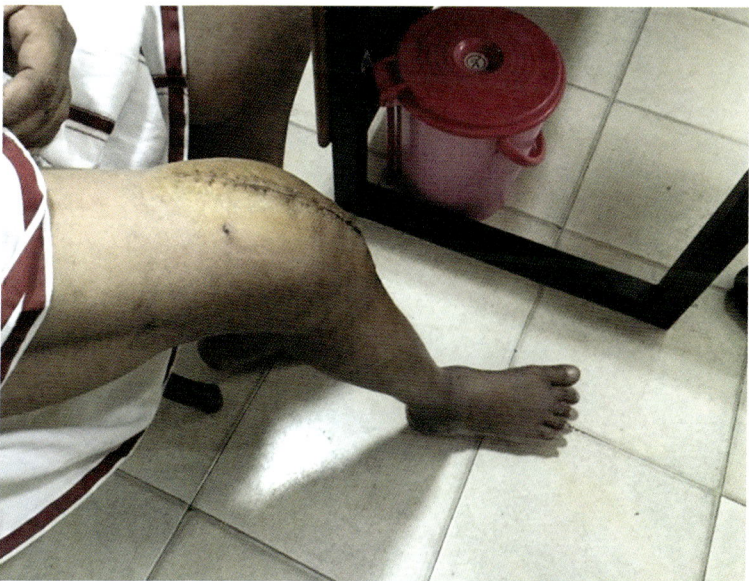

Knee flexion begins on the fifth day.

The patient climbs stairs on the fifth day and if comfortable, is discharged on the sixth. The operated knee is moved first while climbing downstairs and second when climbing upstairs.

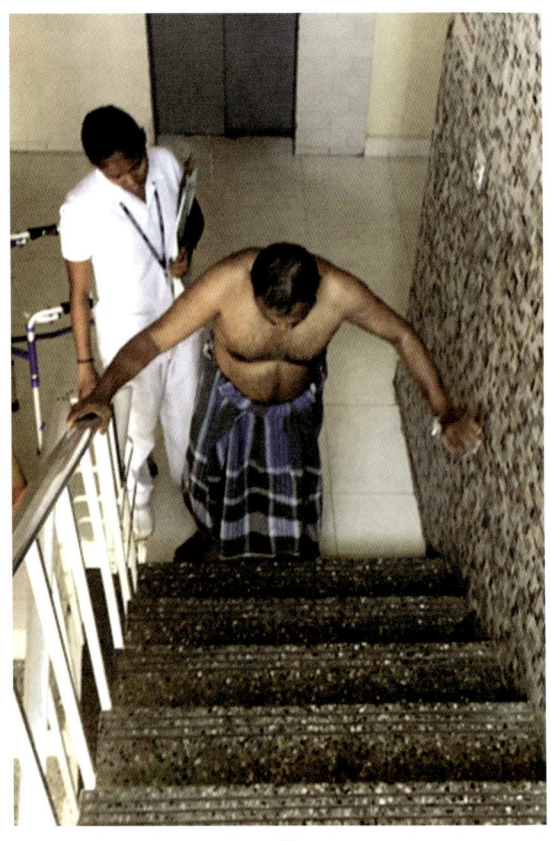

Most patients climb stairs on the fifth day and go home by the sixth.

By the tenth postoperative day, flexion of up to 90° is usually achieved.

Stitches are removed on the 14th day. One X-ray is taken immediate postoperative and another on the 14th day at suture removal.

The patient is called for follow-up at two months, six months and annually thereafter for clinical and radiographic evaluation.

Fixed Varus and Valgus Deformities

It is not possible normally to make a correct assessment of the degree of fixed varus or valgus preoperatively, because the patients' spasms, pain, and apprehension often exaggerate the deformity. Once the patient is anaesthetized, one can make a better assessment of the deformity.

In osteoarthritis, a varus deformity is much more common. Valgus deformity with associated predominant lateral

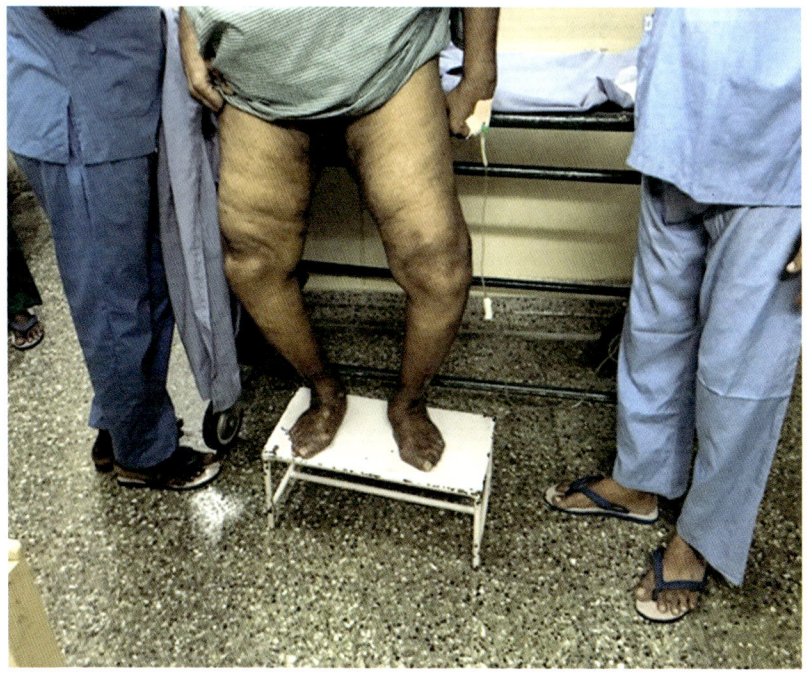

Gross varus on standing.

279

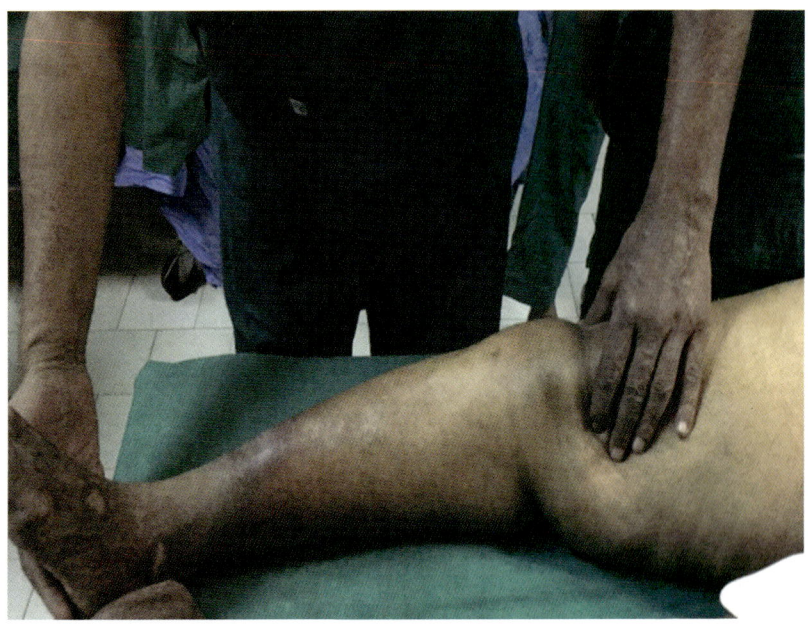

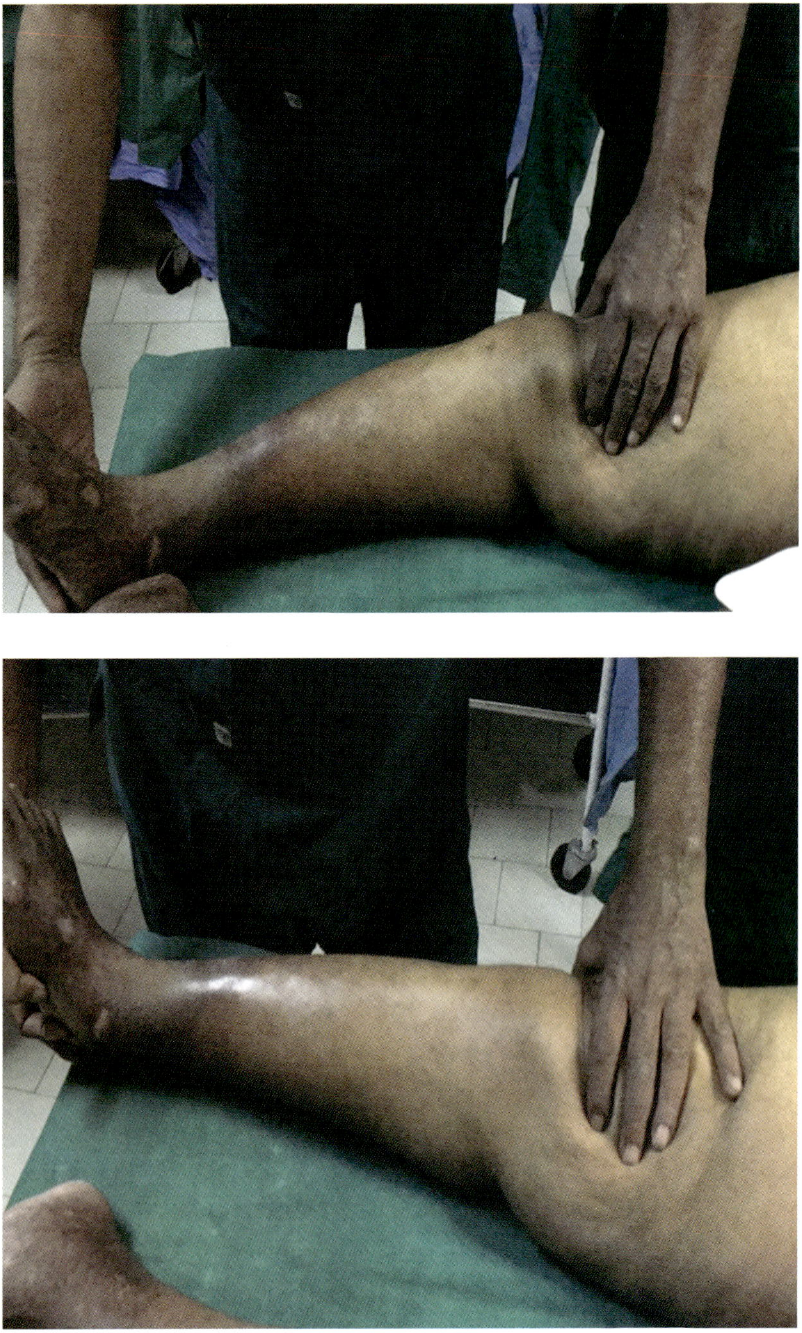

The deformity is correctable to a great extent under anaesthesia.

compartment arthritis may be seen in some OA knees but is not very common. An occasional patient may present with a varus on one side and valgus on the other (windswept knee).

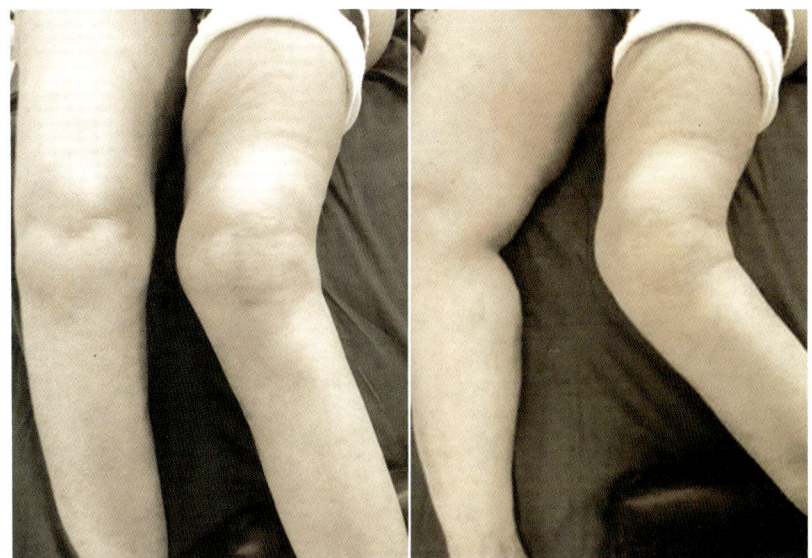

A characteristic windswept deformity.

Rheumatoids may present with varus or valgus with equal frequency!

In rheumatoid and ankylosed knees with a fixed flexion deformity, the varus or valgus component may get camouflaged. To plan for adequate and proper releases, one has to make a very careful assessment once the patient has been anaesthetized.

Fixed varus deformity: The deformity is normally due to a combination of both bony and soft tissue components. Overhanging osteophytes and bone loss contribute to a significant amount of deformity and as the patient bears weight, this deformity exaggerates, causing some laxity and elongation of the lateral structures. Over a period of time, the medial structures tend to contract and will result in a fixed varus deformity.

In rheumatoid arthritis, contracture of the ligaments is less common that in osteoarthritis. But one thing is certain. Even in the most severe deformities, the ligaments do not actually contract too much and we should never cut them. Simple erasure from the bony attachments with a sharp chisel or periosteal elevator will provide sufficient laxity to allow for correction of deformities.

The following steps need to be followed to correct the fixed varus deformity:

1. Exposure as described in the previous chapter.
2. All the osteophytes from the femur are removed using a nibbler. One must ensure that after this is done, the true confines for the distal femur are visible.
3. All the osteophytes from the tibia are now removed as far as the exposure will allow.

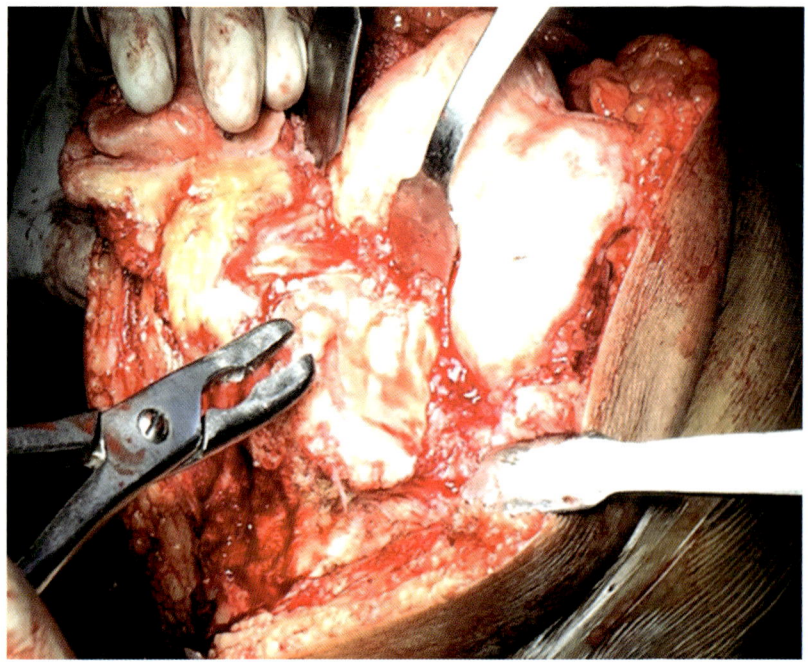

Osteophytes from both tibia and femur are removed.

4. Using the knife, a linear incision is made extending from the tibial tuberosity until the upper lip of tibia. This incision is bone deep; the medial structures are elevated sub-periostealy from the medial to posterior using a cutting diathermy, sharp chisel, an osteotome or a broad periosteum elevator.

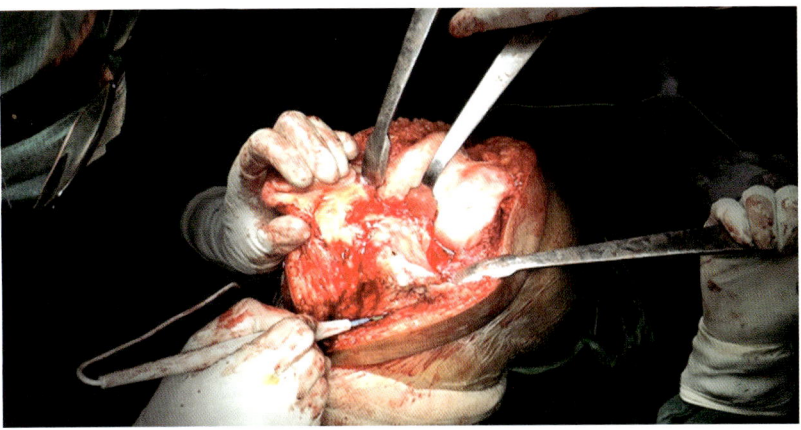

Medial structures are elevated as a single flap.

5. The assistant rotates the limb externally as the release is performed until the tibia is fully externally rotated and the posterior cruciate attachment is visible!

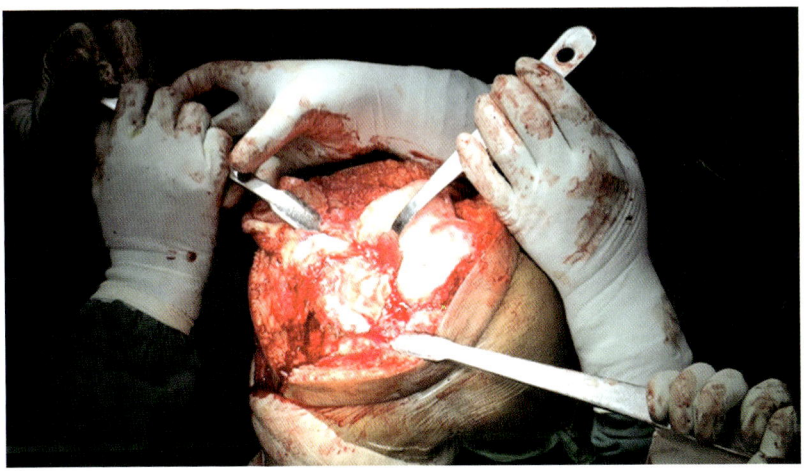

External rotation of the leg translates the tibia forward.

6. At this stage one can identify the remaining osteophytes from the upper border of the medial aspect of tibia and start nibbling them.

7. Sometimes the osteophytes may be overhanging so much that the tibia itself may seem to be very wide. One may have to chisel off these and get a proper picture of the actual size of the tibia!

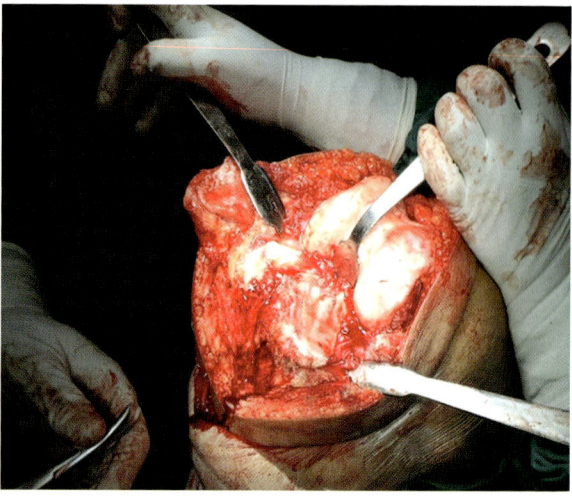

Only after osteophyte removal is the true extent of tibial defect identifiable.

8. The knee is straightened again and checked if the varus is corrected. One must be able to get a 5° to 7° of valgus. This step is very important and should proceed the first bony cut or interference! If the knee is still in varus or just about neutral, we go to step 9.

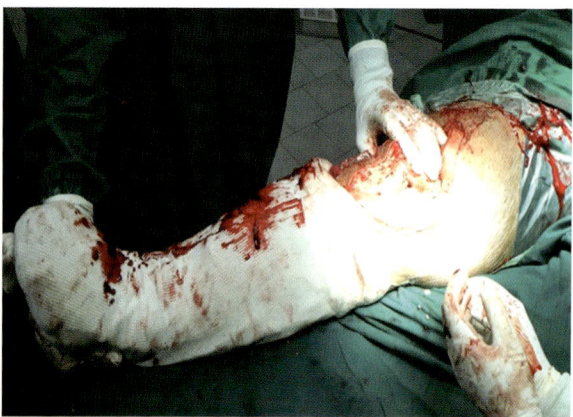

Both flexion and varus deformities should be correctable at this stage.

9. If the knee cannot still be brought into neutral, the next step is to release the posterior cruciate! The assistant keeps on externally rotating the limb so as to bring the taut posterior cruciate into view.

10. The next step depends upon the type of the tibial implant that one plans to use. If using a posterior stabilized implant, one can resect the posterior cruciate ligament with impunity and be at ease.

11. If one is using a posterior cruciate retaining prosthesis, it is better to scrape the posterior cruciate off the back of the tibia!

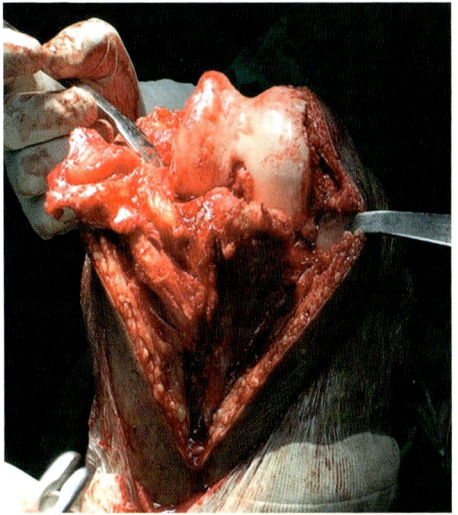

The posterior cruciate is visualized by anterior translation of tibia.

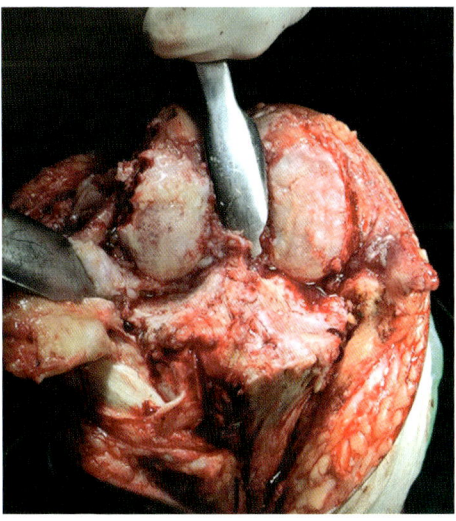

The posterior cruciate is resected and the knee is pulled forward.

12. Many question the wisdom of using a posterior cruciate sparing design in a knee with a deformity severe enough to need a posterior cruciate release. But my personal experience shows that if I erase the attachment of the posterior cruciate using a small sharp chisel, but without actually cutting it, I do get a reasonable amount of correction of the varus deformity; postoperative bracing is seldom needed!

13. On rare occasions, it may be found that even after the marathon efforts described above, it may not be possible to correct the fixed varus deformity! Very early descriptions in the literature, especially by Insall and Freeman, have advocated oblique cuts to the bones to compensate for the residual deformities.

14. But it has been proved time and again that a well-balanced knee is the key to a successful arthroplasty! Bone cuts *cannot and will not* compensate for inadequate soft tissue releases! At the cost of repetition, one must stress that when a resident starts knee replacements, he must not be allowed to buzz along with a saw until all the soft tissues are balanced!

15. *So what does one do if even all the above procedures have failed to get the proper correction?* The controversial answer is a

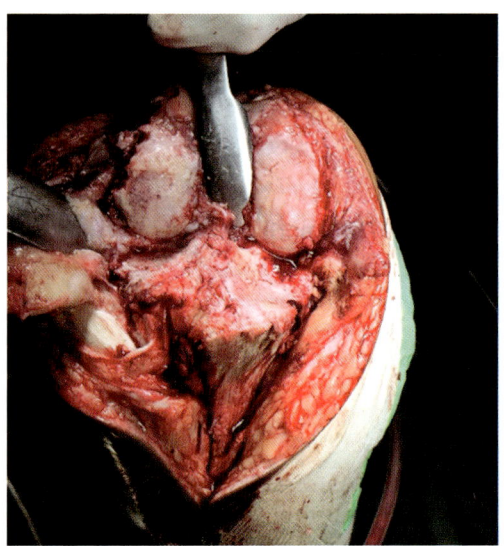

Resection of the medial capsular sleeve to correct final varus deformity.

resection of the medial capsular sleeve! A transverse incision is made in the sleeve distal to the pes anserinus and a valgus strain is applied to the knee! The entire medial flap is erased and allowed to slide proximally, which will invariably correct all the residual varus deformity!

16. One must not accidentally cut the tibial collateral ligament at the joint line level, as this would surely lead to a joint laxity that no bracing or immobilization will correct! As Dr Sancheti always remarks, "Stay close to the bone! Erase and do not cut. Use a periosteum elevator, not a knife and you will be safe!"

17. If all the above steps have been diligently followed, one must invariably have corrected the fixed varus deformity and proceed towards a proper component placement!

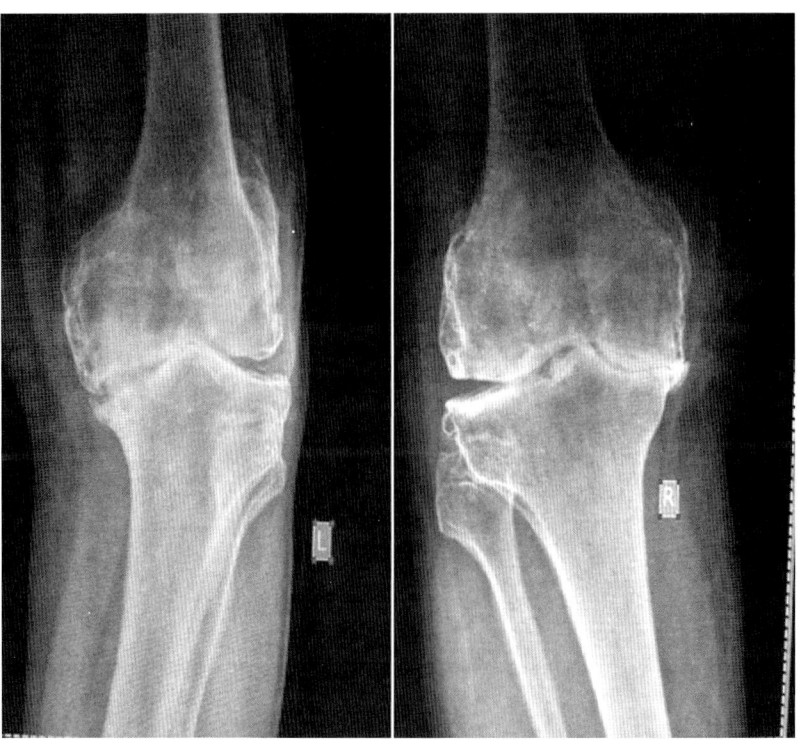

Bilateral varus deformities due to OA knee.

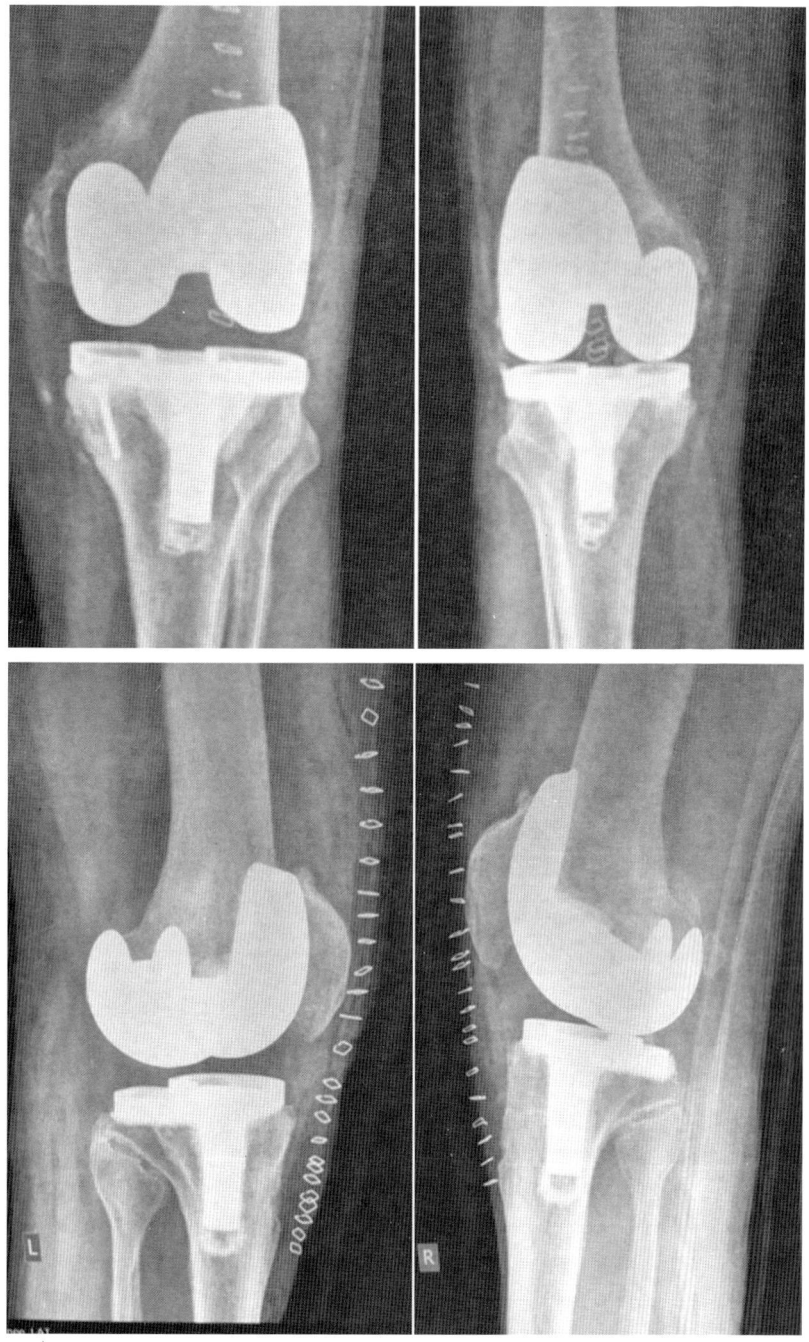

Full correction of the varus knee shown previously.

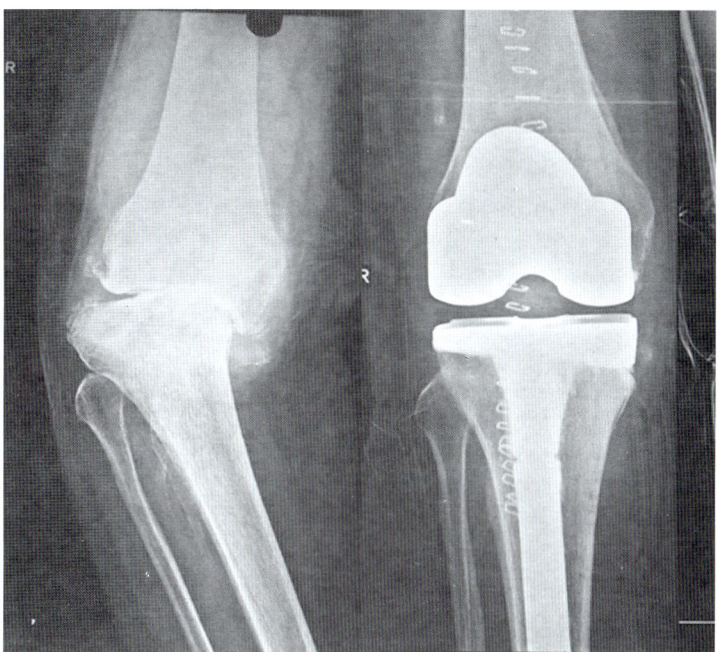

Another case of severe valgus, treated by medial wedges and stemmed tibia.

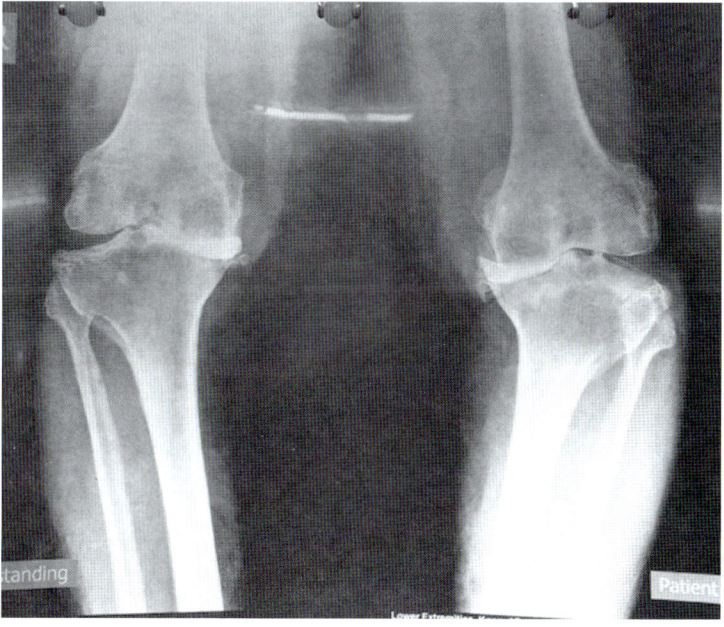

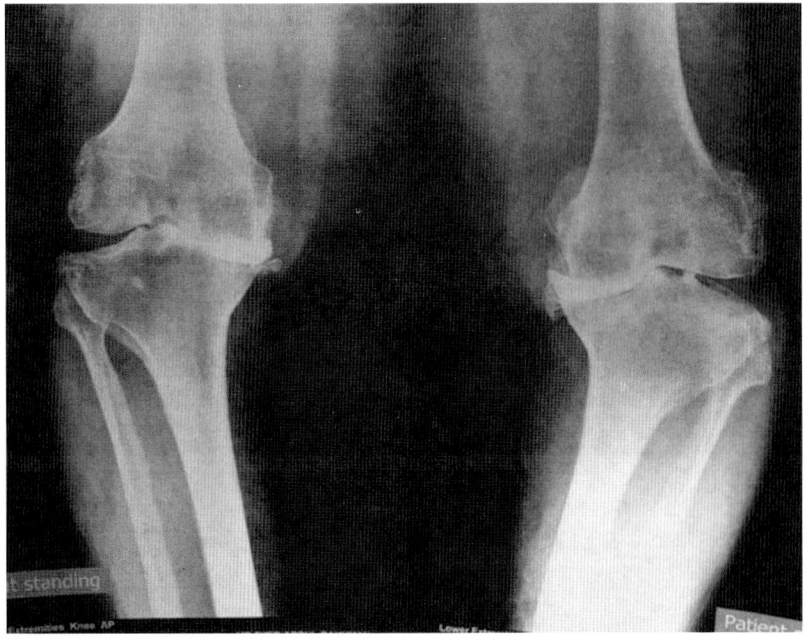

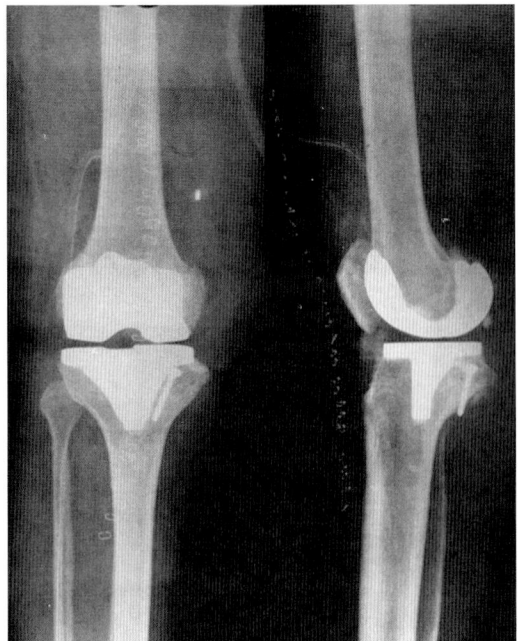

A very gross varus managed with graft and screw, and using an 8 mm insert, avoiding a tibial stem or wedges.

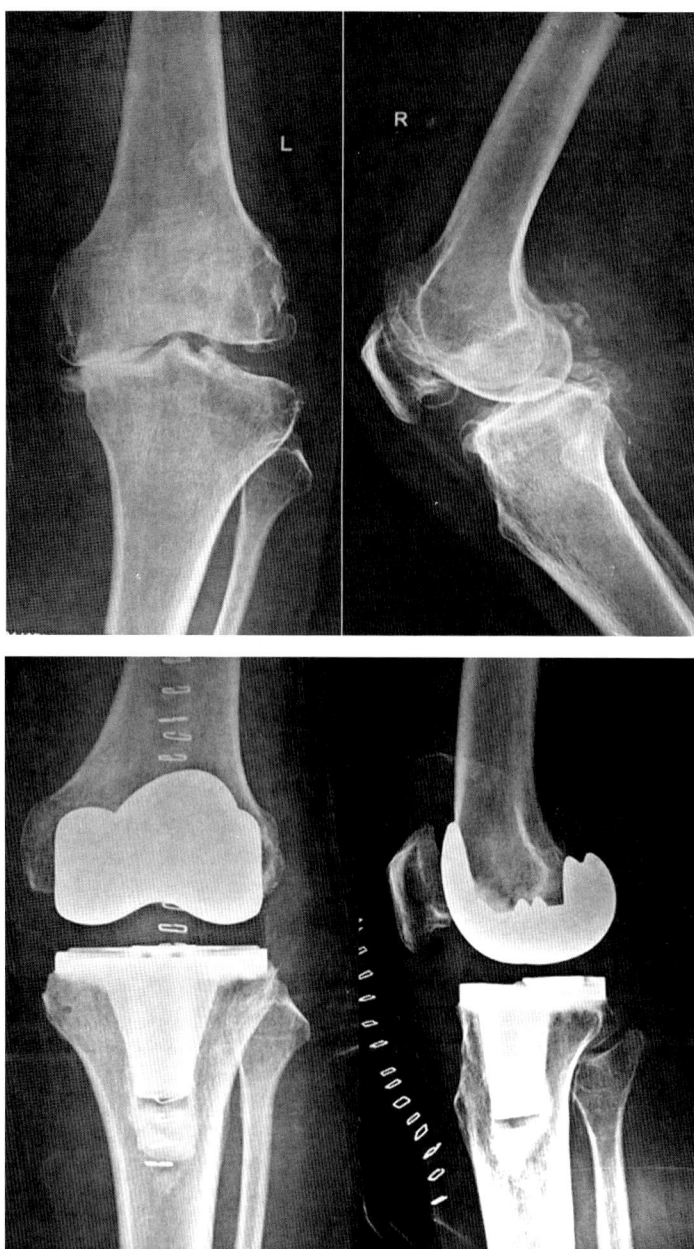

Another knee in gross varus and flexion managed by soft tissue releases and a thin HDPE insert, without wedges or tibial stem.

Fixed valgus deformity: Slightly less common than the former, fixed valgus deformity is commonly caused by a lateral soft tissue contracture associated with a laxity of the medial structures. In many valgus knees, there may be an extensive laxity of the medial side and an associated subluxation or dislocation of the patella. In all cases of valgus, it is better to do a proper release and soft tissue balance to achieve a rectus knee before planning for bone cuts. The sequence of events towards correction of a fixed valgus deformity is:

1. Exposure as described in the previous chapter.
2. All the osteophytes from the femur are removed using a nibbler, after which one must ensure that the true confines for the distal femur are visible.
3. All the osteophytes from the tibia as far as the exposure will allow are now removed. An internal rotation of the tibia will allow for visualization of the posterolateral aspect of upper tibia and a full and clear view of all the osteophytes.

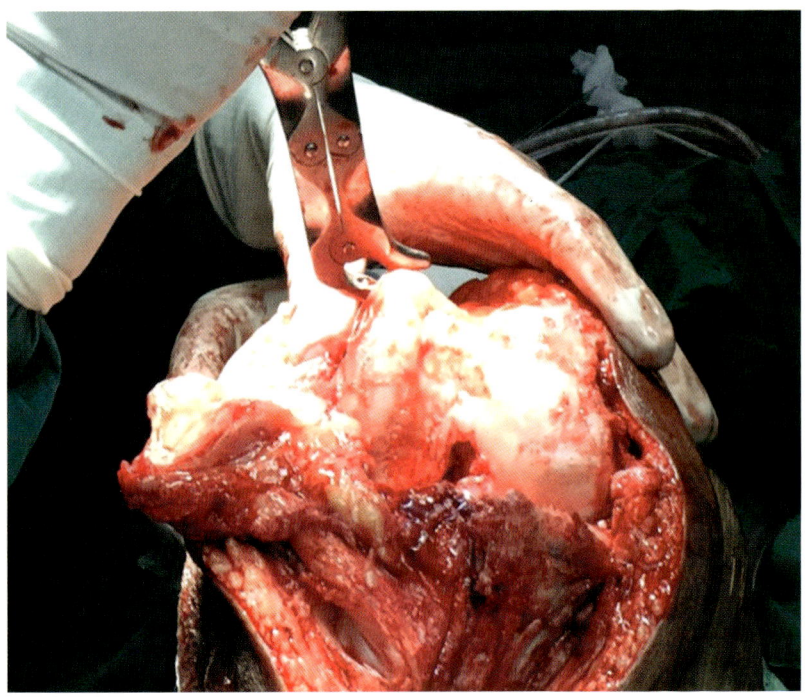

Internal rotation exposes the lateral side and facilitates removal of osteophytes.

4. The patellar fat pad is now excised, and all the capsular attachment from the lateral part of upper tibia is scraped using a sharp chisel or a periosteum elevator.
5. All the attachments and adhesions between the iliotibial band and the lateral tibial plateau are detached. This will allow for freeing of the lateral structures.

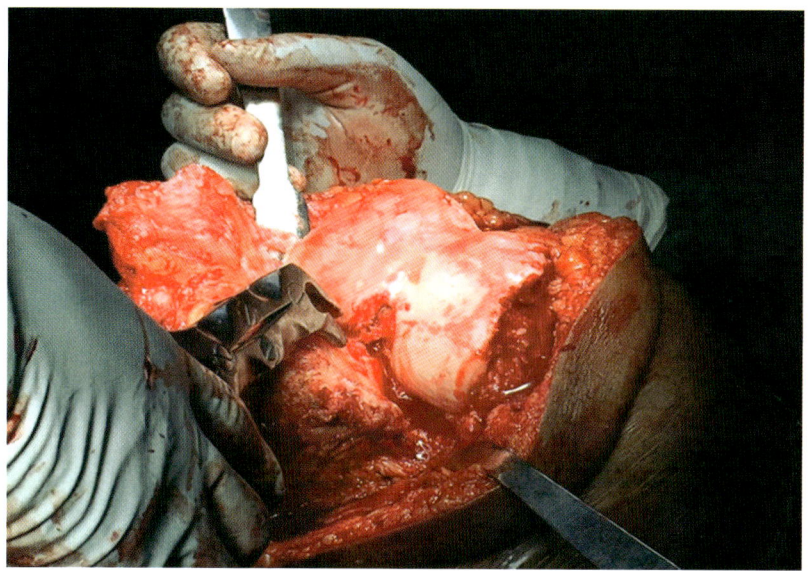

Additional lateral releases are performed.

6. The knee is now extended and a varus strain applied to see if the deformity is correctable and if the knee can be brought to a rectus position.
7. If the above is not enough, then the iliotibial band is released. With the knee flexed and a varus strain applied, the band stands out as a taut chord and is palpable from inside the knee. Using a sharp knife, it can be cleanly cut.
8. If the above procedures are still inadequate to allow for a full valgus correction, a tenotomy of the popliteus tendon and the lateral collateral ligament is done.
9. In all valgus corrections, the lateral popleteal nerve is at risk; hence it is a good idea to visualize it near the fibular head, release it from its sheath and allow it to slide to a comfortable position.

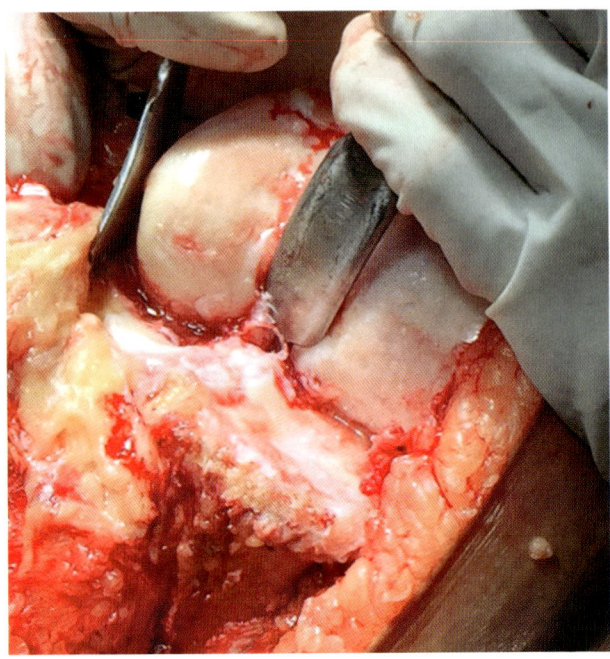

Precise and adequate soft tissue releases will correct the most stubborn deformities.

10. The knee is again extended to check if the deformity is corrected and if a rectus position is achievable. The soft tissue balance can be checked either by the use of spacers, tensioners, or by two lamina spreaders to see if the gaps are equal on both sides.

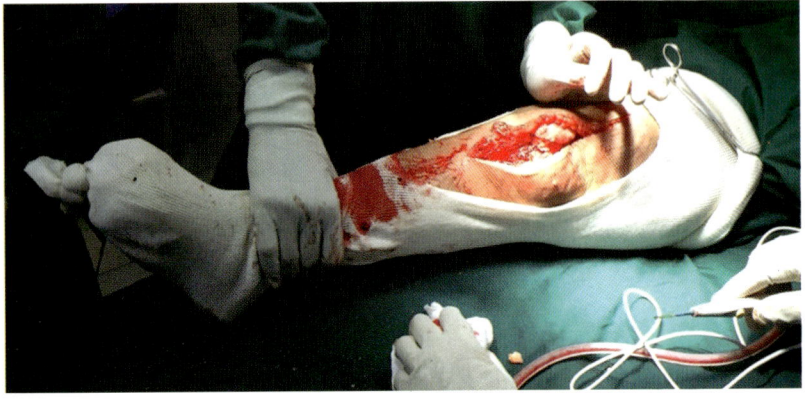

The knee is extended and brought to neutral.

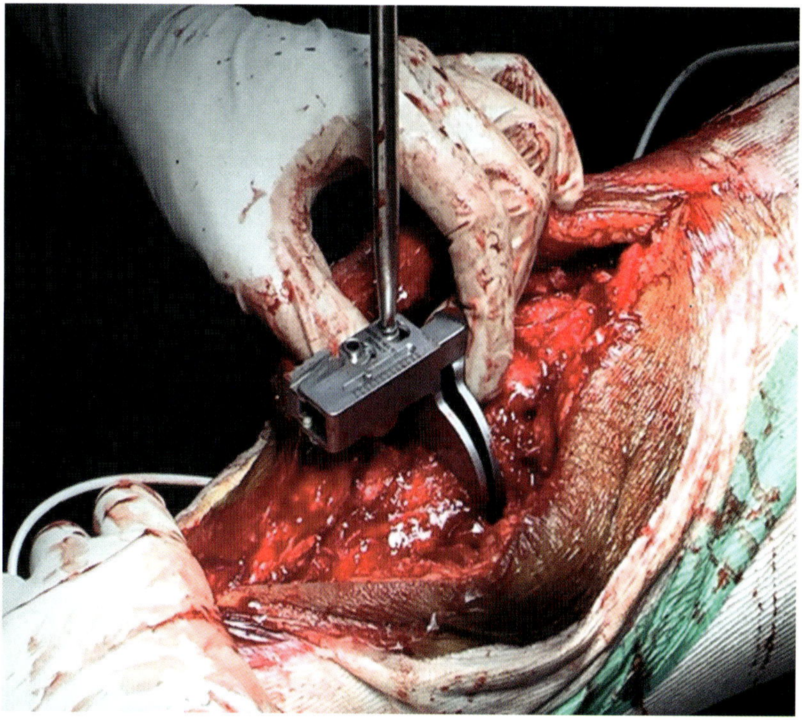

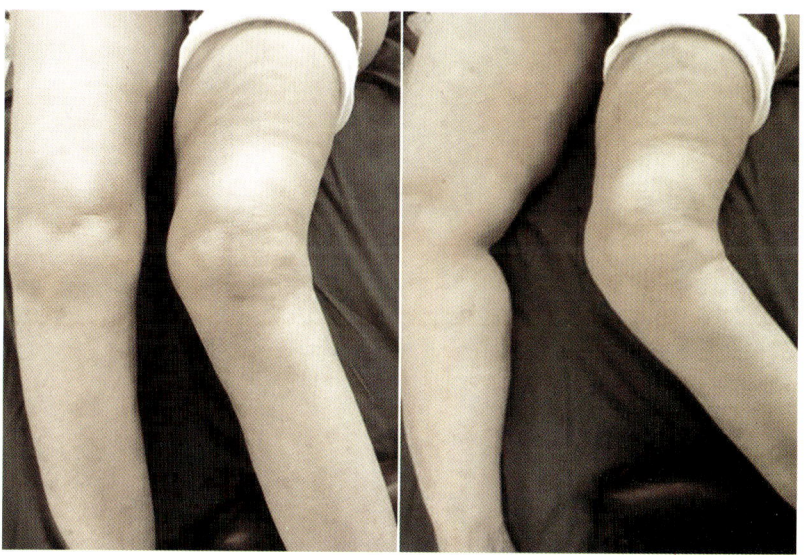

Tensioner will evaluate the degree of deformity correction.

A characteristic windswept deformity.

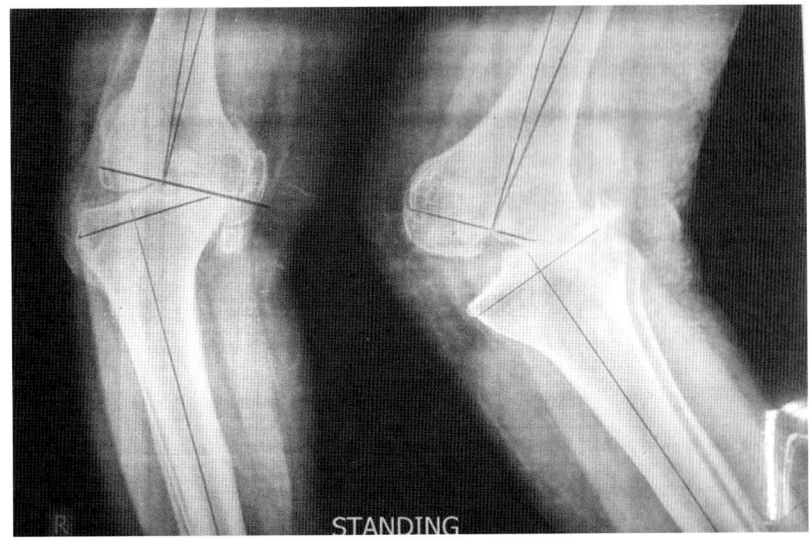

X-ray of the case.

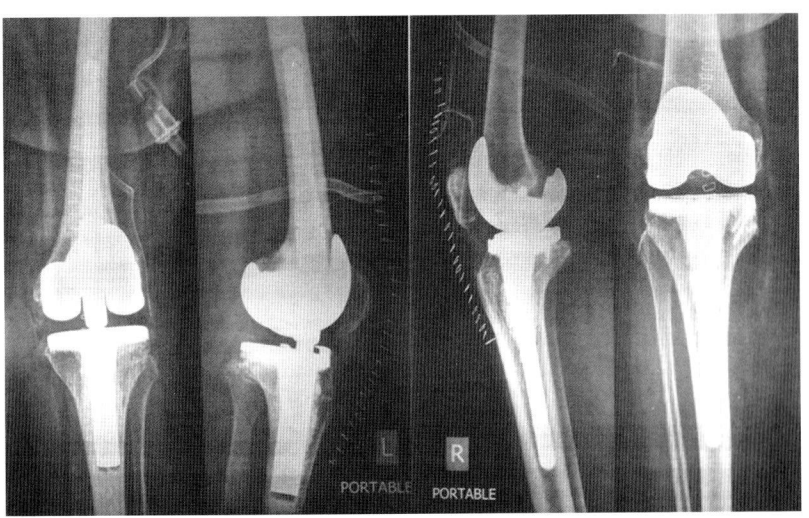

Full restoration of both knees to the correct axis.

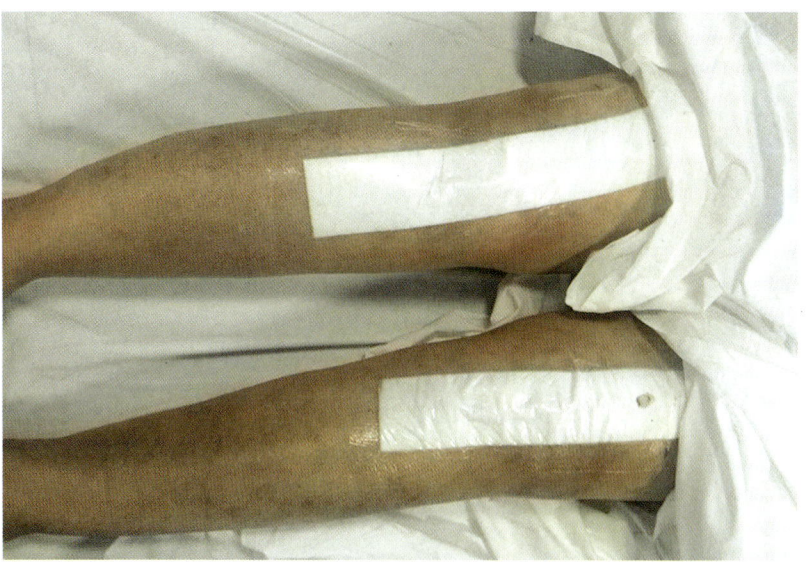

Final clinical picture.

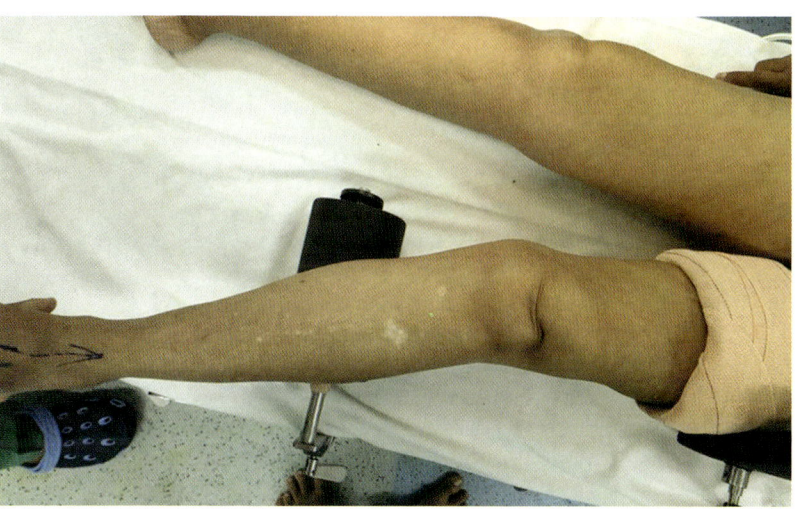

Another case of valgus deformity of the knee.

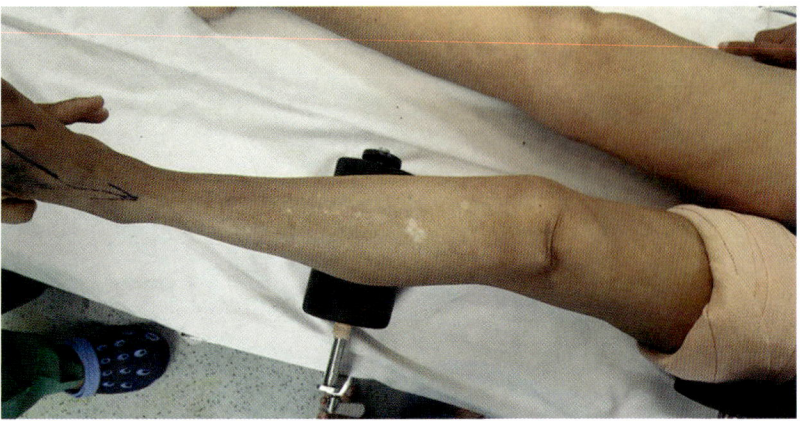

Due to ligamentous laxity, the knee is fully correctable under anaesthesia.

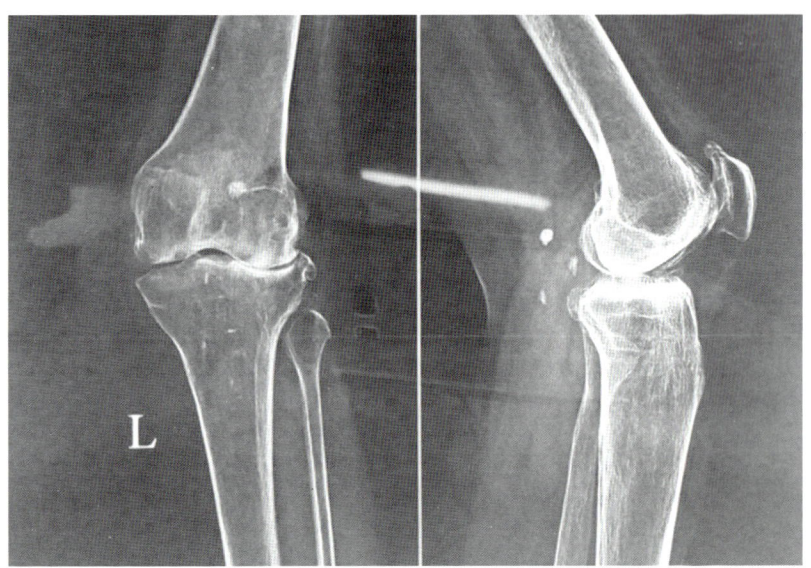

The gross osteoporosis of RA can be appreciated.

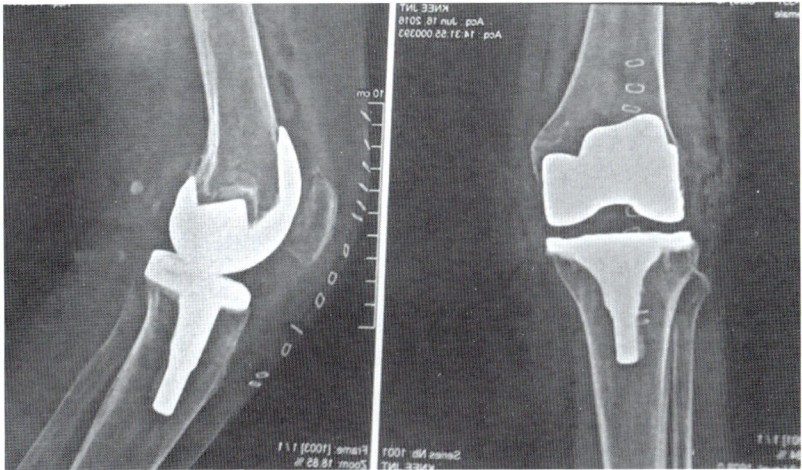

The components and cuts are correct giving a proper correction.

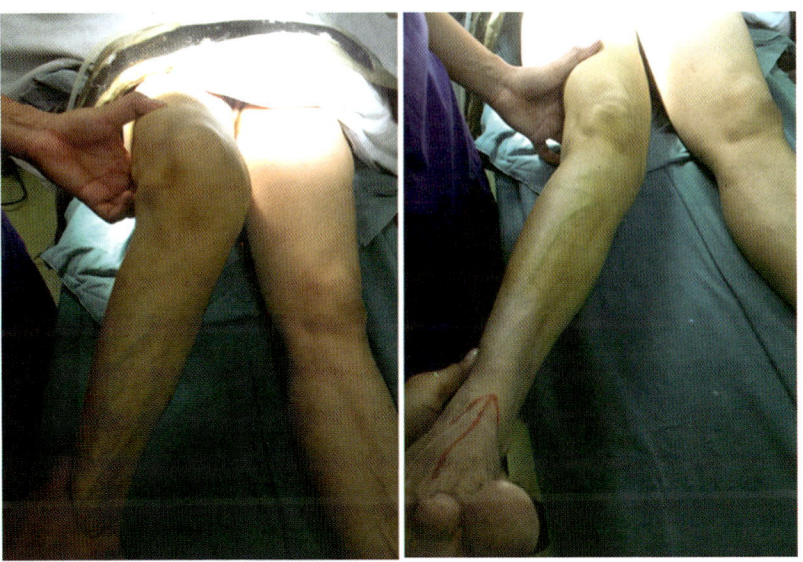

A grossly unstable knee with valgus deformity.

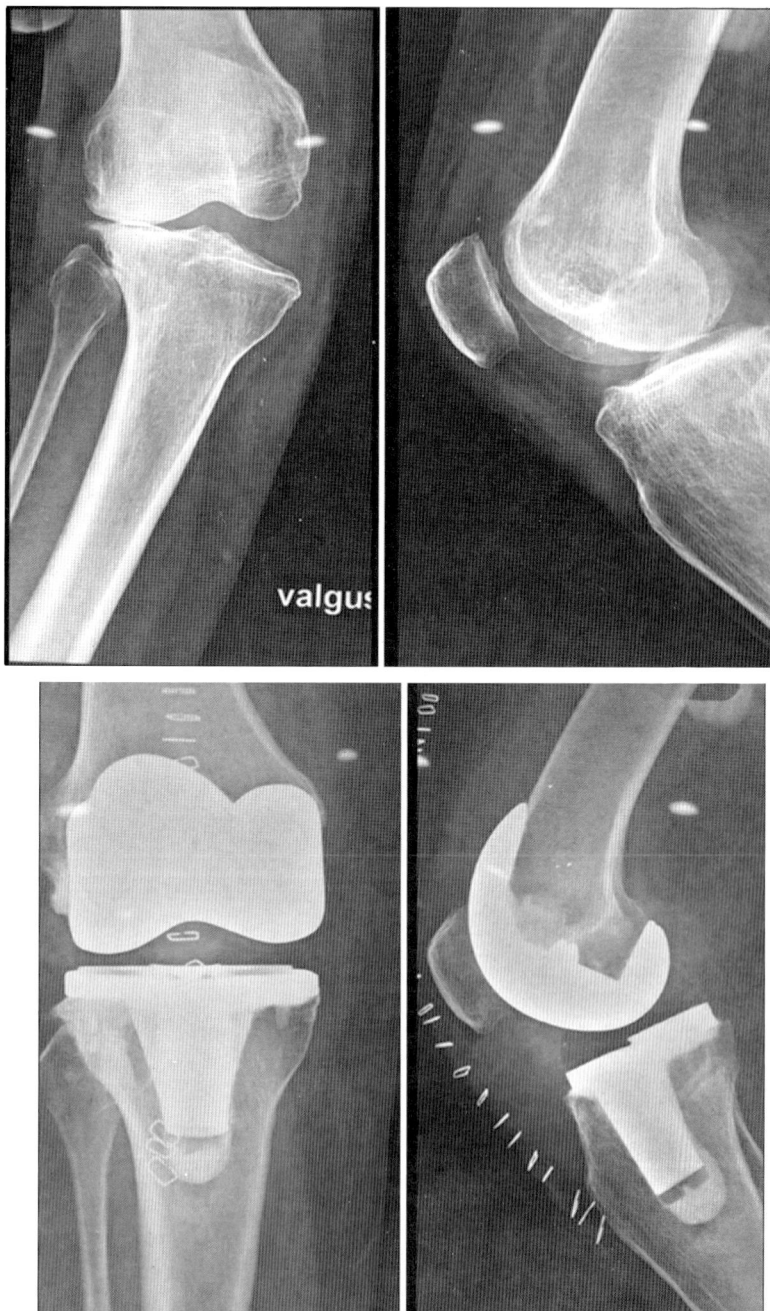

valgus

X-ray immediately postreplacement.

Tricks and Tips with Mediolateral Deformities

1. After the extensive releases mentioned above in severely deformed knees, the gap created may be fairly large. It is thus mandatory that all sizes of tibial thickness are available to get a good fit.
2. If the deformity is very gross, one can do a limited release on the affected side and perform a reefing or tightening of the opposite side. Theoretically this is a possibility that finds use specifically when one finds that the inventory in the theatre lacks extra thick tibial components.
3. Extreme care should be taken in rheumatoid knees whilst performing releases.
4. Be very careful of the lateral popliteal nerve with valgus releases.
5. All valgus knees will need a lateral popliteal release to improve and optimize the patellar tracking.

Fixed Flexion and Recurvatum Deformities

Deformities in the anterioposterior plane manifest as a fixed flexion or a recurvatum deformity. A fixed flexion is much more common than a recurvatum. Most rheumatoids who come for an arthroplasty in our country are severe enough with marked flexion deformities.

Fixed flexion deformity: This is defined as a situation in which there is a block to full extension. The deformity as seen in the clinic may appear markedly more than actual because of a painful hamstring spasm that will keep the knee in flexion for a few degrees more than the actual flexion deformity. The following are the steps for correction of a fixed flexion deformity:

1. The true extent of the flexion deformity is determined under anaesthesia by passively straightening the knee.
2. The knee is exposed as described in the previous chapter.
3. Once the patella is deflected laterally, the superior surface of the tibia is visualized. In most cases with a fixed flexion deformity, there is a large anterior osteophyte which is the main culprit. This is removed with a nibbler or a sharp chisel.
4. The knee is straightened to check if it can be fully extended. In most osteoarthritis with less than 15° of fixed flexion, this manoeuvre alone will straighten the knee. However if it is still not possible to straighten the knee, then the following steps are taken.
5. The tibia is first externally rotated, next, using a sharp chisel or a periosteum elevator, the posterior capsular adhesions are scraped from the posterior tibia. Then the leg is

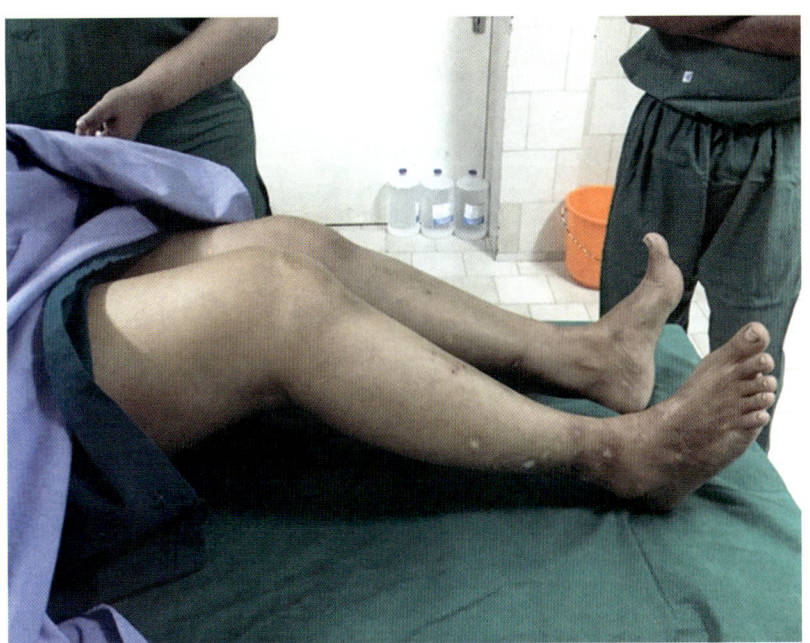

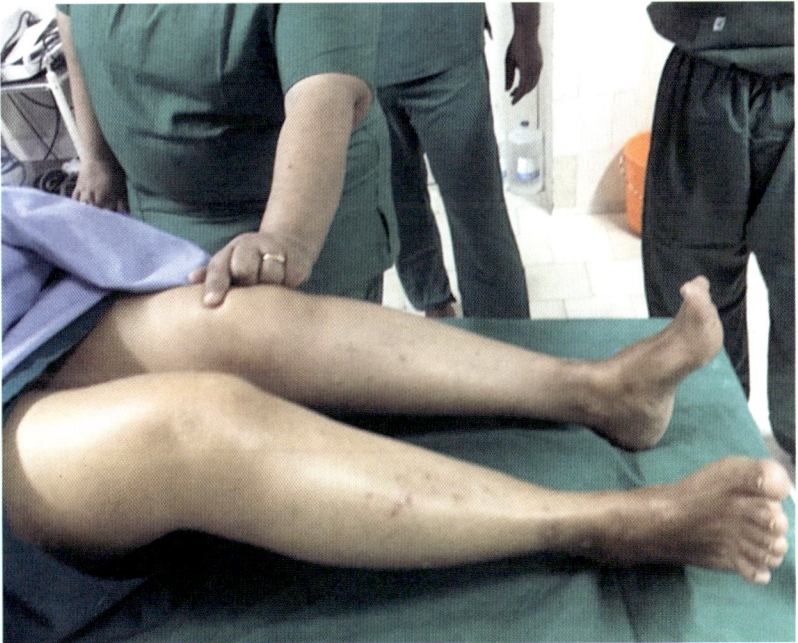

Stretching the knee under anaesthetic will reveal the true extent of fixed flexion deformities.

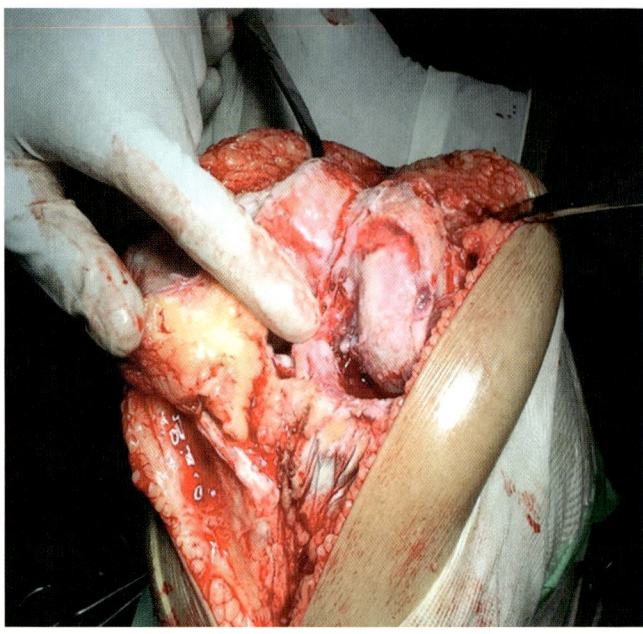

The large anterior osteophyte on the tibia is the main culprit for causing fixed flexion deformities.

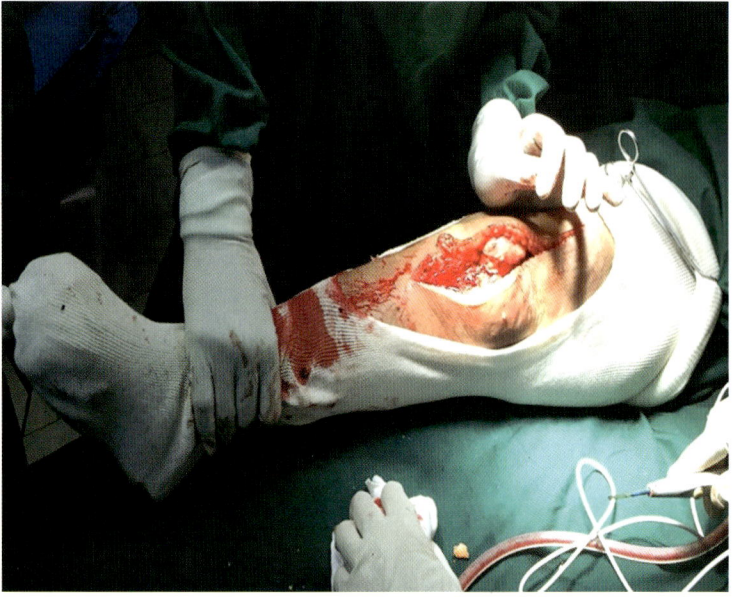

The knee is straightened to see if the deformity is fully corrected.

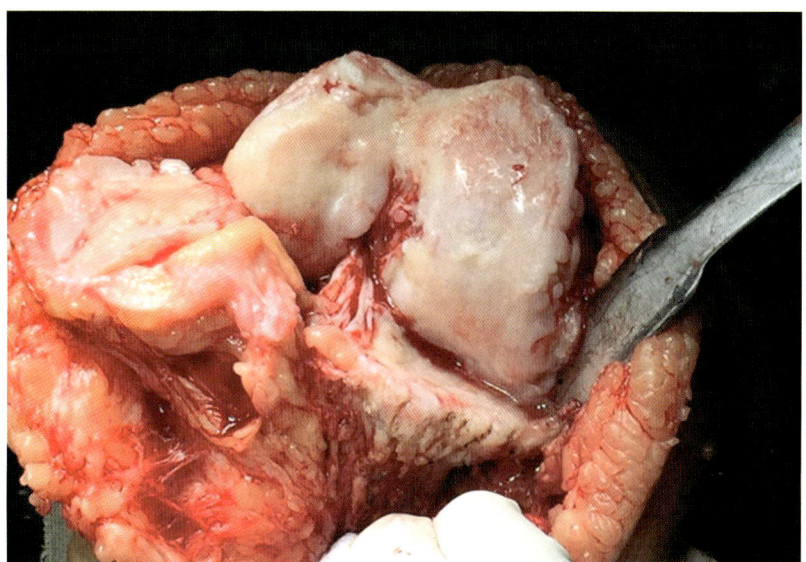

Additional releases are now performed.

internally rotated, and using a Homman retractor placed beneath the patella, the posteriolateral corner of the upper tibia is visualized. The capsular adhesions from this part are now scraped.

6. The knee is straightened to see if a full correction and full extension are achievable.

7. If the above is not adequate, one has to excise the posterior cruciate ligament. If this is done, it is imperative that a posterior stabilized knee is used to avoid instability.

8. If the flexion deformity persists despite resecting the posterior cruciate, one has to erase both the medial and lateral heads of the gastrocnemius. The knee is flexed beyond 130° and the two heads are palpated. Using a periosteum elevator, the two heads are erased. This step can also be performed after the lower femoral and upper tibial cuts to allow easier access to the heads of gastrocnemius.

9. Any residual deformity is corrected by a resection of the posterior capsule. This is done by hyperflexing the knee and allowing the popliteal vessels to fall back. A curved artery forceps is introduced behind the tibia and brought

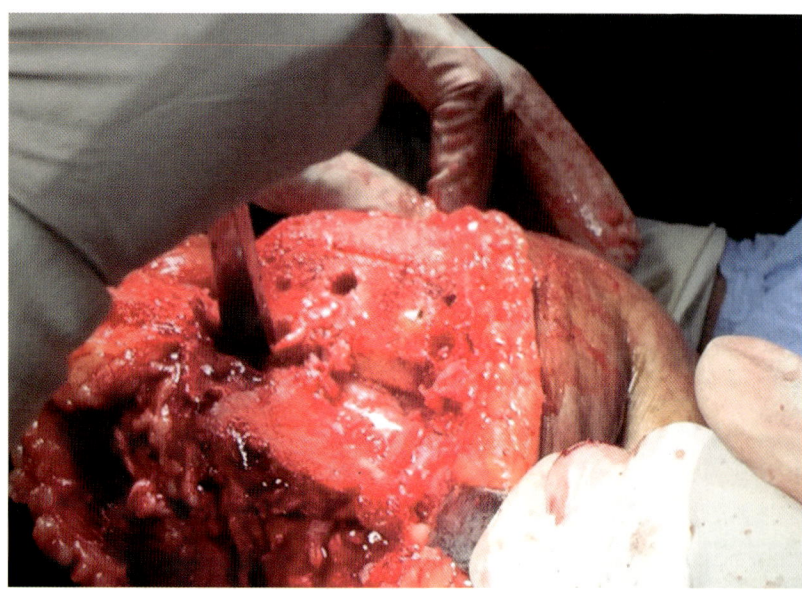

Gastrocnemius head is released after first bone cuts for residual flexion deformity.

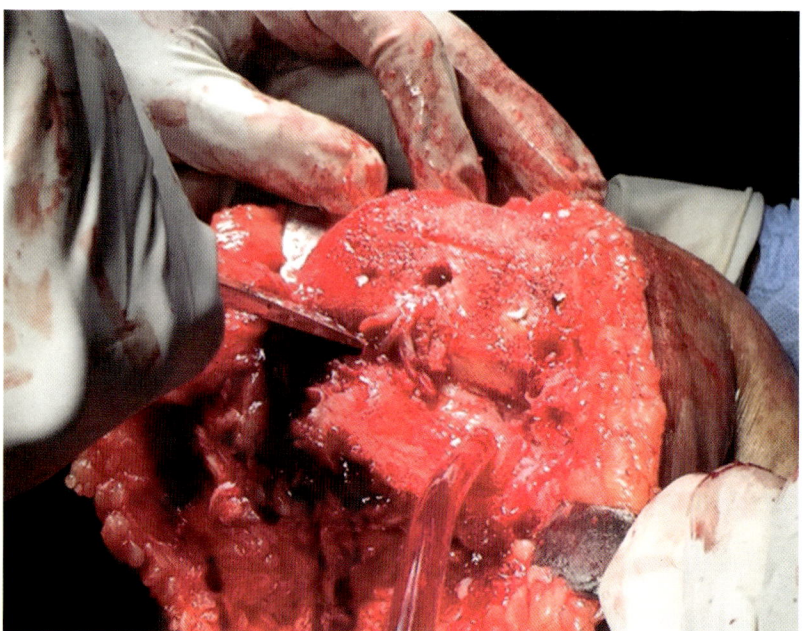

Posterior capsular resection in very severe flexion deformity. This can only be done after the first bone cuts to get space.

out on the other side. This will protect the vessels. The capsule is now resected.

10. The knee is straightened and the deformity correction is assessed. In majority of cases, this is enough to get a full correction. However, if full correction is not achievable, one must resect an extra amount of distal femur. This will result in a superior displacement of the femoral component and will lead to a laxity in the quadriceps mechanism. The resulting extensor lag will take a few months to disappear. This final step is necessary only if the fixed flexion deformity is more than 60° or in nonambulant patients.

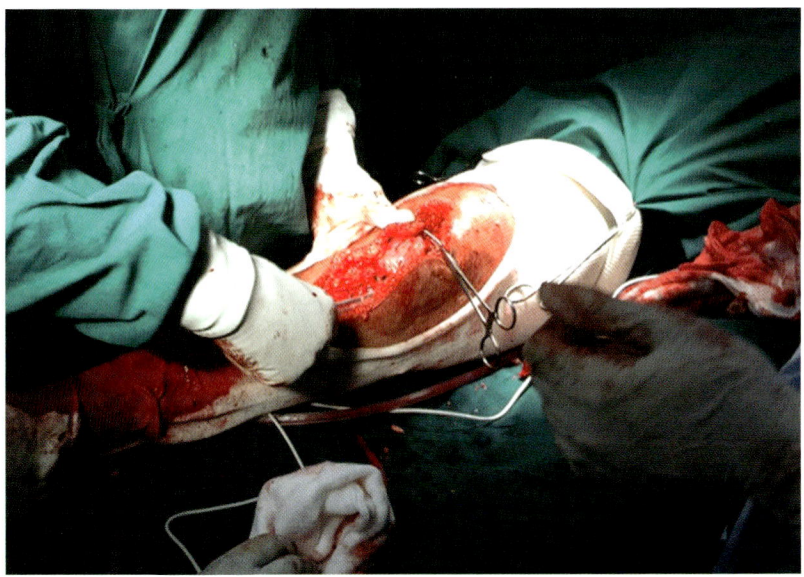

Most stubbornly flexed knees can be straightened out by appropriate soft tissue releases.

In Indian circumstances, where most patients come for surgery as a last resort, we have had quite a few patients with 70° to 90° of fixed flexion deformity. By sequentially following the above steps it will always be possible to straighten out the knee.

Recurvatum Deformity of the Knee

Unlike other deformities where releases will work, with recurvatum one has to resect the posterior cruciate, do an adequate soft tissue balancing and use an implant thick enough to tense the structures after the cuts are made.

Recurvatum knees demand a more constrained prosthesis, and their long-term survival is not assured. Hinges, central pivots or centrally stabilized implants may be needed in these situations.

The beginners to whom this book is addressed are well advised to leave these knees alone and refer them to more experienced colleagues or a centre where complex knees surgeries are being performed regularly.

Knee Replacement in Osteoarthritis

Unlike hip arthritis, knee osteoarthritis is very common in Asian patients. The nonexistent primary OA in the hip is very well compensated in our demography by a preponderance of knee arthritis. Knee arthritis accounts for a large percentage of all orthopaedic outpatients visiting most government and private hospitals. After all first line methods like analgesia, physical therapy, walking and bracing aids, etc. are exhausted, one is left with no option but to consider surgical methods.

Knee replacement is possibly the last resort after treatment by other methods of less invasive surgical exercises are exhausted. The simplest option is an arthroscopic lavage and debridement. This does give some short term relief; at most, it can be called a delaying procedure. A high tibial osteotomy is an excellent operation. Indeed, when performed for the correct indication, may be more rewarding than a total knee arthroplasty itself. A unicompartmental replacement too is an excellent operation, but most of us would consider it a form of replacement arthroplasty with all the associated problems of the same. For predominantly medial compartment arthritis, with varus and a practically normal lateral compartment, I have devised a fibular osteotomy, called the PFO or Prakash Fibular Osteotomy. This is again outside the scope of this book and described in detail elsewhere.

The important points encountered while performing a knee replacement in osteorthritic knee are given pointwise with possible remedies:

1. A varus deformity is much more common than a valgus deformity. Apart from the bone loss that has been discussed

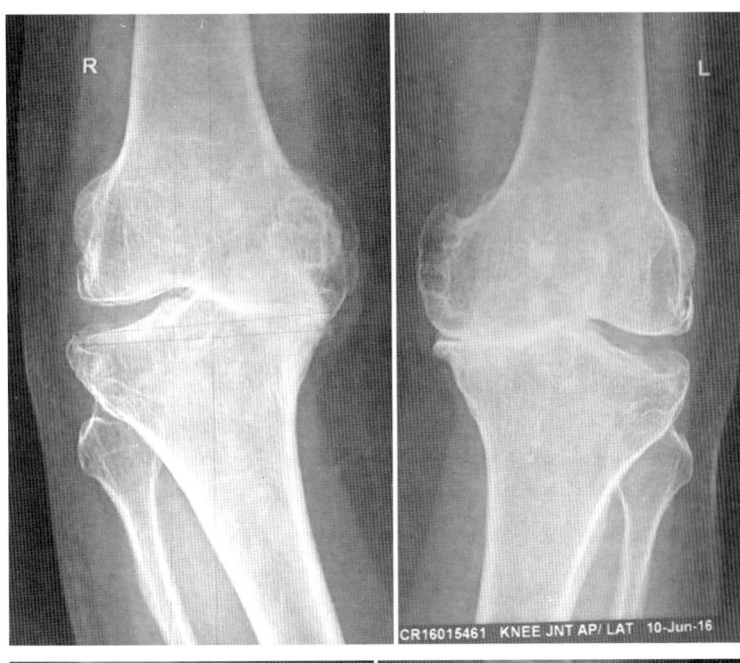

CR16015461 KNEE JNT AP/ LAT 10-Jun-16

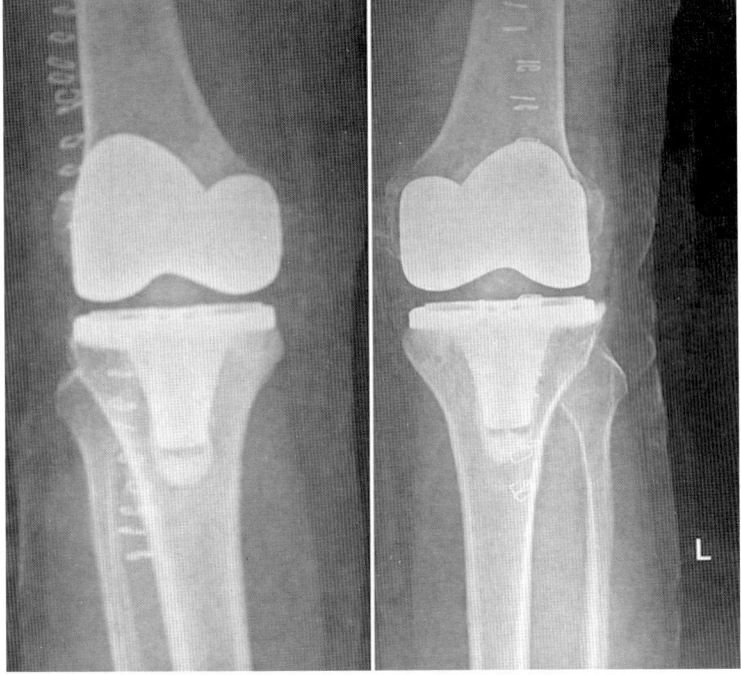

The average OA knee that confronts most of us.

subsequently, it is very important to perform a precise soft tissue release on the medial side. The steps are osteophytes, subperiosteal release, and medial collateral release. No ligaments should be cut. They should be gently erased or scraped from the bony surface of the tibia. An external rotation of the leg by the assistant will allow for a proper visualization of the posterior structures and enable for a thorough medial release. One must not start bone cuts prior to a complete soft tissue release and correction of the deformity.

2. Severe bone loss from the medial side is often encountered. In many cases, there is a corresponding hypertrophy of the medial femoral condyle; after the distal femoral bone cut, all bone should be preserved. In most cases, one can invert this and use it as a graft to fill the defect. When the upper tibia is being cut, be very careful not to cut too much bone! It is always better to cut to a reasonable level of the tibial condyle and fill the gap with grafts, rather than cut too low.

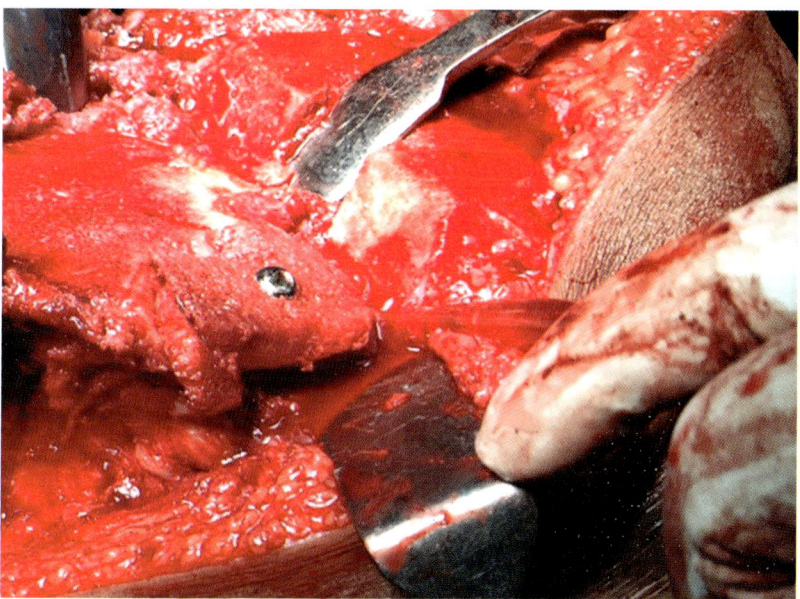

A tibial defect has been grafted with bone from distal femur and affixed with a screw.

3. When enough grafts are not available, up to 6 mm of defect can be compensated by cortical screws! After drilling and tapping a few equally distributed holes on the area of the defect, one can insert a few cortical screws. Their protruding heads will allow for a 6 mm increase and the area in between can be filled with grafts and liquid cement.

4. On occasion, the tibial and femoral surfaces may be very hard and present some difficulty for sawing. This is especially true if the cut is close to the damaged articular surface, and it is a common error to cut the surfaces a bit obliquely (as the saw blade follows the line of least resistance). One has to be extremely careful in these circumstances to maintain an accurate cut to avoid problems.

5. In osteoarthritis, the problem is mostly bilateral, so the choice—whether to replace the two sides one after the other or simultaneously—is entirely based on the facilities available and the interest and experience of the surgeon. In our set up, if both knees need to be replaced, we routinely replace both the knees under a single anaesthetic; to date, we have not faced any significant complications. A double knee replacement has its own advantages and disadvantages. The disadvantages are increased operating time, increased blood loss, and the need for two sets of instrumentation. In addition, the surgeon must be physically fit to perform the two operations simultaneously. However on the credit side, the patient benefits from a single hospitalization, shorter stay, one single episode of pain, a quicker recovery and a much easier physiotherapy.

6. Whilst planning for a bilateral surgery, there are certain important factors to be considered. The two procedures should be treated as independent procedures and separate sets of linen for each side are mandatory. Two sets of instrumentation including power tools are essential. A very well-trained nurse and proper assistance is mandatory, and last of all, a proper preoperative counselling is essential to assess the patient's psychological profile to ensure his/her total postoperative cooperation.

7. The type of anaesthetic employed is very important. In our set up, most cases are done under regional anaesthesia. In the initial stages, we used continuous epidural anaesthetic because of the time taken. However, as the procedure became routine and common, we switched over to a spinal anaesthetic. Most cases, including bilateral knees, are presently routinely replaced under a spinal anaesthetic, unless there is a specific contraindication for administering it.

8. Unlike rheumatoid arthritis and ankylosing spondylosis (where the patient is bedridden and unable to walk), patients with osteoarthritis are invariably more independent and have greater expectations. It is imperative to counsel such patients preoperatively and assess their habits and social circumstances. If the disease has been progressive enough to cause limitations of movements and make the use of an Indian toilet impossible, it does not matter much. However, if the patient uses an Indian type closet despite difficulties, one has to be very particular in counselling the patient regarding the change in toilet habits and the need to use an European closet thereafter.

9. Obese patients are another risk element who have to be tackled with due diligence and care. A body weight of over 100 kg is a definite risk factor to the extent of being a contraindication. Very short and extremely obese patients are asked to come back after they have shed appropriate weight after diet, medication and exercises. However, a borderline overweight patient should not be denied the benefits of the operation, because the immobility due to the pain may be a cause of lethargy and overweight.

10. In the Asian circumstance, there may be patients with gross arthritis but surprisingly good range of motion. These patients are often accustomed to using Indian toilet and squatting. It is essential to counsel them preoperatively, and tell them that after replacement, both squatting and use of Indian toilet is prohibited.

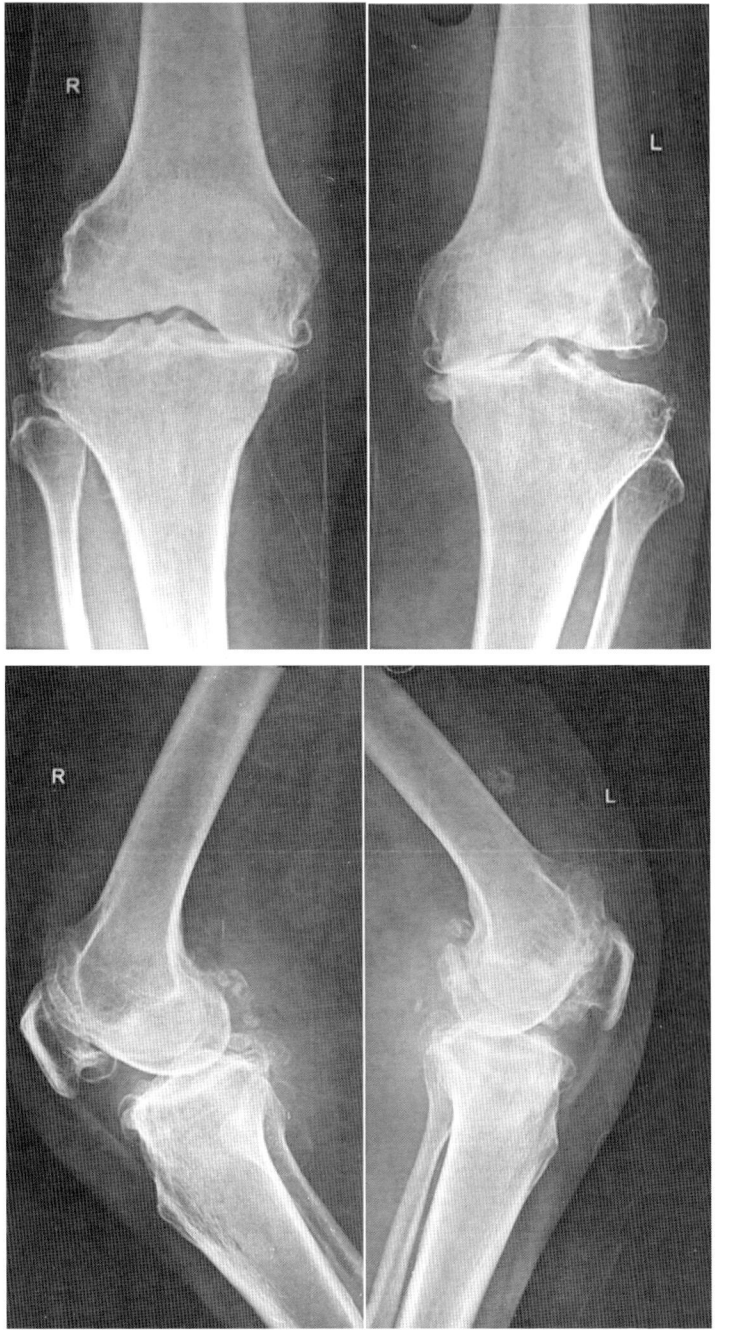

A typical OA knee.

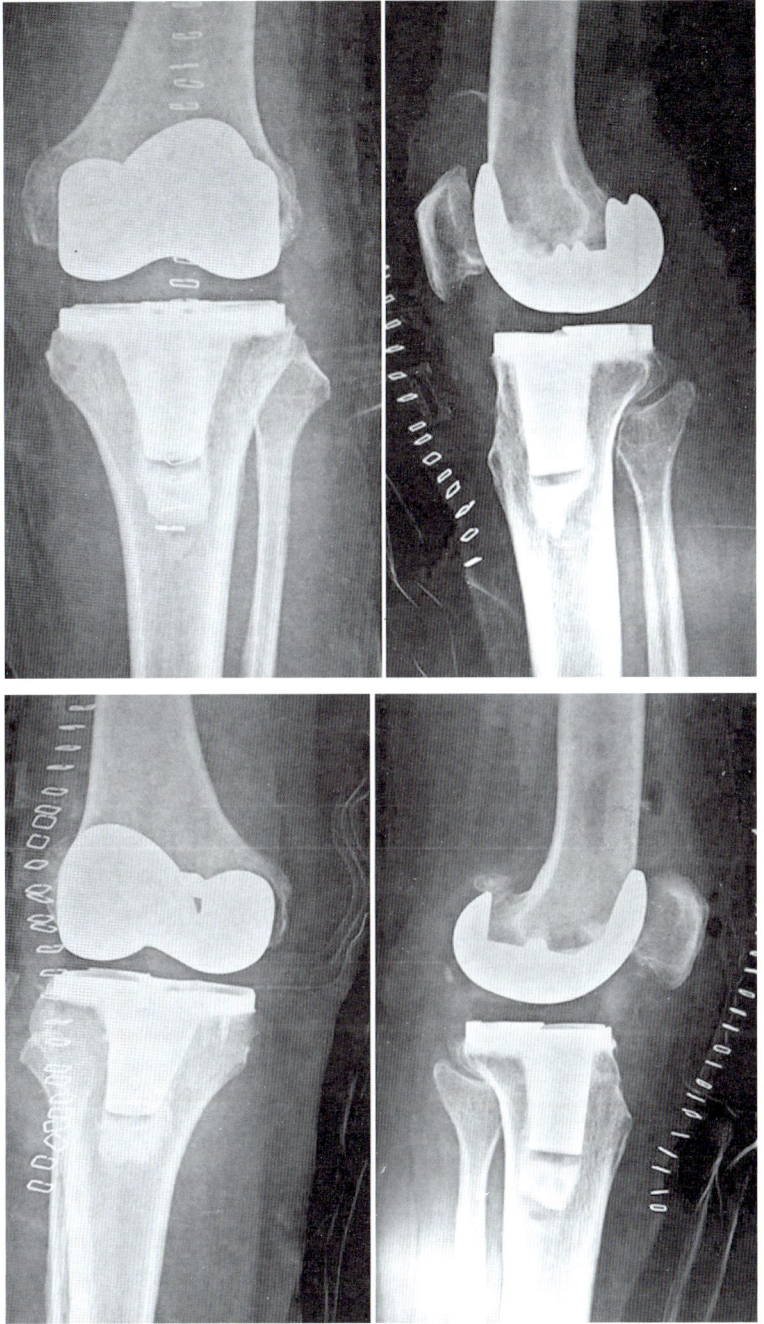

Treated with a typical cemented TKR.

Knee Replacement in Rheumatoid Arthritis

Total knee replacements have heralded a new era in relieving the pain, stiffness and deformity of patients with rheumatoid and allied disorders. The rheumatoid family includes Still's disease, psoriatic arthropathy and other collagen disorders. Most of these patients are generally disabled with multiple joint involvement and may be immobile. Because of the disease being long-standing, there may be gross destruction of bones, joints and a distortion of the normal anatomy. If hips and knees are involved simultaneously, one must replace the knees before attempting to replace the hips, because extreme flexion needed for making the cuts during a knee replacement might dislocate the hip. The following points are important while planning a replacement in these patients:

1. A complete assessment of the whole patient, including skin condition, musculature and psychological status is needed prior to planning an operation.

2. Most of these patients have a severe degree of anaemia and this will have to be corrected by repeated blood transfusions prior to performing a procedure.

3. The disease might involve the cervical spine leading C1, C2 subluxation and the anaesthesist should be made aware of this fact if he plans to give a general anaesthesia and intubate the patient.

4. The bones are grossly osteoporotic and one must be extremely careful in all manoeuvres. Whilst subluxating the patella laterally, enough soft tissue must be released so as to not avulse the tibial tuberosity.

5. Extreme care should be exercised while drilling the pilot hole for the intramedullary alignment rod. The very soft bone will yield very easily to the power drill. After this, extra caution should be exercised while inserting the intramedullary rod, as a slight deviation could cause the rod to perforate the lateral or anterior cortex.

6. There is usually a degree of osteoporosis varying from moderate to marked, which might lead to fracture of the shaft of femur or tibia while the knee is put through various manoeuvres. After soft tissue balance, while one tries to correct the varus or valgus and attempts to see the degree of correction, it is possible to accidentally crust the articular surface.

7. The diseased synovium may on occasions be very proliferative and extensive. This may present difficulties in proper identification of the entire bony surfaces of the femur and tibia. Thus a proper and extensive synovectomy should precede bone cuts and the use of other instrumentation.

8. Once the exposure has been made and the steps proceed towards bone cuts, extra care should be used whilst using the oscillating saw. The blade may cut like a knife through butter and may accidentally damage soft tissues. Also, if the direction of the blades is even slightly oblique, one will end up with improper cuts.

9. In rheumatoids, the ligaments becomes very lax. Hence, one will end up using much thicker tibial components to keep the ligaments tight. Thus it is imperative to have the entire range of components, including thicker ones.

10. Occasionally, these knees will have very gross deformities. Further, due to the poor quality bone stock and gross osteoporosis, enough grafts will not be available. In such circumstances, a proper preoperative evaluation is essential and if needed, implants with bone defect wedges should be used.

11. It is a good idea not to go on extensively with the chamfer cuts. After making the distal, anterior and posterior cuts, just inserting the femoral component will squeeze the soft cancellous bones into the perfect shape of the interior of

the femoral component. Likewise, it is not essential to make big holes or rasp the area for the tibial stem. A gentle push of the tibial component over the upper tibial surface will compress the cancellous bone and achieve the desired tight fit.

12. While performing trial reductions, one must avoid fracturing the femoral or tibial shaft by not using any aggressive manoeuvre.

13. As these patients are usually on steroids, special care must be taken to maintain steroids therapy pre- and post-operatively to avoid steroid withdrawal shock.

14. As the skin and soft tissues are very delicate and fragile, one must take special care while inserting powerful retractors to avoid bruise or tearing of the skin. If one is not careful with the skin edges and with the soft tissues, there may be a wound dehiscence or a delayed healing of the soft tissues.

15. Rheumatoid tissues are non-elastic and non-retractile and hence have a tendency for considerable oozing and bleeding. Soft tissue handling should thus be very meticulous, a thorough cautery of all the bleeders should be performed and adequate drainage employed to avoid postoperative haematoma formation.

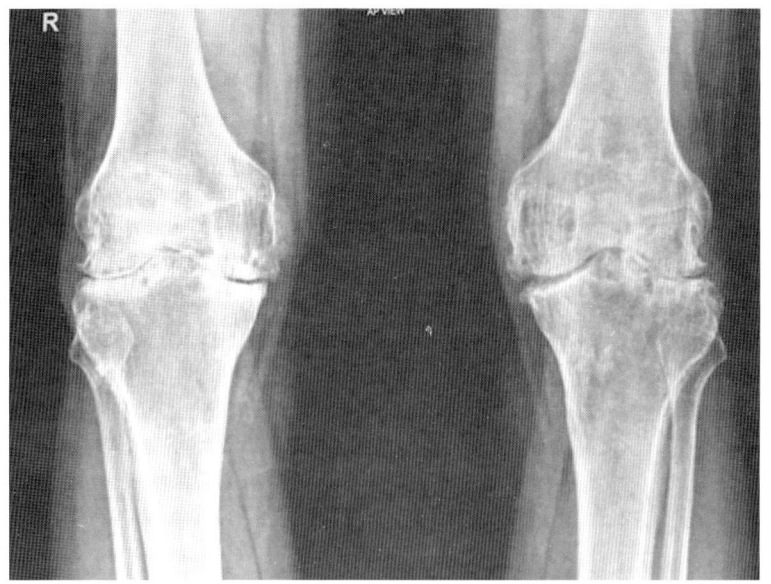

A typical case of rheumatoid knee.

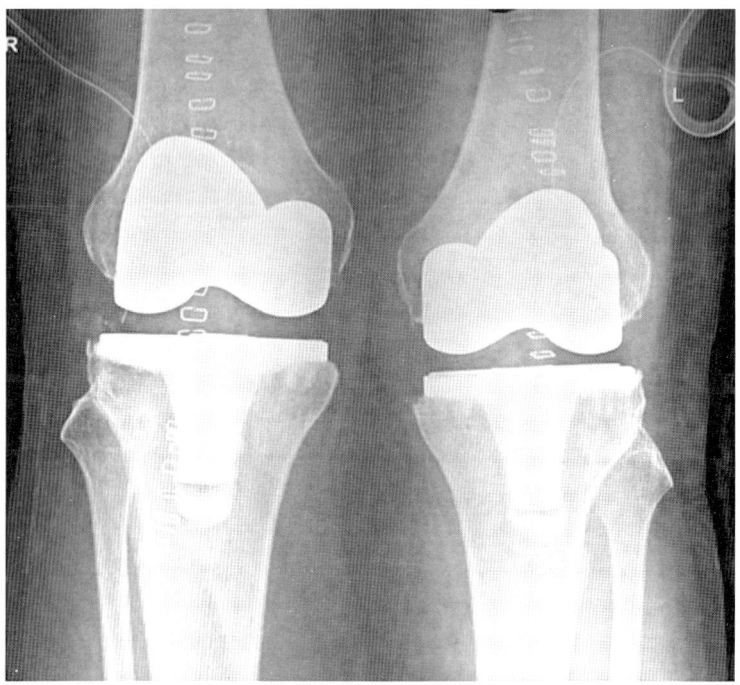

Bilateral replacements done and correct balance achieved.

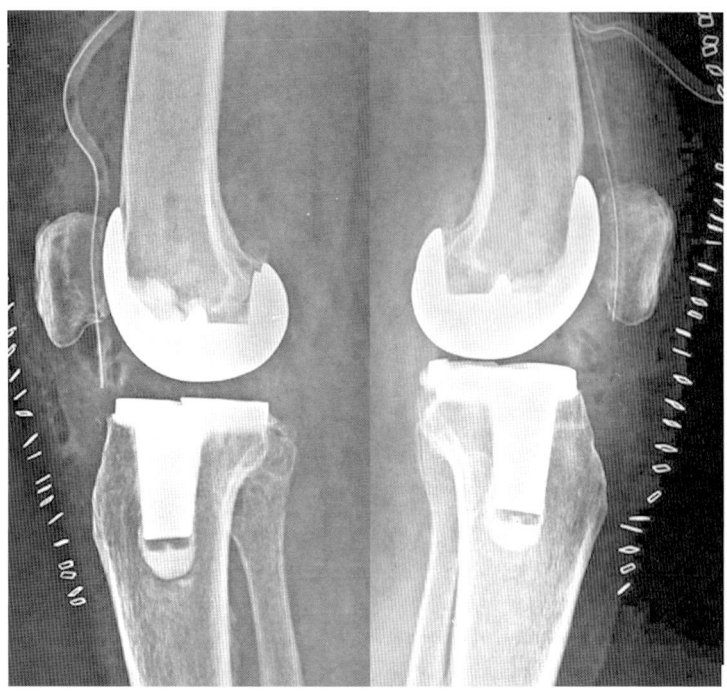

Fixed flexion deformities on both sides have been fully corrected.

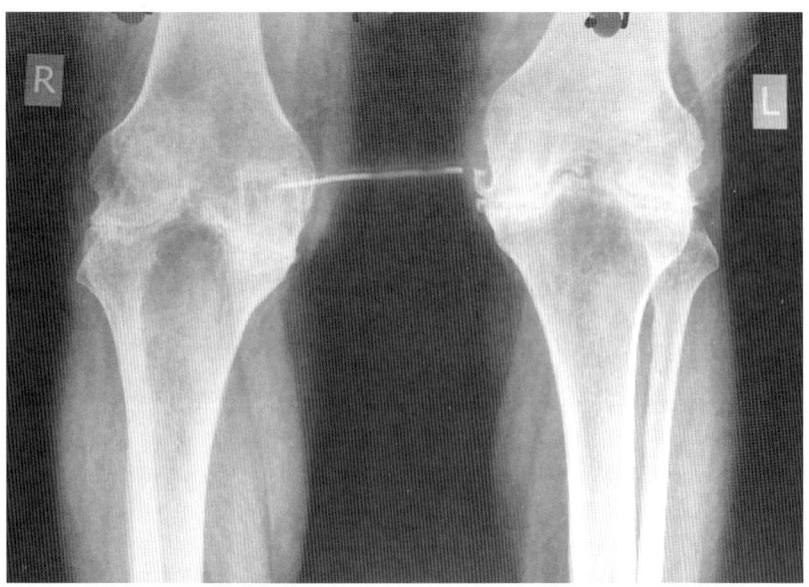

Another typical case of rheumatoid arthritis.

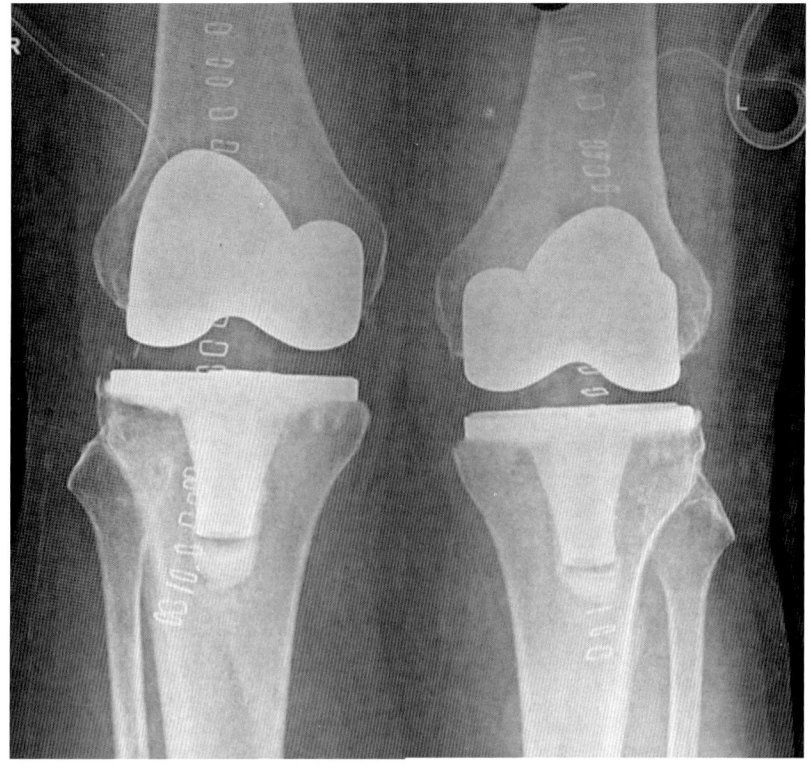

Properly placed components and deformities are fully corrected.

The following case operated by Dr Vijay Sharma in a single sitting clearly demonstrates that even the most grotesque rheumatoids can be managed wonderfully with a little planning and attention to meticulous detail.

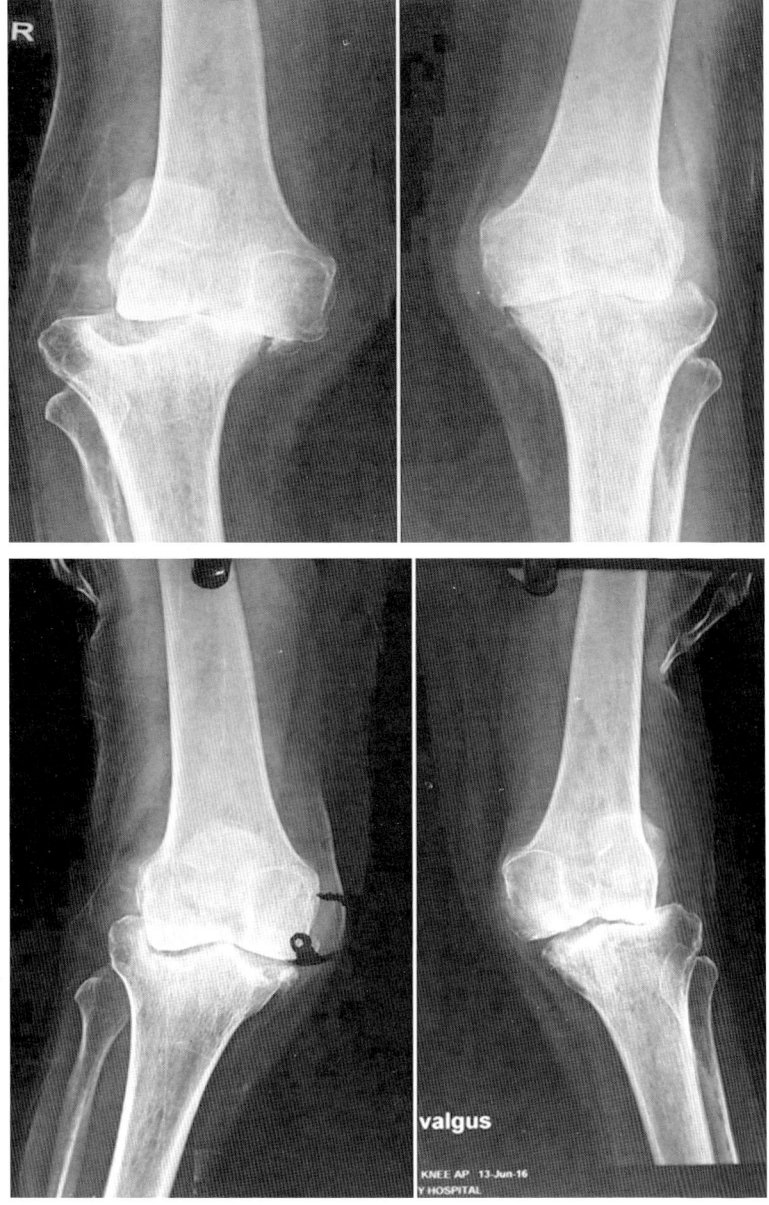

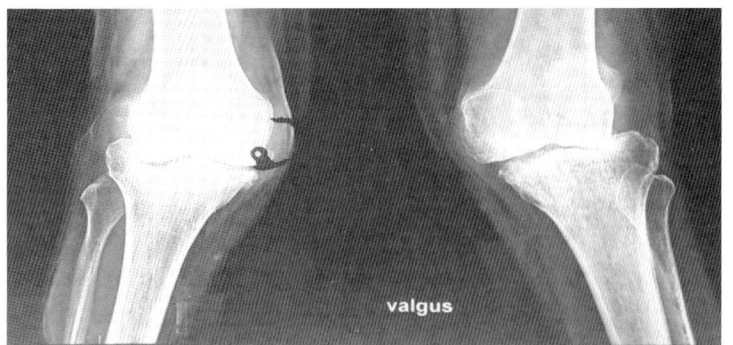

valgus

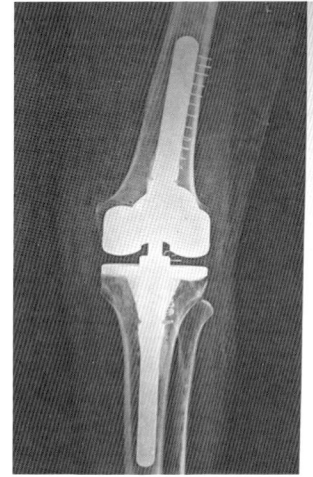
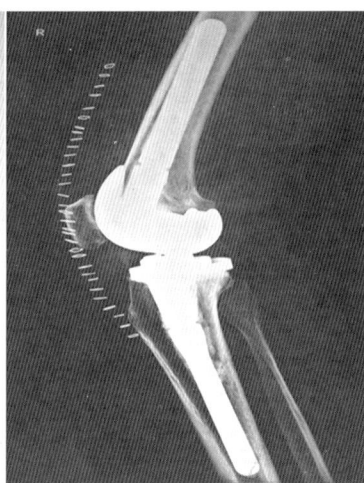

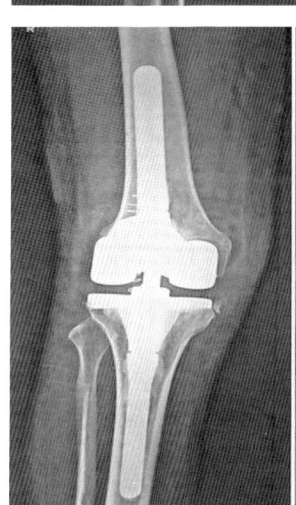
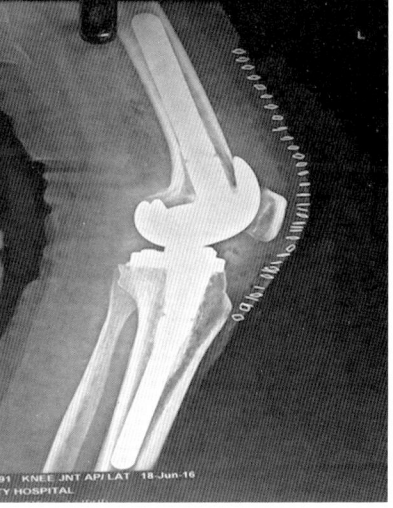

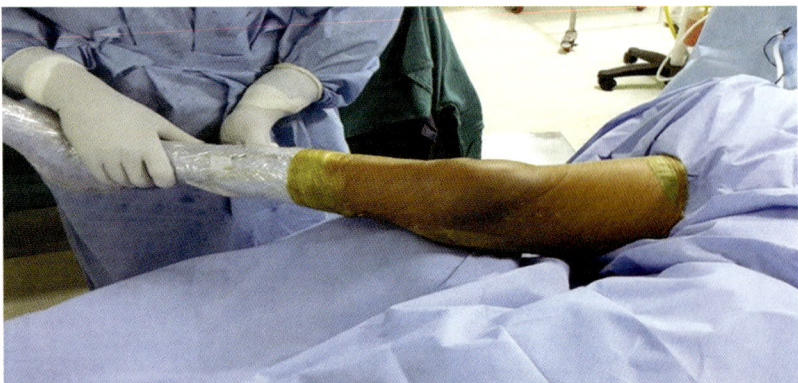

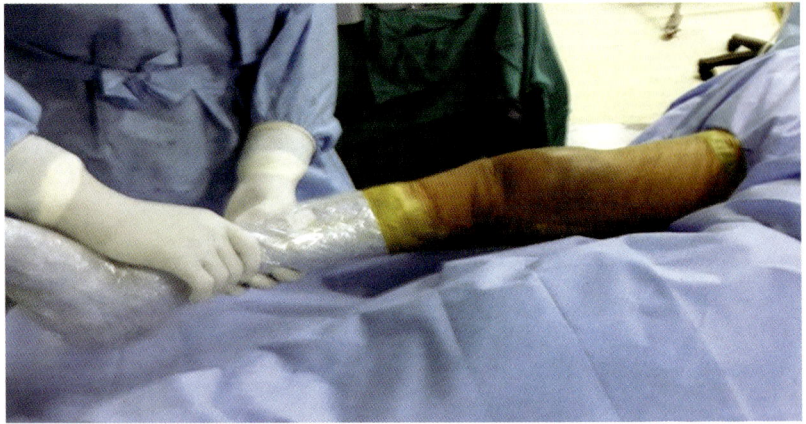

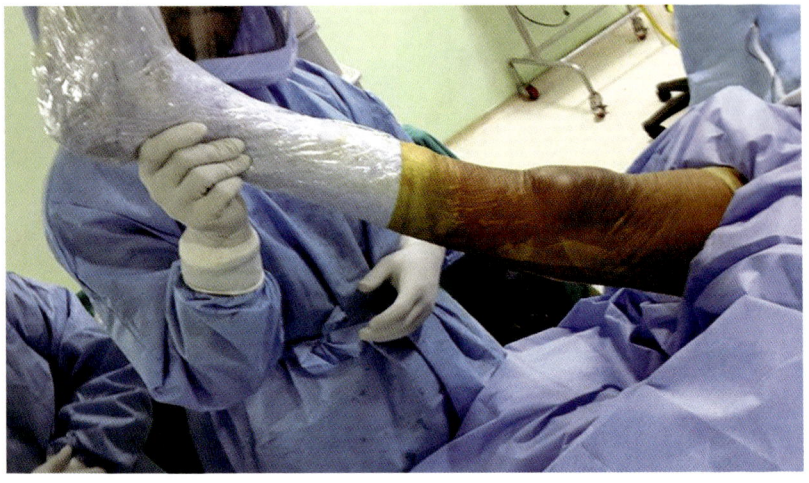

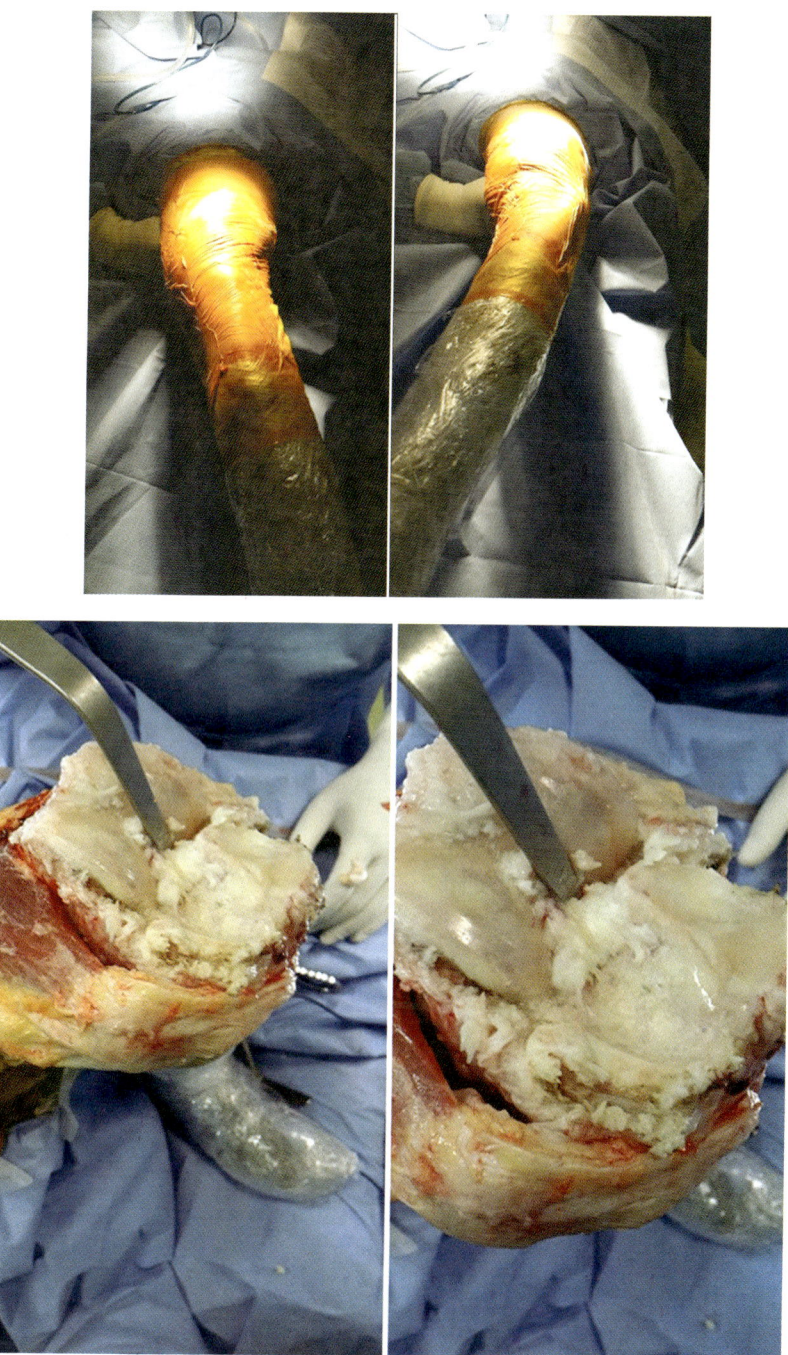

Total Knee Replacement in Old Tuberculous Knees

Though the role and value of knee replacement in burnt out tuberculosis is meagerly covered in Western literature, encouraging reports have been given by various Asian surgeons. In our institution, the indications for replacing the joint in patients with tubercular arthritis of the knee are:

a. Stiff painful knees in patients aged above 40.

b. Incomplete fusion leading to restricted motion and pain.

c. Fusion (or failure of fusion) of long-standing duration presenting a severe back or hip pain.

d. Solid fusion in a functionally unacceptable position.

e. With evidence of active disease, we prefer to administer anti-tubercular treatment for at least three months prior to replacement.

The following points are to be noted while attempting to replace knees with old or existing tuberculosis:

1. Intensive chemotherapy using a four-drug regime is necessary.

2. The chemotherapy should be started four weeks before surgery and should be continued up to nine months after surgery.

3. Knees with evidence of superinfection with non-tubercular organisms (as evidenced by positive cultures of knee aspirate) should not be taken up for replacement.

4. The bones are osteoporotic and soft; hence due care must be taken to avoid fracturing of the tibia or femur, or splitting the patella while dislocating it.

5. Usually there is some amount of synovial and pencapsular thickening and hypertrophy around the joint. This must be generally exercised prior to soft tissue releases.

6. In cases where there is an apparent subluxation of the joint or a very gross valgus or varus, adequate soft tissue releases must be performed as described in the chapters on soft tissue releases and deformity corrections.

7. We routinely add 2 gm of streptomycin powder to the cement polymer while mixing the cement. Experimental studies in our laboratory show that the drug continues to leach out of the cement for up to 18 months. Addition of streptomycin to the cement does not significantly hamper its strength.

The following pictures demonstrate a case of one such problem managed by a well-done TKR. This case is from Dr. Anuj Agarwal.

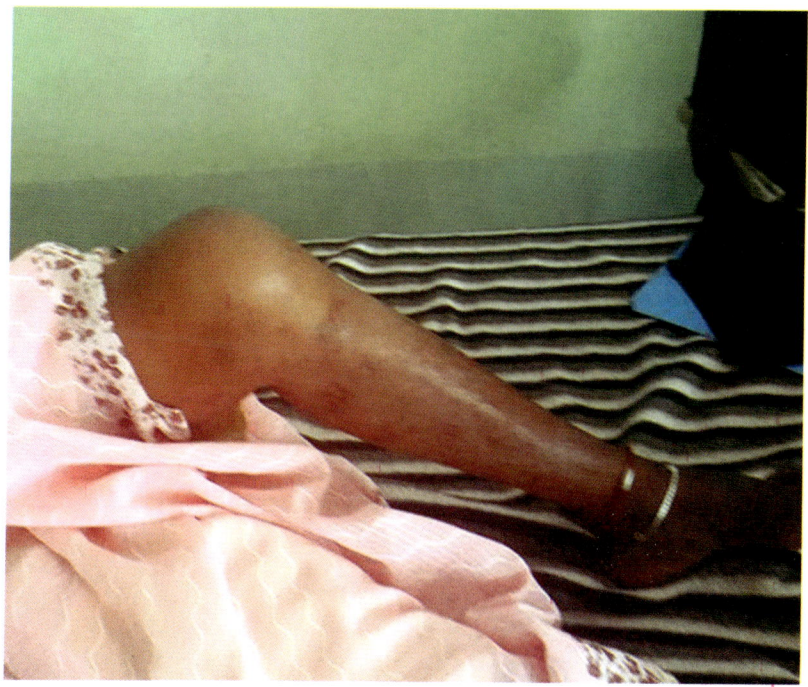

A case of burnt out tuberculosis of knee with fixed flexion deformity of 70°.

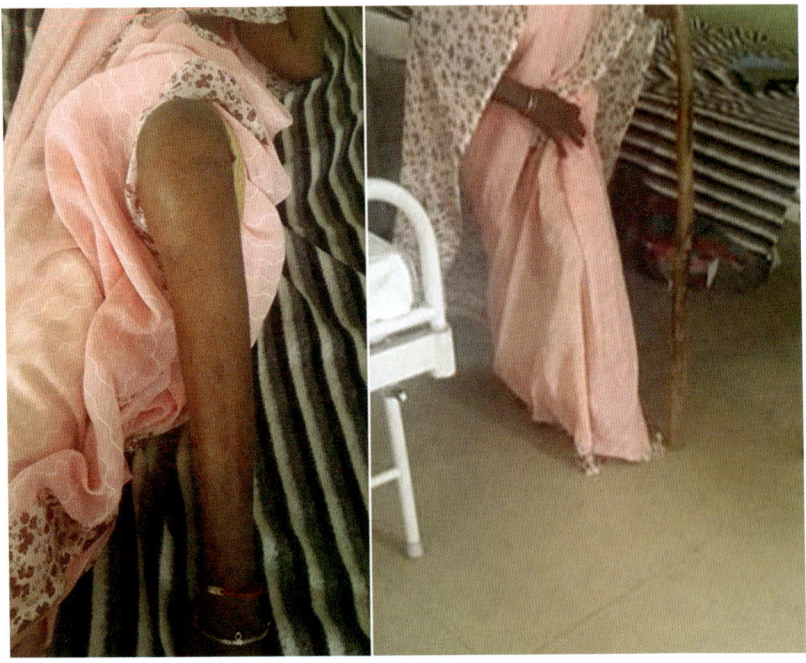

The fixed flexion deformity has handicapped the patient to a considerable extent.

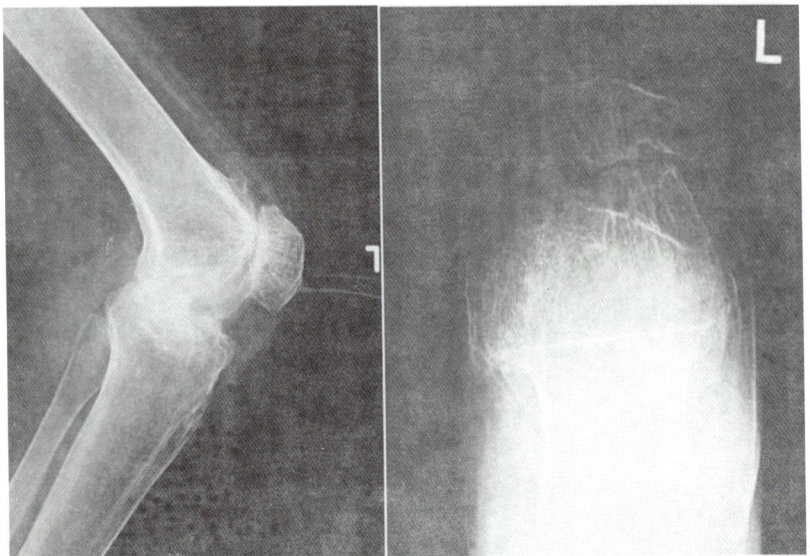

See the extensive tricompartmental disease and the almost absent joint line. Even the patella has a degree of fibrous ankylosis.

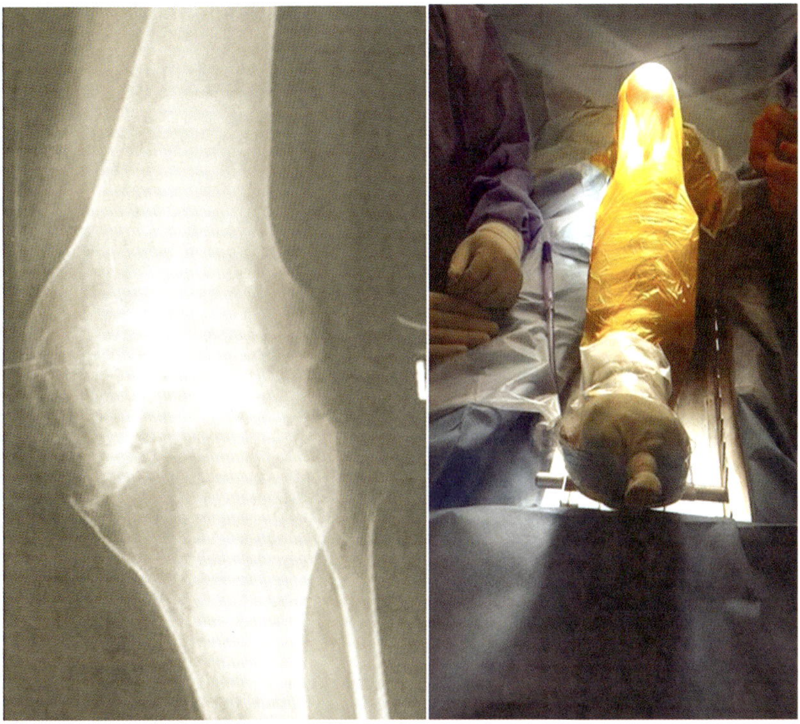

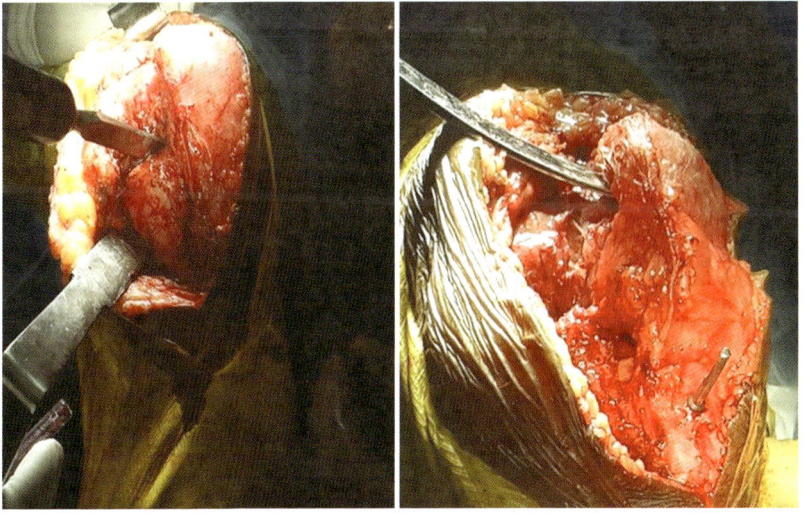

One can appreciate that the joint is practically fused.

An osteotomy was needed to separate femur and tibia.

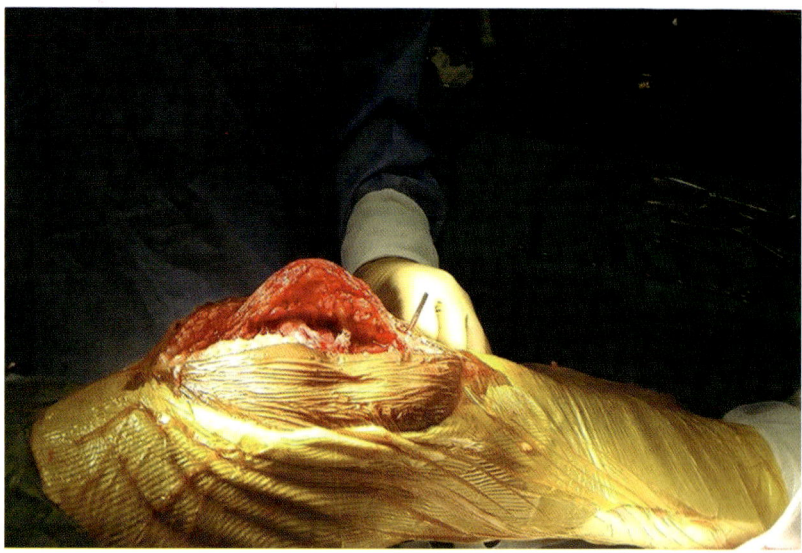

After releases, the deformity was corrected and a posterior stabilized knee implanted.

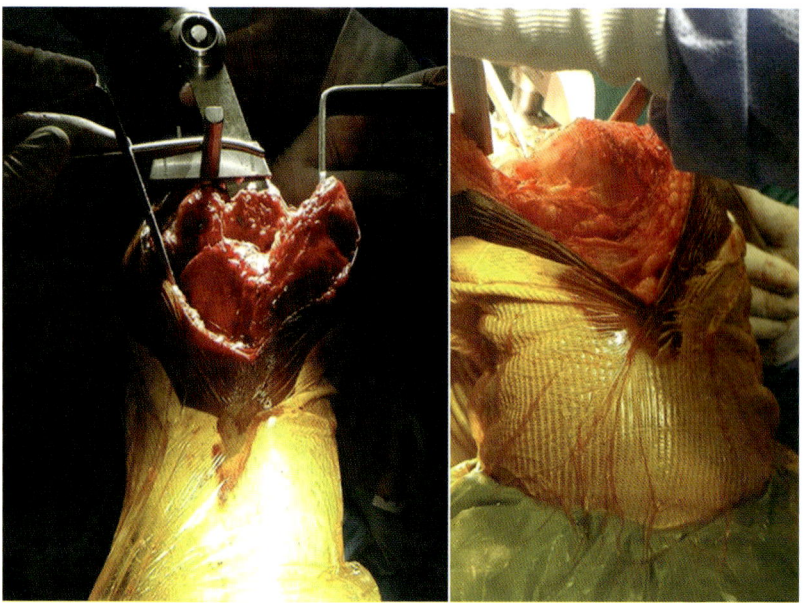

To prevent joint line errors, anatomical references are strictly followed.

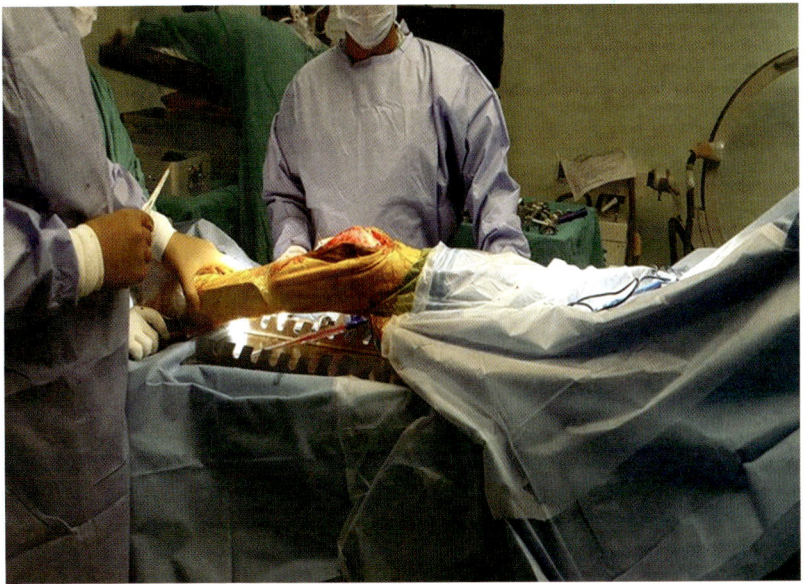

A near complete correction is achieved on the table.

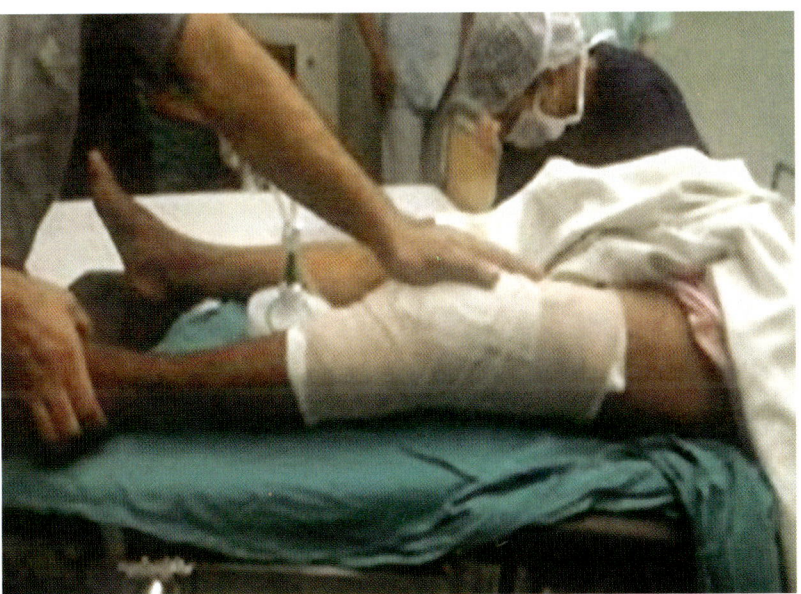

Immediate postoperative picture.

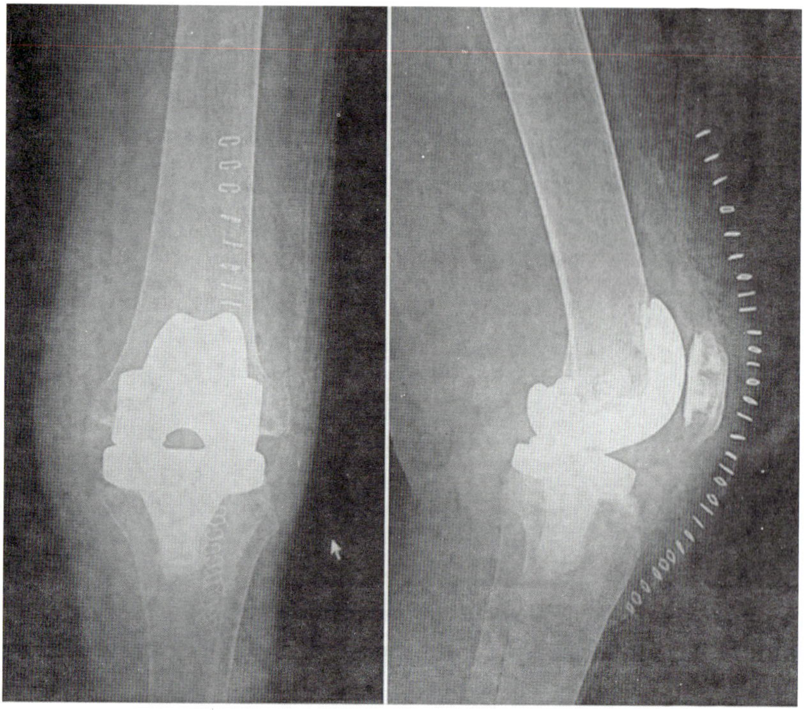

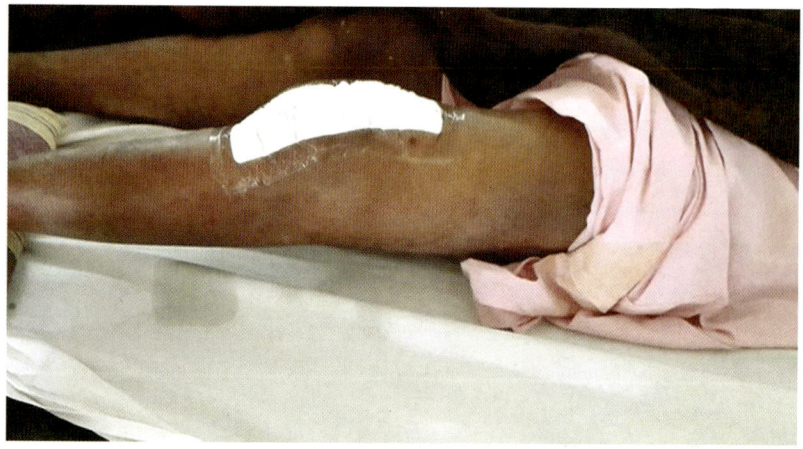

Postoperative radiograph.

Clinical picture at two weeks.

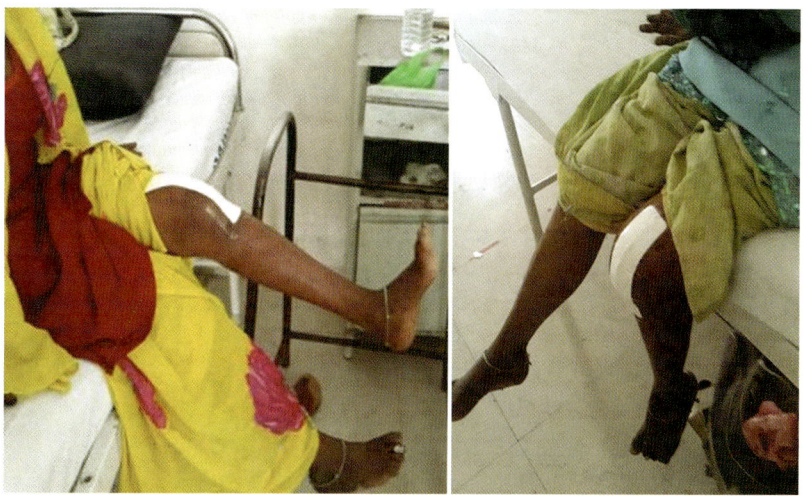

Gradually improving flexion.

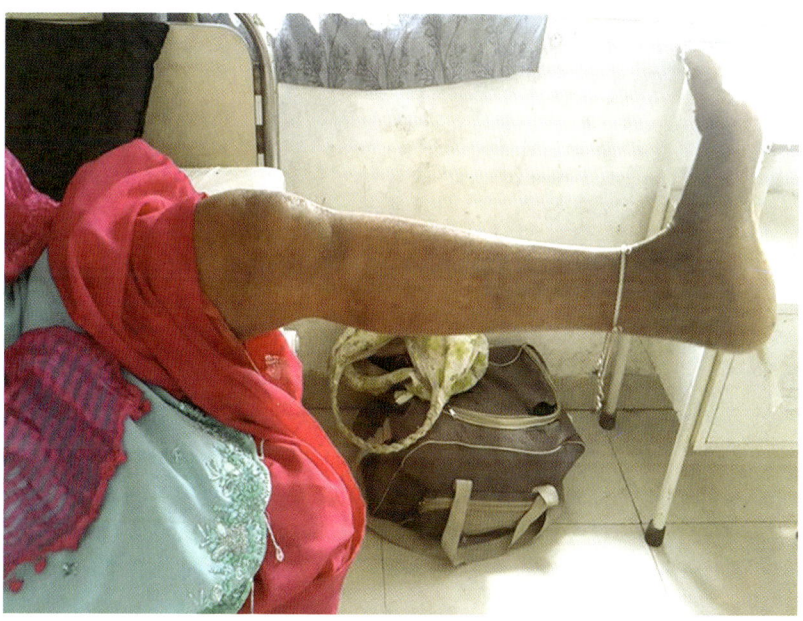

Good power and ability to straight leg raise within a few days of surgery.

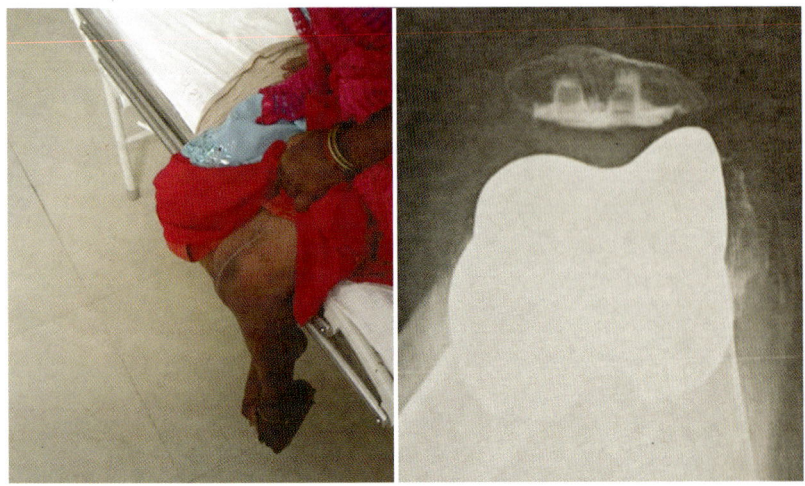

Clinical result. See the correct patellar tracking.

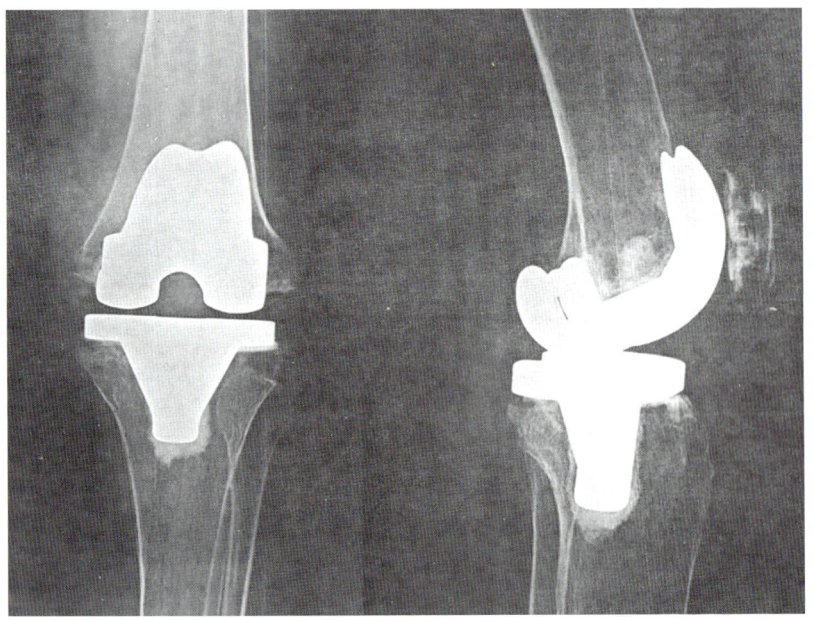

Final postoperative X-ray.

Total Knee Replacement in the Haemophillic Knee

Haemophilia causes severe damage to the articular surfaces of joints into which recurrent and regular bleeding occurs. Being the largest joint, knee is usually affected in haemophiliacs surviving beyond middle age. In haemophillics, knee arthritis is quite a crippling disability.

There are centres abroad that have extensive experience of total knee arthroplasty in the haemophiliac patient. However, in my series of just four cases with very limited experience, I have found this a very gratifying and satisfying procedure for the patient as well as the surgeon.

I apologize if this chapter seems anecdotal and does not teach you anything new. (Readers with this opinion may seek deeper knowledge from other orthopaedic literature.)

About 20 years ago, I was referred a patient with haemophiliac arthritis of the knee. This patient had come from very far off and the condition of his knee warranted a replacement clinically and radiologically. However, the mere thought of doing such a major operation on a haemophiliac was a nightmare. I phoned the haematologist, who was aghast! He opined that the large cancellous areas left after bone cuts would surely make the patient bleed to death!

I then called the pharmacist of a leading local medical shop which is famous for stocking imported and rarely available drugs and medicines. He told me that anti-haemophiliac factors are available in plenty. All we need is to give factor eight for haemophilia and factor nine for Christmas disease.

I then referred to Campbell, where it was mentioned that even patients with 50% normal factor level can withstand surgery.

Pronto came the factor and the surgery went on well. The first patient was followed up for nine years and did well.

After that I have had three more patients—two classical haemophiliacs and one with Christmas disease—and all have gone home without problems, except one patient with Christmas disease who had a large haematoma that had to be drained. The re-operation caused some infection in the knee and this persisted for some time. The patient eventually ended up with an arthrodesis after removal of the implants.

Total Knee Replacement in the Grossly Unstable Knee

Knee instability occurs due to various factors. The patient with degeneration associated with instability loads the knee to the direction of least resistance, leading to gross deformities; eventually this may result in a massive bone loss and major bony defects. This in turn stretches the ligaments on the opposite side, making them very lax. Conditions like Charcot's joint (neuropathic osteoarthropathy) in themselves present with joint laxity. Certain important points should be considered whilst planning for a knee joint with laxity:

1. Conditions like Charcot's joint are an absolute contraindication to this procedure.
2. Most wobbly knees present with an absence of both cruciate ligaments. It is imperative that a posterior stabilized type of implant is used with a fairly thick tibial component which will stretch the loose ligaments.
3. In case the knee is very loose, one may elect to use a hinge or a rotating platform type of knee to confer stability to the joint.
4. Soft tissue balancing is very important. With the judicious use of spacers or lamina spreaders, the joint space on both sides is to be essentially equalized. After stretching the ligaments on both sides, a correct assessment of the appropriate thickness of the tibial component is to be made.
5. With bone defects and bone loss, one must not cut to the parallel level of the defect. Rather one must cut to the level of the healthy bone, and build up the deficient side with the correct use of wedges or grafts.
6. If a constrained implant is being considered, its limitations and disadvantages should be communicated to the patient so that he/she is well prepared.

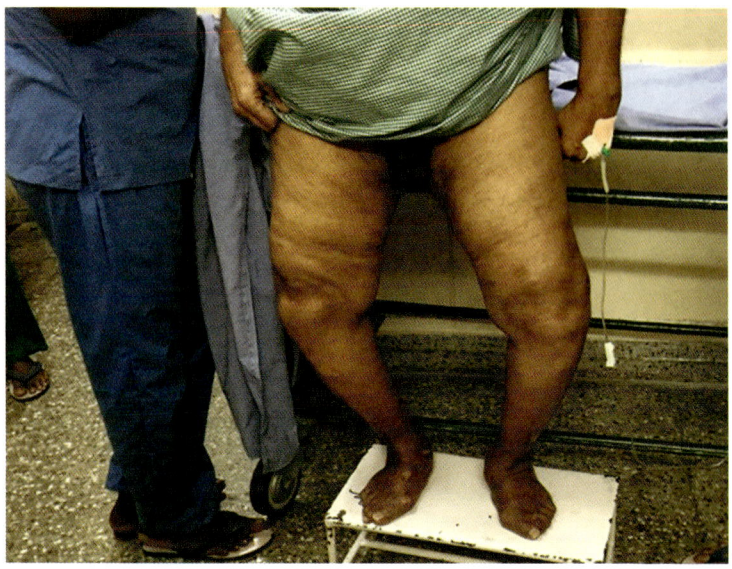

An unstable knee due to severe osteoarthritis.

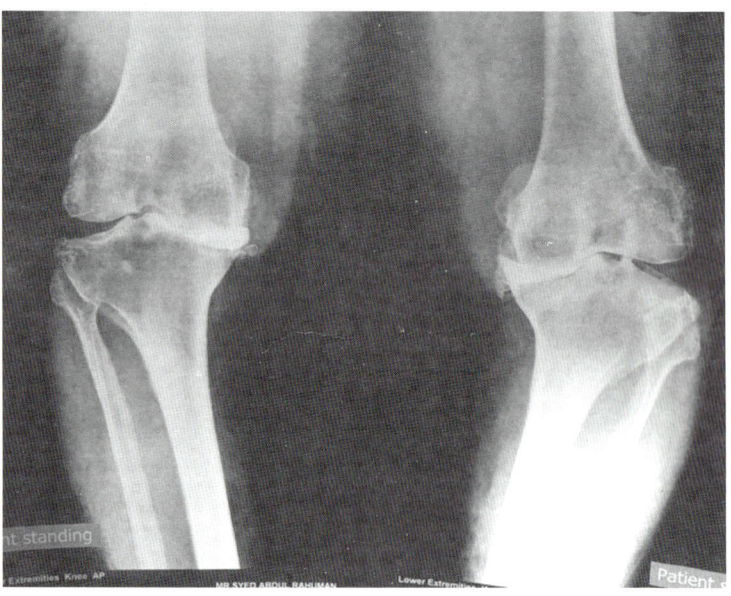

The varus is about 25° on either side.

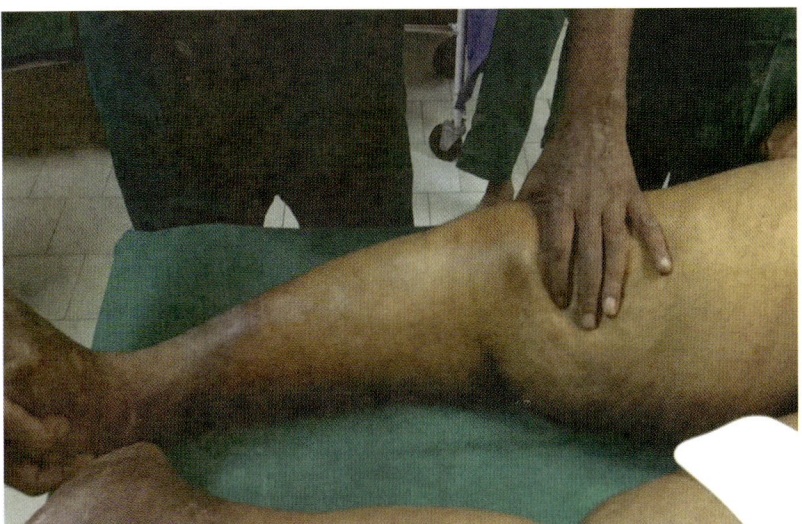

Under anaesthesia the deformity is correctable to a large extent.

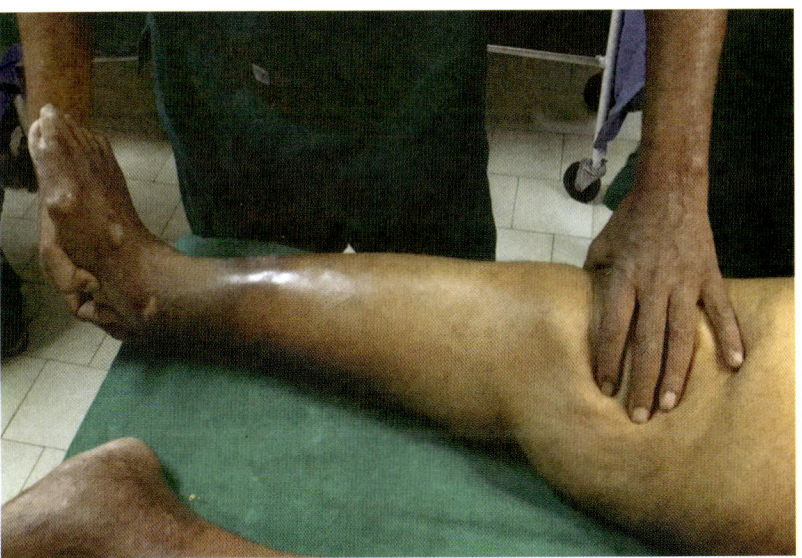

See the residual varus, which needs to be corrected by medial releases.

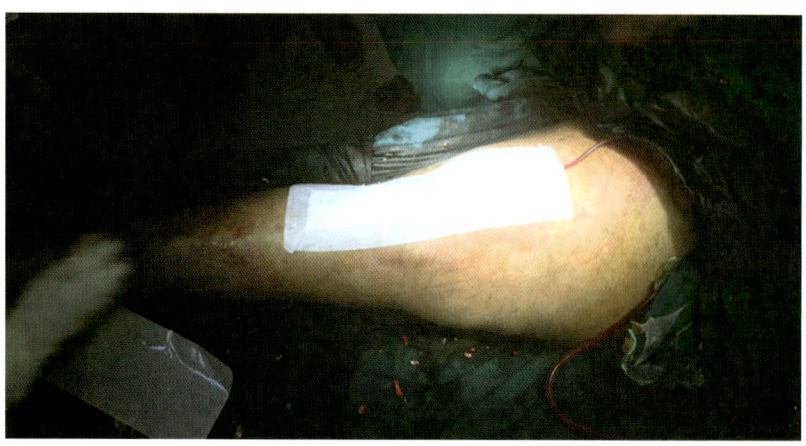

Deformity is fully corrected and the knee is stable.

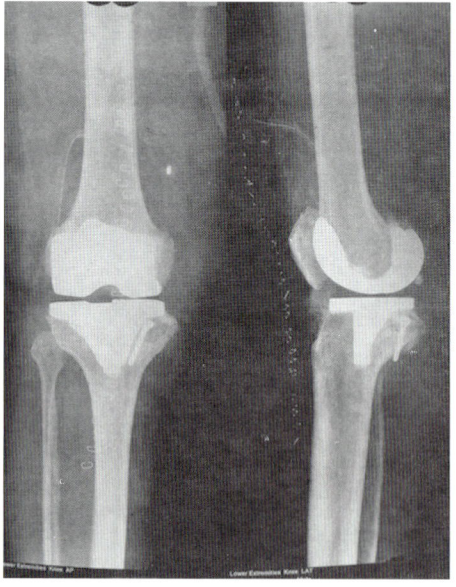

Postoperative radiograph. The defect in tibia is managed by bone grafting and a screw. Standard implants were used, avoiding wedges and stem.

21

Unicompartmental Knee Arthroplasty

Introduction

In most cases, arthritis of the knee first starts in one compartment. Depending on the axis and loading, an uneven force distribution across the joint will cause one-half of the joint to wear out first. This will secondarily lead to a deformity on the side of degeneration and consequently exaggerate the wear to that side. As a consequence, the degenerated side continues to wear; in the initial stages, the eccentric loading of the joint actually protects the opposite compartment! Once the cartilage on medial side is fully worn off, the opposite side starts wearing too and the arthritis proceeds from a uni- to a bi- and tri-compartmental damage!

The idea of just replacing the damaged compartment seems very attractive in theory and looks more sensible than osteotomy and realignment to bring the forces to act upon the undamaged side. However, a protracted and difficult history of unicompartmental knees with a lot of initial failures has put this procedure into disrepute!

Relevant Biomechanics

The knee joint, unlike the hip, is a very complex articulation indeed. To simplify our understanding, we can consider the knee as made up of three different joints: the medial compartment, the lateral compartment and the patellofemoral compartment.

The medial compartment has the medial collateral as its medial stabilizer and the anterior cruciate as its lateral stabilizer, with the patella and the posterior structures as the sagittal anteroposterior stabilizers.

Likewise, the lateral compartment has the posterior cruciate as its medial stabilizer and the lateral collateral as its lateral stabilizer, with the patella and the posterior structures as the sagittal anteroposterior stabilizers.

The patellofemoral articulation has the quadriceps mechanism at its front. If we analyse the loading pattern, both the tibiofemoral articulations are loaded whilst walking and the patellofemoral articulation is loaded from extension to flexion, the maximum load being in extremes of flexion.

In an anatomical model of the knee, the articular surfaces are polycentric and no two surfaces show the same radius of curvature. While acting as mobile cushions, the menisci also increase the curvature radii of the flat tibial upper surface! Thus an eccentric loading of the joint consequent to degeneration in one compartment will cause tightening and contracture of the structures on the concave side and will also lead to a stretching and laxity of the structures on the opposite side!

Consequently, whatever the attempts made to either realign or resurface the damaged compartment, one must ensure that all ligaments are balanced to achieve success. The balancing of ligaments in a unicompartmental arthroplasty is indeed more important and essential than in a total knee arthroplasty!

OSTEOTOMY VERSUS UNICOMPARTMENTAL REPLACEMENT

High tibial osteotomy is indeed an excellent operation for a single compartment disease. It has a sufficiently long follow-up and predictable results to allow for its continued advocation. However, it is very important to select the cases very carefully to get the best results. As both an osteotomy and unicompartmental replacement are performed for more or less similar indications, one has to know the potential advantages and disadvantages of both the procedures.

Advantages of a HTO:
1. Simple procedure that can be performed in most setups.
2. Good to excellent short term to medium term results as far as pain relief is concerned.

Disadvantages of a HTO:
1. Very meticulous preoperative planning and execution to avoid under- or over-correction.

2. Loss of 5° to 10° of flexion.
3. It takes six weeks with internal fixation and four months without fixation for the patient to get to normal activities.
4. Not suitable for bi- or tri-compartmental arthritis.
5. Not suitable for the very elderly.
6. Better results with a varus knee rather than with a valgus knee.
7. Long-term results are not very satisfactory.

Advantages of unicompartmental replacement:
1. Excellent pain relief.
2. Loss of flexion is practically nonexistent.
3. Excellent ligament balancing is achieved.
4. Mechanical realignment of the joint with the large number of tibial bearings available.
5. Easy conversion to a total knee at a later stage.
6. Equally suitable for both medial and lateral compartment arthritis.
7. In a bi-compartmental disease, two joints can be used.

Disadvantages of unicompartmental replacement:
1. Complex procedure needing sophisticated instrumentation.
2. Not suitable in all district hospital level operation theatres.
3. Exacting and critical procedure.
4. Not suitable for the grossly overweight patient.
5. More expensive than a high tibial osteotomy.

Studies in Oxford and Bristol reveal that as the indications of both the procedures are more or less similar, the choice of procedure is more surgeon dependant than the patient's condition. These studies also found that a uni-compartmental replacement has a little edge over HTO as far as pain relief and motion is concerned.

Surgical technique: As the commonest indication is medial compartment arthritis in a varus knee, the following steps give the procedure for a medial compartment replacement. Isolated lateral compartment osteoarthritis is rare and I do not have much experience of isolated lateral compartment replacement.

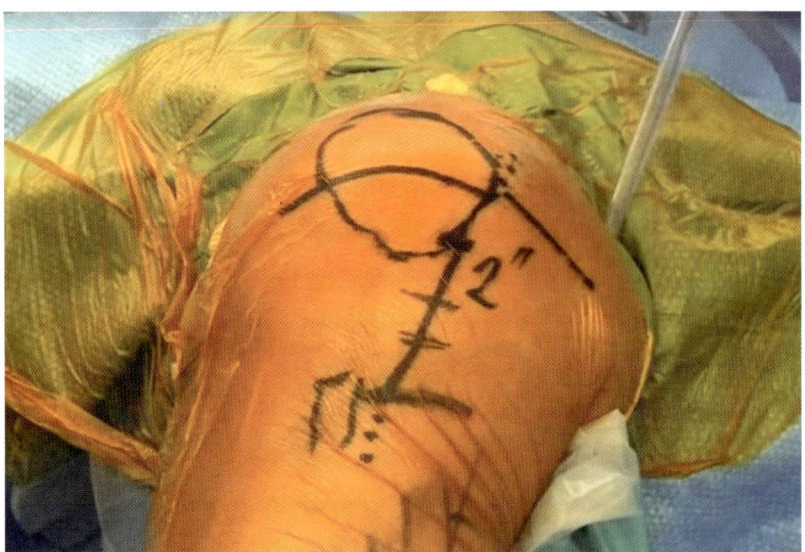

The incision is medial and begins from the medial part of lower pole of patella and extends to the medial border of tibial tuberosity.

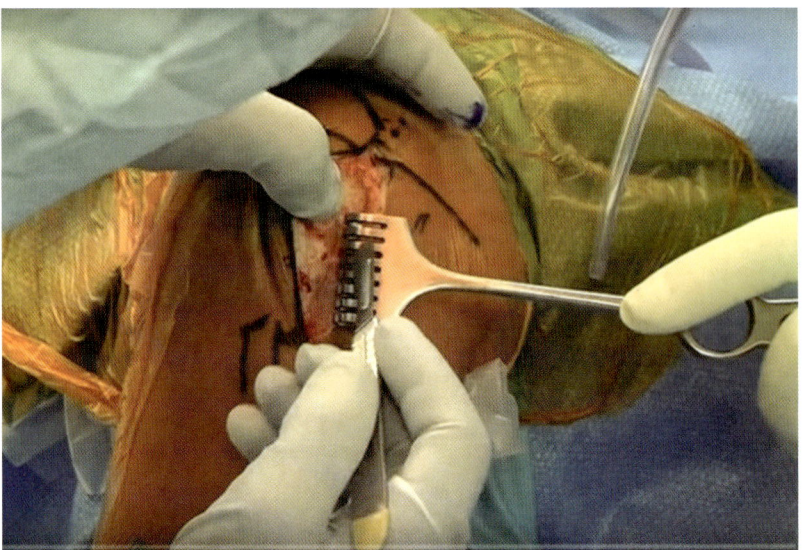

Once the skin is incised, the fat and the subcutaneous tissue are separated by a pad to allow for a correct and proper visualization of the patellar tendon and the patella.

Now an incision is made in the patellar tendon to allow a proper visualization of the medial border of patella. Using an oscillating saw, a small strip of the medial patellar border is cut.

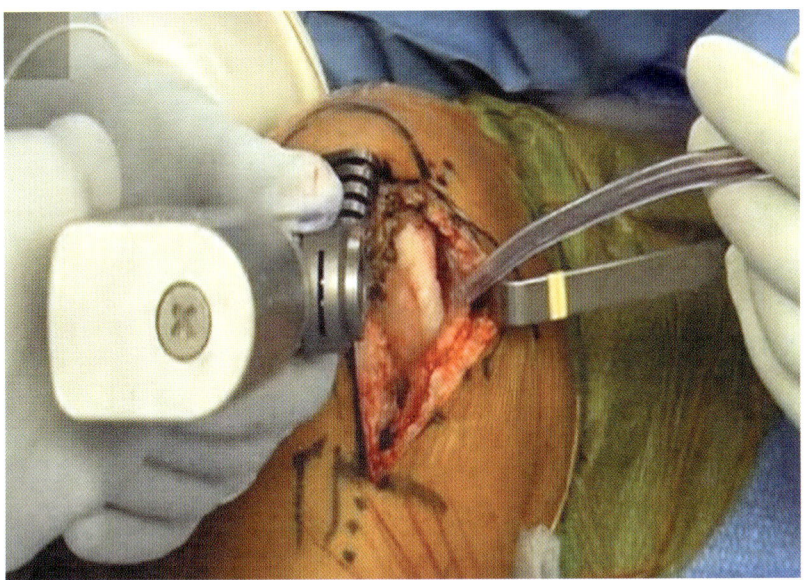

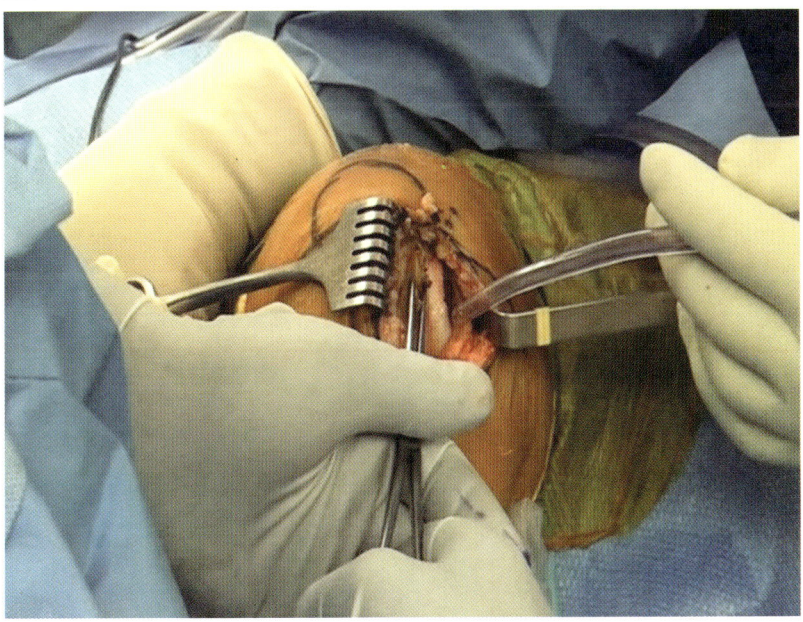

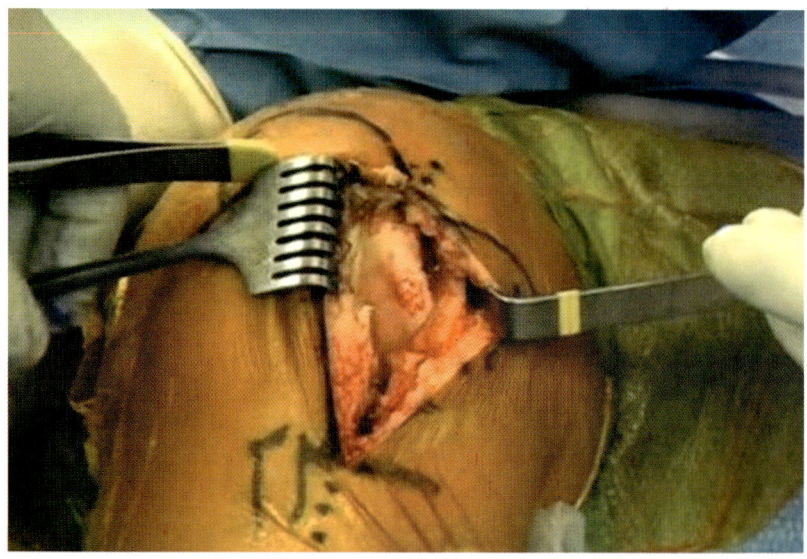

Removal of the patellar strip exposes the medial compartment more fully.

The joint is spread with lamina spreaders to expose the medial compartment of the knee.

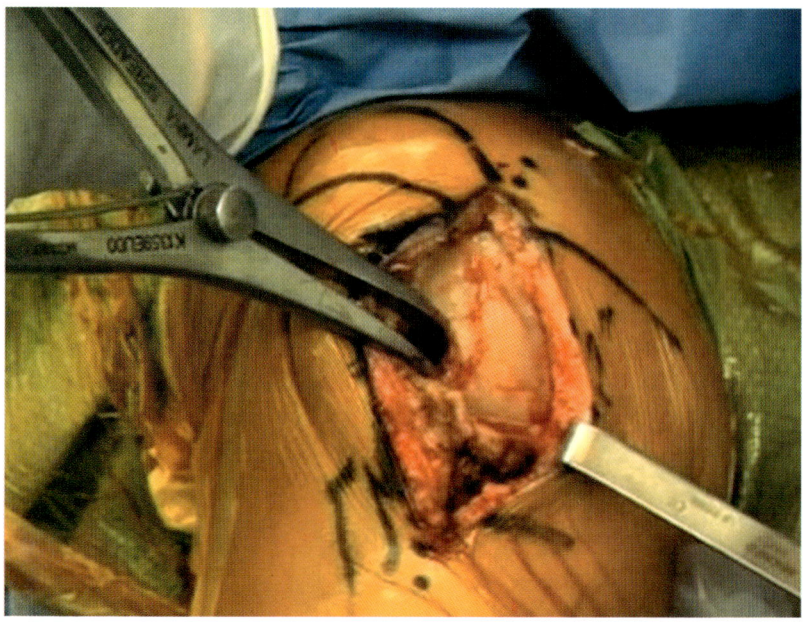

The upper tibial guide is pinned in place. The design ensures that no more than 5 to 6 mm of upper tibia are cut.

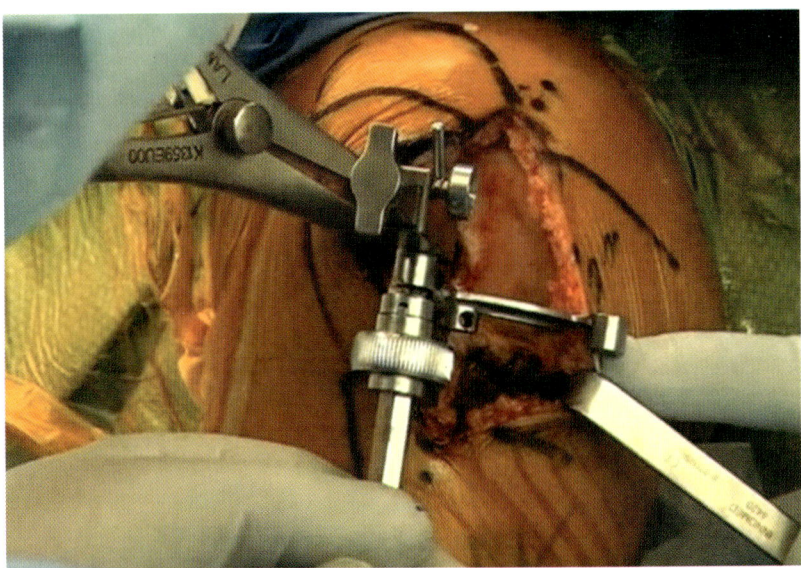

This guide ensures that the medial portion of the upper tibia is cut exactly parallel to the floor in mediolateral direction and in a 3° posterior slope.

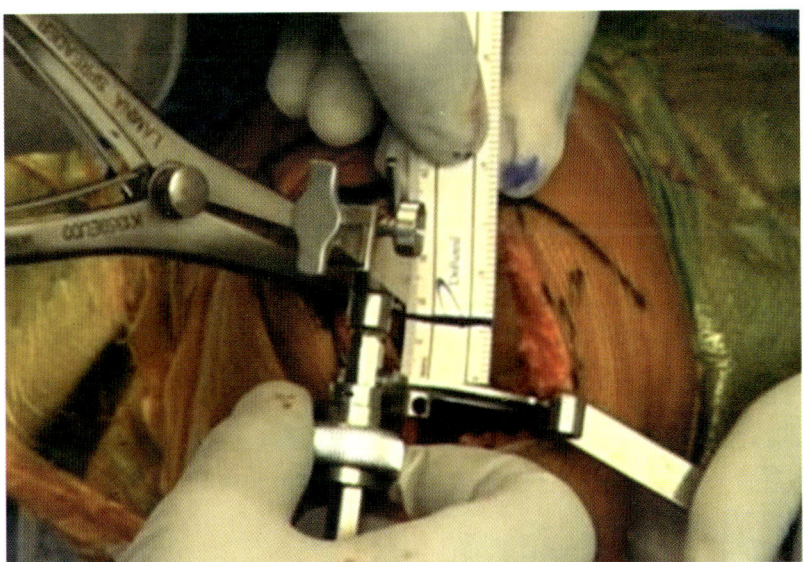

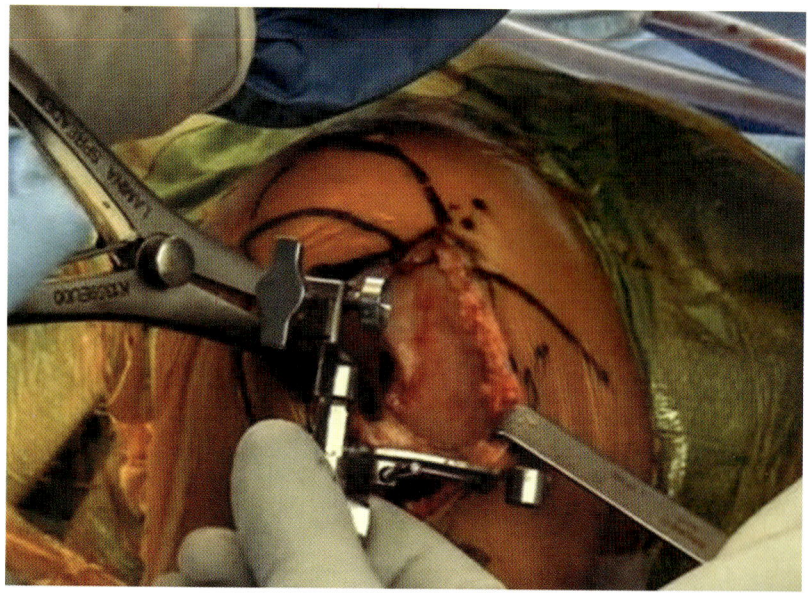

With an oscillating saw, the upper tibial cut is made.

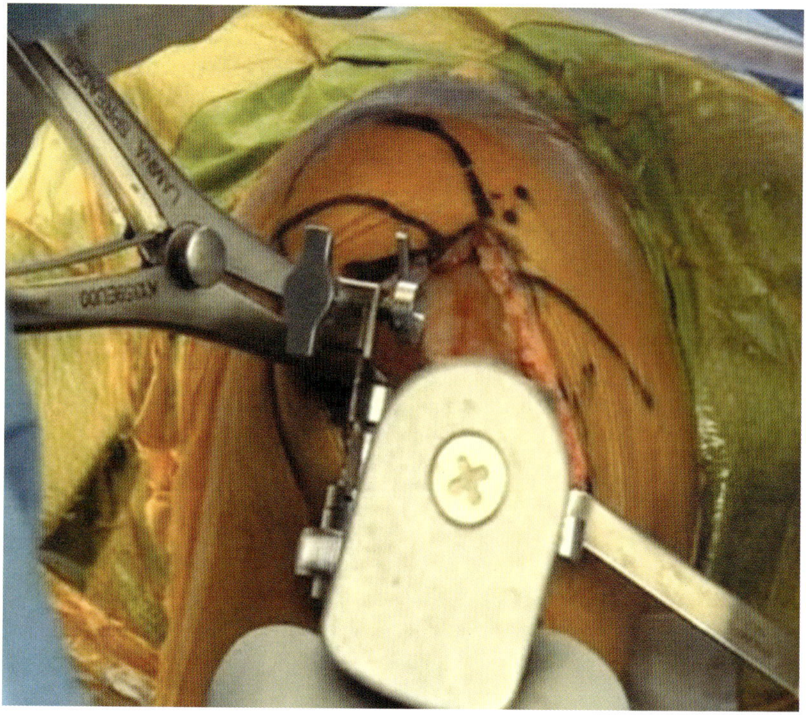

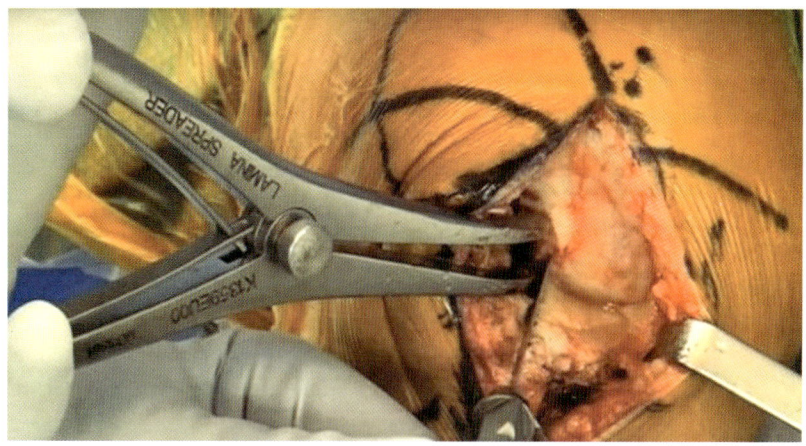

Using a reciprocating saw. the lateral edge of the medial compartment is cut deep enough to join the upper tibial cut. Care must be taken not to injure attachment of cruciates.

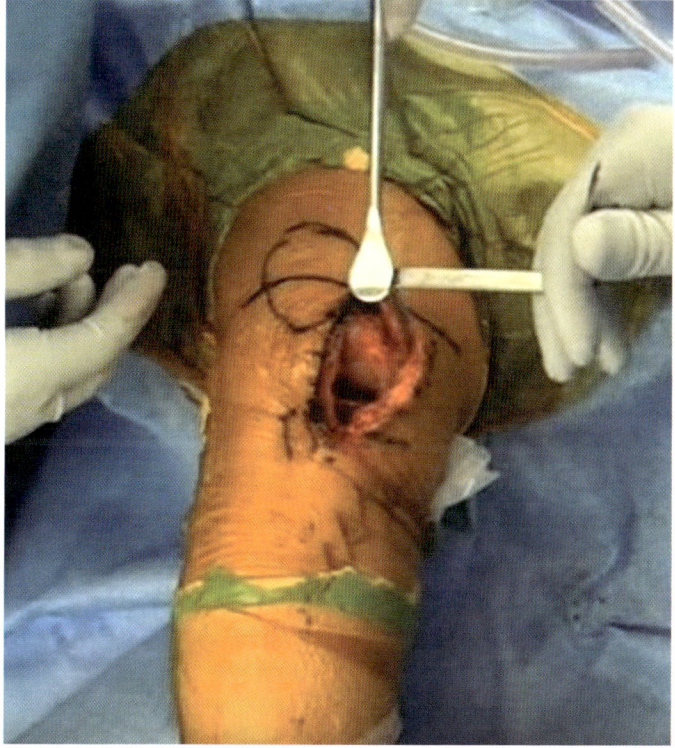

The knee is straightened and the gap inspected.

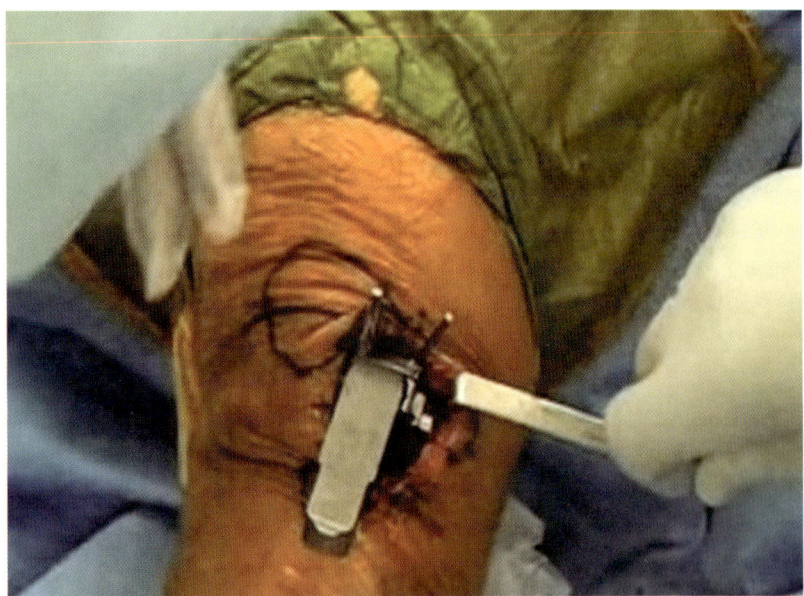

The distal femoral cutting block is pinned in place and the distal femoral cut is made. As this has an attachment to a plate resting on the cut surface of tibia, this cut becomes exactly parallel to the tibial cut.

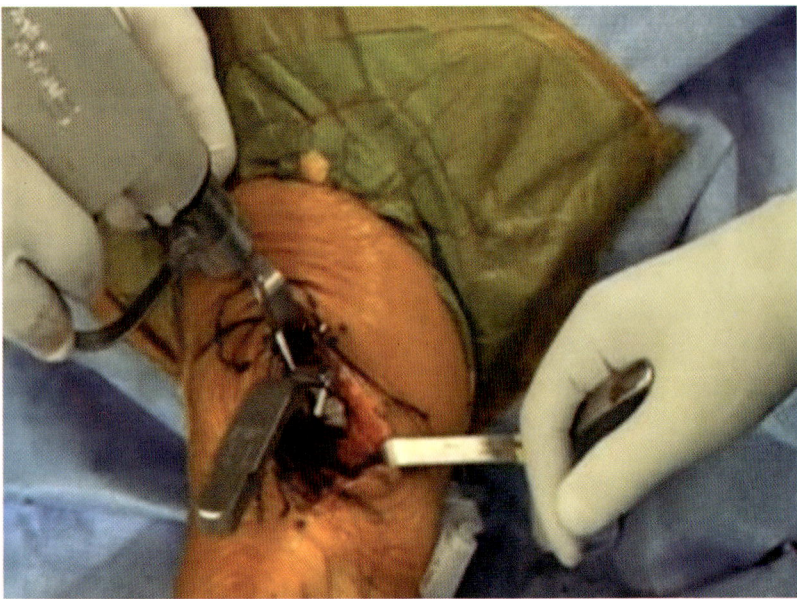

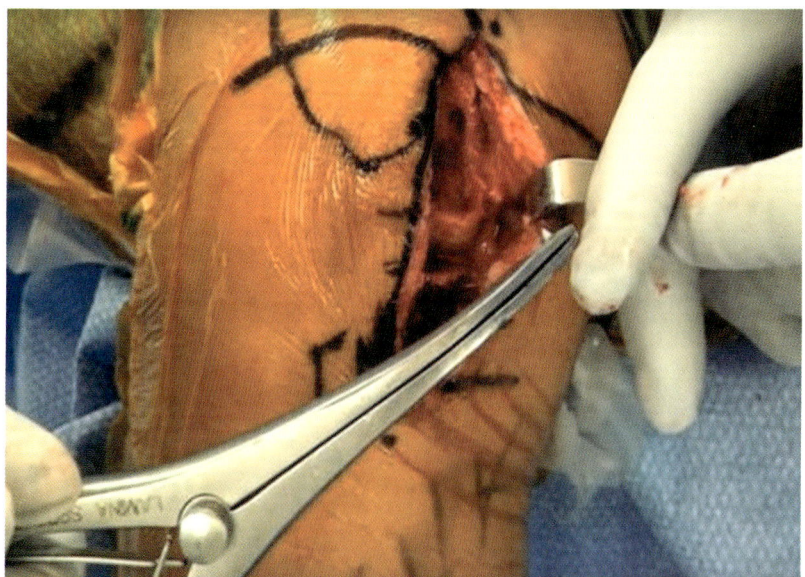

The cutting block is now removed.

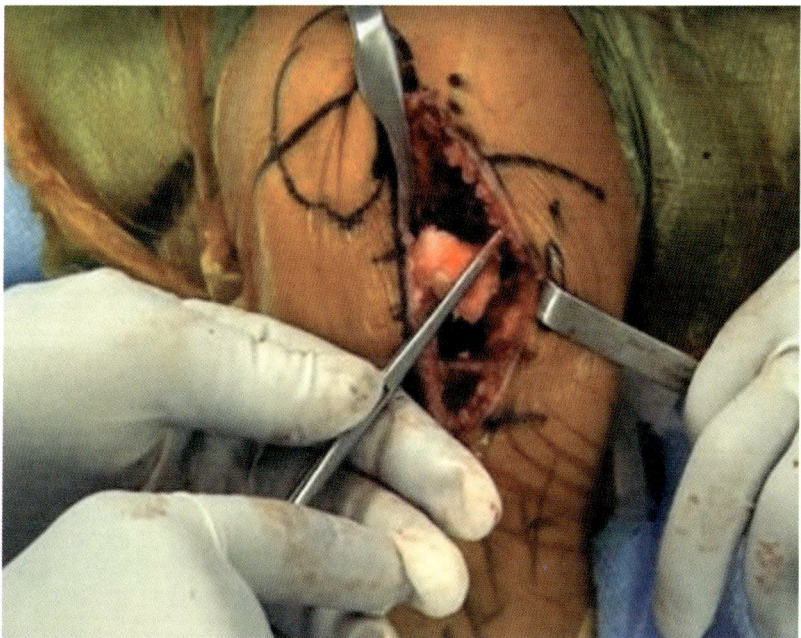

It can be seen that only a thin (5 to 6 mm) flake of bone has been removed.

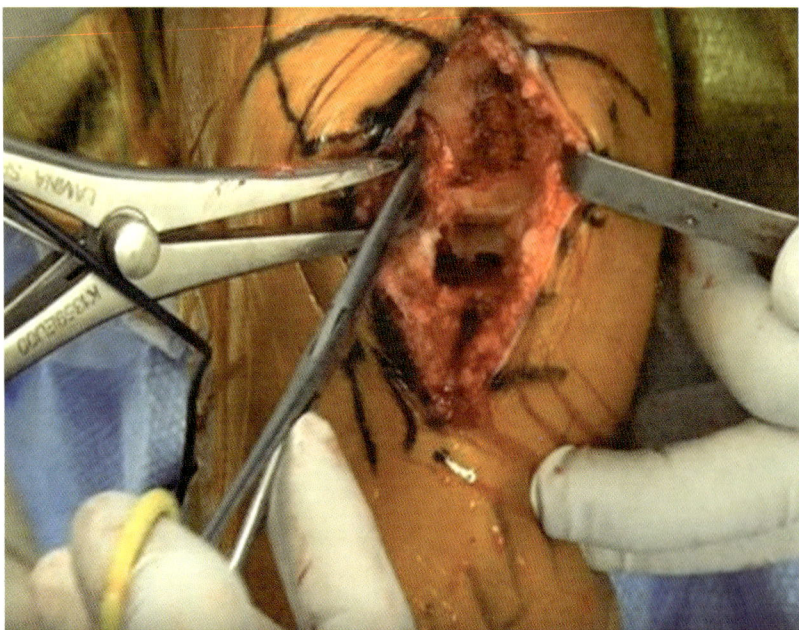

Homman retractors on either side expose the lower end of femur for placement of the anterior and chamfer cutting block.

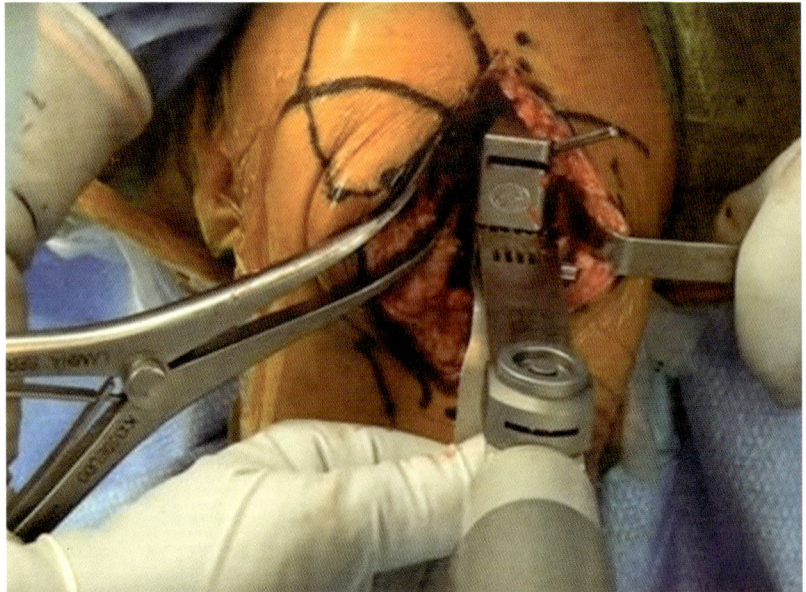

The anterior and chamfer cuts are now made.

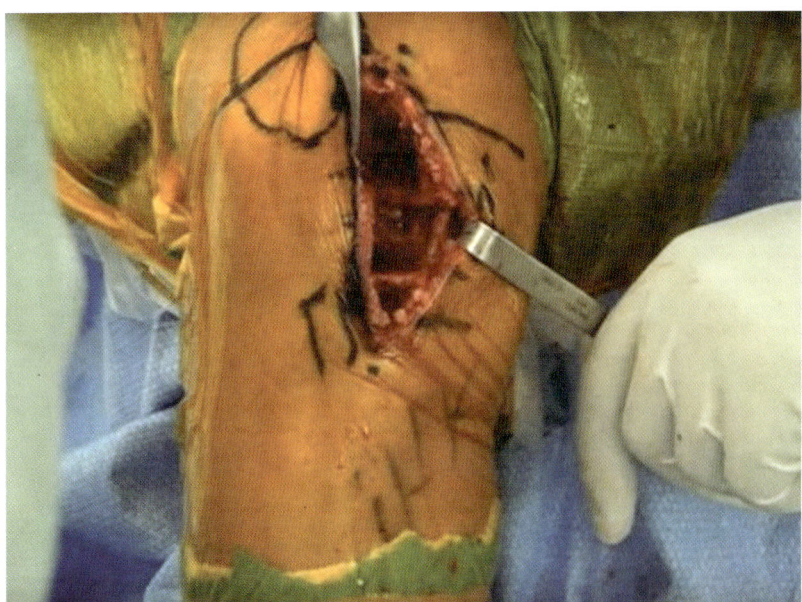

The posterior soft tissues are excised, taking due care to ensure that the medial collateral and anterior cruciate remain undisturbed.

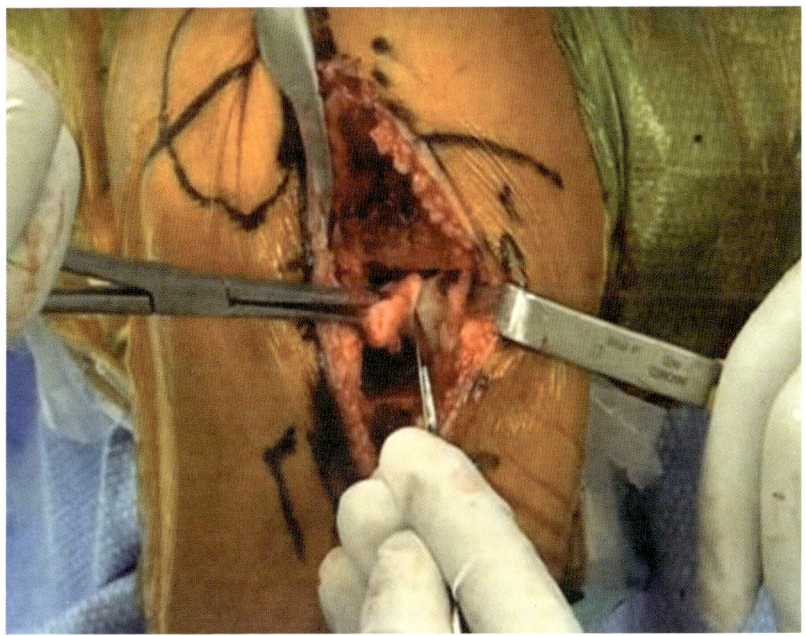

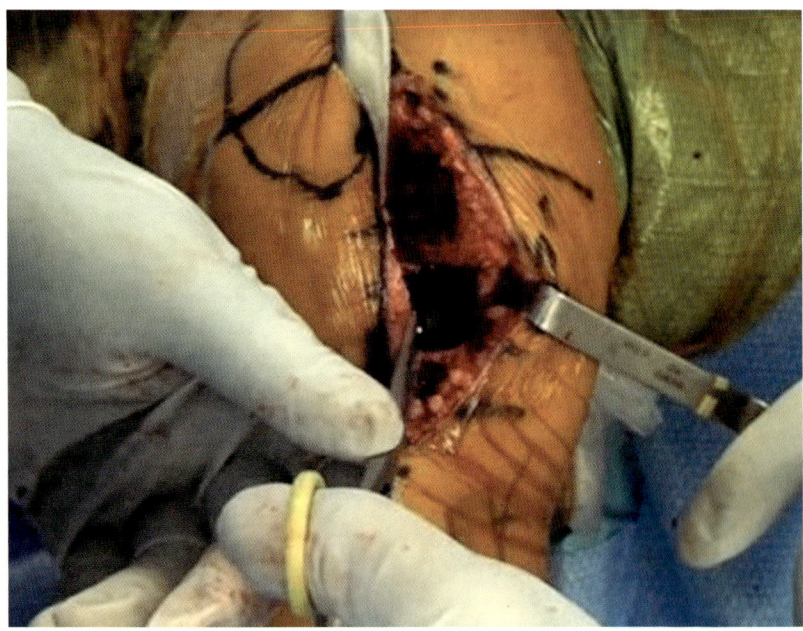

Trial femoral and tibial components are now placed over the cuts. It is ensured that the undersurfaces of both components exactly match the bone cuts and the components seat perfectly.

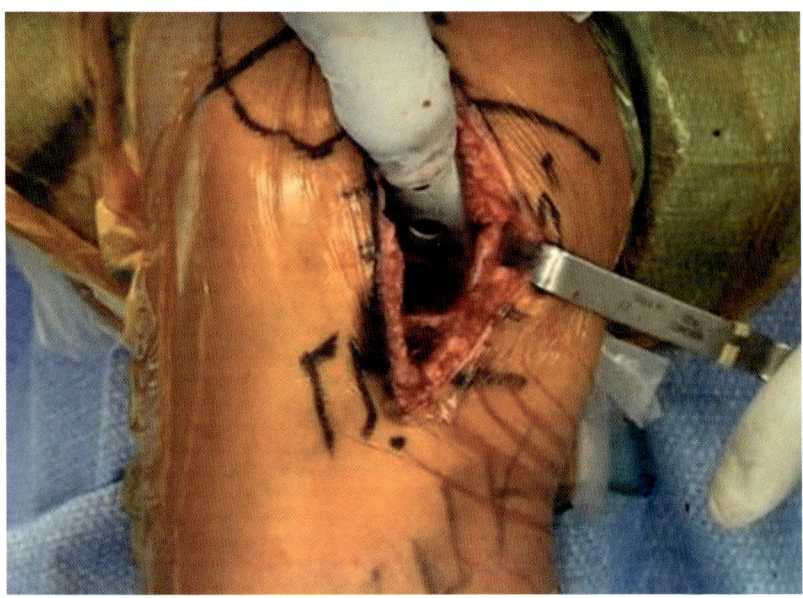

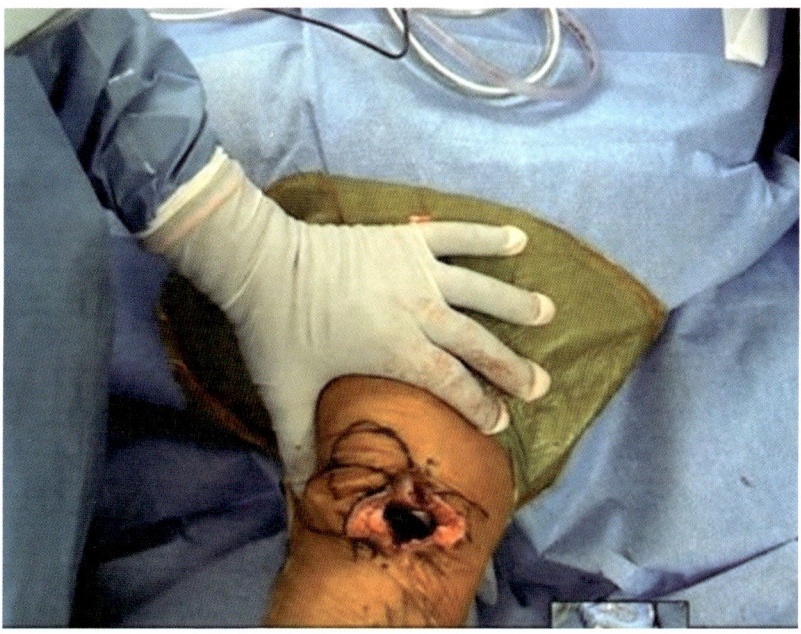

The ligament balance is assessed in both flexion and extension. In extension, the knee should be in 5° of valgus.

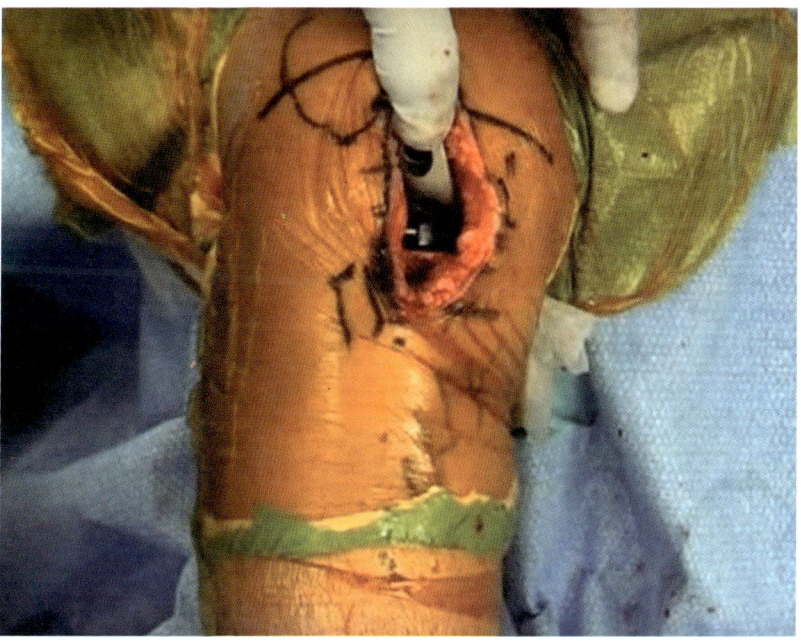

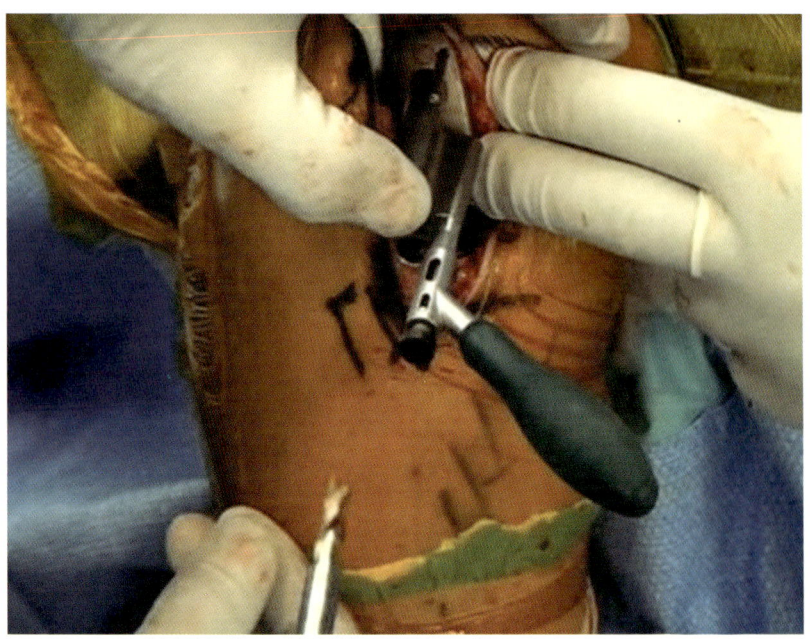

Femoral anchorage holes are now made using the special jig.

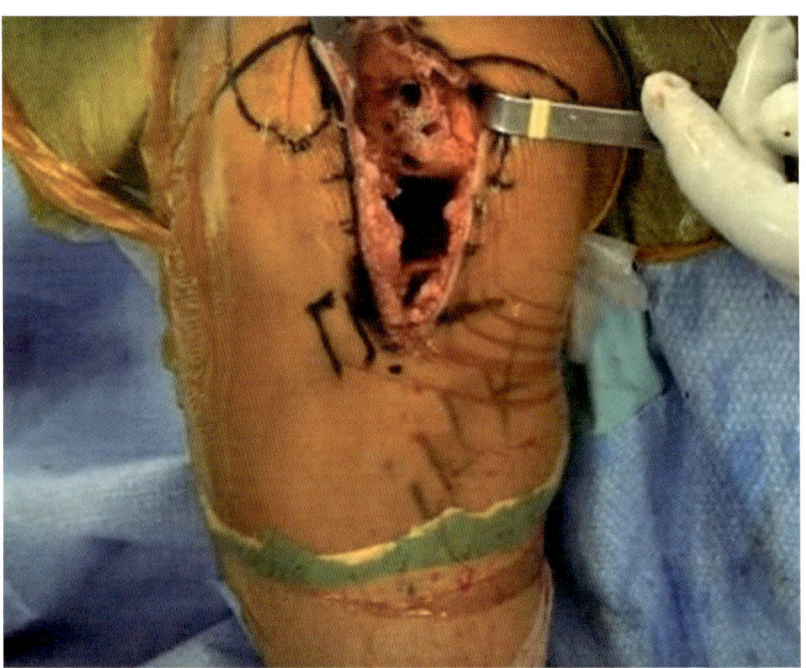

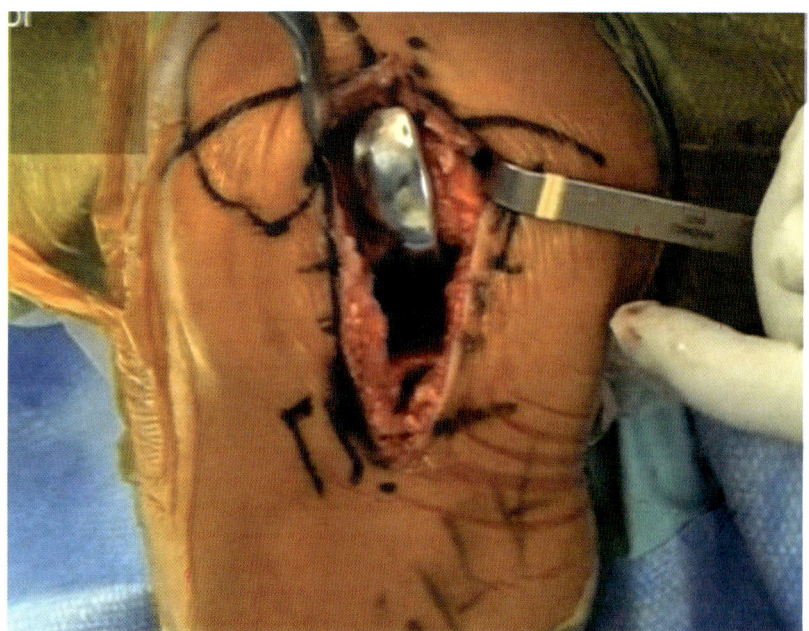

Femoral prosthesis is placed over the cut surface once again and its seating is checked.

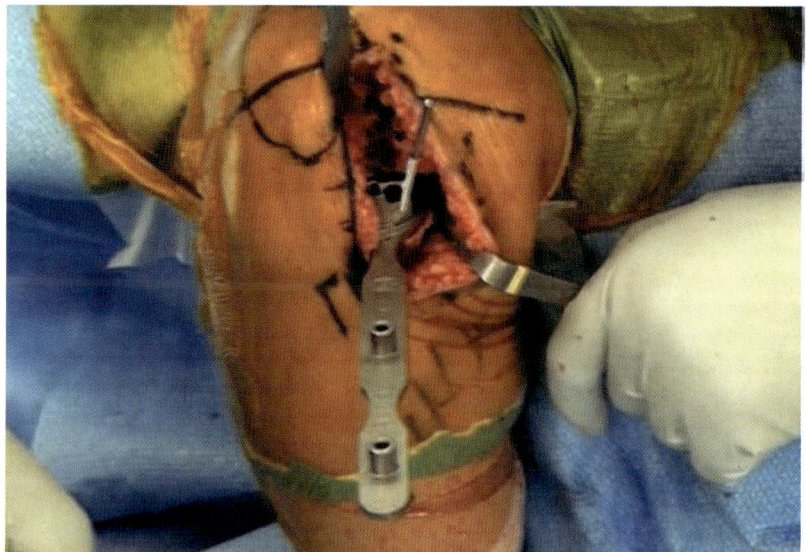

The tibial template is positioned and appropriate drill holes are made.

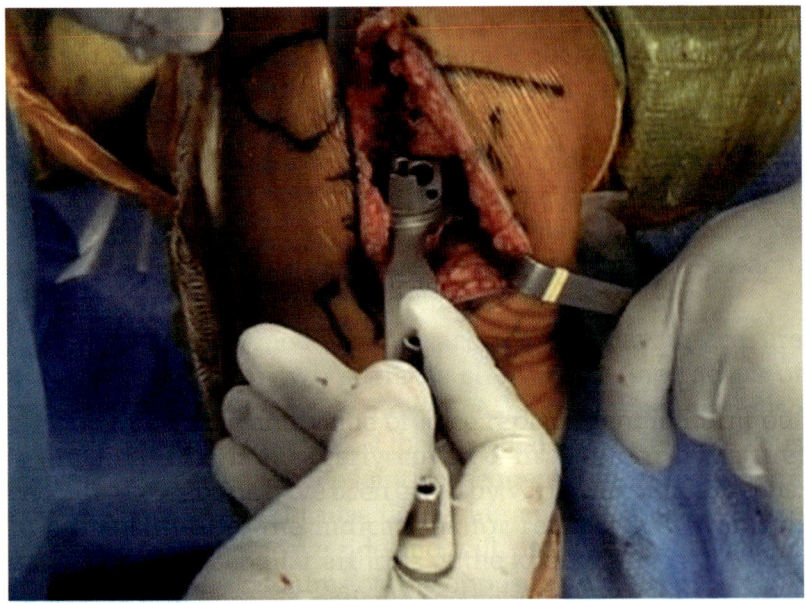

The jig ensures that the pegs on the underside of the actual tibial metal-back seat perfectly on the cut surface of upper tibia.

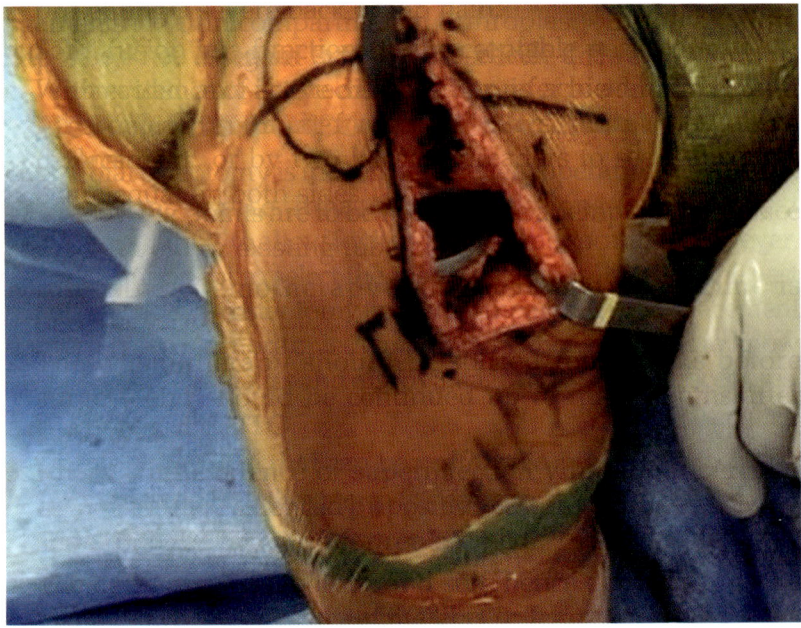

The actual component is placed and its seating is checked.

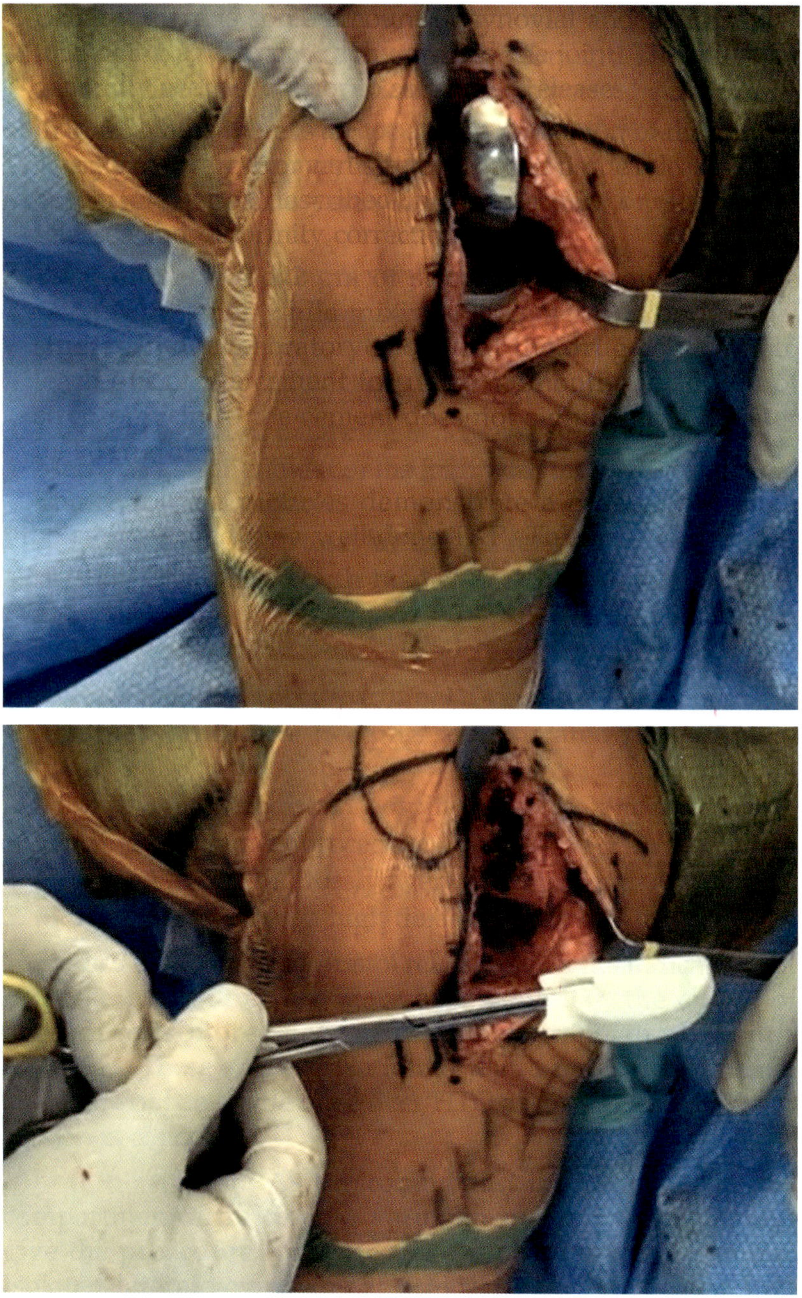

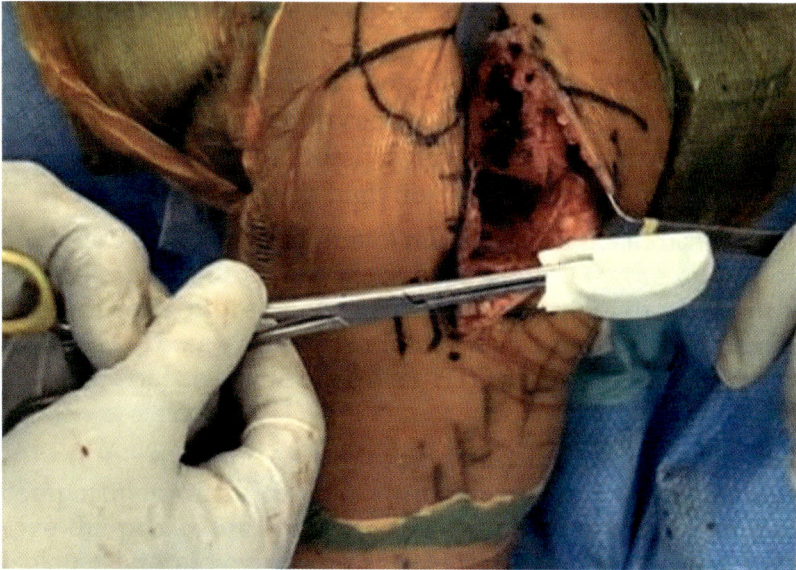

A plastic piece wrapped in a small stockinette held in a needle holder forms a cement pressurizing trowel.

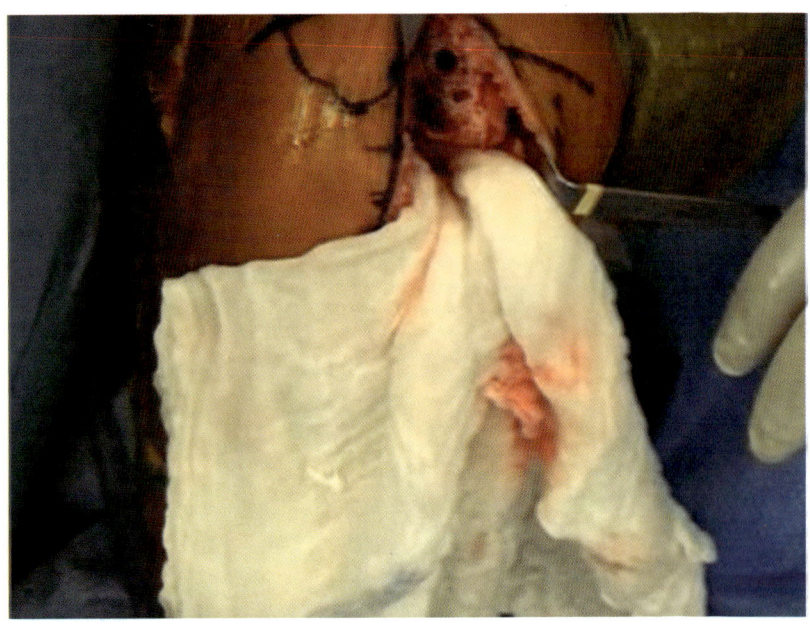

The joint is packed with adrenaline soaked gauze.

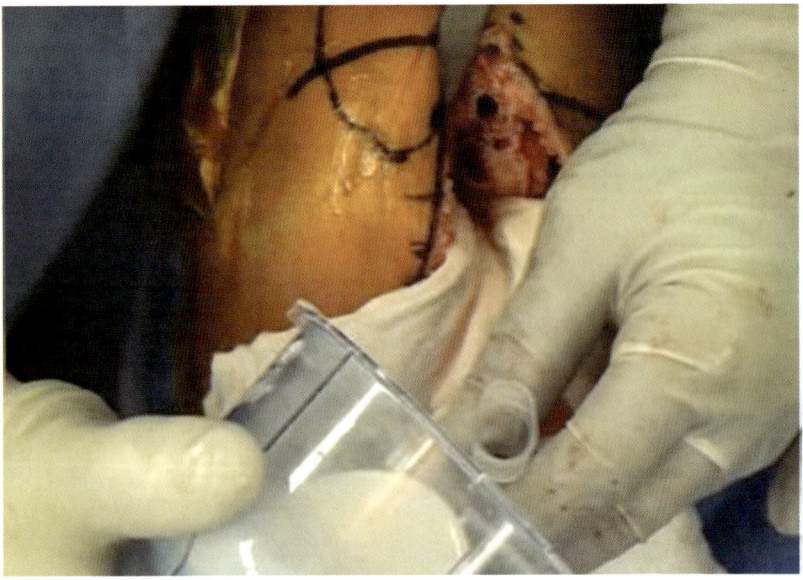

As liquid cement penetrates well into the cancellous area, it should be used as far as possible. When the cement is in a liquid state, it is poured into a 10 cc syringe.

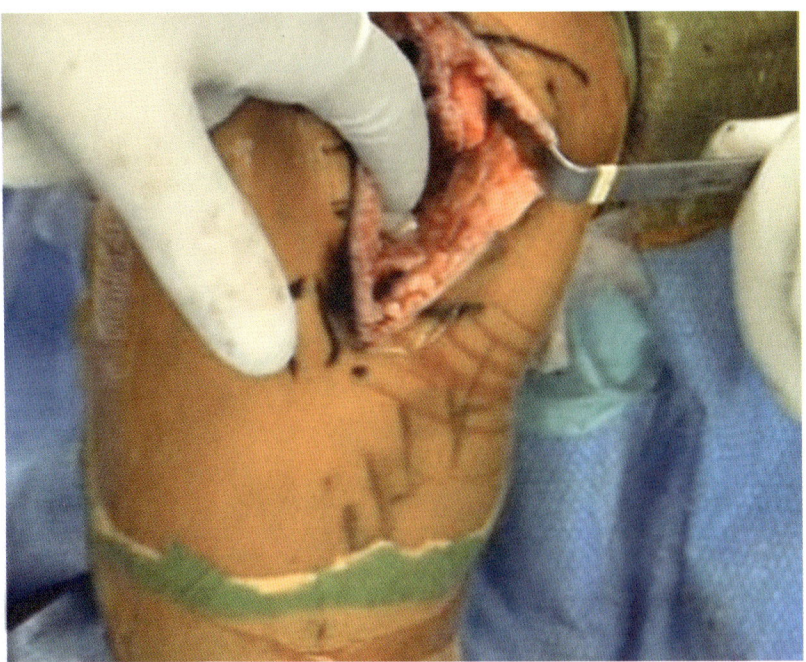

Cement is now injected over the upper cut surface of tibia.

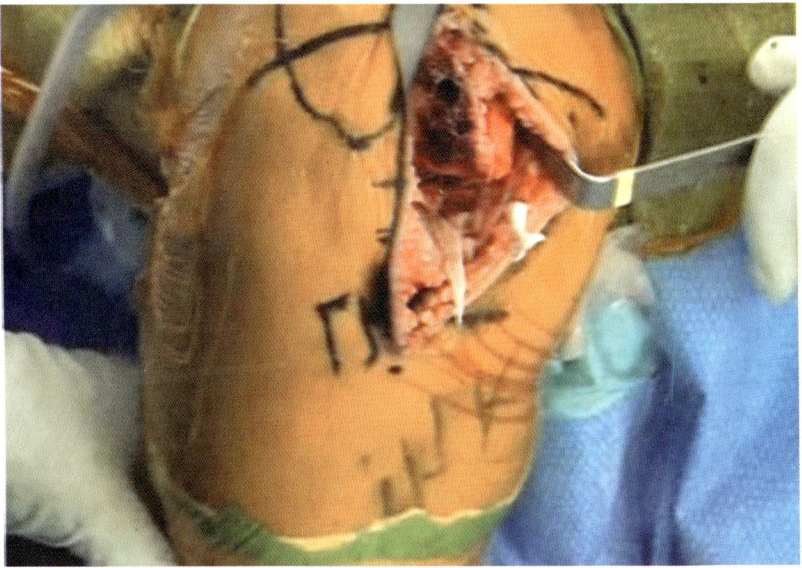

Excess cement is now removed with an artery forceps or a small curette.

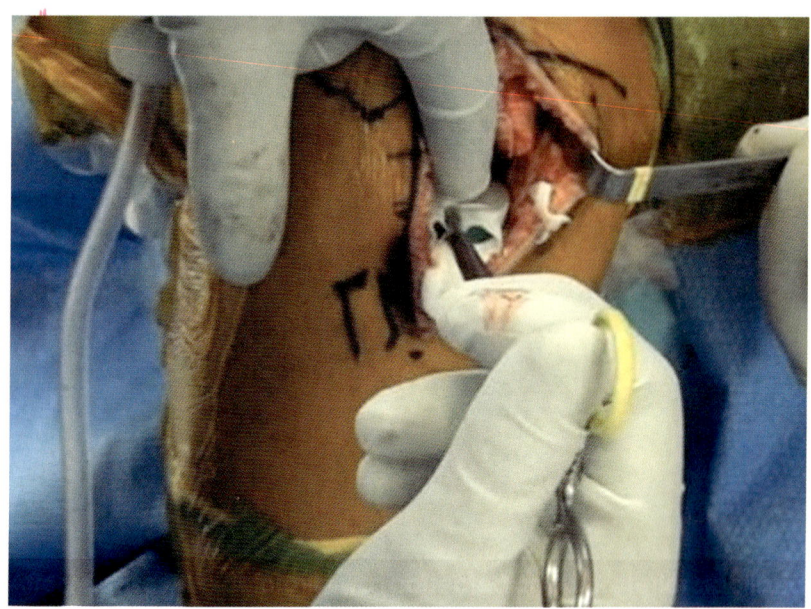

The cement is now pushed home with the trowel fabricated earlier.

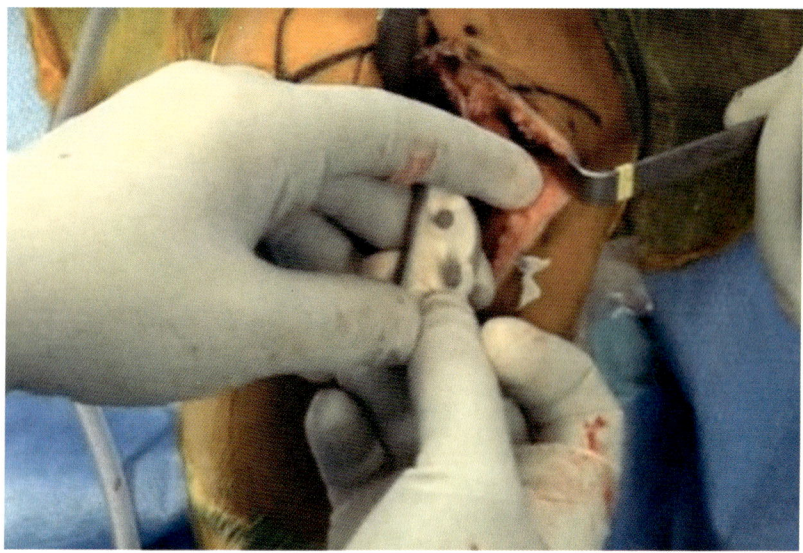

Additional cement is now applied to the under surface of the tibial component. This is now placed over the tibial surface and pressed home.

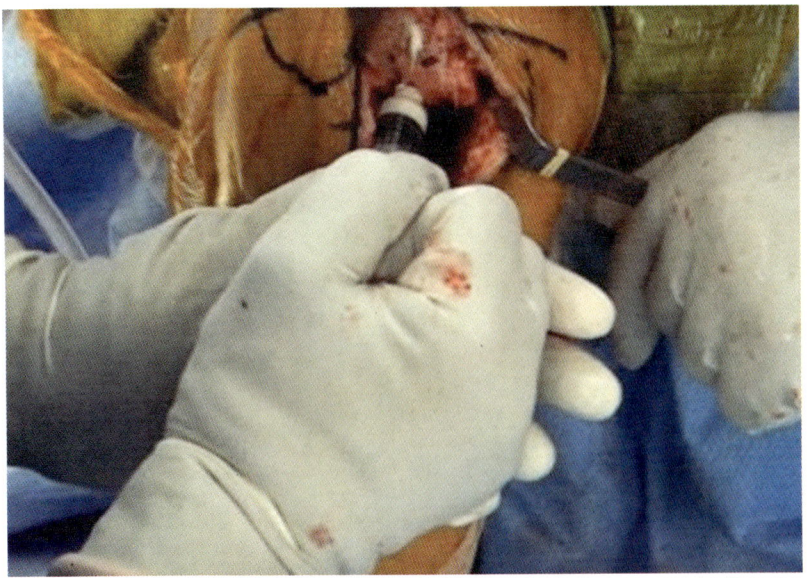

Liquid cement is now injected over the cut femoral surface and pressed back with the trowel to push it into cancellous areas.

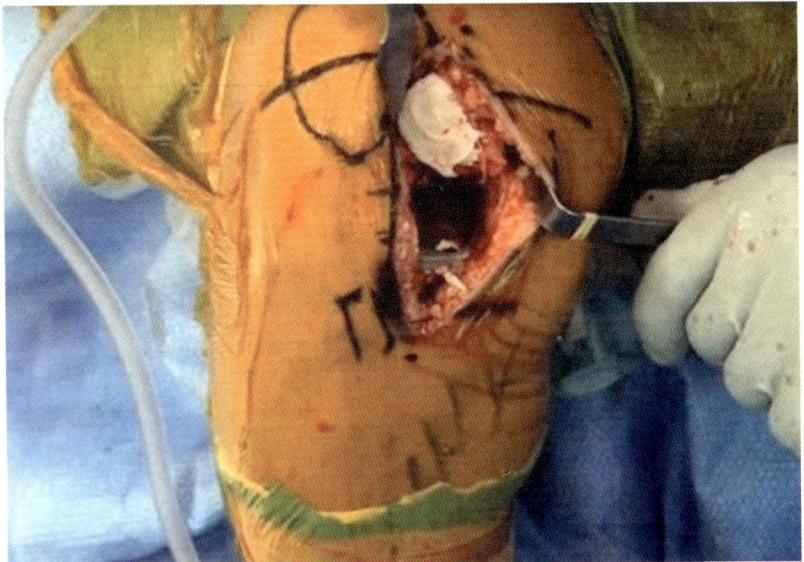

We must ensure that the cement mantle is uniform all around the femoral cut surface.

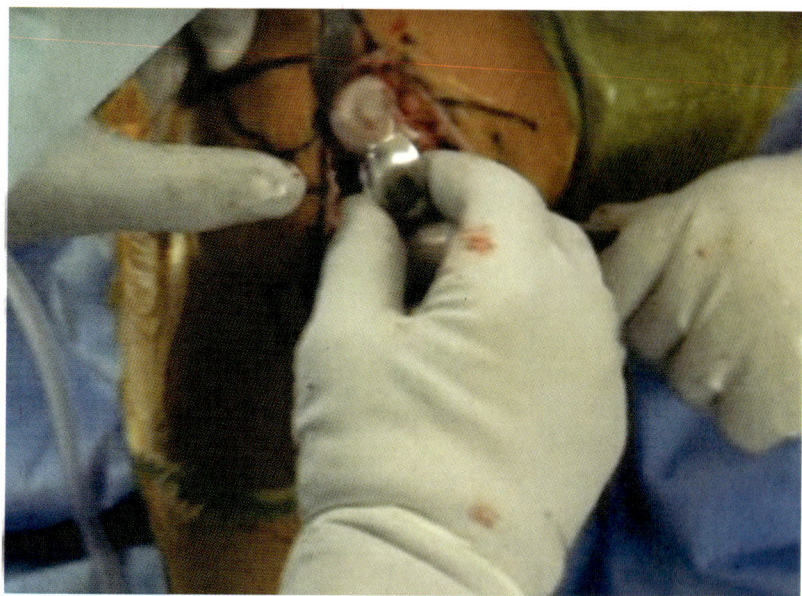

The prosthesis is now pressed home, taking care to ensure that it seats in its correct position.

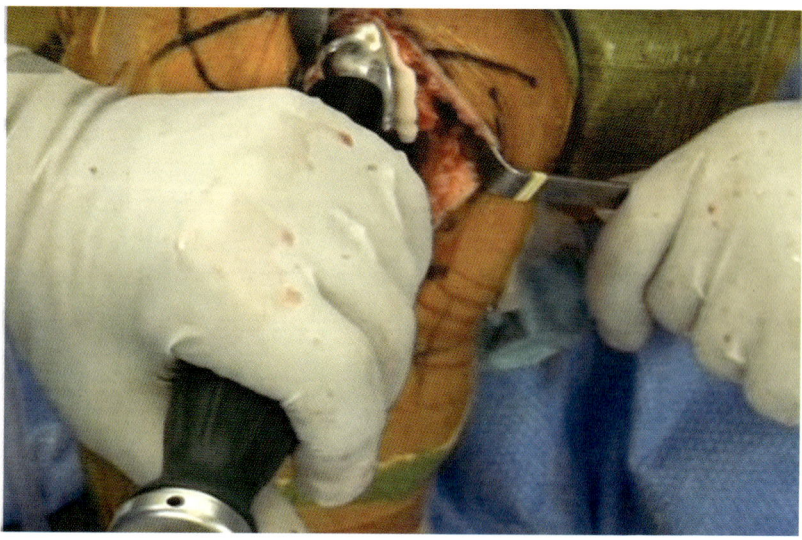

Using an impactor, the prosthesis is pushed home and sustained pressure applied till cement sets. A cement which is setting should never be hammered. Sustained pressure is the key to successful cementation.

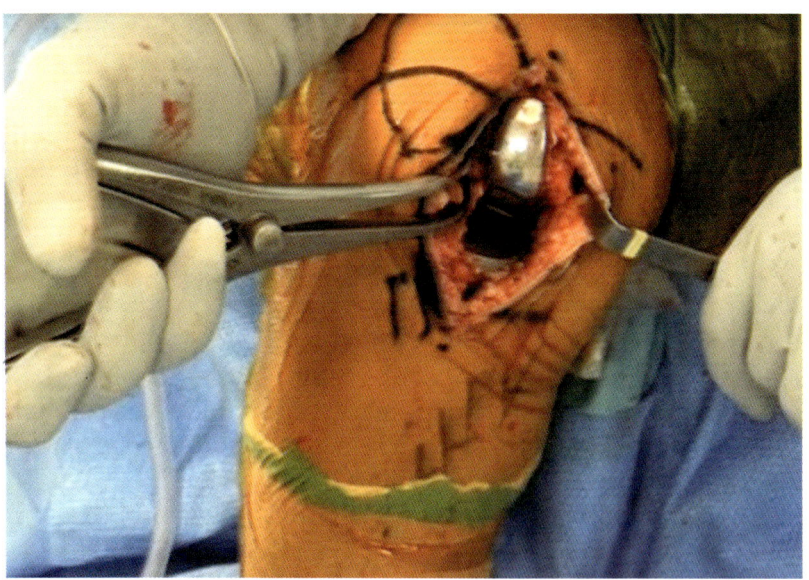

The joint is now washed to remove all loose cement bits.

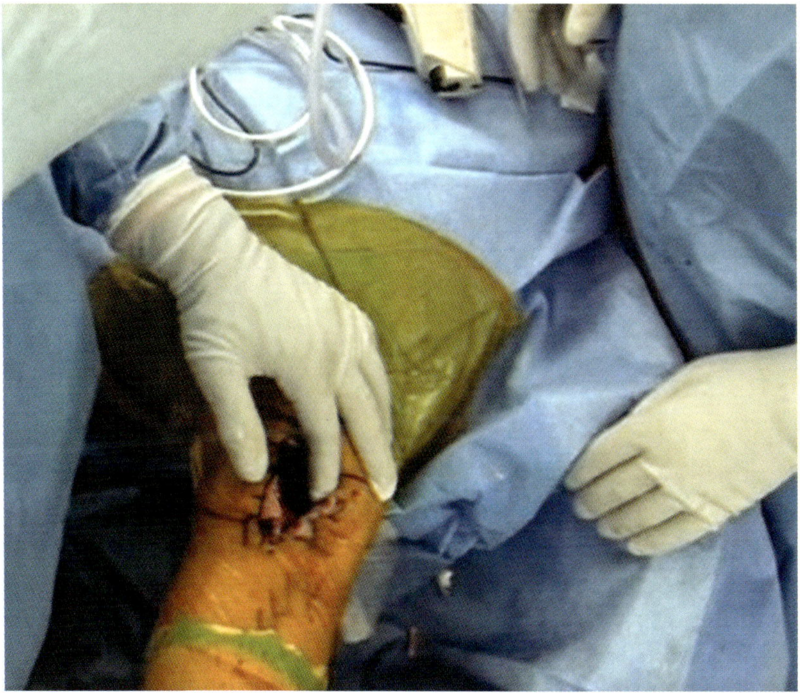

A spacer is now inserted into the cemented components.

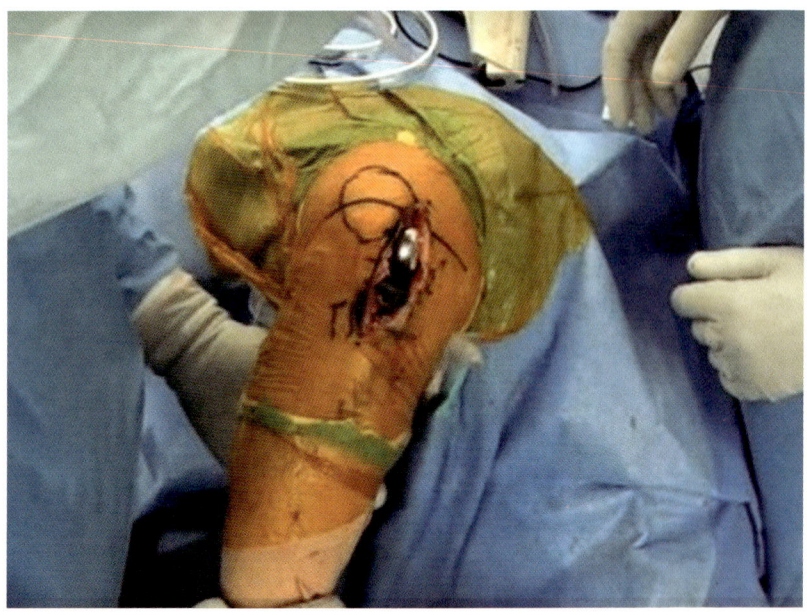

The joint is now put through the full range of motion and its stability checked in flexion, extension and mid-range.

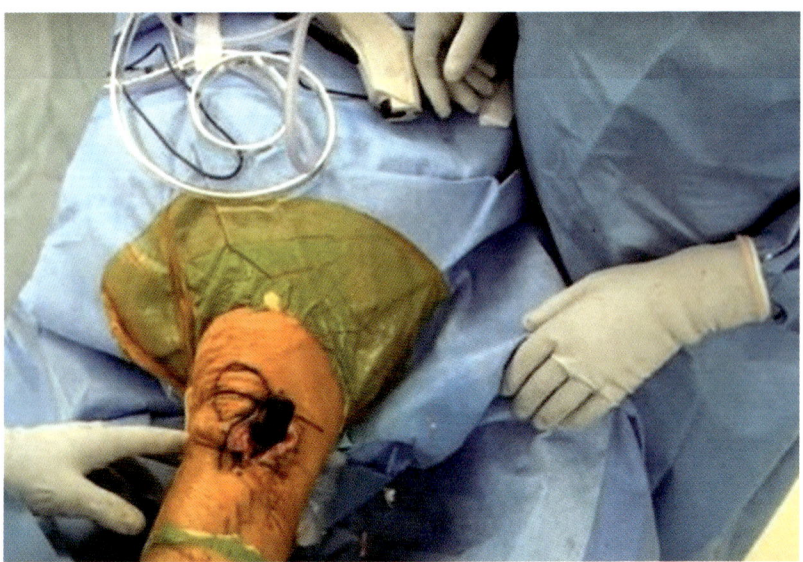

The knee should be in varus, and rock solid in extension, while permitting a small mediolateral rock in mid-flexion. At this stage the spacer thickness is decided.

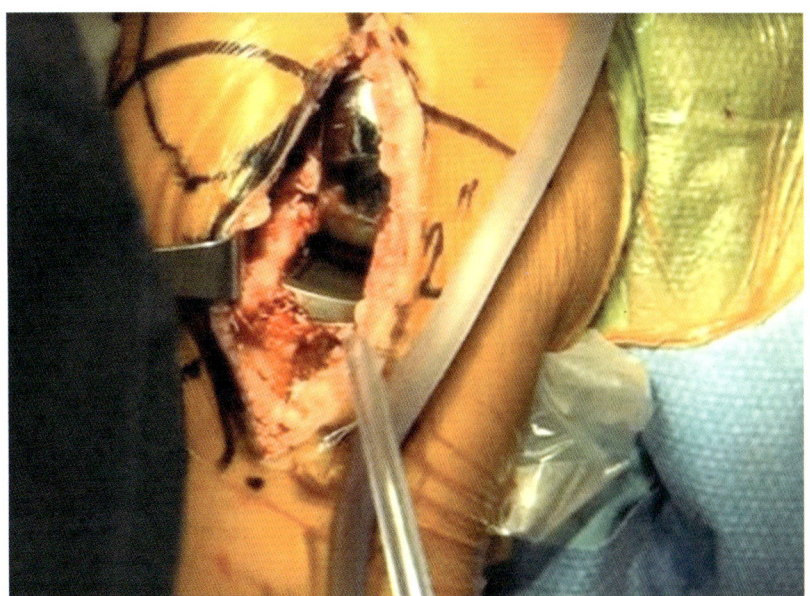

The joint interior is washed thoroughly to clear it of all cement bits.

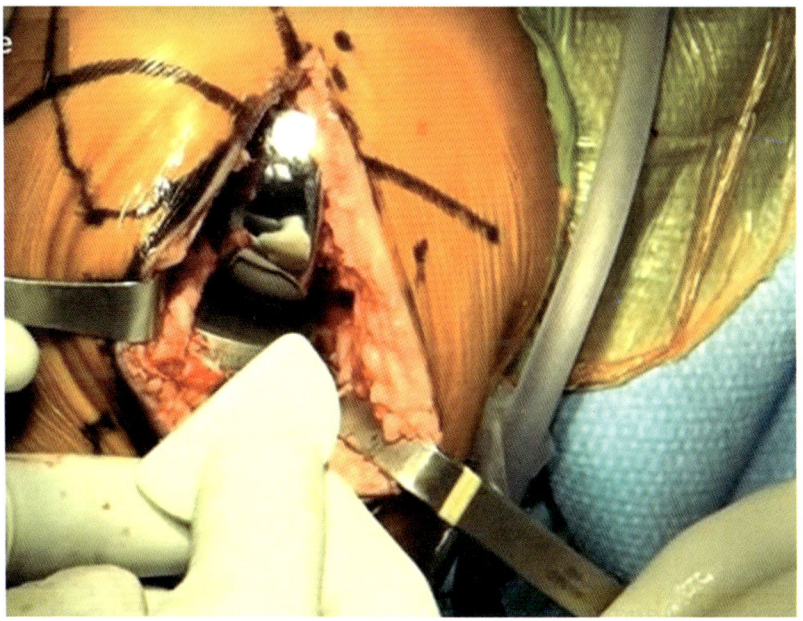

Appropriate sized HDPE insert is removed from its packing.

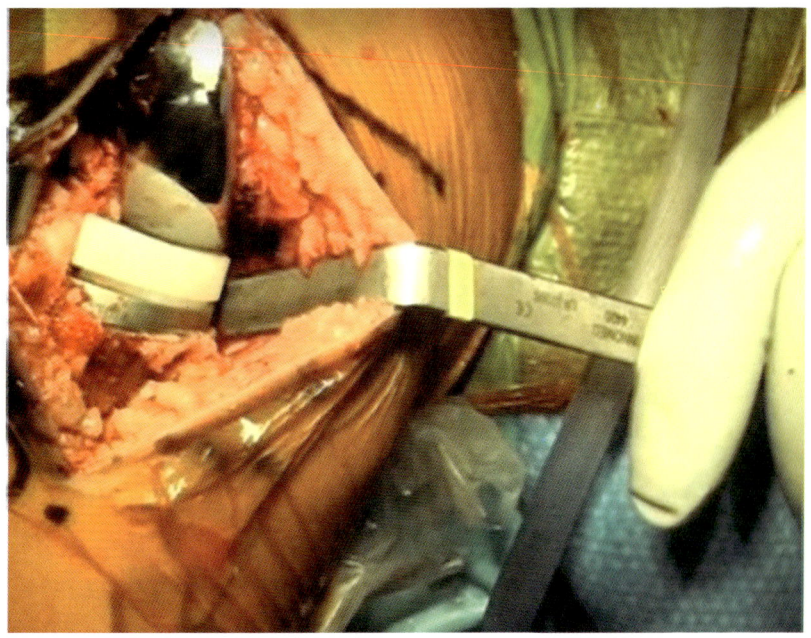

The insert is pushed into position and hammered for a snap fit.

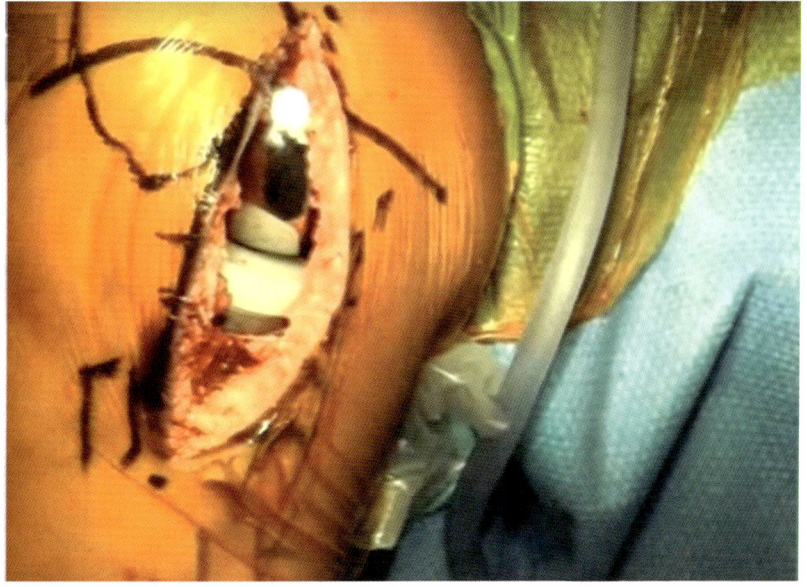

The knee is once again put through the full range of motion.

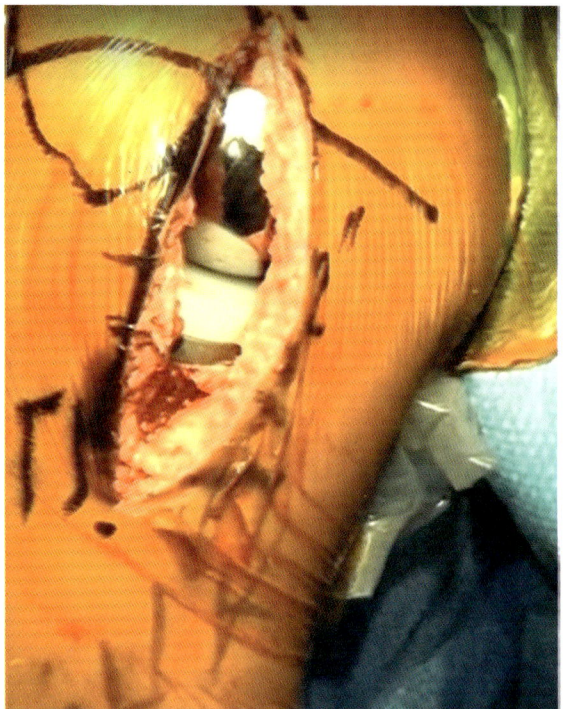

The incision is less than 100 to 125 mm and a drain is usually inserted.

The wound is closed in layers and compression bandage is applied.

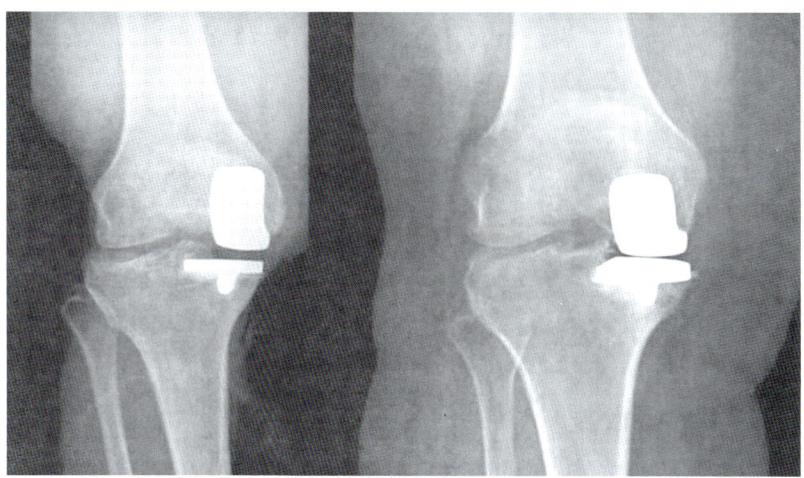

The postoperative radiograph should show the following: The knee should be in 4° to 6° of valgus.

The joint line should be parallel to the ground with the patient standing.

The components should be seated properly.

Steps for cementation of unicompartmental knees:

These steps are essentially similar to those for cemented knees. For the sake of completeness, the correct cementation technique is described once again.

The correct implants are removed from their sterile wrappings and inserted without cement. The knee is put through full range of movements after the patella is put back. In case there is a laxity, the next higher thickness is chosen. Likewise, in case of a knee with a flexion deformity on extension, a thinner component is chosen.

The cut surfaces are thoroughly washed with saline. Using a nylon brush mounted on a pneumatic drill, the cancellous area is scrubbed and washed once again. The complete cementation area is packed dry with a swab soaked in adrenaline and kept dry until cementation.

Cement is mixed. It is better to start cementation while the cement is semi-liquid. About 30 cc are poured over the flat surface of the tibia with a spoon, else it is poured into a syringe and injected over the tibial surface.

There should be no blood on the gloved hands of the surgeon or the assistant. The component is shoved in and sustained pressure applied with a tibial pusher. A small pad is kept on the posterior aspect of the tibia to avoid thermal necrosis and damage to popliteal vessels.

By this time the cement gets a bit more tacky and is dabbed on the interior of the femoral component. The remaining cement is applied as a single layer over the cut surface of the femur. Some surgeons prefer to use a second mix, and while liquid, pour it into the syringe and inject it under pressure into the femoral holes. The prosthesis is now inserted, and sustained pressure applied to compress the cement and remove air bubbles.

A curette is used to scrape off all overflowing cement from both surfaces and the knee is reduced with a trial spacer in place.

The knee is pushed into hyperextension, by which both components will pressurise each other. Sustained pressure is applied until the cement sets.

Once the cement is fully set, the knee is flexed again, the spacer removed and the interior inspected for the presence of loose cement bits. Overhanging cement from either the tibia or the femur is gently tapped off using a small sharp chisel. The interior of the knee is washed thoroughly, and the knee extended.

A drain tube of size 12 is inserted. The patellar tendon is sutured with a good absorbable suture like 1 Vicryl or 1 Daxone. Subcutaneous and skin closure is routine. The drain tubes are connected to a closed suction drainage system. The skin is closed with a 1 nylon or 1 zero proline. A sterile dressing is applied over the sutured area and cotton and crepe are applied in two layers.

The patient is shifted to the ward. In case a spinal anaesthetic is used, and for elderly patients with a history of prostatic or urinary symptoms, it is usual to catheterize in the theatre itself.

On the first postoperative day, the catheter is removed. If the patient has a good pain threshold, one can make him stand. Walking with a walking frame is started on day two and the bandages are loosened on the fifth day and knee flexion is started. Using a smooth mica board with talcum powder on it, the patient is encouraged to rub the heel on the board allowing gradual flexion.

The patient climbs stairs on the fifth day and if comfortable, is discharged on the sixth. By the tenth postoperative day, flexion of up to 90° is usually achieved. The operated knee is moved first while climbing downstairs and second when climbing upstairs.

Stitches are removed on the 14th day. One X-ray is taken immediately postoperative and another is taken on the 14th day at suture removal. The patient is called for follow-up at two months, six months and annually thereafter for clinical and radiographic evaluation.

Complications of Knee Replacement and their Management

Knee replacement is a major surgical procedure and consequently subject to various complications that may occur from any procedure of this magnitude. The fact that such a large amount of foreign body is implanted into a joint so superficially, and the fact that the circumferential soft tissue coverage is so less, leads to certain complications that really trouble the surgeon and the patient.

The commonly occurring complications are given below. The list, by no means exhaustive, should not scare away the beginner from attempting to perform this procedure. Rather, these should make the surgeon forewarned and forearmed, so as to prevent these; should these complications occur, he should be well knowledgeable and prepared to overcome the problems.

Early complications:
- Thrombosis and thromboembolism.
- Skin problems and poor wound healing.
- Superficial and deep infections.
- Joint instability
- Fractures
- Patellar tendon rupture

Late Complications:
- Delayed infection
- Fractures
- Patellar problems
- Loosening
- Wear and deformation
- Component breakage

Thrombosis and Thromboembolism:

Clinical evidence of DVT is between 1 and 10%, but routine fibrinogen scans and venography show a much higher incidence (up to 60%). Most of these studies have been conducted in the West and published in the western literature. There have been no publications of the incidence or fatalities due to pulmonary embolus in Indian patients.

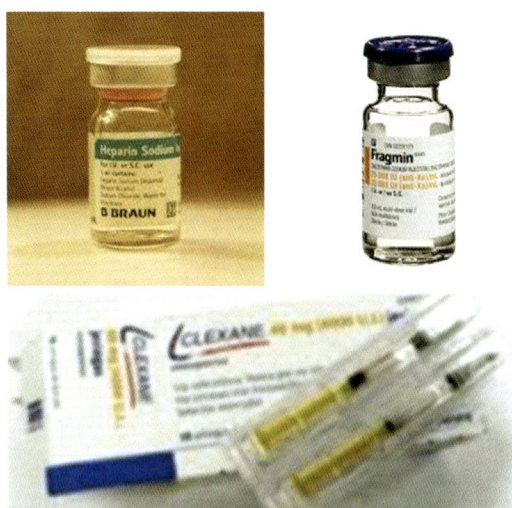

Various anticoagulants and regimes are in use.

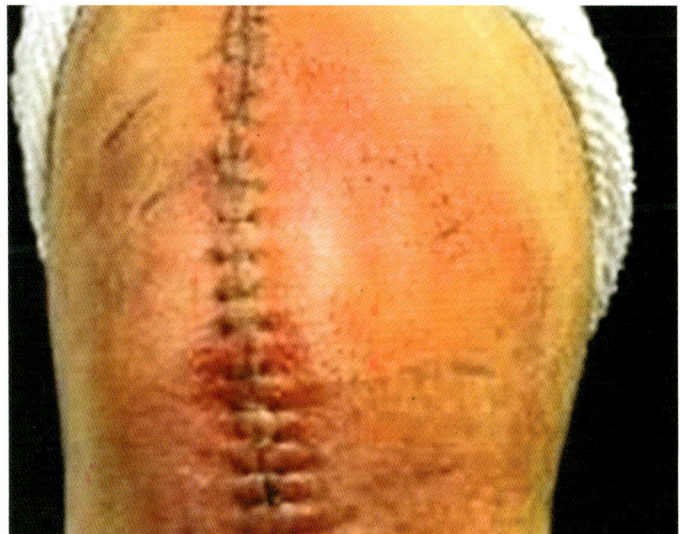

Using anticoagulants to a therapeutic level is indeed riskier with a knee replacement than in a hip because of the larger implant size and closer proximity to the skin. Thus the complications of poor wound healing and haematoma formation are much higher with anticoagulated patients. In the West, most centres use a protocol of partial or total anticoagulation using Heparin, Minihep, Warfarin, etc. In my centre, however, I do not use anticoagulants at all. A specific tailored regime is used ONLY for high risk patients and those with a proven history of associated problems.

Skin problems and poor wound healing:

Up to this point, all the clinical pictures in this book are from my own patients, and drawings drawn by me. The radiographs are either those of my patients or belong to my coauthors.

It is a fortunate coincidence that I have not faced any of the complications described below. So I had to depend on the internet to download these photos. But it is essential to know about these problems, so that they can be solved with confidence if they occur.

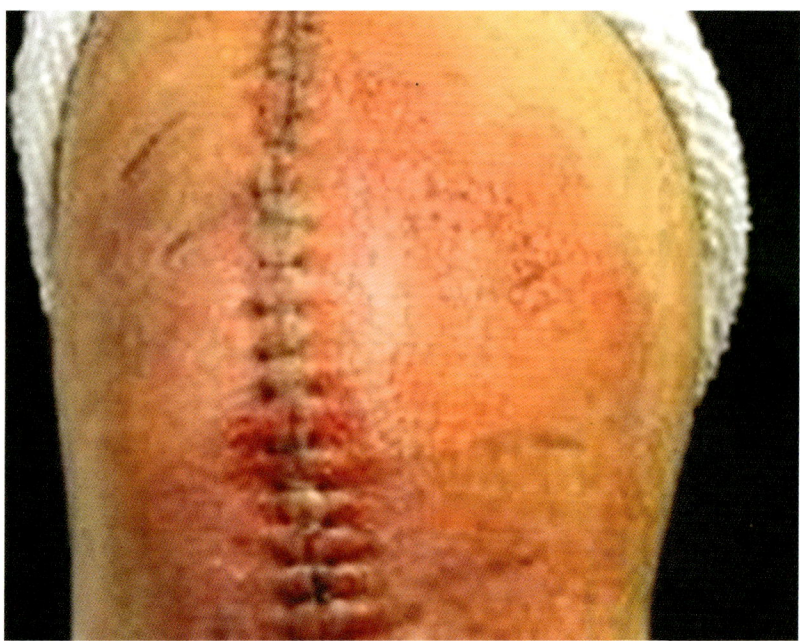

Signs of inflammation, the earliest sign that all is not well.

The commonly found skin problems are:

1. Marginal skin necrosis
2. Extensive sloughing of the wound
3. Complete sloughing of the entire operated area
4. Partial healing with a sinus formation
5. Small haematoma
6. Large haematoma

At this stage, one must not delay in trying to diagnose and solve the problem. Early infection is imminent in the above picture. It needs opening up, a thorough wash, lavage, cultures, antibiotics and intense efforts to prevent it from becoming a deep infection and needing removal of the implant.

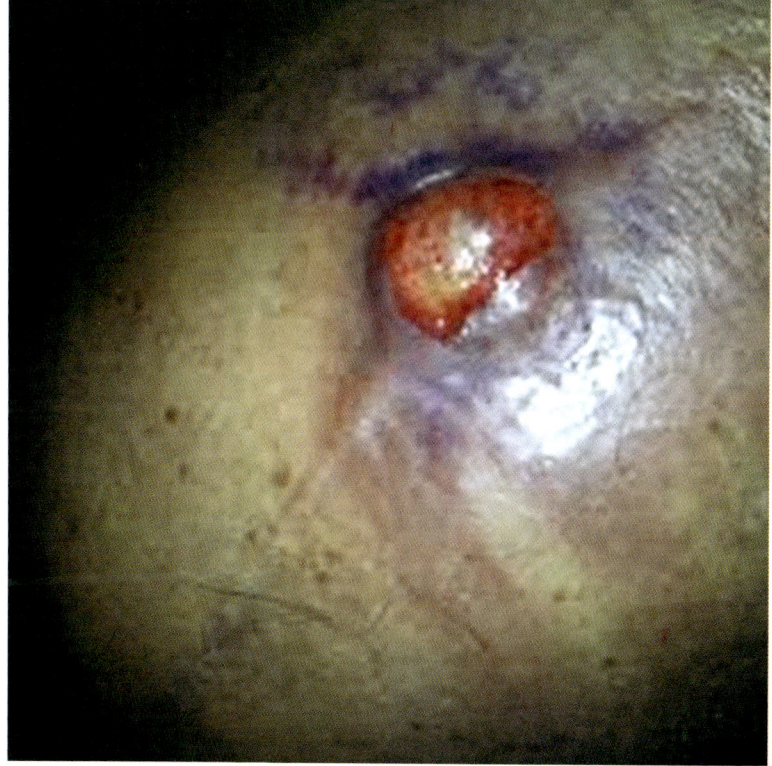

Superficial infection, if left unattended, will become deep and then need more extensive management. All infections or suspected infections need aggressive treatment from the earliest point of diagnosis.

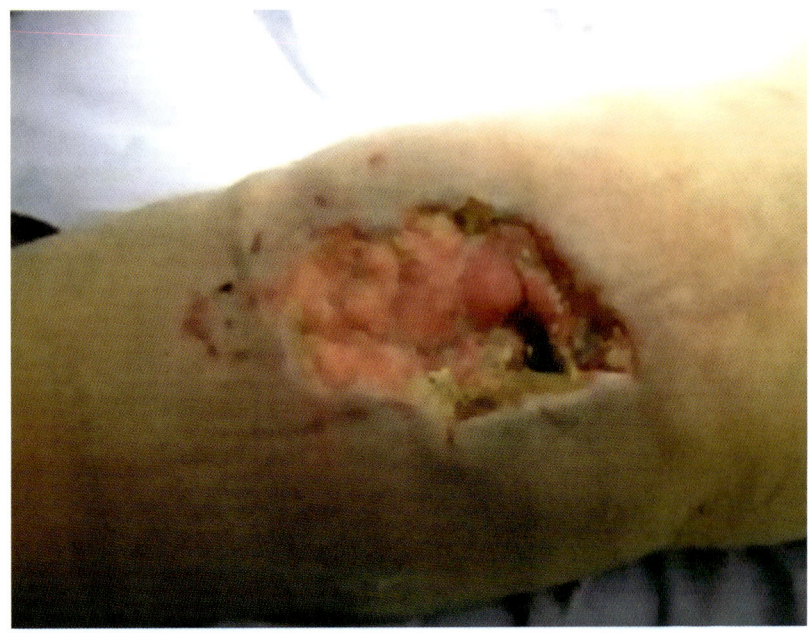

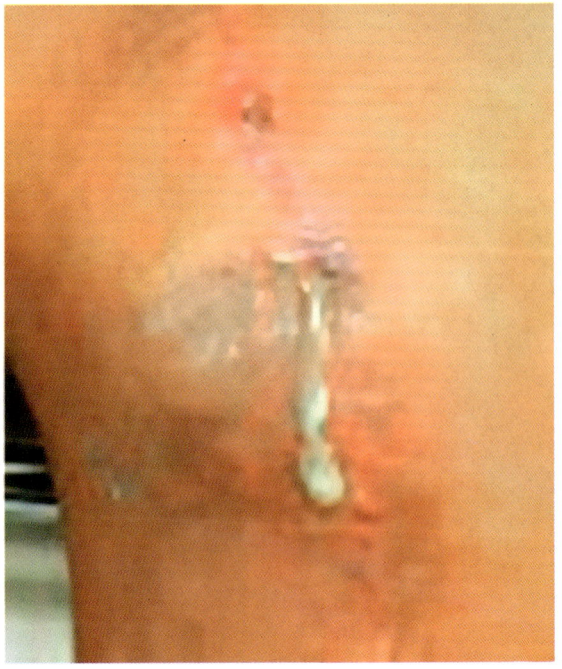

Culture of the discharge and appropriate antibiotics sometimes settles the fulminant stage of infection.

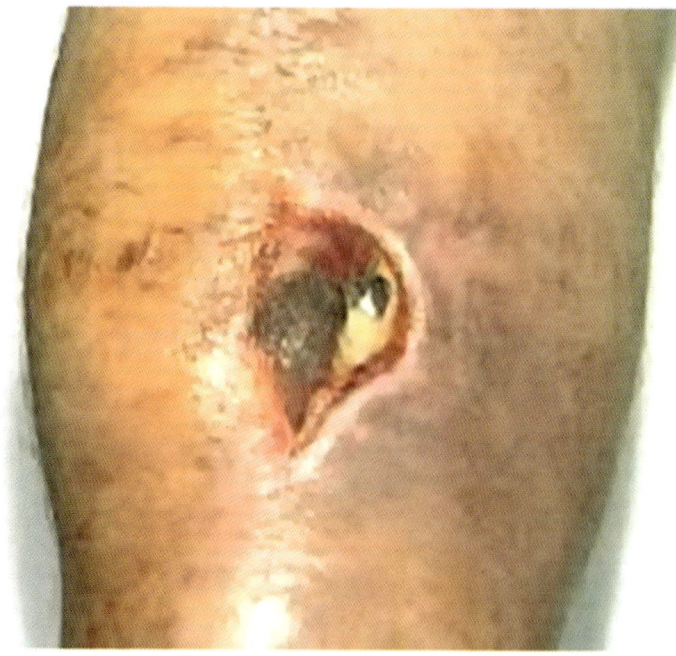

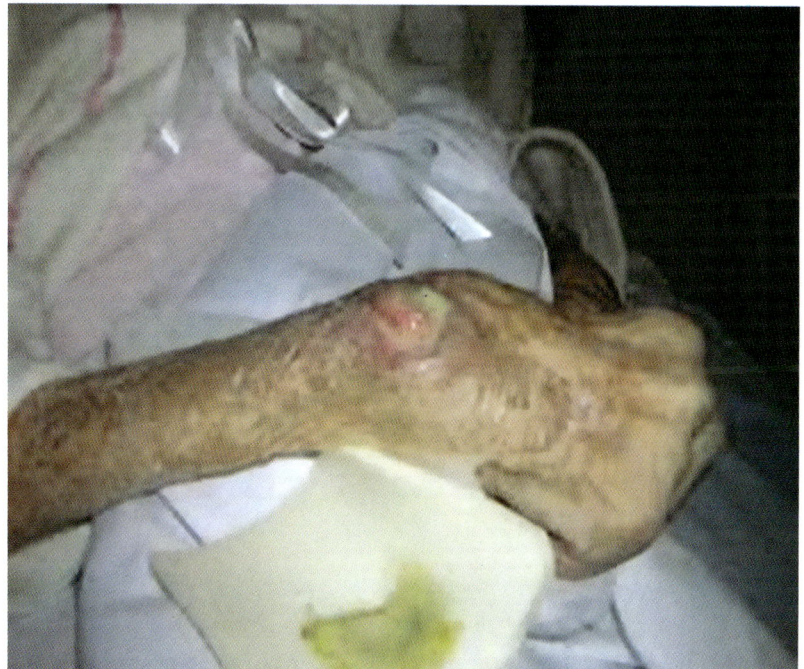

Superficial infection eventually healing with antibiotics.

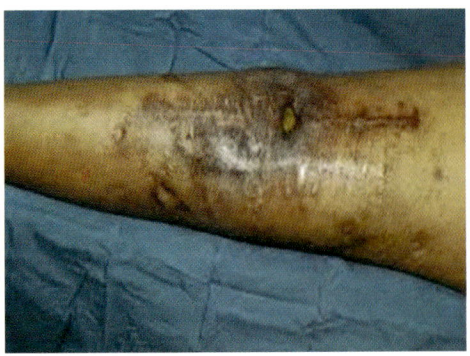

It is better to prevent these complications. When they occur, they warrant very aggressive management to prevent deep infection and disastrous results.

The following are the methods to avoid the problems:
1. Avoid tourniquet as far as possible, especially in rheumatoid arthritis.
2. Gentle soft tissue handling is the key.
3. Avoid excessive use of diathermy.
4. Avoid crushing of soft tissues.
5. Take thick skin flaps and whilst performing soft tissue releases, elevate bone deep, thick periosteal and capsular flaps.
6. Meticulous water-tight skin closure is mandatory.

If problems develop, their management has to be aggressive and thorough. Simple marginal dehiscence demands a wound debridement and closure. Larger areas will necessarily need split or full thickness skin grafts.

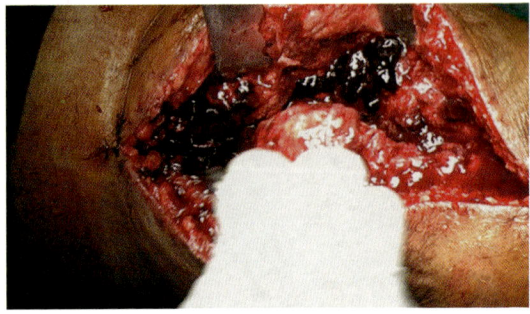

A large anticoaglant induced haematoma, needing evacuation and a thorough wash on the sixth postoperative day.

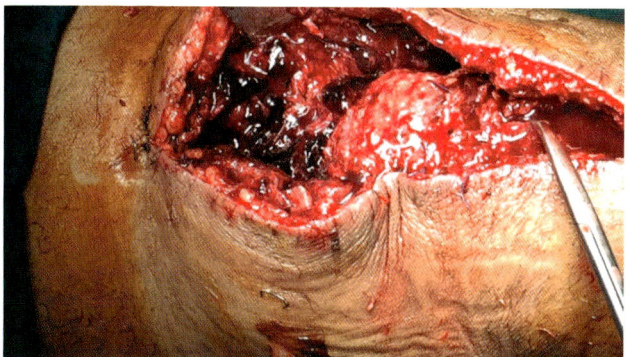

Small hematomas may be managed conservatively, but large ones will need evacuation in the operation theatre under sterile conditions. Sinuses should be excised and closed, and occasional large defects will warrant the help of a plastic surgeon for a thorough skin closure.

Superficial and deep infection: The most dreaded complication that can occur, both from a surgeon's and patient's point of view, is infection. An infection in arthroplasty is catastrophic, painfully disabling, and may require removal of implants. In a patient with an elective surgery, such a complication will result in either a fused knee or a loose, unstable, painful and short limb with the associated mortality and morbidity.

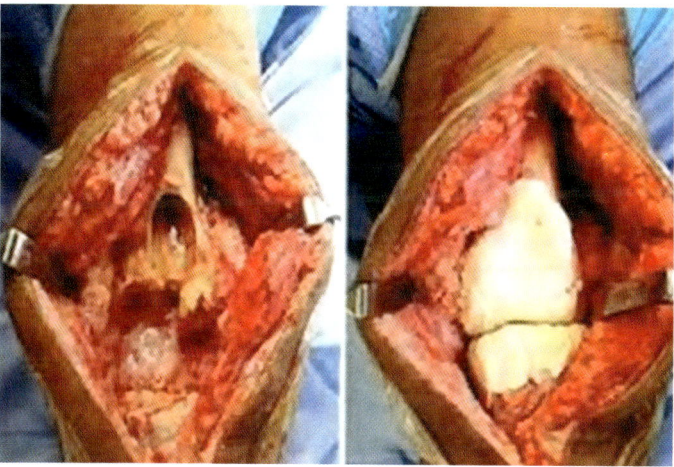

A knee with deep infection treated by removal and cement spacer application.

Sir John Charnley was the pioneer who contributed extensively towards the prevention of infection in joint replacements. In the early era of arthroplasty, the rate of infection was well in excess of 6 to 10%, a major problem to be reckoned with. Later developments have resulted in a substantial reduction, and present figures work range from 1 to 2%.

Primary infection is usually airborne and results from contamination of the operating field at the time of surgery. The host responses determine if this bacterial contamination will result in infection or not. Wroblewski in 1984 reported that the incidence of infections in patients undergoing arthroplasty and with no antibiotic prophylaxis was 0.3% in osteoarthritis, 1.2% in rheumatoids, 6.2% in patients who had undergone a TUR prostate, and 5.6% in diabetic individuals. Thus it is evident that whereas there are controllable factors—asepsis and surgical technique—that the surgeon can tackle, there are also some host dependant factors to be considered.

There are various precautions that a surgeon can take to avoid or at least reduce the chances of infection; these are listed in a combined order of priority and practicality. Some are very easy; others are cumbersome and difficult. Some cost practically nothing; others are far too expensive to be implemented in an average Indian hospital. What is required is a balance between practical and affordable steps necessary to reduce infection. The measures include:

1. Preoperative evaluation of infective foci.
2. Avoid shaving the skin and causing abrasions.
3. Avoid preoperative hospitalization above two days.
4. Atraumatic surgical technique, double gloves, hemostasis, quick efficient surgery.
5. Prophylactic antibiotics.
6. Ultraviolet light and good fumigation of theatres.
7. Large thick impervious drapes, bio-occlusive clothing and impervious headwear and masks.
8. Reduction of airborne bacteria in the operating room by reduction of personnel.
9. Laminar or vertical airflow with a number of air changes per minute.
10. Space suits with body exhaust system.

The first eight are reasonably easy to achieve and affordable. The last two may be a little out of the budget of the average hospital. In a multi-centre trial done by the British Medical Research Council for the study of infection in hip arthroplasty, it was found that clean air, antibiotics and impervious clothing all play equal parts and *are independent of each other in reduction of the infection rate*. Thus it was found that without any of the three, the rate of infection was in the order of 6%; this fell to 3% with any one of the methods used. Using two of these together, the infection rate fell to about 1 to 1.5%.

Combining all the three reduced the rate of infection to less than 0.6%. Antibiotics and reasonably impervious clothing are easy to achieve and do not cost much. Laminar flow on the other hand is a tad expensive to install. In my centre, I routinely operate in a standard air-conditioned theatre, and have an infection rate of less than 1%.

The purpose of the above statement is not to dilute the value of air flow systems, but to emphasize that even without such sophisticated systems, knee replacements can be performed with a reasonable outcome. If facilities exist, it is always of great advantage. The other methods outlined above are very easy to achieve and are detailed in the section on surgical procedure and techniques. But in any case, it is quite easy and safe to follow all the protocols and methods that one has at his disposal to avoid infection, rather than attempt to treat it once it occurs.

Once infection occurs, its management involves one or more of the following:

1. Antibiotics
2. Incision and drainage and wound lavage
3. Removal of components and an arthrodesis
4. Revision arthroplasty
5. Very rarely, excision arthroplasty with external bracing

Infections present from day 4 to up to day 70 after surgery usually result from wound contaminants or due to seeding of the haematoma with secondary infection from the bladder or some other focus. In our set up we do not open the dressings until 14 days after the operation. We believe that unnecessary opening of the operated site predisposes the wound to secondary contamination by hospital bacteria which are resistant to antibiotics.

A good rule of thumb is to not remove the sterile dressings applied in the theatre until suture removal, unless there is a pressing reason to remove them and inspect the wound. Unless the patient complains of very severe pain at the operation site accompanied by a rise of temperature and a raised ESR, we do not recommend removal of dressings in the ward. Surgeons are usually complacent and do not like to accept that operations done by them can ever get infected. Thus a sensible balance has to be struck between the temptation to open all wounds post-operatively and to allow them to rot even if they unfortunately happen to get infected.

The diagnosis of an early postoperative infection is not difficult as the classical symptoms of fever, local warmth, increased pain and a raised ESR are all present. At this stage, rather than hope for some other cause for these findings, the surgeon must suspect infection and immediately start the patient on a broad spectrum antibiotic.

The response to this administration will reveal if the infecting pathogen is susceptible to the antibiotic administered. If the symptoms have started prior to suture removal, it may be a good idea to inspect the wound and see if the edges are inflamed, if there is tension in stitches, and if there is any ooze; in the last case, a swab is taken for culture.

If the infection is in the superficial planes only without the deep haematoma being infected, there may be a good prognosis. But if the infection extends deep down, right up to the prosthesis, the prognosis is guarded at the least and might even be disastrous. In our set up, we have not had many infections, hence the management outlined subsequently is based on our experiences abroad and other references. A panic reaction and sudden removal of implants should not be done immediately. There are 6 progressive steps:

1. Antibiotics alone.
2. Superficial drainage, swabs and antibiotics.
3. Limited drainage, wash, and closure or grafts.
4. Complete opening right up to the implant, irrigation with antibiotic solutions and leave it packed and allow the wound to granulate from inside out. Follow this by plastic surgery procedures.

5. Complete removal of all the implants and cement, and immediate replacement under massive antibiotic cover.
6. Complete removal of the implants, A spacer application to retain the gap and prevent arthrodesis, followed by a second stage revision after the infection has been controlled.
7. Complete removal of all the implants and cement followed by arthrodesis.
8. Complete removal of all implants and cement, converting it into a loose joint and either leaving it alone, or exchange operation after an interval of a few months.

If step 1 fails, go to step 2, and so on. If the first 4 steps (followed in the same order) eliminate the infection, both surgeon and patient are lucky. However, if these steps fail, the choice lies between a resection arthroplasty with an orthosis, arthrodesis or an exchange revision, immediate or delayed.

Arthrodesis is a good salvage procedure and must be attempted if the patient is anaesthetically fit and willing. However as per the literature, the rate of fusion is in the range of 70 to 85% only.

The advent of Ilizarov's methodology has increased the chances of fusion to almost 100%. The following examples show knee fusion by both Ilizarov and conventional railroad fixators. The cause of fusion failure is either persistent infection or gross loss of bone stock. Ilizarov's methodology has caused a considerable improvement in the success rates of the procedure.

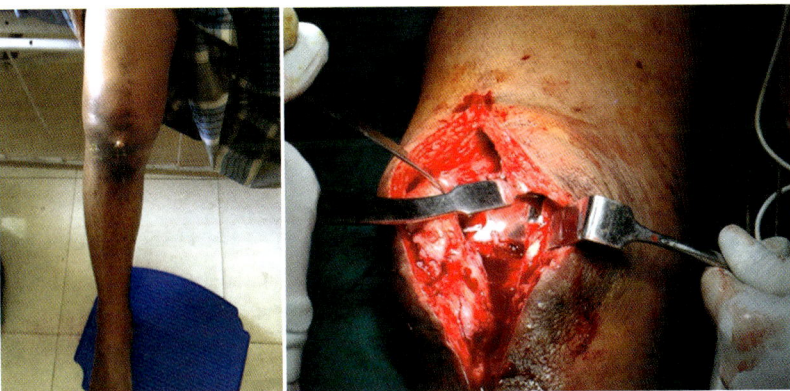

An infected knee, treated by implant removal and arthrodesis by a railroad fixator.

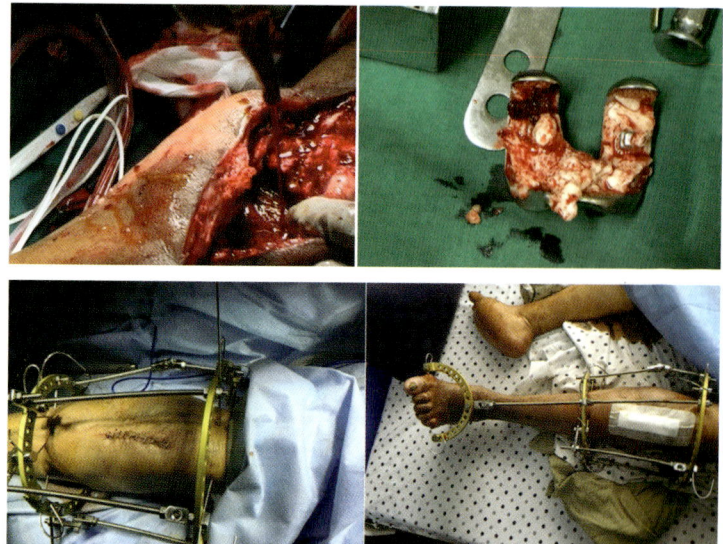

Ilizarov fixator gives a three-dimensional compression and helps joint fusion.

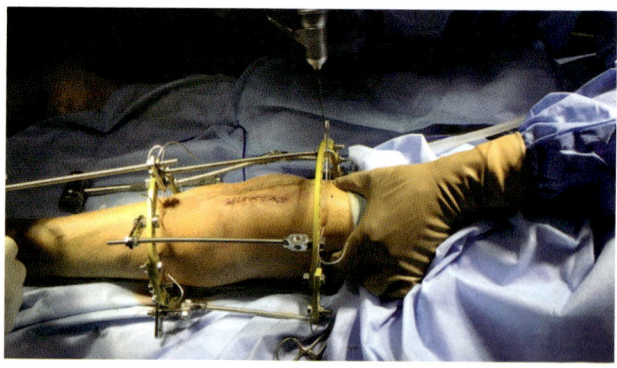

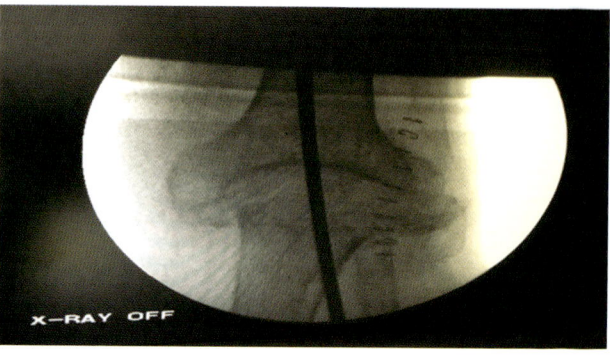

A recent advent in management of deep infections is a two stage exchange procedure. In the first stage, the prothesis is removed and PMMA spacer inserted. This spacer mimics the original knee prosthesis, gives some movement, keeps the joint well stretched, and encourages function during the waiting period between the two stages.

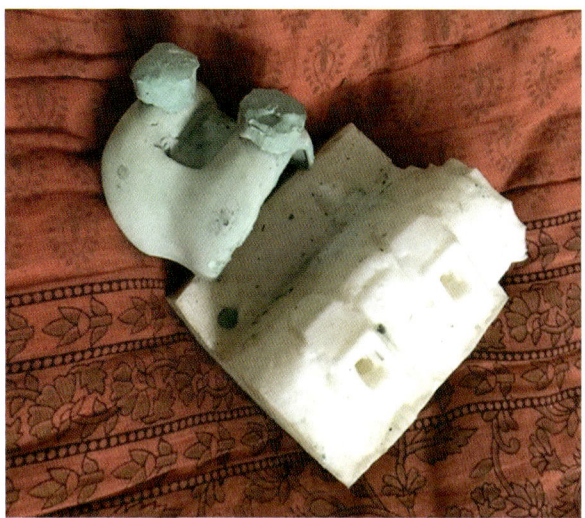

A bone cement spacer and silicone rubber mould (author's design).

The spacers are either fabricated on the table or are available readymade. The most common antibiotic impregnated into the cement is gentamicin. However, additional or different antibiotics can be mixed, depending upon the culture result of the aspirate.

The spacer method and two-stage revisions are now being recognized as producing better results than one-stage revisions. The advantages are:

1. A thorough infection clearance is achieved before proceeding to the next step.
2. The joint space is maintained.
3. Ligaments kept under proper tension avoids the need to cut the bone during definitive surgery.
4. Mobility and stability (most important ingredients of restoring function) are provided, allowing the patient to be more comfortable and self-sufficient.

Elderly, ill, and those with multiple joint involvement can safely be persuaded to undergo a resection arthroplasty, but they will need to use a knee foot ankle orthosis for the rest of their lives.

The operative procedure is quite simple. The implants, cement and all the necrotic and infected tissue are removed and the wound is closed under a couple of drains. Intravenous antibiotics are administered for four weeks and the knee encased in a plaster cylinder for six weeks. Occasionally, the knee might fuse up, but even when it does not, enough scar and fibrotic tissue will develop to give the knee a reasonable amount of mediolateral stability. However, the patient will need a knee foot ankle orthosis for the rest of his life for weight bearing stability.

Reimplantation or exchange revision is an ideal option, provided it works. A one-stage revision is probably less successful than a two stage-revision. In a small series Insall and colleagues have reported a 100% success with a two-stage revision.

The current concept regarding revision for infected knee arthroplasty involves the following steps:

1. Removal of all components and cement, through debridement and wash.
2. An Ilizarov or other fixator to distract the joint and stabilize it whilst maintaining the joint space. Else an acrylic cement spacer constructed in a shape and size similar to the components is implanted and retained until the infection is fully controlled.
3. Complete antibiotic administration parenterally until the infection is completely eliminated.
4. Re-operation under antibiotic cover.
5. Use of antibiotic loaded acrylic cement.
6. Careful and meticulous follow-up to assess the state of recurrence, if any.

Joint instability or persistent deformities: The reported incidence of these complications is between 1 and 6% and the origin of these complications can be directly traced to technical errors, either in the technique or the choice of implants.

Laxity: Laxity commonly occurs due to the following factors:
1. Too thin a tibial component.
2. General joint laxity needing a more constrained prosthesis, where a surface replacement prosthesis has been employed.
3. Absent anterior and posterior cruciates, where a nonposterior stabilized knee has been used.
4. Charcot's or neuropathic joint where the joint replacement was contraindicated in the first place.

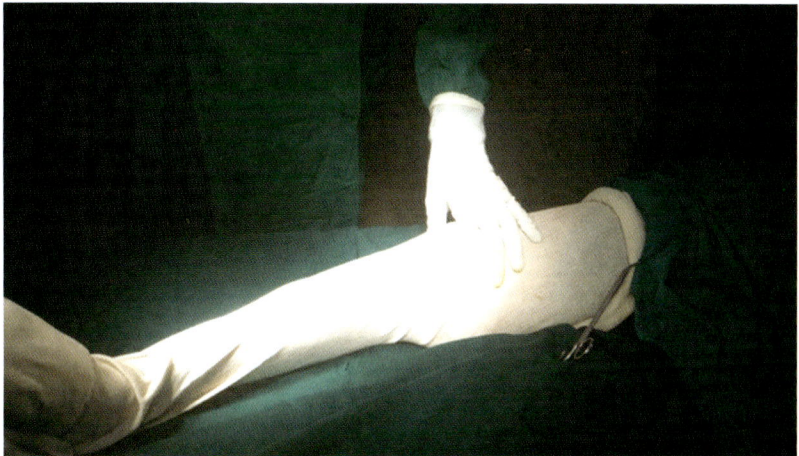

The gross side-to-side movement is clearly visible in the above lax knee.

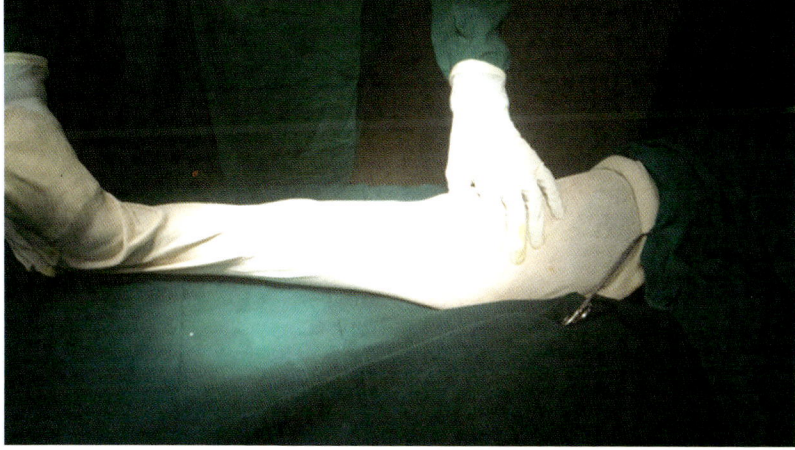

Laxity can be avoided by choosing the correct type of constraint in the implant that is being employed. On the table, after the trial components are inserted, it is essential to test the stability of the joint in all directions, and to ensure that the joint is tight and stable. If not, one must elect to use a thicker tibial component or a more constrained type of implant.

But if this complication is manifested in the postoperative period, the knee has to be braced permanently in minimal laxities and revised in gross laxity to prevent abnormal wear of the components due to tremendous amounts of uneven loads distributed across the unstable joint.

Persistent deformity is a calamitious complication that can be directly attributed only to poor surgical technique. A residual flexion deformity is invariably due to (a) an obliquity of the bone cuts in the coronal plane or (b) too tight a tibial component. A varus or valgus deformity is either due to one or a combination of oblique bone cuts and/or insufficient soft tissue releases. These should not occur; if they occur, they would rightly be termed technical errors rather than complications!

Fractures and patellar tendon rupture:
Acute fractures and patellar tendon ruptures may occur in very soft and osteoporotic bones or frail soft tissues, especially in rheumatoid knees. The treatment is operative and depends upon the type and site of fracture. Displaced fractures are internally fixed, after which the implant is cemented. Adequate

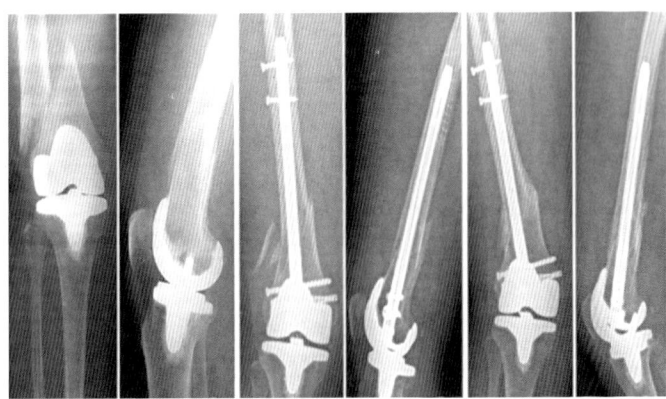

Distal femoral fracture managed by a revision with a locking stemmed implant.

immobilization is needed until the fracture heals. An acute rupture of the patellar tendon usually occurs by forcibly flexing the knee and everting the patella in frail tissue rheumatoids without reasonable release. It is better to prevent this complication, but if it does occur, the same should be repaired with strong non-absorbable synthetic suture material and the knee immobilized properly and adequately.

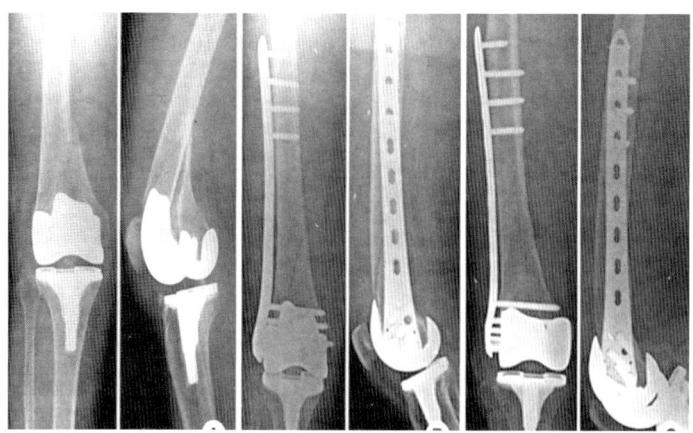

A similar fracture managed by a distal femoral locking plate.

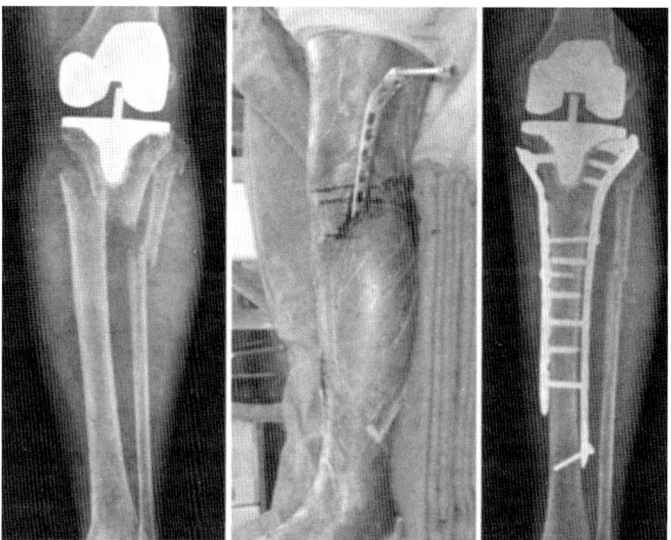

Proximal tibial fracture managed by dual plating. The pictures below show the final outcome.

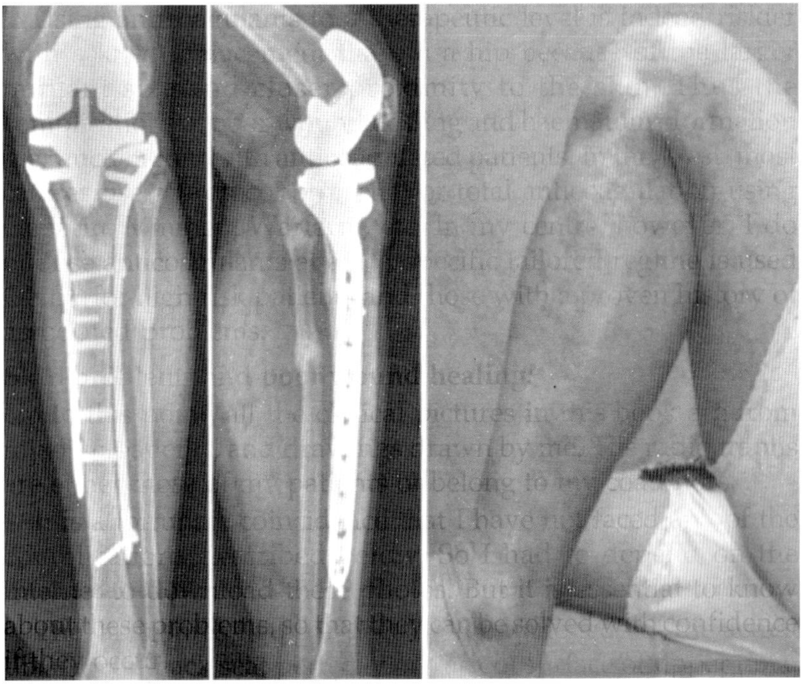

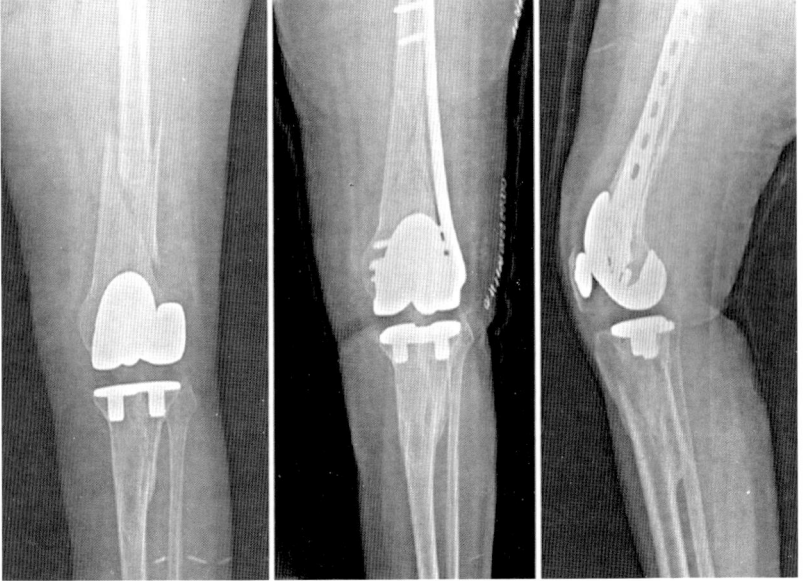

An injury due to a fall producing a spiral fracture with a large butterfly, treated by minimally invasive plate.

LATE COMPLICATIONS

Delayed infection: These occur spontaneously months or years after the replacement in a normal and functioning knee. The source is usually haematogenous and secondary to throat, chest, tonsils or bladder infection. The patient suddenly develops severe pain and swelling. The function is dramatically affected and initial radiographs may not present any abnormality. It is very important to diagnose the problem early by an aspiration under aseptic conditions in the operating theatre, and start an aggressive management after proper cultures have been done. The sequence of events in managing late infections is identical to that of early infections and the same steps should be followed.

Fractures: Delayed fractures occur due to trivial trauma in osteoporotic bones, especially with stemmed or constrained implants. A femoral fracture may occur near the tip of the stem in a stemmed implant. Most of these fractures occur in the bone just adjacent to the prosthesis as the bones here are markedly weaker than the ones embedded with prosthesis and cement. Whether to treat these fractures conservatively or operatively depends on their location and type. Most will heal well when treated conservatively. However, in the interests of early mobilization, they are usually fixed with a suitable implant.

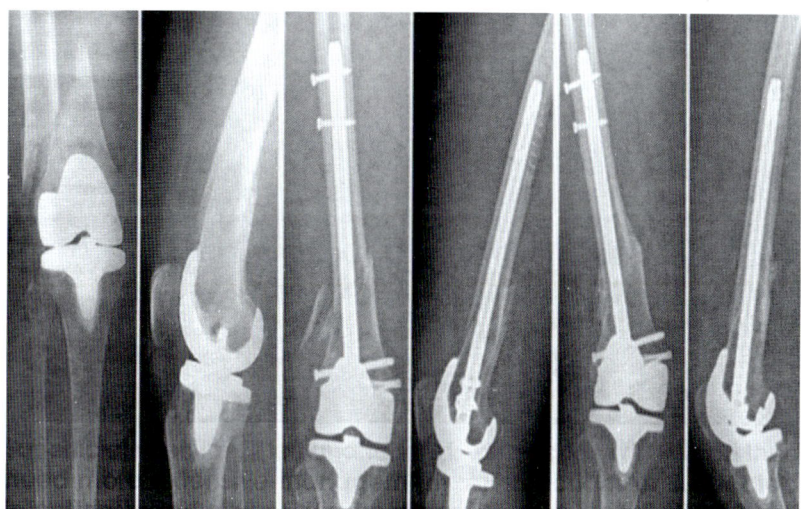

A delayed fracture managed by an exchange revision.

Patellar problems: Delayed patellar problems occur both in knees with and without patellar replacements. However, these constitute the largest number of complications after a total knee arthroplasty and the literature reports 10 to 40% complication rate. Commonly seen complications are:

- Subluxation
- Dislocation
- Articular surface erosion
- Fracture
- Component loosening
- Separation of metal-back from the HDPE
- Retropatellar pain

To avoid patellar problems, it is imperative that the post-replacement thickness of the remaining patella and the implant should be equal to the prereplacement thickness of the entire patella. A lateral release should be performed whenever deemed necessary. Prior to closure, it is essential to see the patellar tracking, to strictly adhere to the 'no thumb rule' and ensure there is no tendency for the patella to snap out laterally. A metal-backed patella should not be used. The positioning should be critical. Once this complication occurs, its management depends on the specific condition.

Loosening: Aseptic loosening of the tibial component is much more common than femoral loosening in the unconstrained knee. Loosening in the constrained knee occurs with equal frequency both femoral and tibial components. Loosening was very common with earlier designs, but improvements (in shapes and sizes, precision of instrumentation to give accurate reproducible positioning, improvements in cementation techniques, etc.) have resulted in much lower incidence of aseptic loosening.

Current literature talks about a 5 to 7% loosening rate for a 5-year follow-up. Clinically, the presentation is pain and some instability, which is manifested radiologically as a radiolucent line of more than 2 mm in the entire area of contact between the tibial component and the cancellous tibial area. As the condition progresses, there is a rapid loss of bone stock, which in turn increases the rate of loosening.

These knees have to be revised to alleviate the symptoms; if the condition is identified early before much loss of bone stock and absence of gross instability, it can be revised with a semi or unconstrained implant. However, if the bone loss is severe or the laxity is gross, one may need a more constrained knee like a rotating hinge!

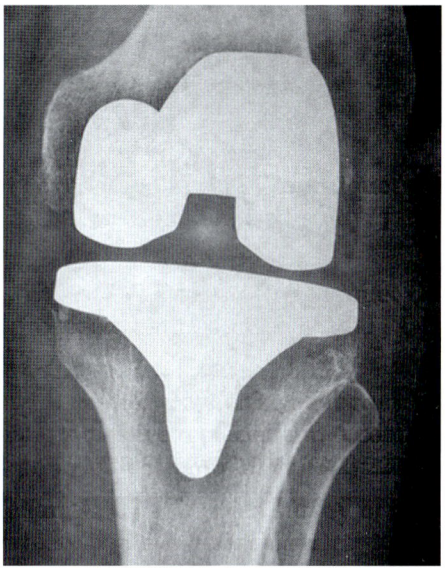

Radiolucent lines at the prosthesis bone interface are always indicative of loosening and should be tackled aggressively.

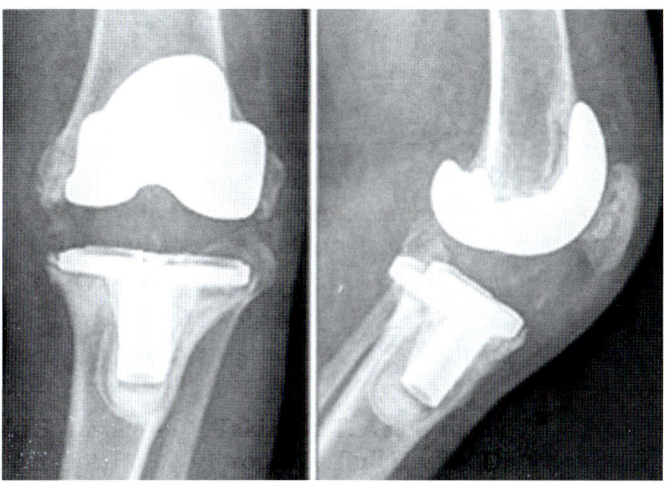

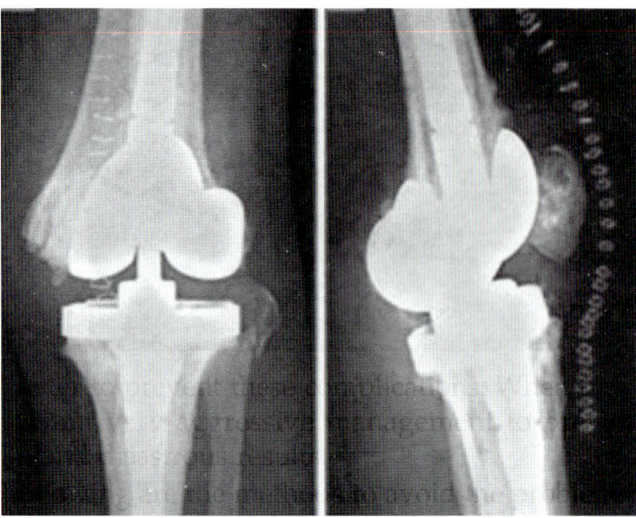

A knee loose at 19 years, revised by stemmed semi-constrained prosthesis.

Wear

The wear in the total knee components represents a problem that is fairly recently envisaged because long-term follow-up of knee replacements is only now being reported. As would be apparent, wear in the metallic components would seem to pose a lot less problem than wear in the plastic components. The following points are of relevance and shall be individually discussed later:

1. Entrapment of cement particles between the components.
2. Shape of the articular surfaces and their relation to wear.
3. Stress shielding and cold creep.
4. Metal-backing, metallosis and metallic attrition.
5. Optimal HDPE thickness and the relationship of the same to wear.
6. Gamma sterilization, plastic oxidation and wear.
7. Management of wear and wear related problems.

Cement particle entrapment: Though the friction and wear between metal and HDPE is quite low and this combination has proved to last pretty comfortably for a long period, the joker in the pack is the cement particles. Entrapment of cement particles is a rule rather than an exception. Despite meticulous lavage and cleaning, small cement particles (which invariably remain behind in most cases) cause problems. The joint tends to attract these pieces which will eventually gravitate into the joint and get entrapped between the surface of the joint. The rough particulate cement abrades the plastic and generates wear debris. Also secondarily it will cause irregularity in the plastic, that will wear badly with the metal and cause increasing wear. The vicious cycle continues; the debris causes a wear particle granuloma and giant cell formation, leading to osteolysis. Fortunately, the good cancellous bone of the tibia is less prone to osteolysis than the hips, where the upper femur almost disintegrates. Apart from a meticulous cleaning, lavage and a committed effort to eliminate all cement particles before closure, one must also make diligent efforts to chop off all overhanging bits of cement and look deep back into the posterior aspect of the joint to ensure that no loose bits remain.

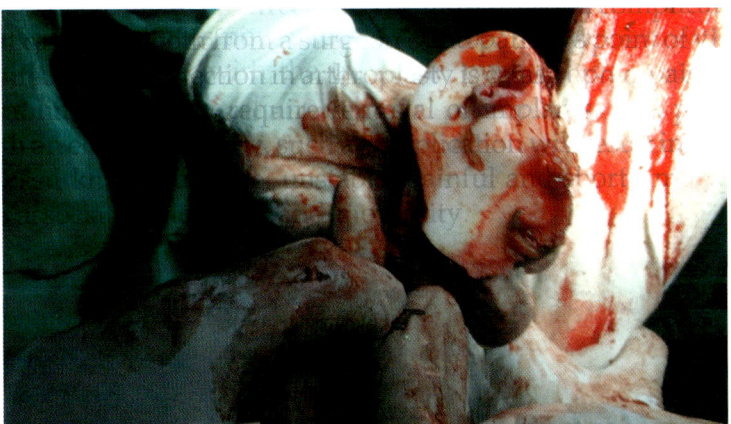

Gross wear of the medial plateau and deformation of the HDPE insert (after 16 years).

Shape of the articular surface and their relation to wear: Unlike a congruous hip joint (where there is a full conformity between the two surfaces), an artificial knee is a large complex asymmetrical joint with minimal constraint and consequently low contact! The possibility of increased wear between the contact points is real because of the minimal surface areas of contact. As the surfaces adapt to the worn-out shape and get more congruous, the irregular areas become more prone to wear.

The more modern knee designs eliminate this problem by a scientific and congruent design including the recent meniscal designs. However, design-related wear problems still remain very real with older designs.

Stress shielding and cold creep: Experimental studies show that stress shielding and cold creep are very relevant and important parameters whilst assessing the wear patterns of a total knee replacement. There have been several studies about the role of metal-backing a polyethylene component; over the years, it has remained a very controversial topic. Though experimental studies have shown that the metal-backing is beneficial in allowing a more uniform stress distribution across the surface of HDPE (especially in the flatter surfaces), this has not been proved to be very accurate in the human body!

The failures with metal-backed acetabular cups and metal-backed patellar components have resulted in a switch towards an all-polyethylene tibial component in recent times. The long term (20 years) follow-up of all unprotected poly cups of the Charnley hip system have proved that stress shielding is not a big problem per se!

In the laboratory, it is indeed a fact that a backing of metal for polyethylene does result in a much more uniform distribution of stresses across the plastic and hence theoretically results in significantly less wear. However this has not been proved correct in actual practice, because in actual follow-up studies over 10 years, there has been no significant difference in the wear rates of all poly- and metal-backed tibial components! 2 points do stand out very significantly:

1. *Thin* HDPE should not be metal-backed. Especially patellar components thinner than 4 mm will result in a premature wear of the plastic and a disastrous metal-on-metal rub and debris as the metal-back grinds across the femoral component!

2. For the tibial component, a metal-back is not mandatory to reduce wear. Meniscal and rotating platform designs necessarily need to have a metal tibia and femur and a plastic meniscus to glide in between. However, for a fixed metal-backed HDPE component, a metal-back allows for some degree of stress shielding.

However, if the plastic is very thin and there are entrapped cement particles, the early wear of the plastic may result in a direct articulation between the femoral component and the tibial metal-back with disastrous results!

Gamma sterilization, plastic oxidation and wear: The relation between gamma radiation for sterilization of plastic and wear has caught the attention of surgeons and bio-medical engineers in the very recent past. Sterilization by gamma radiation in an atmospheric ambience will allow 30% of atmospheric oxygen to remain inside the sterile wrapping. Over a period of months and years this will cause the plastic to oxidize, resulting in increased wear susceptibility. Sir John Charnley used to remark anecdotally (as oft repeated by Wroblewski, his assistant) that in the initial stages when we sterilized plastic by either chemical or gaseous means, they seemed to last much longer than when we used gamma radiation. To combat the problem of oxidation and plastic weakening, a lot of American companies manufacturing knee implants either sterilized the plastic with ethylene oxide or started packing the HDPE in argon or nitrogen prior to gamma radiation to prevent the damaging effects of radiation!

Management of wear and wear related problems: Unlike hip replacements where it is an easy matter to assess wear radiologically, the large flat tibial surfaces do not lend themselves to such a form of radiological diagnosis. However, the particle related problems will become symptomatic and the bony changes and osteolysis (as a result of wear debris) will manifest radiologically. Once they are evident clinically and radiologically, it is imperative that the patient has to undergo a revision surgery. Extensive bone loss is compensated either by bone bank bone or bone cement. Revision components with stems and wedges are used. In addition, some form of constraint in the knee is needed in view of the knee becoming wobbly as a result of loosening and wear.

Deformation and Breakage: Plastic deformation is commonly seen as a result of constant stresses under body temperature; in engineering terms, it is called cold creep or cold flow. This deformation results in an irregularity. Plastic contained within a metal-back or shell tends to dissipate the forces more uniformly across the surface, which will protect against deformation and creep. However, non metal-backed components are much more prone to this deformation. Once the component gets out of shape, the contact between the surfaces is no longer maintained, resulting in stress raisers and wear. So in many cases, deformation may be a precursor to wear.

Breakage of components is commoner with older designs of all metal or constrained knees where the maximum loading occurs at the junction or the hinge. With minimally constrained knees, this phenomenon is not very common. Breakage of the plastic may follow its wear when it becomes very thin and some shear stresses will crack the plastic. Breakage of the femoral component of an unconstrained knee on its own is practically unknown.

The management of wear and breakage is again revision. After a correct assessment and preoperative planning, all the components are revised. Extensive bone loss is compensated either by bone bank bone or bone cement. Revision components with stems and wedges are used. In addition, some form of

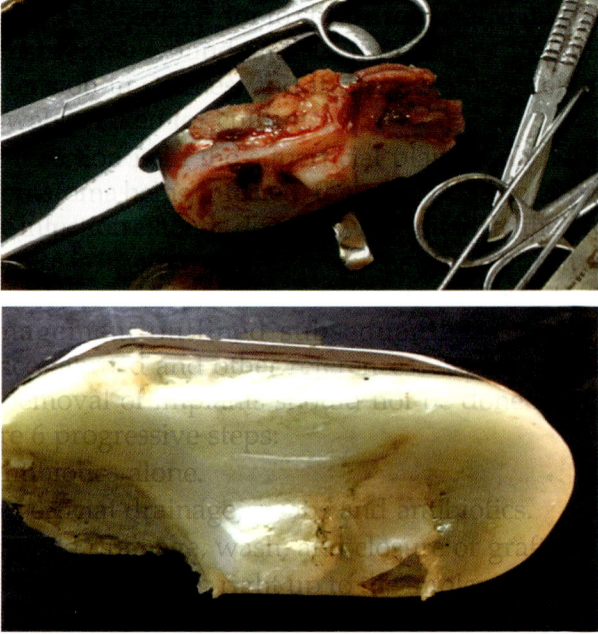

Plastic deformation, component wear and breakage after 19 years of implantation.

constraint in the knee is needed in view of the knee becoming wobbly as a result of loosening and wear.

Certain important points that will help while doing a revision of a knee are:

1. A comprehensive preoperative planning and a thorough clinical and radiological examination. Special emphasis is to be laid on the degree of instability in the knee, the amount of bone loss, available bone stock, angular and plateau deformities in both anteroposterior and side-to-side axes.

2. A decision on the type of knee to be used has to be made preoperatively; in most cases, this will be with a constraint greater than the current knee implant.

3. Because of significant bone loss, a much greater thickness of tibial plastic will be needed. Thus one has to have a good inventory of thicker tibial sizes.

4. Occasionally after removing the femur, there will be so much bone loss distally, that it would be almost impossible to delineate the shape of the condyles. This will also make it extremely difficult to plan for a valgus seating of the femoral component. These cases will need femoral components with an intramedullary stem that will help in a proper valgus alignment.

5. One must have enough allografts or bank bone to fill in the defects if this is the planned method of filling the defects; if one plans to use bone cement, again adequate stocks are necessary.

6. For asymmetrical bone loss on the tibial side, it is necessary to have metal wedges that will compensate for the defects. These wedges may either be built into the revision tibial stem or may be of the design and type where the wedges are fixed on the table after assessing the degree of the defect.

7. On occasion, one may elect to use a stemmed tibial component for revision.

8. It is a good idea to use an antibiotic loaded cement, because revision surgery, especially a superficial joint like knee, is very prone for infection.

9. After repeated surgeries, patients have a low morale; one must also counsel them psychologically and explain all the risks involved in the procedure.

Revision Knee Replacement

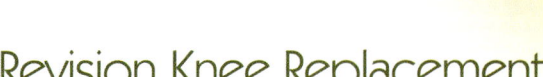

Revision knee replacement is a complex subject and deserves a book of its own, but for the sake of completeness, I have outlined the basic steps and also added appropriate photographs. However, the following points are very important and have to be kept in mind before embarking on revision knee replacements:

1. Unless the surgeon is well versed with primary knee replacement, it is better not to venture into revisions.
2. Revision knee replacement is not only a technically demanding operation, the results are never as good as primary replacements.
3. Complication rate of a revision knee is much higher than for a primary replacement.
4. The expenses involved in using the range of revision instrumenting and implants makes this procedure quite unaffordable for the average Indian patient.
5. The patient who has already suffered tremendously, physically, mentally and financially from the failed first surgery must be presented with a realistic view of the probable results of revision.

CHECKLIST OF POINTS TO BE CONSIDERED WHILE PLANNING A REVISION KNEE REPLACEMENT

Certain important points that will help while doing a revision of a knee are:

1. A comprehensive preoperative planning and a thorough clinical and radiological examination. Special emphasis is to be laid on the degree of instability in the knee, the amount of bone loss, available bone stock, angular and plateau deformities in both anteroposterior and side-to-side axes.

2. A decision on the type of knee to be used has to be made preoperatively; in most cases, this will be with a constraint greater than the current knee implant.

3. Because of significant bone loss, a much greater thickness of tibial plastic will have to be used. Thus one has to have a good inventory of thicker tibial sizes.

4. Occasionally after removing the femur, there will be so much of bone loss distally, that it would be almost impossible to delineate the shape of the condyles. This will also make it extremely difficult to plan for a valgus seating of the femoral component. These cases will need femoral components with an intramedullary stem that will help in a proper valgus alignment.

5. One must have enough allografts or bank bone to fill in the defects if this is the planned method of filling the defects. On the contrary, if one plans to use bone cement, adequate stocks are necessary.

6. For asymmetrical bone loss on the tibial side, it is necessary to have metal wedges that will compensate for the defects. These wedges may either be built into the revision tibial stem or may be of the design and type where the wedges are fixed on the table after assessing the degree of the defect.

7. On occasion, one may elect to use a stemmed tibial component for revision.

8. It is a good idea to use an antibiotic loaded cement because revision surgery, especially in a superficial joint like knee, is very prone for infection.

9. After repeated surgeries, patients have a low morale; one must also counsel them psychologically and explain all the risks involved in the procedure.

In normal circumstances, an average surgeon will need to perform knee replacements for three distinct conditions:

1. A grossly mal-positioned knee that is sure to fail if not exchanged immediately. This problem is quite frequently seen in our country after first timers put the components in a grossly unacceptable position.

2. An aseptic loosening of a knee that has been in place for some time.

3. An infected knee, either immediate or delayed. This would represent possibilities in the form of alternatives to replacement, a single stage or a two-stage procedure, the entire plan wholly dependant on the condition of the knee as well as the experience of the surgeon!

This chapter is not meant to transform an average orthopaedist into an expert revision surgeon! The advice that can bear repetition is: *Unless fully confident, stay away! Refer when in doubt!*

Malpositioned knee and immediate revision: Probably one of the simplest revisions, it can be safely done by a beginner. The patient may be your own or that of another surgeon. The time gap between presentation and the original operation is about six weeks to six months. The following are the presentation symptoms:

1. The knee does not look right! The legs are too bandy or too crow legged. This is the patients' way of telling us that there is an excess of varus or valgus deformity.
2. The patient cannot straighten the leg fully. One has to carefully assess the residual flexion deformity.
3. The leg hyperextends. There is recurvatum.
4. The knee is very wobbly.
5. Of course, there will be associated symptoms like pain, stiffness, clicks, etc.

One has to know well at this point that once it has been established that there is a component malpositioning, apologetic and conservative treatment is of no use. An immediate revision is mandatory! Splints, braces, etc. will only satisfy the surgeon but will not benefit the patient! One must have sufficient courage to tell the patient that the components are not perfectly placed. Left alone, this will cause a dramatic eccentric loading of the components and the resultant failure will have an accompanying bone loss that may need more exacting procedures if the revision is deferred.

The following are the standard steps for revising a knee with component malpositioning:

1. A preoperative assessment of the exact degree of malposition and an identification as to whether it is in the femur or tibia and in what axis!

2. A provisional plan as to what has to be done.
3. The knee is exposed in the standard manner, going right through the previous incision if the situation warrants.
4. The patella is deflected laterally and the knee is hyperflexed to see the interior of the knee joint. At this juncture it is understood that the revision is not being performed for patellar problems. If the same is being done for this, the patella can be replaced and the knee closed.
5. If the previous tibial cut is in too much varus (as often happens in these cases), one must translate the tibia far forward to enable removal of the tibial component without scratching the femoral articular surface.
6. A small chisel is introduced between the tibial component and the bone and with gentle tapping the tibial component is extracted. Either one is lucky that the component comes out along with the full cement mantle or the component alone comes out, leaving the cement mantle inside the cancellous tibial area.
7. If cement is left in the tibia, it is painstakingly removed using a small chisel and curettes until the entire cement mantle is removed.
8. Using an extramedullary or intramedullary guide, the proximal tibial surface is cut again, to get a position of exact parallelity to the floor with a 3° to 5° posterior slope!
9. A thicker trial prosthesis is now inserted and the knee straightened. Three things are looked for:
   a. The knee when straight should be in valgus to rectus to an acceptable degree.
   b. The tibial component should be in a slight 5° posterior slope.
   c. The knee should freely be put to a good range of movement with an uniform soft tissue tension from flexion to extension.
10. If the above criteria are met, the correct-sized prosthesis is now removed from the sterile wrappings and cemented!
11. A thorough wash to see that there are no loose cement bits, a proper haemostasis and a closure complete the procedure.

12. If the malpositioning has been in the femoral component, the same is removed in exactly the same manner. Proper recuts are then performed using the appropriate instrumentation sets and cementation of the femoral component is done!

Delayed revision for aseptic loosening: This will be a future problem which our younger surgeons are going to face with increasing frequency.

The knees may be earlier hinged versions, or the modern unconstrained versions. They may have been cemented primarily or may be cementless versions. All present with a period of satisfactory functioning in the patient's body for years, then initially start as small niggling pains or wobbliness.

The radiograph taken immediately when the patient comes may show some radiological evidence of component wear, and many radiolucent lines in both the femoral and tibial components. A decision to revise should be made early before too much of a bone loss makes it an unsalvageable situation. In most cases, one will need to use a component with a constraint greater than that of the originally implanted prosthesis.

The following steps outline the brief steps, but one must be well aware that each loose knee is an individual situation and the exact operative details will differ from case to case!

1. The choice of exposure depends upon the earlier scars and surgeries, but the straight anterior incision is preferable if it is usable!
2. One must be very careful to take out as thick a flap as possible and include skin, fascia, fat and all the old scars in one thick unit to avoid skin problems at a later date.
3. Retain as much of the patellar fat pad as possible as this is an insurance against skin necrosis and pads the revision prosthesis!
4. Most loose knees are wobbly. It is an easy matter to translate the tibia far anteriorly to visualize its entire surface. After inspection for wear, debris plastic deformation and breakage, one has to extract it.
5. Occasionally, the prosthesis is loose enough to be pulled out very easily. On other occasions, it is indeed a very difficult proposition with a hard metallic prosthesis firmly

adherent to stiff cement properly glued to the soft bone and all violence directed at the implant and cement will have to be borne by the soft osteoporotic bone.

6. Flexible or thin osteotomes can be inserted between the prosthesis and the cement and gentle taps will loosen the implant. After a careful extraction of the same, all loose cement is diligently removed. One must point out at this stage that unlike hip revisions (where one works down a poorly illuminated cortical tube of the femur), cement extraction from the tibia is much easier and simpler.

7. The next step is removal of the femoral component. Again insertion of a flexible or small chisel between the cement and the implant will do the trick. However, one must be very careful not to remove large chunks of bone along with the implant. Whenever the old implant resists removal, please be patient. Do not hurry! Do not use force-Patience and gentleness will succeed when force and strength will fail. Remember the axiom: Do not cause damage!

8. The patella, if used previously, can now be removed. All the cautions mentioned above stand true for patella as well. Do not fracture the patella and do not avulse the patellar tendon. Be careful!

9. Once all components and cement have been removed, a thorough wash with saline is done. All loose cement bits are painstakingly removed. If available, a pneumatic powered wire brush is used to roughen all the cancellous area so that good bleeding surfaces are obtained!

10. Irrespective of the implant design or instrumentation used, the following points are very relevant:

    a. The flexion and extension gaps should be equal. Use spacers, lamina spreaders or any other tensioning devices that are available. The key is to have the same gap in fill extension, 45° flexion and 90° flexion.

    b. If the gaps are unequal, it means that the soft tissue balance has not been adequate. Correct soft tissue releases as described in the previous chapters are essential to get the gap right throughout the entire range of motion!

    c. Once the gap is equalized, one has to assess the status of the limb with all the soft tissues fully tensed. With the pardonable error of repetition, l have no hesitation in stressing that the knee should be in VALGUS!

11. If the joint is not in valgus, one must find where the fault lies. Correct valgus is achieved by giving appropriate cuts either to the femur or tibia.

12. All the above procedures will invariably result in a much thicker tibial component. A preoperative preparation to keep the appropriate sizes is mandatory for the smooth progress and full success of the procedure!

13. The rest of the steps in using the correct trials, an assessment of the range of motion, the actual implants, their cementation and drainage and closure have been covered already.

The following photographs show two revision scenarios and describe the procedure step by step.

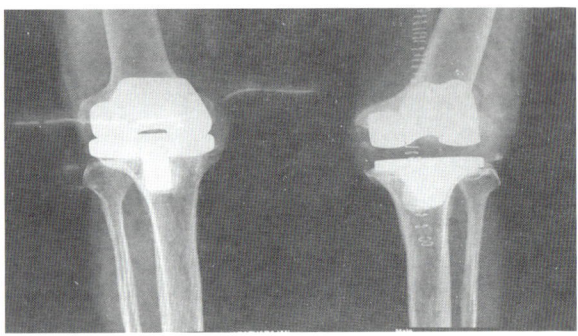

Revision for wear and aseptic loosening. This is a 60-year-old male with bilateral replacements done by me 19 years ago. The left side has been revised 5 days ago and the right side revision steps are shown here.

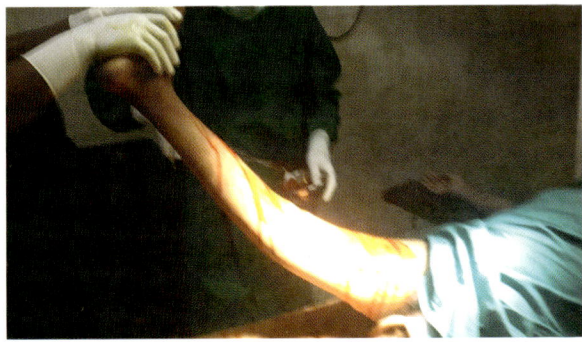

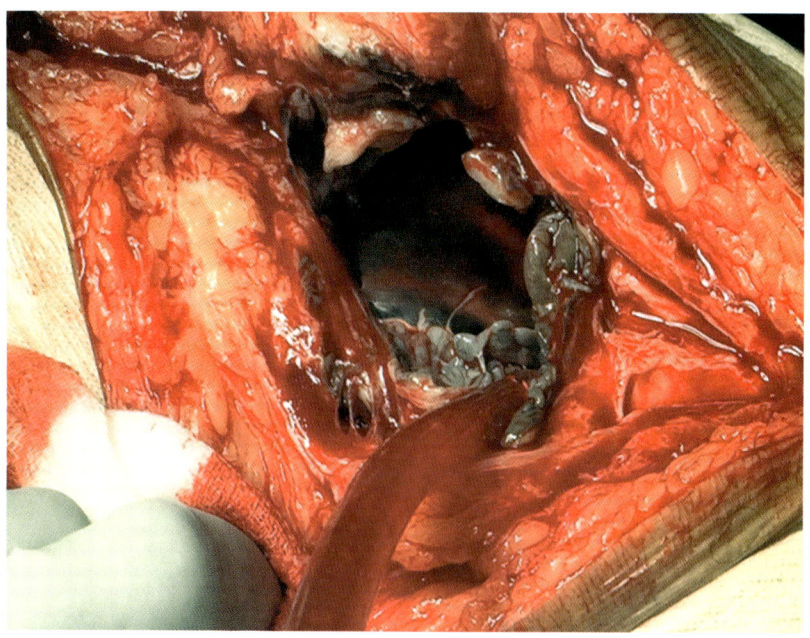

Approach here is though the same incision used for primary surgery. We can appreciate severe metallosis and black tissue.

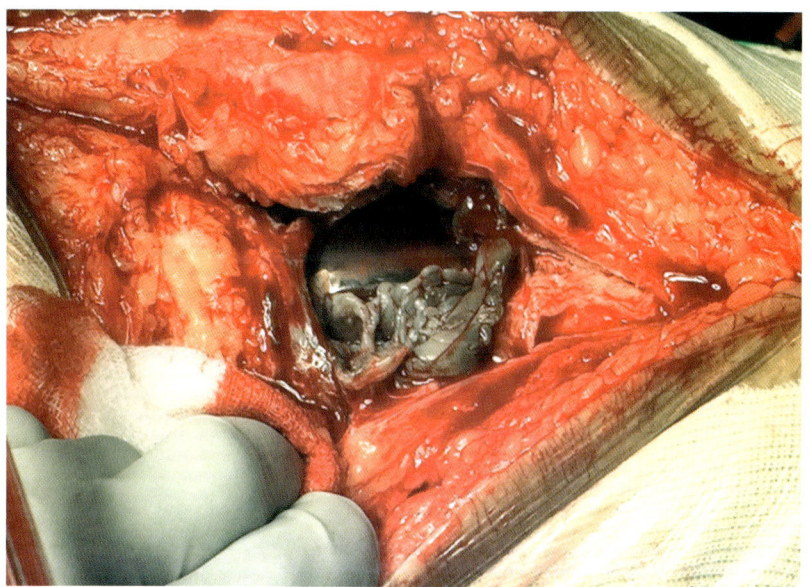

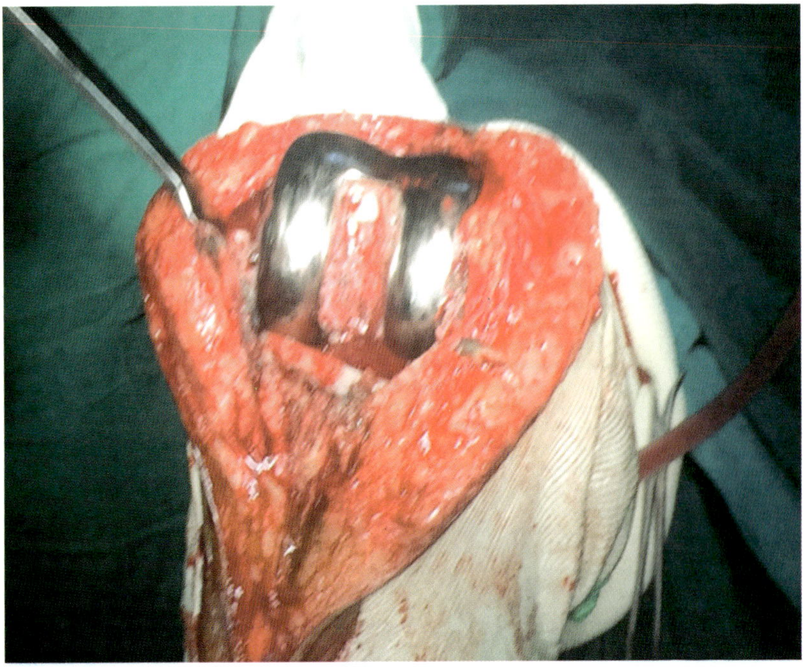

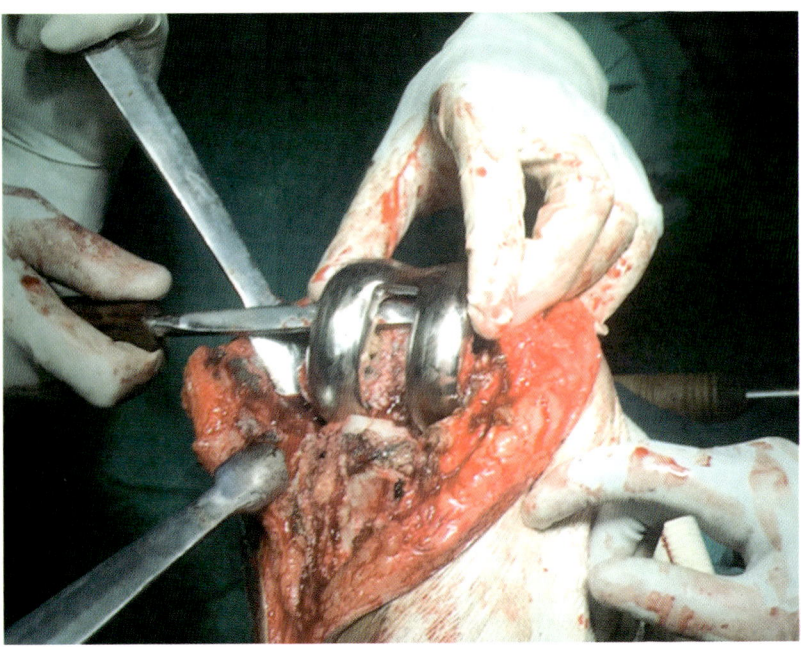

The femoral component is levered out with a small chisel.

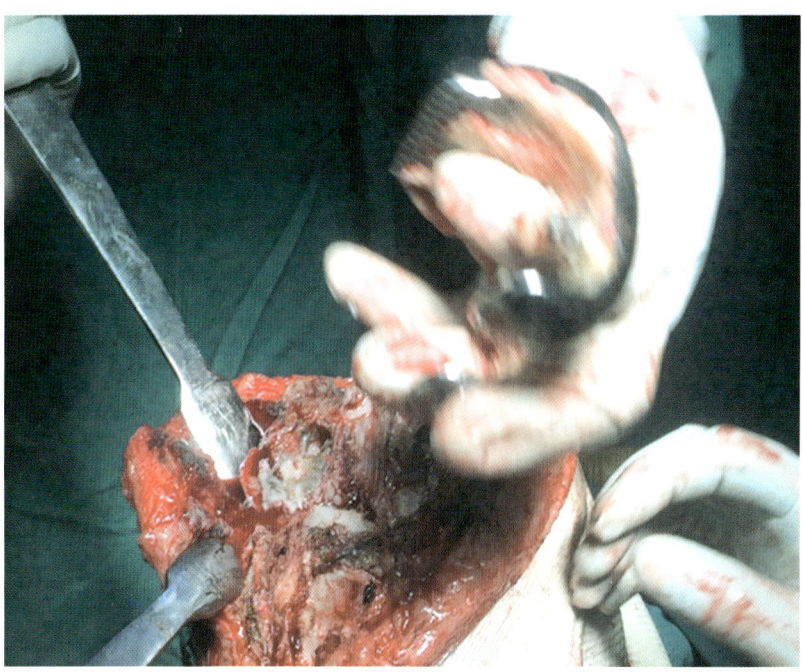

All the cement comes out with the femoral component. The worn out tibia can be appreciated below.

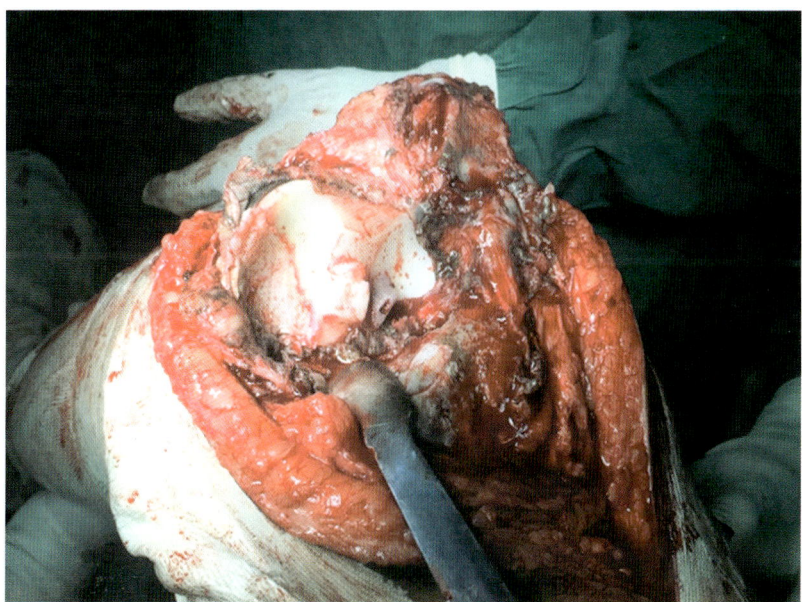

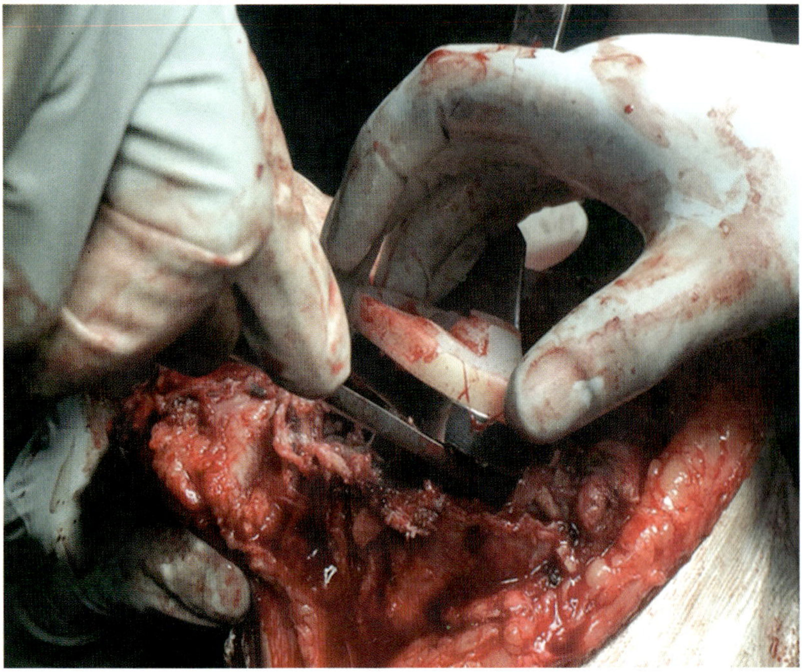

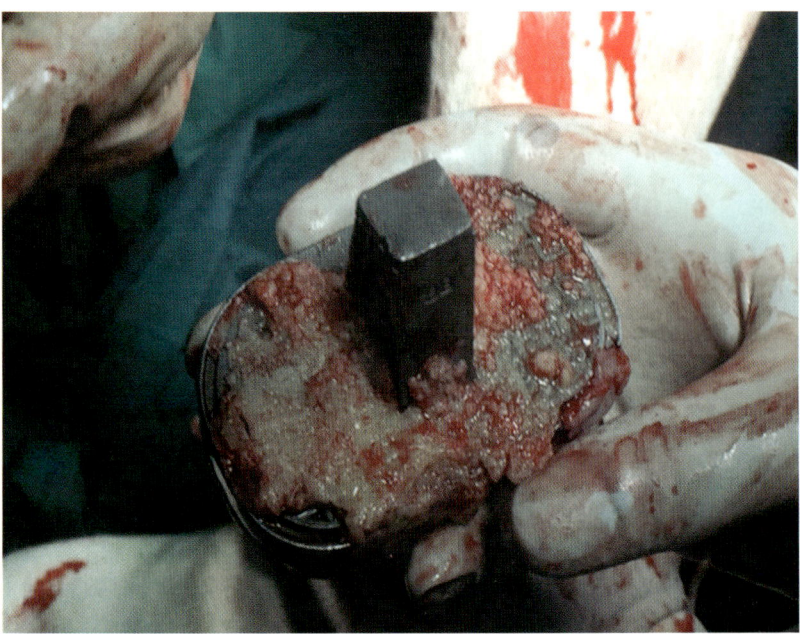

Next, the tibial component is levered out.

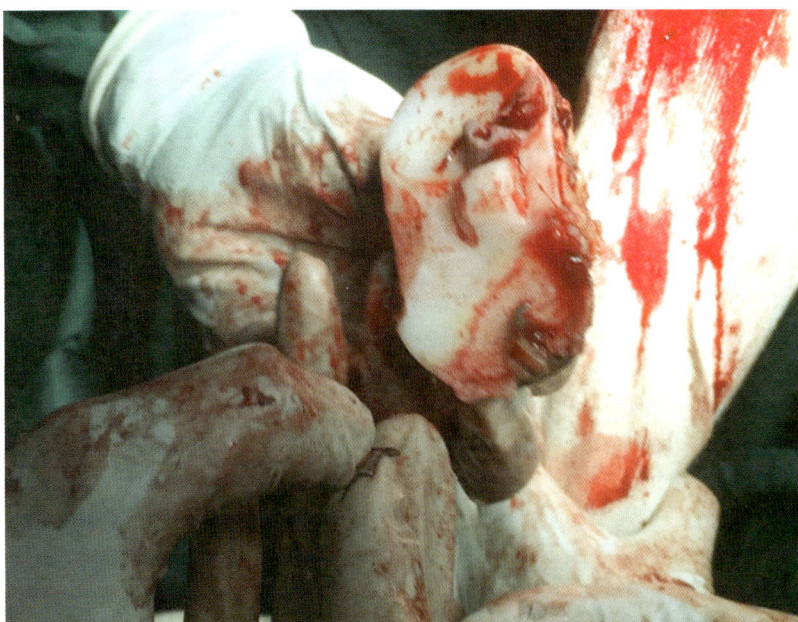

It can be seen that the tibial component has worn down considerably and the metal most aspect has rubbed down right up to the metal.

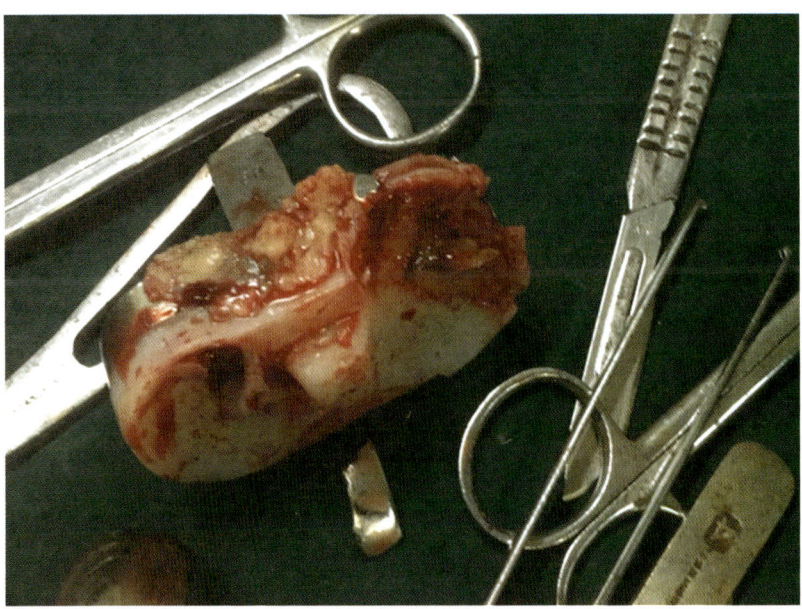

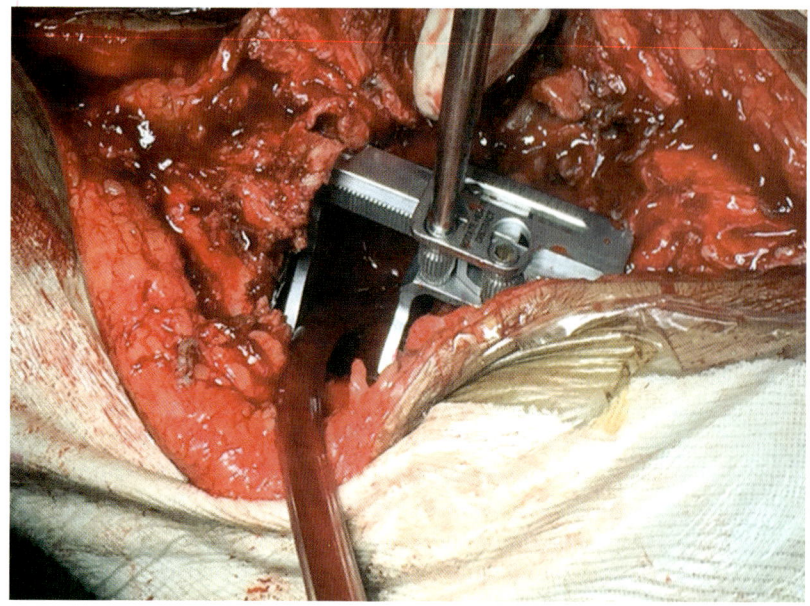

The granulation and fibrous issue is removed and the joint gap measured.

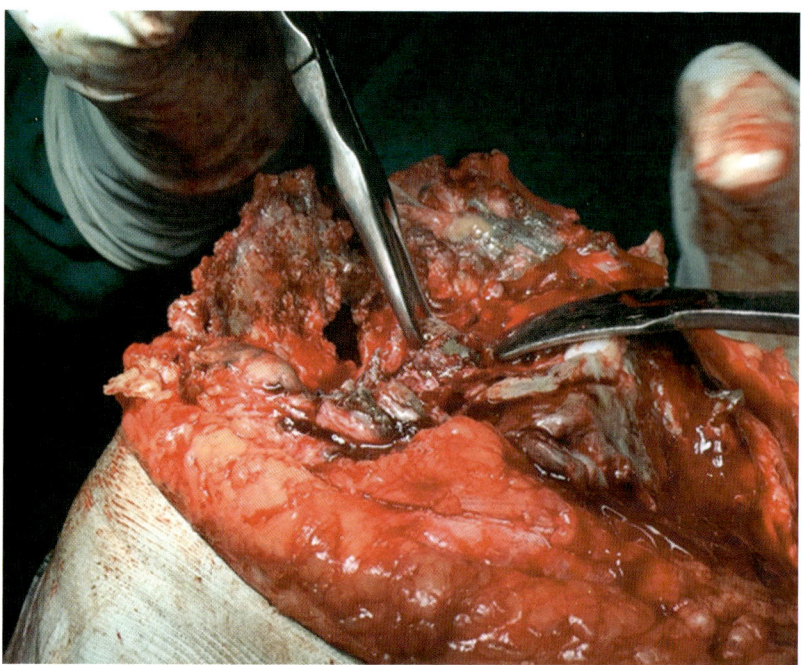

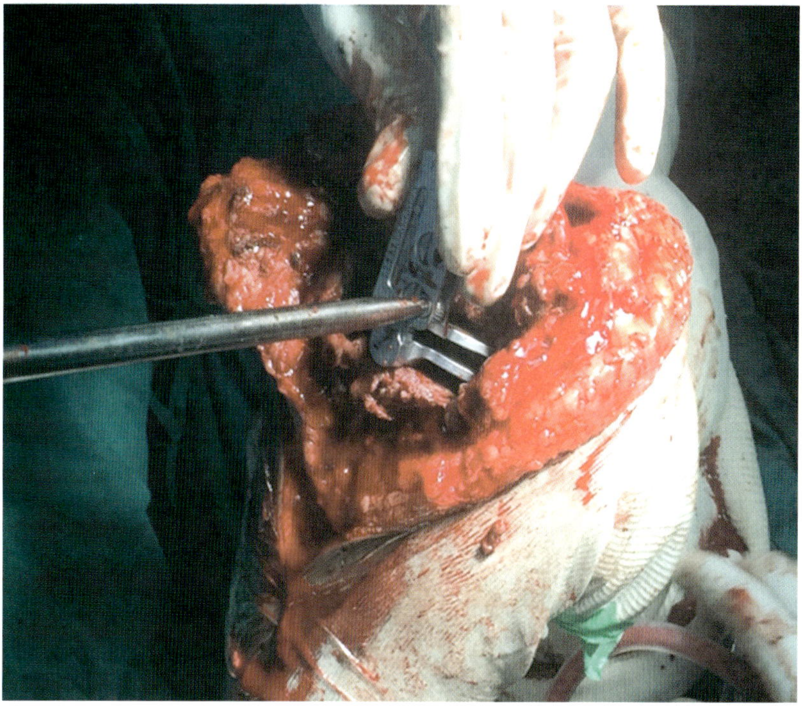

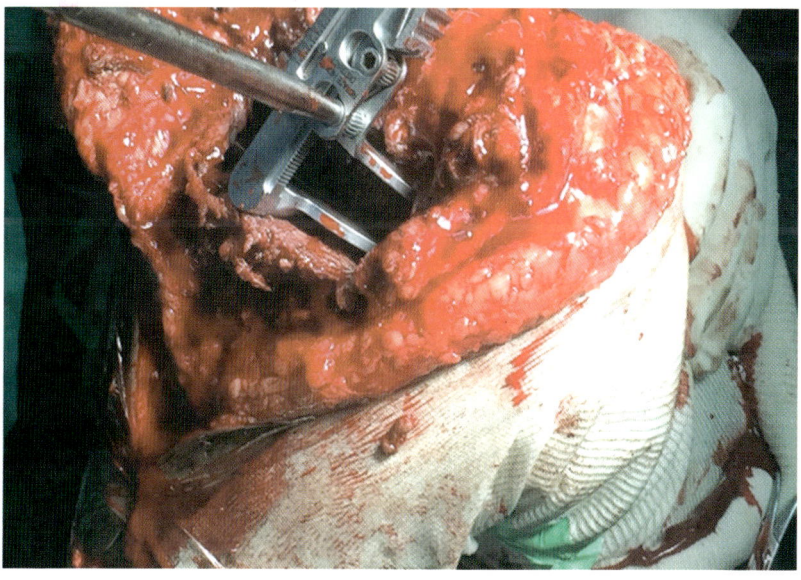

It is essential to balance the flexion and extension gaps; soft tissue releases are done to ensure that they are equal.

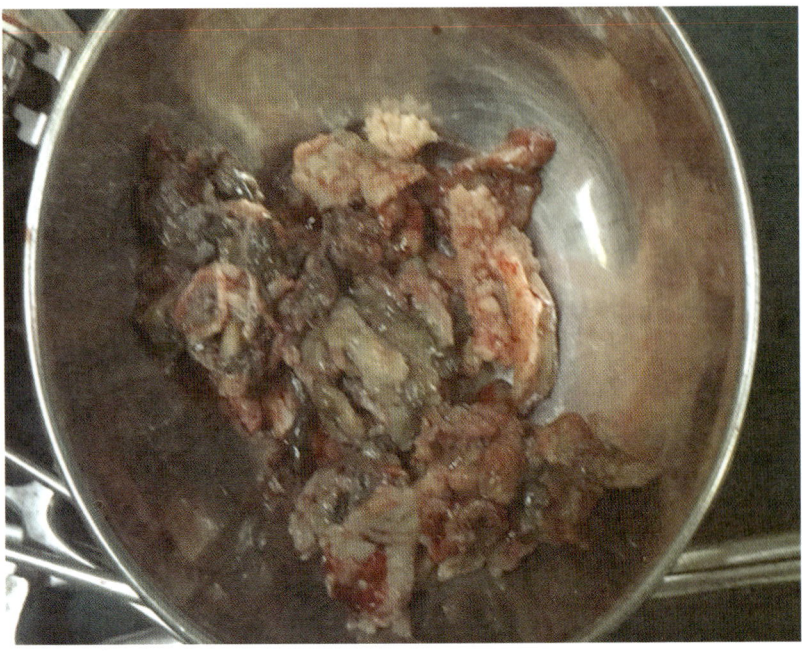

The granulation tissue removed. As a posterior stabilized knee is planned, the bio-cutter is used to cut the notch.

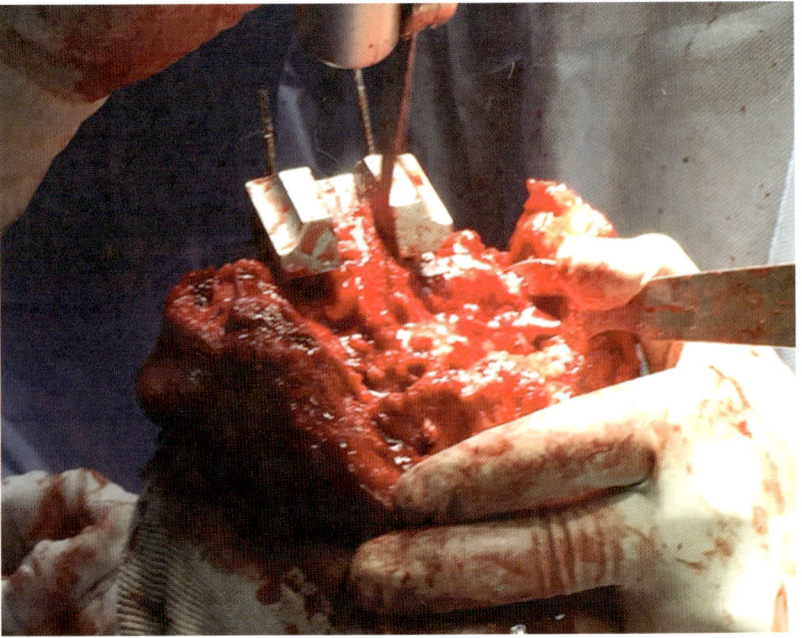

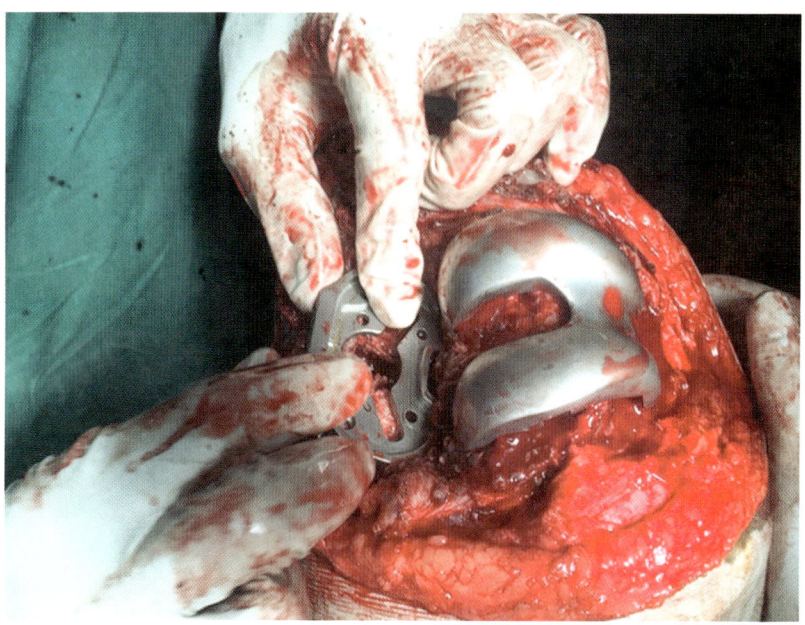

Trial femoral and tibial components are now placed over the surfaces after proper measurement.

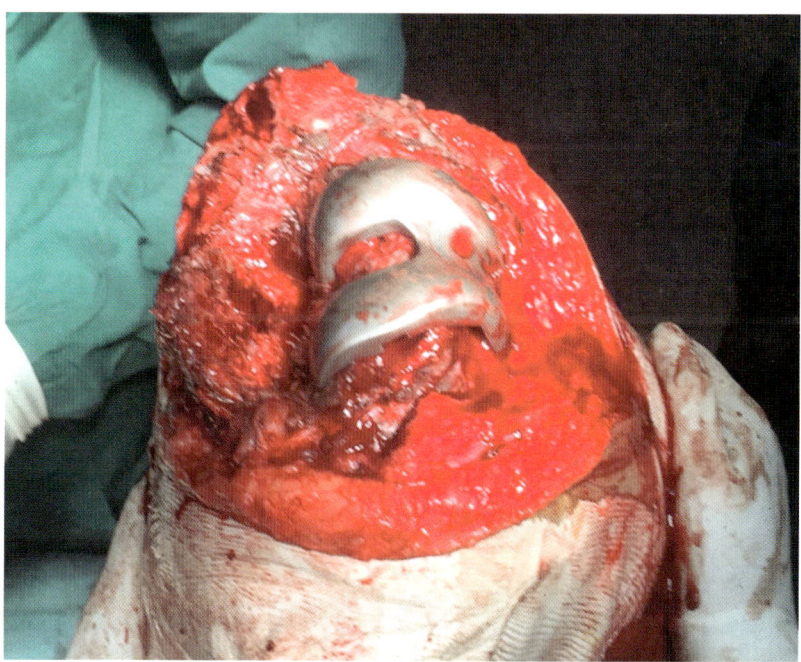

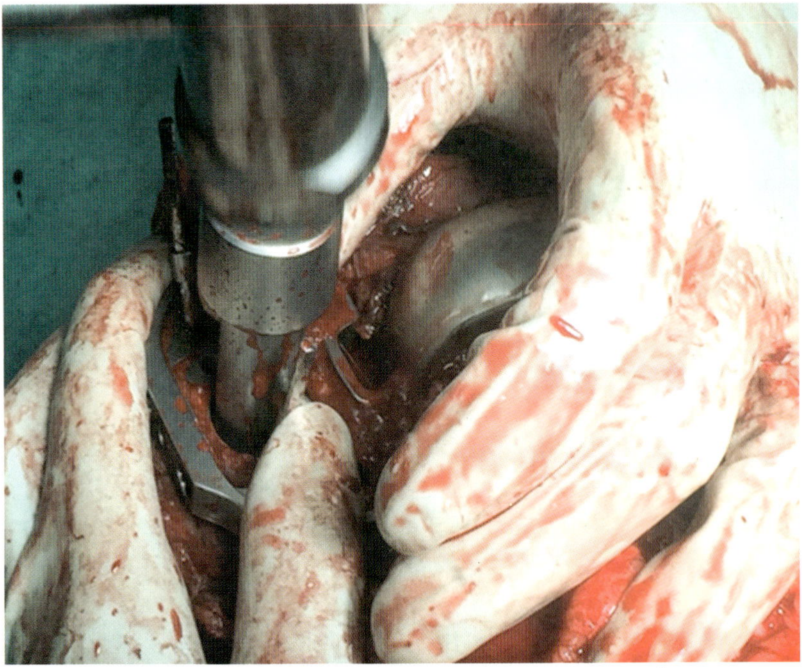

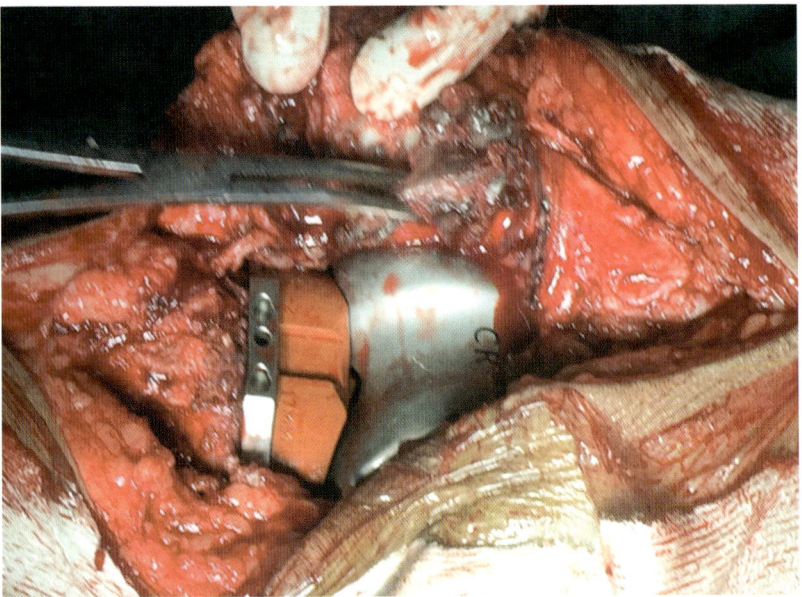

The tibial surface is prepared and the insert of appropriate thickness is pushed home.

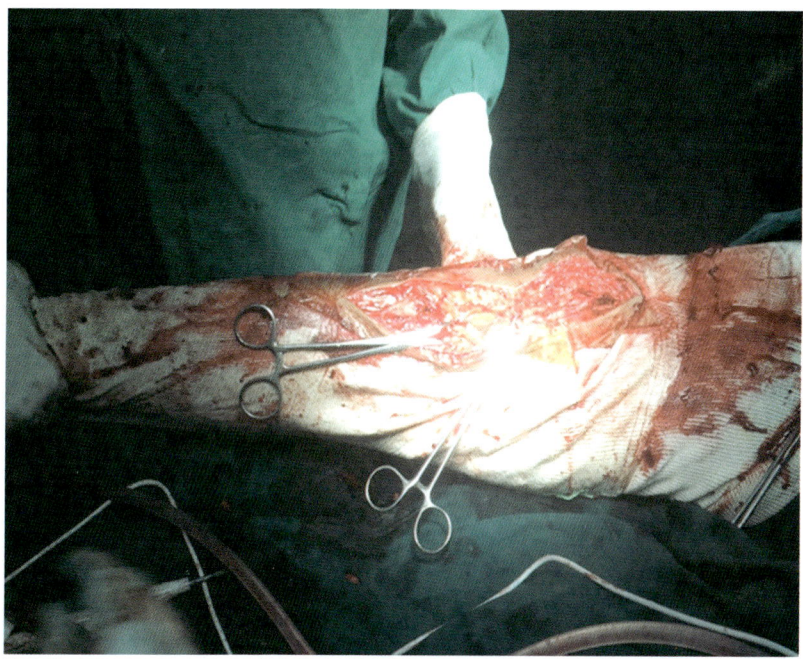

The knee is put through full range of motion; stability mobility and patellar tracking are checked.

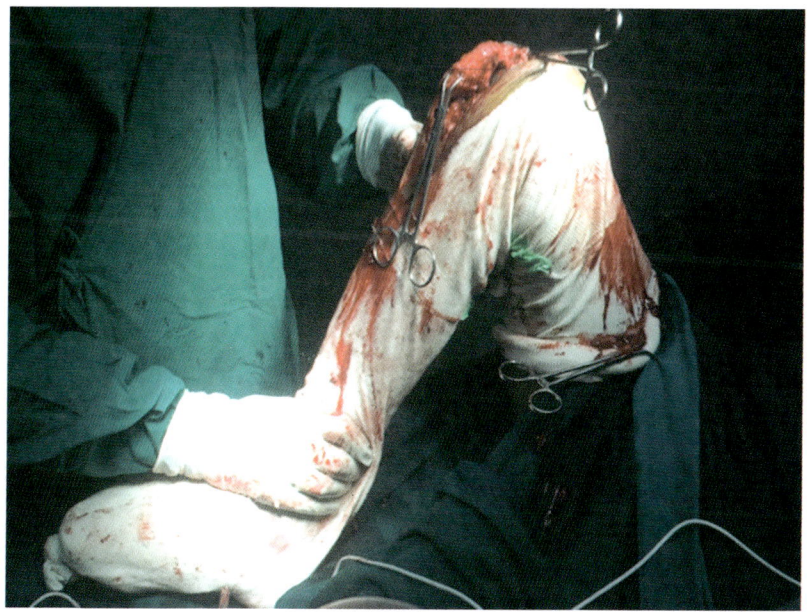

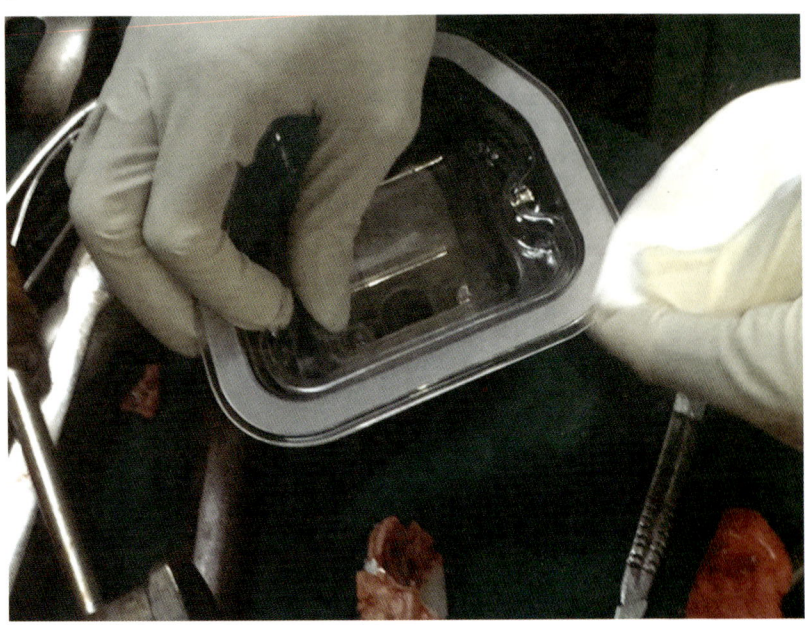

The actual implants are now unpacked.

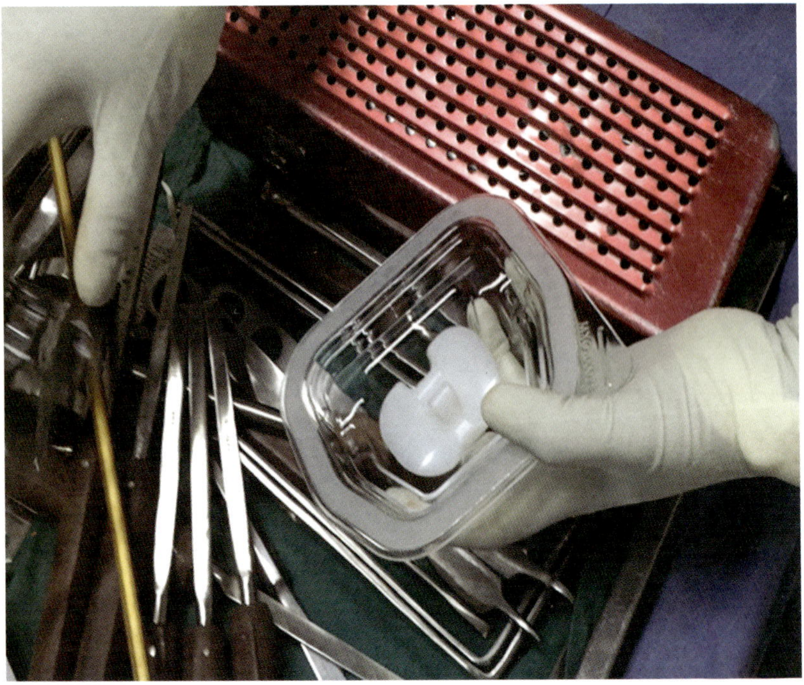

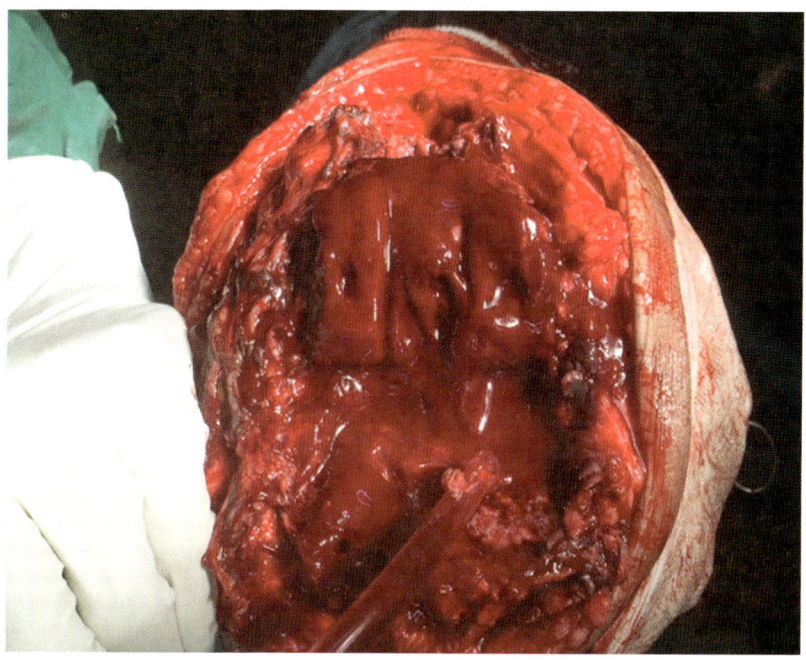

The bony surfaces are washed and packed with adrenaline soaked gauze or pads.

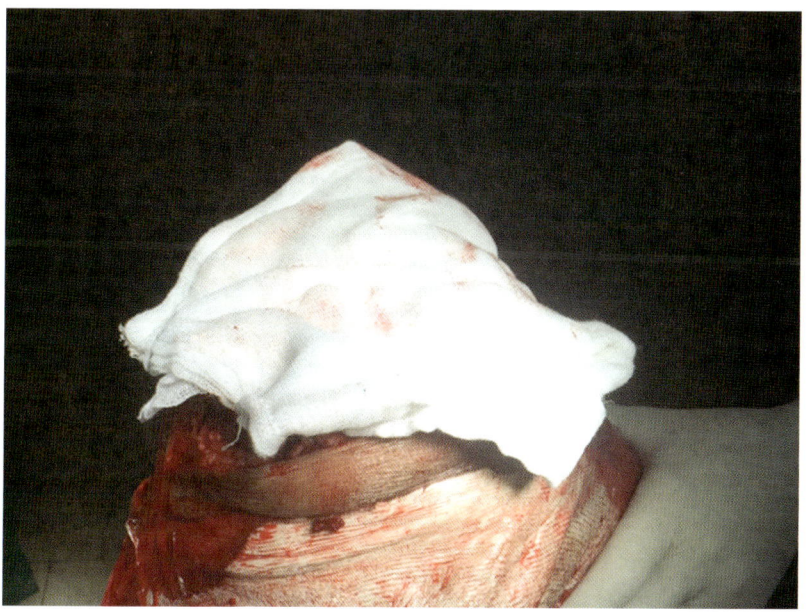

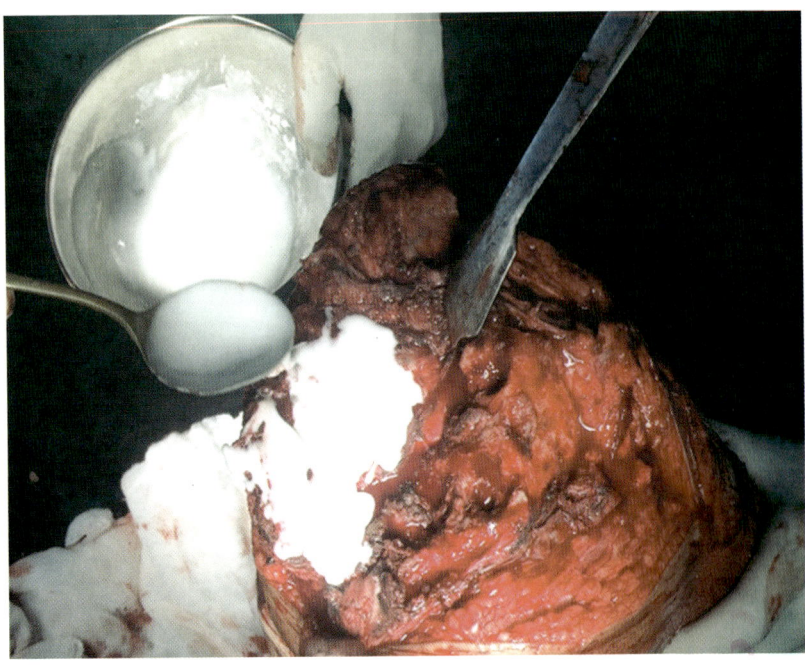

Cement is applied to tibial surface and the inside of the femoral component.

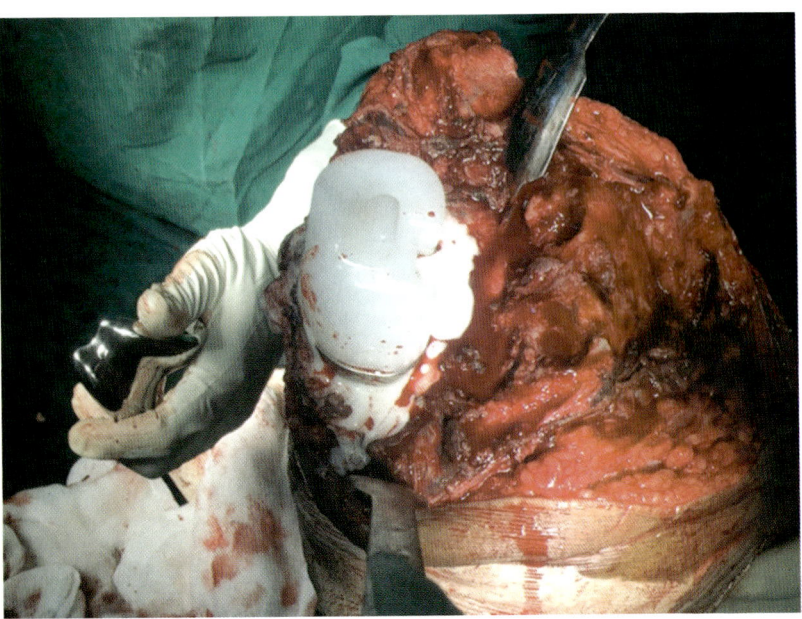

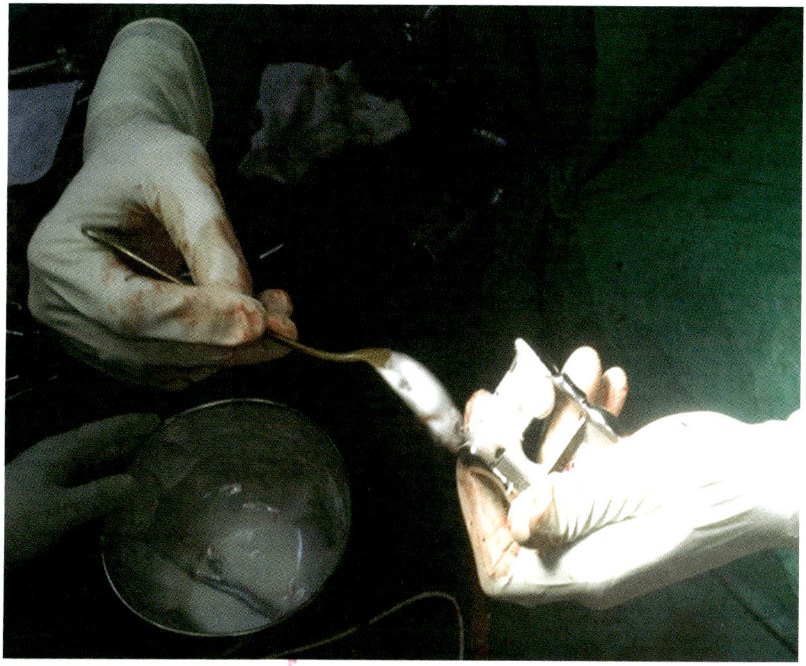

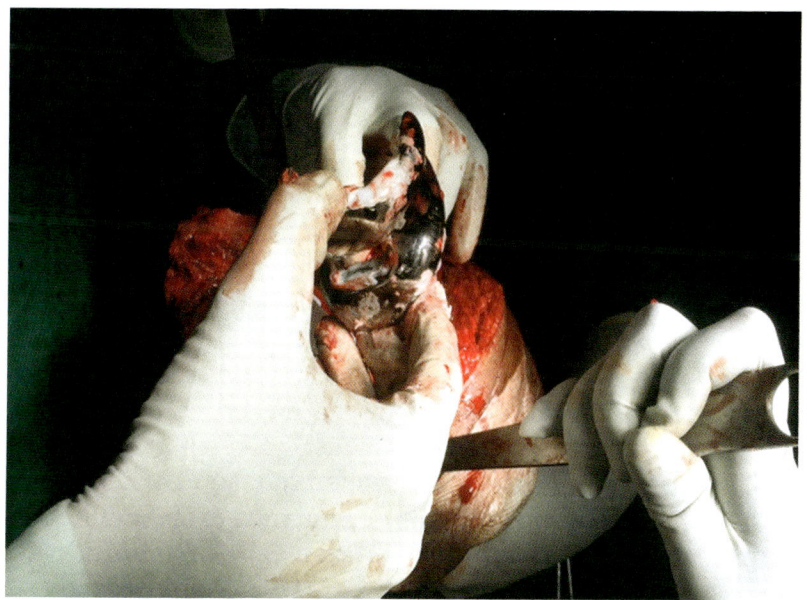

It is important to apply cement to the inner side of the lower femoral condyle.

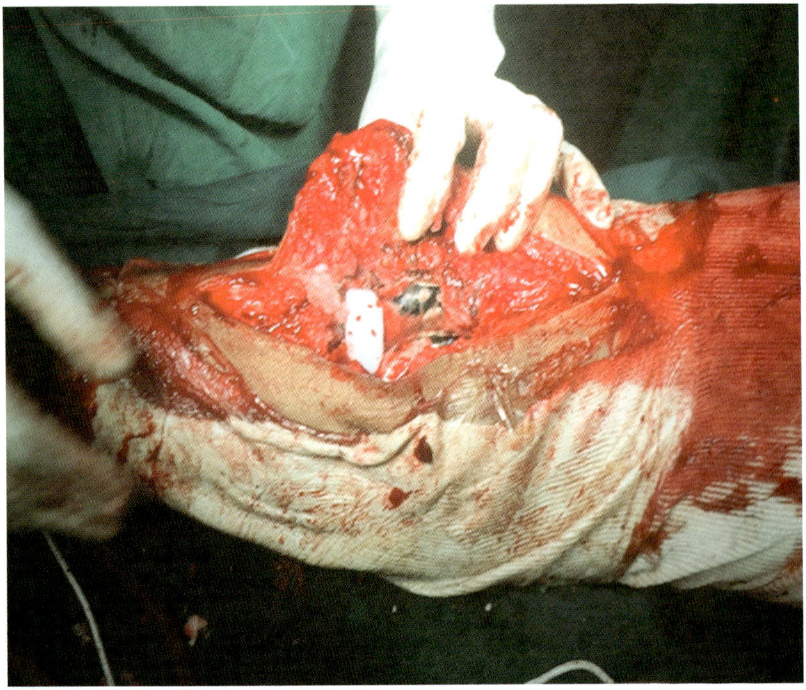

The components are pressed home and the knee is kept in full extension.

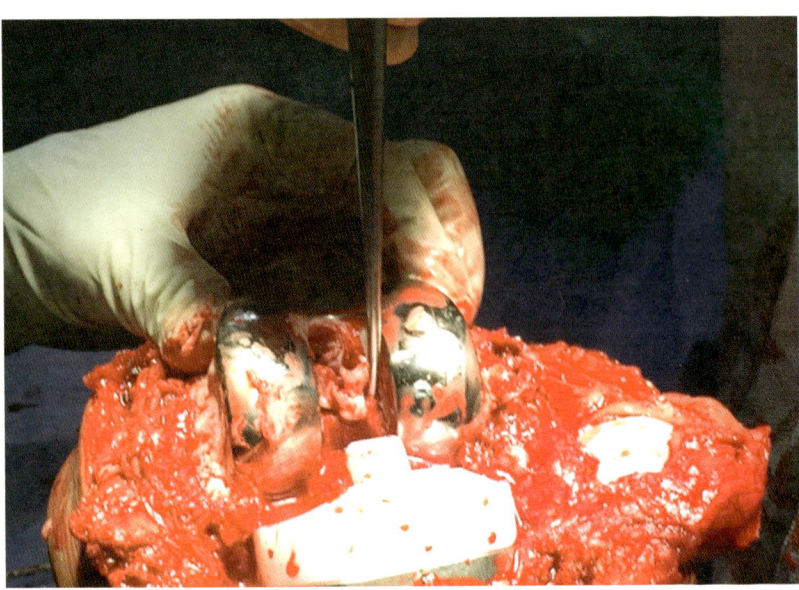

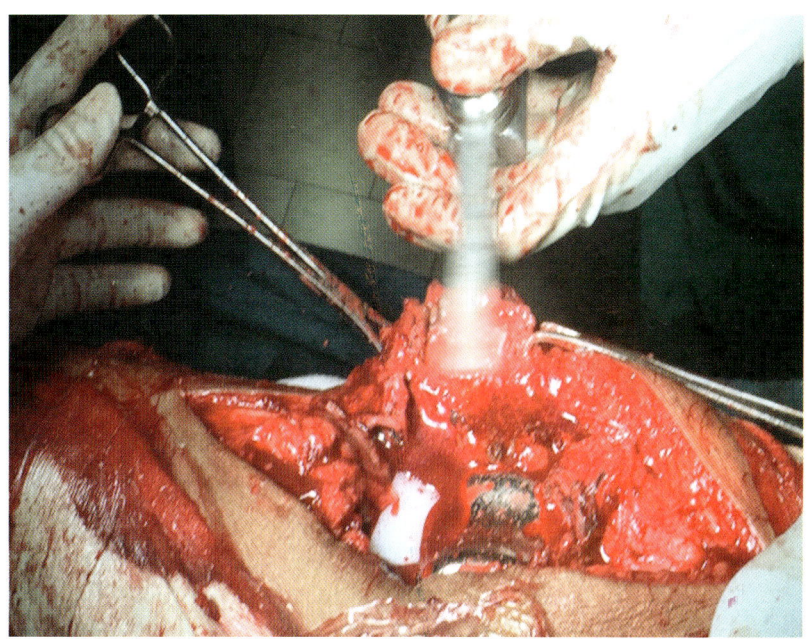

Patelloplasty and excess cement removal.

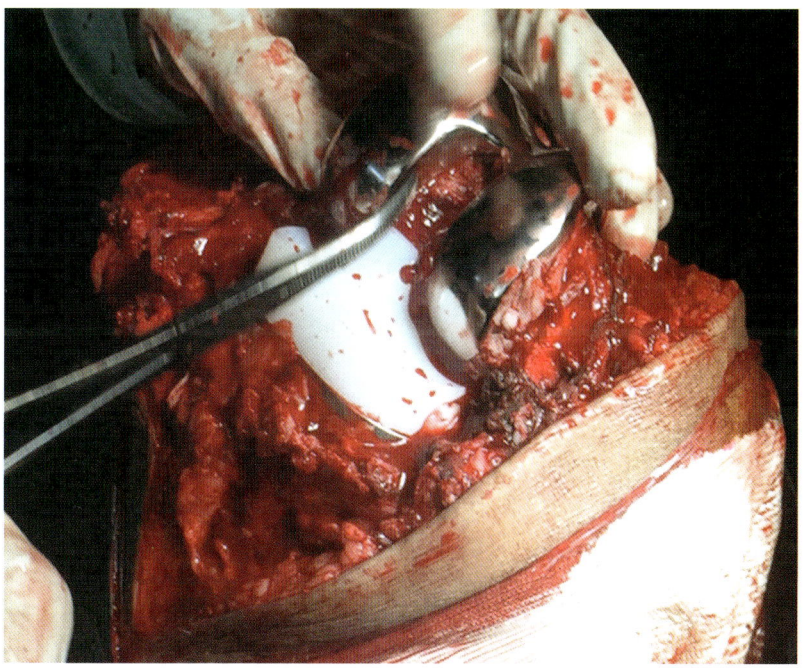

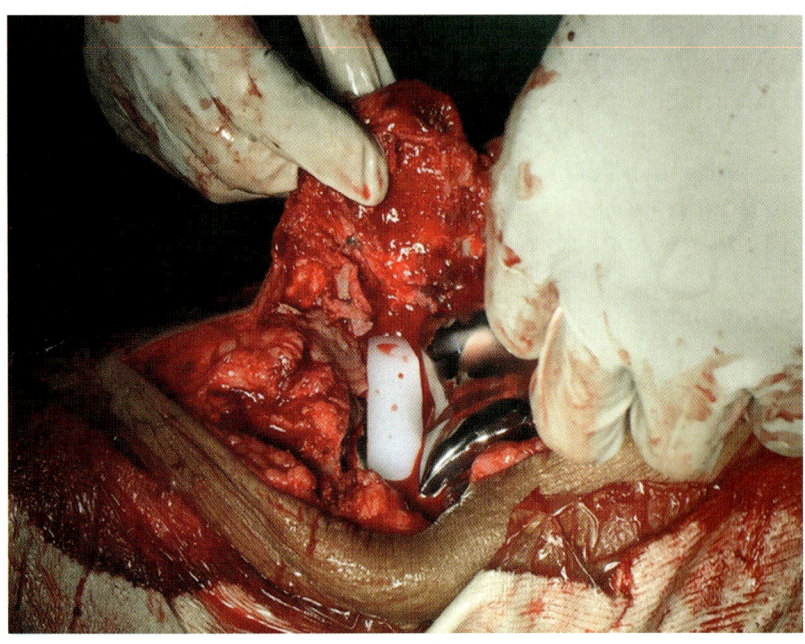

Final wash and suction drain.

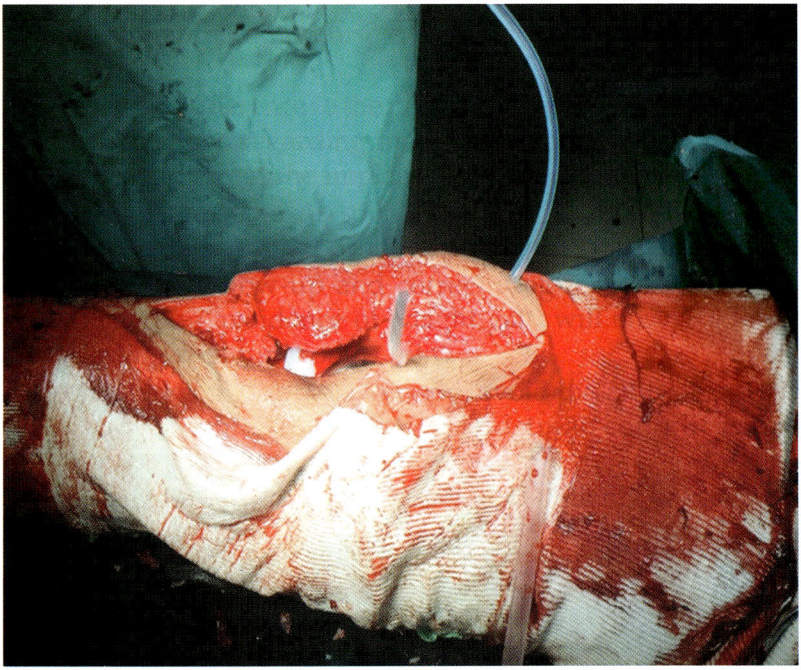

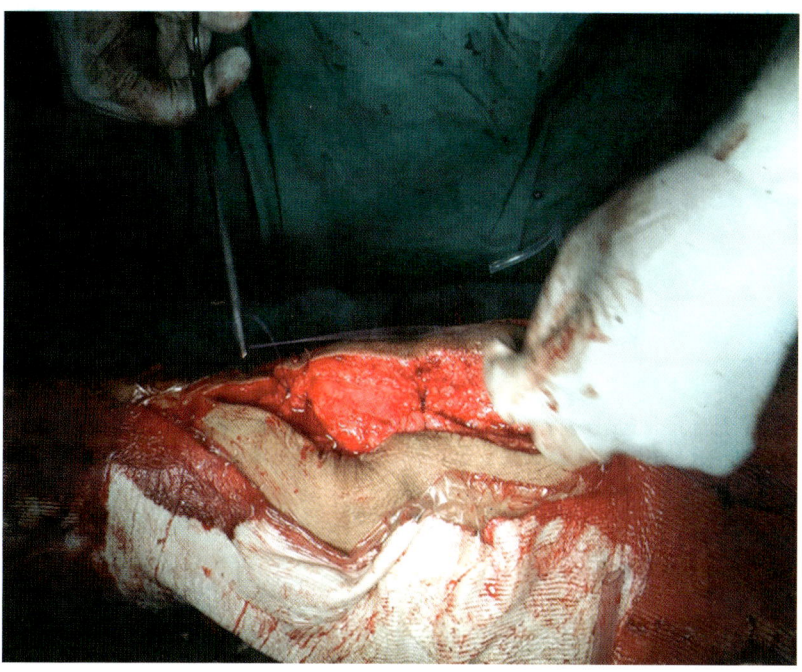

Closure in layers.

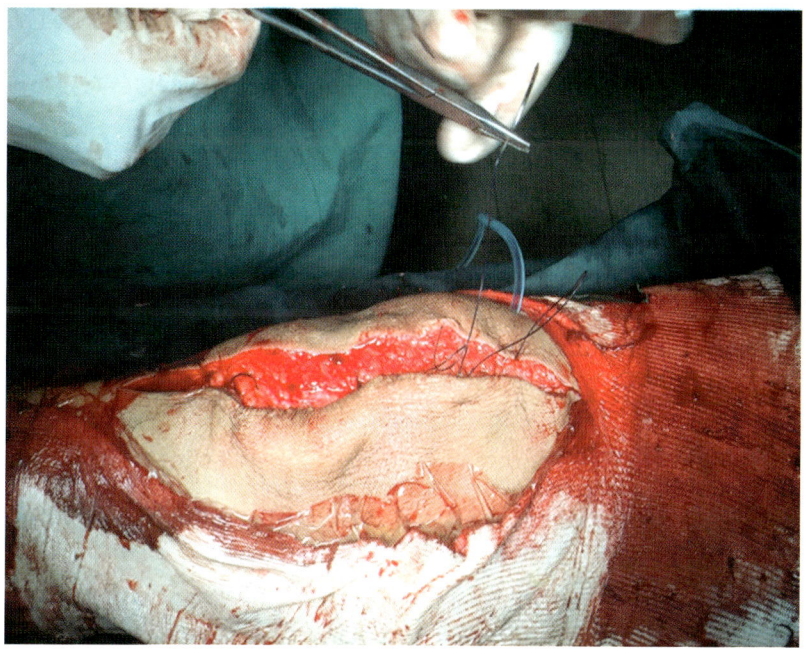

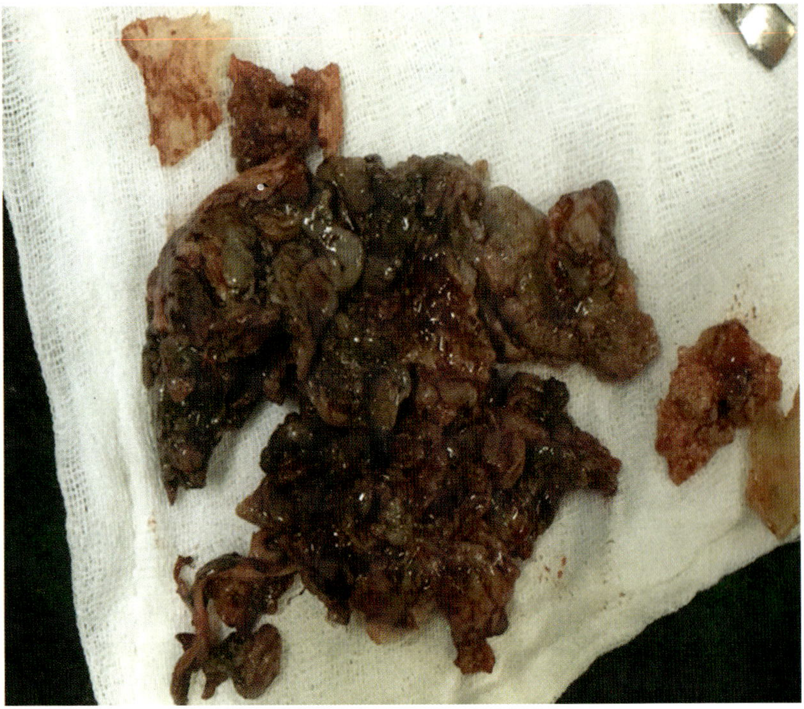

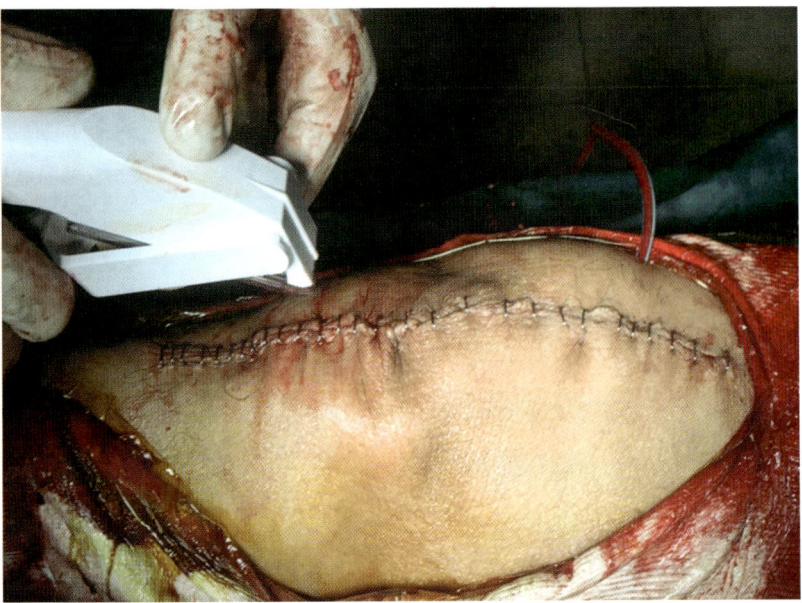

Skin stapling.

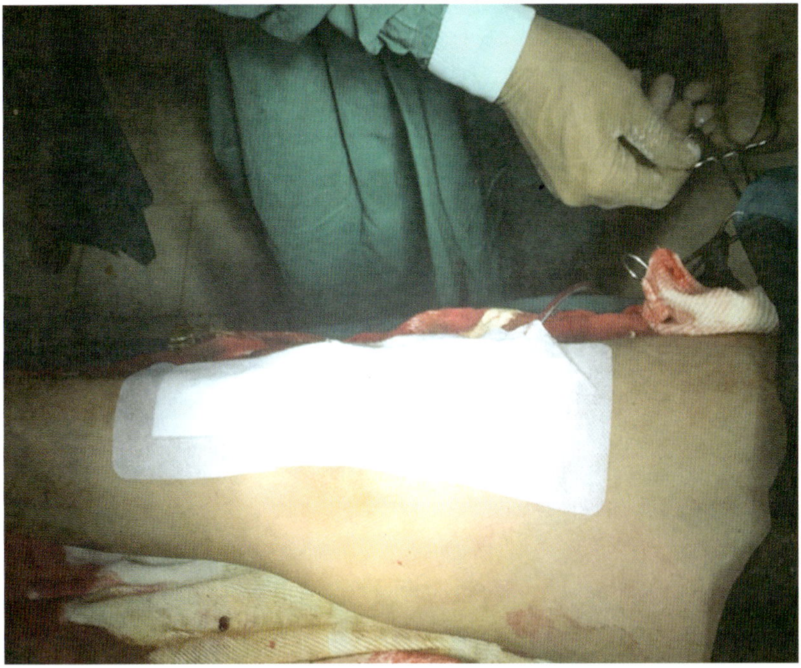

Check that the deformity is corrected.

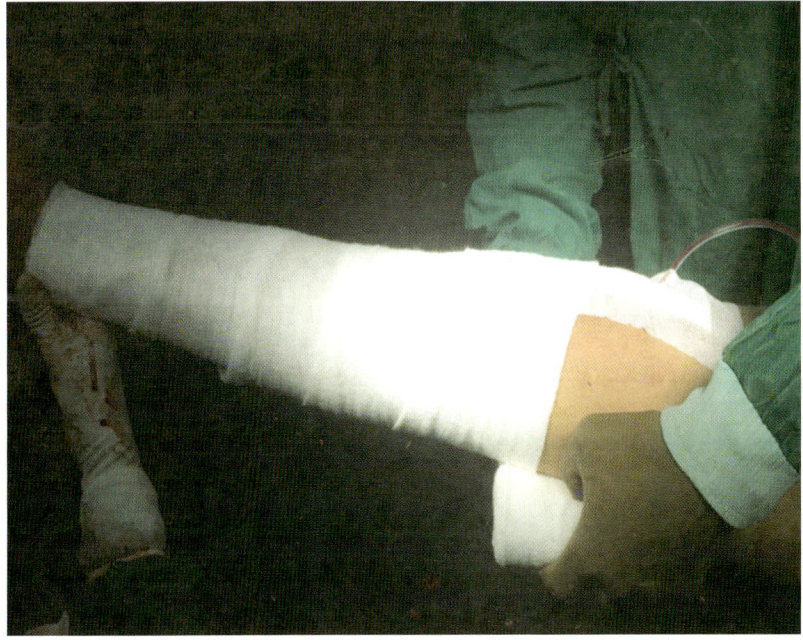

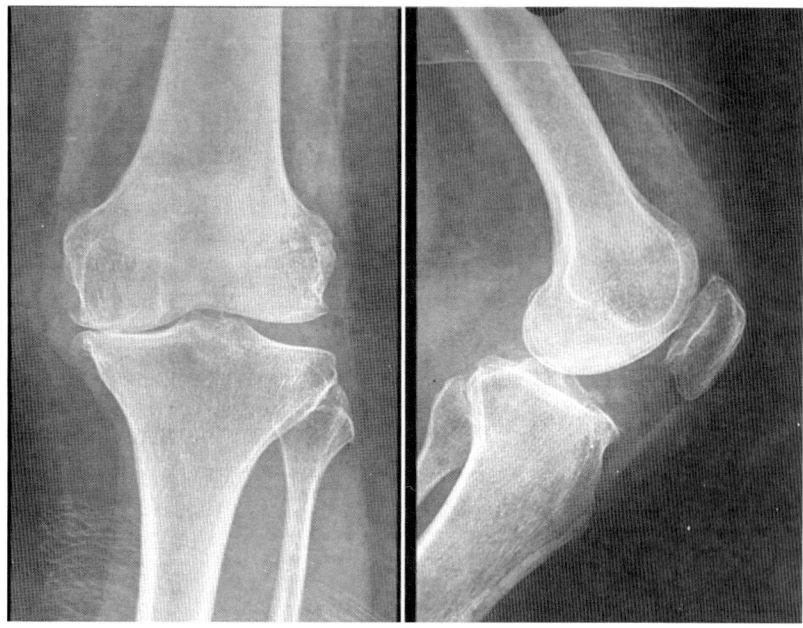

A case of severe medial compartment arthritis, treated by medial unicompartmental Oxford mobile bearing knee.

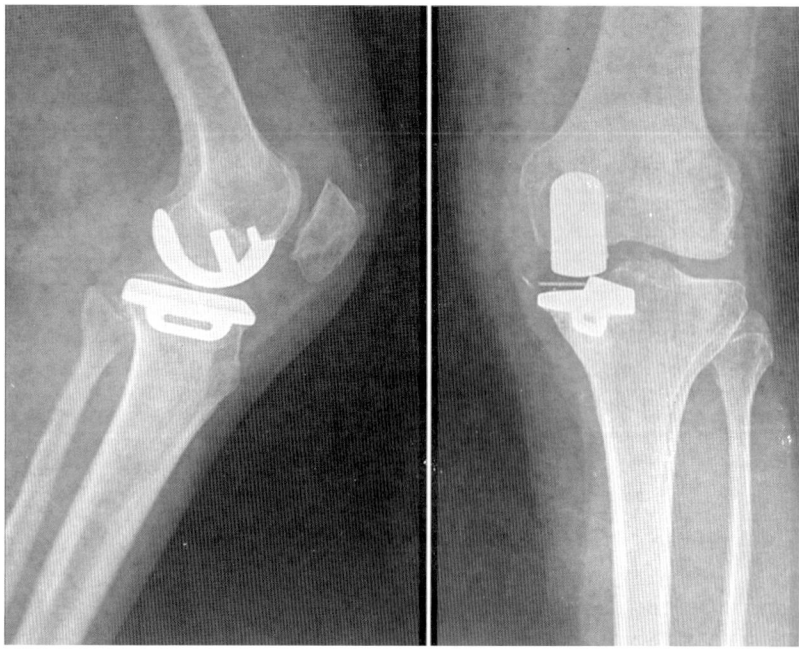

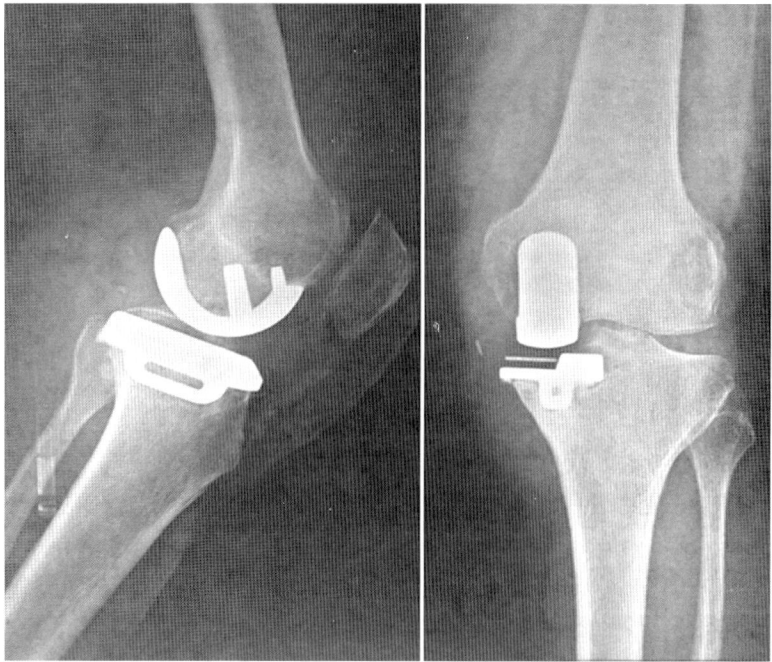

Failure within two years because of component malpositioning.

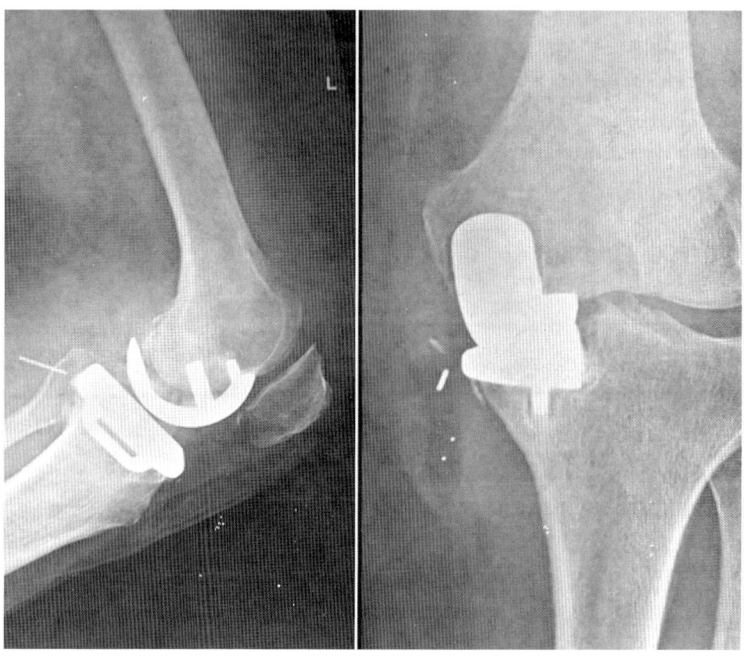

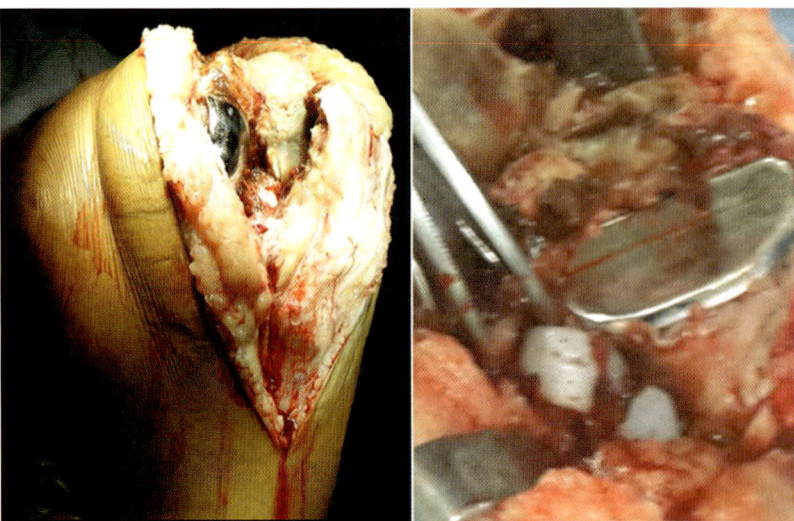

Standard incision and exposure. The meniscal bearing is dislocated and slipped. This is removed.

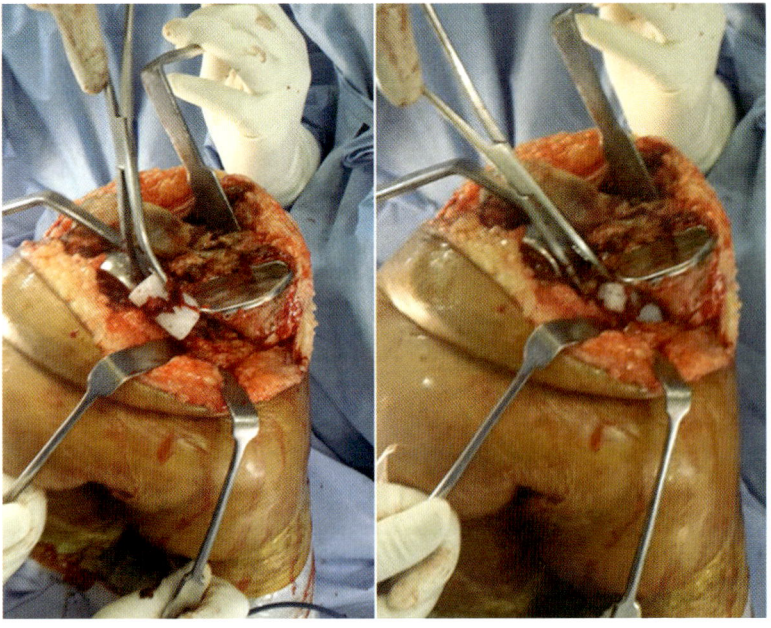

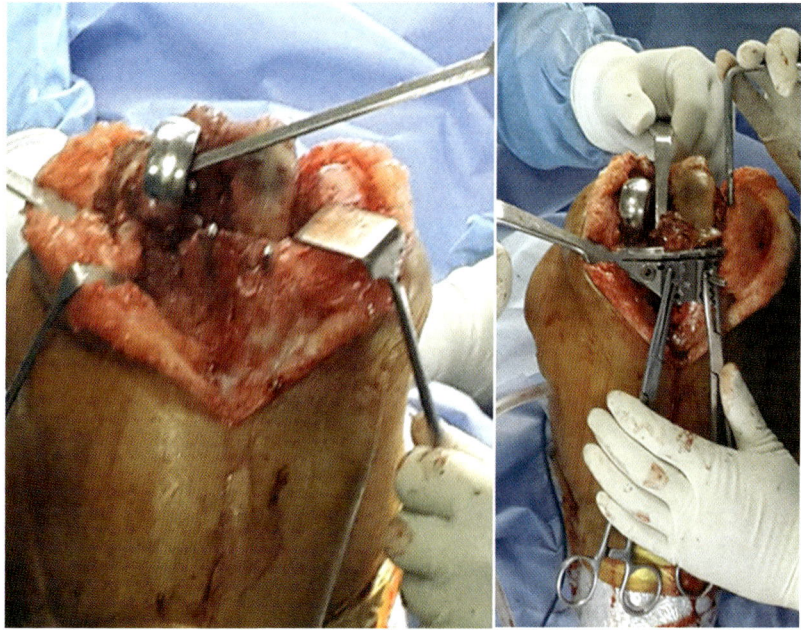

Components are removed and fresh bone cuts performed.

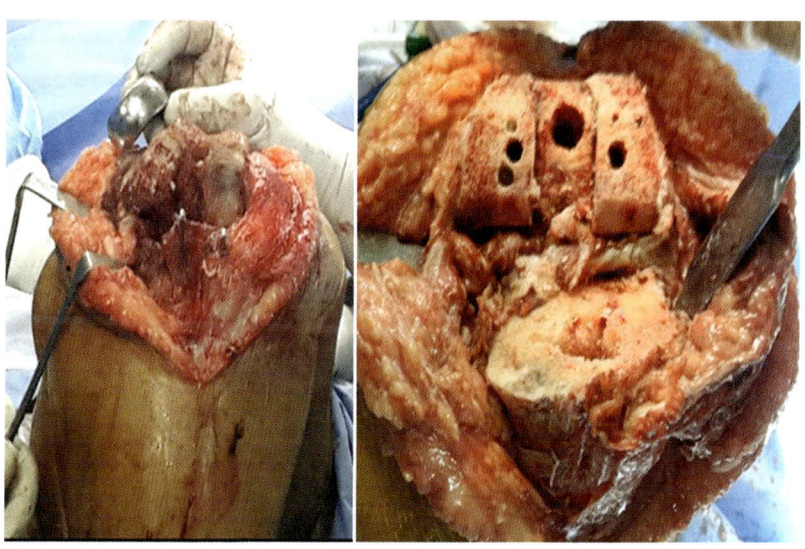

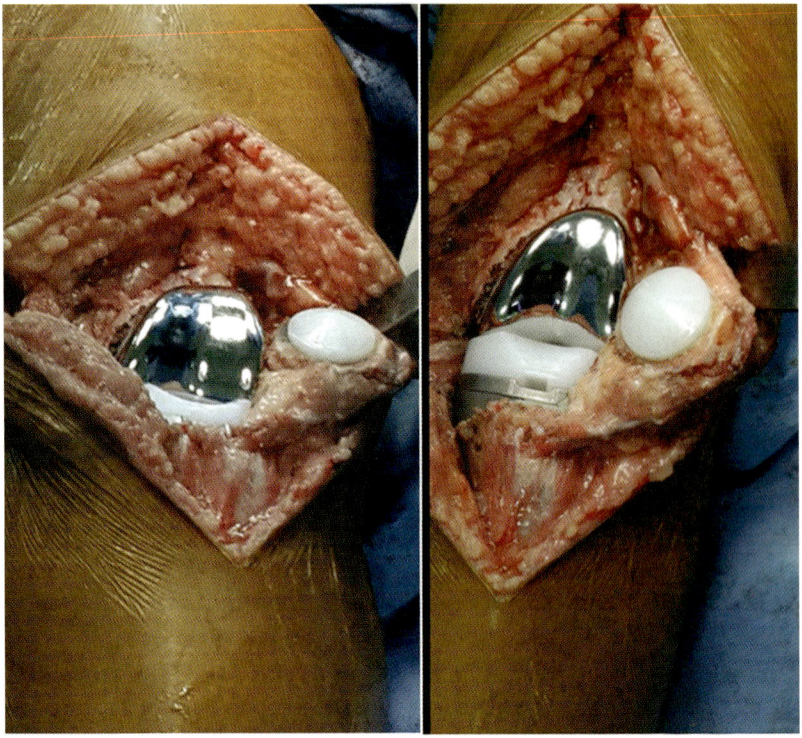

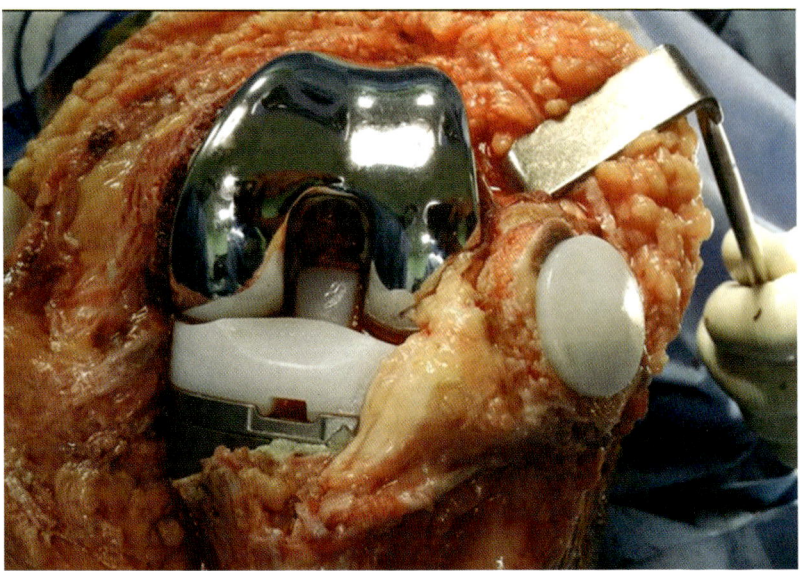

Cementation of all the three components.

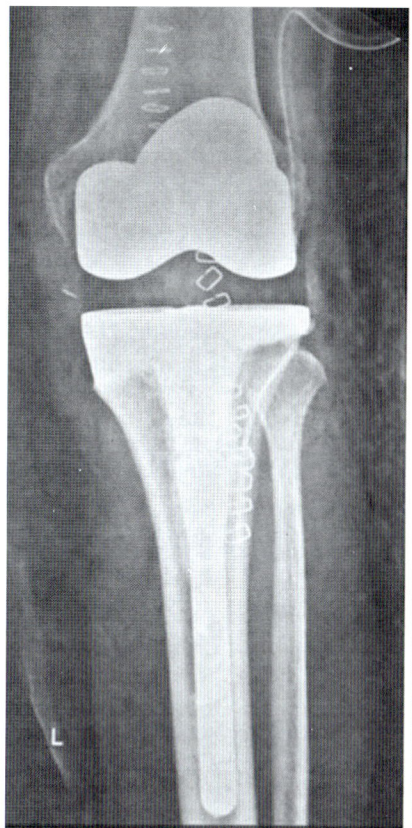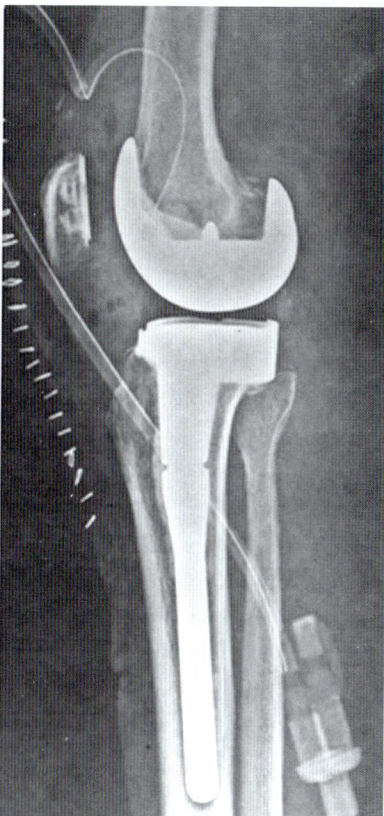

Postoperative X-ray.

REVISION FOR A SEPTIC LOOSENING

A knee that has failed due to a primary or secondary infection and needs revision can either be revised as a one-stage procedure or a two-stage procedure. The choice of the method depends on various factors. The surgeon, patient, the clinical and radiological picture and organizational and infrastructural facilities—all play an important part in choosing the procedure to be employed.

A two-stage procedure involves thorough removal of the implants, cement, and all dead and necrotic material, followed by a bone cement block as a spacer. At a later stage this cement block is removed and a fresh prosthesis is implanted.

In a single stage procedure, the removal, clearance and reinsertion are completed in one session. This beginner's guide is hardly the place for details about such an exacting procedure, hence the reader may refer to more detailed publications on this aspect.

REVISION SURGERY FOR AN INFECTED KNEE

Infection, whether immediate or delayed, is a serious problem. The steps for tackling the infection are:

1. Diagnosis, clinical and radiological.
2. Bone scan.
3. Aspiration and bacteriology.
4. Plan for revision
5. Single stage revision or
   a. Removal of components, cement spacer and delayed revision or
   b. Removal of components, space retention with an external fixator followed by revision or
   c. Component removal and arthrodesis.
6. Special care for soft tissue handling.

The above is a generalized sequence that can be tailored to each patient individually, depending on the severity of infection, bacterial nature and virulence, antibiotic sensitivity, sinuses and scarring, type of original implant used, and patient profile and make up.

One must inform the patient that there is a high risk of these revisions failing, and consequently he/she must be prepared for an arthrodesis if the revision does not succeed in clearing up the infection or giving an satisfactory function. In very rare and severe extremes, the patient may also end up with an amputation.

The process of decision making in an infected knee:

The first step is diagnosis. As mentioned above, the clinical picture is very important. The following points are noted:

1. Pain and inflammation.
2. Swelling and haemarthrosis, pyarthrosis.
3. Discharging sinuses and scars.
4. Limitation of movement.
5. Laxity and instability.

X-ray is then analysed to see the degree of bone loss, sequestra and radiolucent lines. A very careful note is made of the shift and tilt of the components, breakage of the cement mantle, subluxations and deformities.

A radio isotope scan is done in doubtful cases to distinguish between infection and aseptic loosening.

This is followed by aspiration of the knee and sending the aspirate for culture and cytology. A careful note is made of the type of growth in culture and the antibiotic sensitivity of the organisms grown.

Based on the above parameters, one chooses among the following options:

1. Removal of the prosthesis, lavage, clearance of the remaining cement, and arthrodesis.
2. A two-stage procedure consisting of removal of all components, space retention by a cement block spacer or an external fixator followed by a later revision.
3. A single stage revision.

Arthrodesis: This is a simple option and likely to give a reasonable long-lasting result and must be discussed with the patient in all cases. Unlike a single or double stage revision (with a limited life span and a high chance of failure and recurrence of infection), arthrodesis offers a pain-free stable knee with a high chance of eradication of infection. However, a good percentage of patients may not accept a stiff knee; those who have had a good run with their primary knee and now have a delayed infection are a bit difficult to convince. However, if a decision has been made to remove the components and arthrodesis the knee, the following are the steps:

1. A preoperative culture and antibiotic sensitivity is mandatory. The patient is started on appropriate antibiotics before surgery. A combination of antibiotics must be used depending on circumstances and a consultation with the bacteriologist will be of significant advantage.
2. The incision is straight midline. In case there are any sinuses, these are excised. A thick flap, including the skin, subcutaneous fat and soft tissues, is removed in one piece to avoid postoperative sloughing and necrosis.

3. All components are removed as described under revision for aseptic revision. Soft tissue bits and pieces of synovium and fat are removed and sent for culture and histology.
4. All cement is removed and the surfaces are now washed thoroughly. All loose cement bits are removed. All adherent cement mantle is painstakingly removed. Using a wire brush, the cancellous surfaces are scrubbed until fresh bleeding cancellous bone is visible.
5. The entire interior of the knee is washed with copious amount of saline and dried thoroughly. The femoral and tibial surfaces are apposed and checked if the two out surfaces match. There should be no gaps, and the unevenness of the surfaces should be smoothened by minimal shavings of cuts using an oscillating saw.
6. On apposition of the two out surfaces, there must be a 15° of flexion, and a 5° to 7° of valgus. This is the acceptable position for arthrodesis. Anything short of this needs to be corrected with additional bone cuts. One must desist from making large bone cuts, which may lead to an unacceptable shortening of the arthrodesed knee.
7. The choice of fixation device depends of the preference and experience of the surgeon. As a rule, internal fixation is avoided. The external fixator used can either be an Ilizarov type of ring fixator, a Charnley type knee arthordesis clamp or an AO type of fixator. A modified Hoffman frame is also acceptable.
8. After cleaning and apposing the surfaces, the fixator is applied if a good fit is present. However, if there are gaps, they are filled with cancellous bone from the iliac crest before applying the fixator.
9. The fixator is applied, the surface compressed and a routine closure performed after adequate drainage.
10. Appropriate antibiotics are administered postoperatively, and the patient is mobilized in the standard manner.
11. The fixator is tightened and additional compression is given depending on the situation. The fixator is removed after radiological and clinical evidence of solid fusion.

Double-stage revision: This is the preferred method where there is a fulminant infection with large sinuses, a bad skin and a lot of slough and scars. The space between the femur and tibia is preserved, either with a blob of antibiotic-loaded cement or with an external fixator. The following are the steps:

1. The patient is informed that the first stage is meant to eradicate infection. If there is incomplete eradication, the patient may have to undergo an arthrodesis rather than a knee replacement.
2. The exposure and component removal are standard as described above. All the sinuses are excised, and scar tissue is removed. One may need the assistance of the plastic surgeon for a good flap coverage in case there is a large skin loss.
4. The two surface are stretched as far apart as possible using lamina spreaders. Bone cement mixed with appropriate antibiotic is kneaded to a doughy consistency and packed into the space. It is a good idea to keep the flat handle of the Hohman retractor behind the cement blob as the cement sets. This will prevent thermal damage to the popliteal vessels.
5. In case an external fixator is to be used, the same steps are employed. But the fixator is used to distract the two joint surfaces to retain maximum gap. I always prefer the thin pins of the llizarov type frame to thick Stienman pins.
6. The interval between this and the second surgery depends on complete eradication of all signs of infection. Once this is achieved, the second stage is put into action.
7. The steps of reimplanting a fresh knee are similar to those described for revision of an aseptic loosening. The post-operative and follow-up are also identical.

Single stage revision for infection: This is the method of choice in cases with doubtful sepsis, minimal signs of inflammation, delayed infection, good skin, and absence of bad scars and sinuses.

After a thorough preoperative assessment, the following steps are employed. These steps are similar to those for revising an aseptic loosening:

1. The skin incision is straight midline. A thick skin flap is taken. The debridement of the knee and removal of all infected material follows.
2. Removal of components and cement is done in a manner similar to that described under revision for aseptic loosening.

3. Acrylic cement loaded with an appropriate antibiotic is used for cementing the components. The bone loss present at the time of surgery may necessitate the use of a prosthesis either with a larger constraint or a hinged implant.

4. Closure and postoperative management are routine.

This chapter only offers a brief description of the outlines of management of an infected total knee prosthesis. However, it must be reemphasized that the operation is not an easy one and that the chances of failure are high. It is mandatory that all facilities, proper instrumentation and adequate stocks of all sizes of implants with a larger constraint are available in the operation theatre. It is also essential that the surgeon has adequate experience before undertaking this surgery.

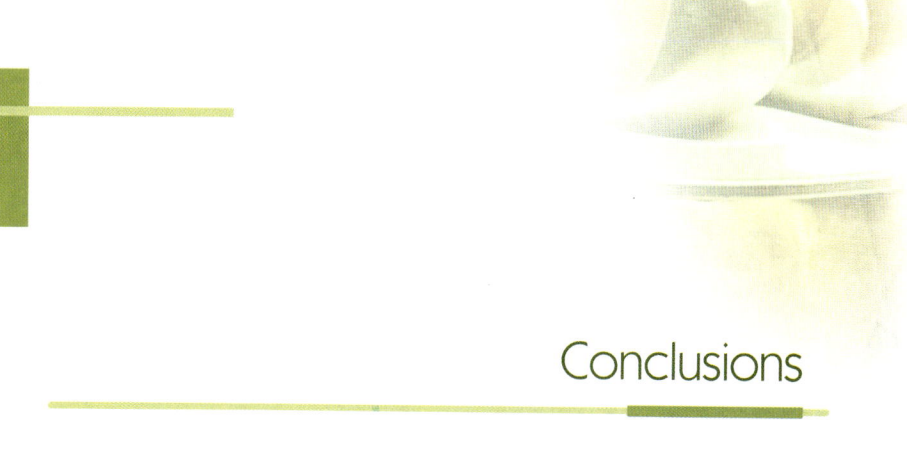

Conclusions

It is with a feeling of immense pleasure that an author reaches the last chapter of his/her book! The feelings can be compared to those of successfully delivering a child! Now that I look through the 700 plus pages I have penned over the last 18 months, I find a lot of omissions and commissions. At a glance the book reads like a manual for a self assembly IKEA furniture. On occasions and in some pages, the impression is that of a simple carpentry or electronic assembly. It is quite apparent that the pages of technique and "how to do" far exceed the descriptions on "when not to do" and "what not to do".

This chapter is not a summation of the merits and advantages of knee arthroplasty. I have laid all emphasis on the salient aspects of pitfalls and trouble spots of this form of surgery in the Asian circumstance. You, dear reader, are warned that the operative part may seem (and in most cases is) really easy! However, the difficult parts (patient selection and counselling, avoiding of undue promises and preoperative enthusiasm and a meticulous adherence to systems and procedures) are indeed is the key to this aspect of orthopaedic surgery.

The following observations regarding knee replacement surgery sum up the pitfalls, things to do and things to avoid:

1. Patients who have good movements and are accustomed to squatting and Namaz prayers are not good candidates for knee replacement unless they are willing to give up these activities and demand the operation.
2. Results for rheumatoid knees with crippling disability are much more gratifying than for knees with osteoarthritis.

3. Obese patients are a taboo and 85 kg is the upper limit. Ask for a weight reduction before picking up the knife.
4. A very careful preoperative evaluation is mandatory and all aspects of the patient demand very careful scrutiny.
5. If the theatre is not adequate, do not take chances! Please try to have an exclusive operating theatre for orthopaedic and arthroplasty work; avoid sharing the OT with the general surgeon and gynaecologist!
6. Choose your system of implants and instrumentation very carefully.
7. Have the complete range of instrumentation on hand, including all trials. Ensure that your saw and drill work. Keep all instrumentation ready.
8. A complete range of implants is mandatory. All sizes, all thicknesses, good stock of cement!
9. Do the soft tissue part of the operation before the first bone cut. The tendency of the resident to start whizzing away with the saw should be discouraged.
10. Be careful in closure and take adequate precautions to handle the soft tissues gently and meticulously.
11. Antibiotics, bio-occlusive clothing and clean air (in that order).
12. A strict adherence to the postoperative regime and correct instructions regarding mobilization and weight bearing (depending on the implant type) are essential.
13. Discharge soon. As soon as patient is comfortable! This will avoid hospital contamination and infection.
14. Regular follow-up and correct long-term instructions, including avoidance of weight gain will ensure a long-lasting well functioning joint.
15. Should complications develop, avoid the attitude of wait and watch. Be aggressive and treat complications immediately and properly.
16. Maintain records for your sake and patients' sake.

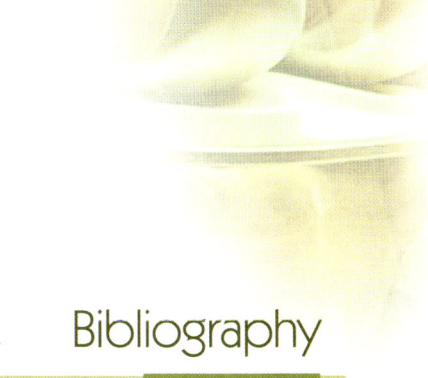

Bibliography

Abdel-Salam A, Eyres KS. Effects of tourniquet during total knee arthroplasty. A prospective randomised study. J Bone Joint Surg Br 1995; 77(2):250–3.

Abdel-Salam A, Eyres KS. Effects of tourniquet during total knee arthroplasty. A prospective randomised study. J Bone Joint Surg Br 1995; 77(2):250–3.

Abernethy PJ, Robinson CM, Fowler RM. Fracture of the metal tibial tray after Kinematic total knee replacement. A common cause of early aseptic failure. J Bone Joint Surg Br 1996; 78(2):220–5.

Acheson RM, Collart AB. New Haven survey of joint diseases. XVII. Relationship between some systemic characteristics and osteoarthritis in a general population. Ann Rheum Dis 1975;34(5):379–87.

Ackroyd CE, Whitehouse SL, Newman JH, et al. A comparative study of the medial St Georg sled and kinematic total knee arthroplasties. Ten-year survivorship. J Bone Joint Surg Br 2002; 84(5):667–72.

Adili A, Bhandari M, Petruccelli D, et al. Sequential bilateral total knee arthroplasty under 1 anaesthetic in patients > or = 75 years old: complications and functional outcomes. J Arthroplasty 2001; 16(3): 271–8.

Ahl T, Dalen N, Jorbeck H, Hoborn J. Air contamination during hip and knee arthroplasties. Horizontal laminar flow randomized vs. conventional ventilation. Acta Orthop Scand 1995; 66(1):17–20.

Akagi M, Nakamura T, Matsusue Y, Ueo T, Nishijyo K, Ohnishi E. The Bisurface total knee replacement: a unique design for flexion. Four-to-nine-year follow-up study. J Bone Joint Surg Am 2000; 82-A(11):1626–33.

Akizuki S, Yasukawa Y, Takizawa T. A new method of hemostasis for cementless total knee arthroplasty. Bull Hosp Jt Dis 1997; 56(4): 222–4.

Alemparte J, Johnson GV, Worland RL, et al. Results of simultaneous bilateral total knee replacement: a study of 1208 knees in 604 patients. J South Orthop Assoc 2002; 11(3):153–6.

Alexander R, El-Moalem HE, Gan TJ. Comparison of the morphine-sparing effects of diclofenac sodium and ketorolac tromethamine after major orthopaedic surgery. J Clin Anesth 2002; 14(3):187–92.

Alibhai A, Saunders D, Johnston DW, et al. Total hip and knee replacement surgeries in Alberta utilization and associated outcomes. Healthc Manage Forum 2001; 14(2):25–32.

Alicea J. Scoring systems and their validation for the arthritic knee. In: Insall JN, Churchill SN, eds. Surgery of the Knee. 3rd ed. New York: Livingston; 2001:1507–15.

Amadio PC, Naessens JM, Rice RL, et al. Effect of feedback on resource use and morbidity in hip and knee arthroplasty in an integrated group practice setting. Mayo Clin Proc 1996; 71(2):127–33.

Anders MJ, Lifeso RM, Landis M, et al. Effect of preoperative donation of autologous blood on deep-vein thrombosis following total joint arthroplasty of the hip or knee. J Bone Joint Surg Am 1996; 78(4): 574–80.

Anderson DR, Gross M, Robinson KS, et al. Ultrasonographic screening for deep vein thrombosis following arthroplasty fails to reduce posthospital thromboembolic complications: the Postarthroplasty Screening Study (PASS). Chest 1998; 114(2 Suppl Evidence):119S–22S.

Anderson JG, Wixson RL, Tsai D, et al. Functional outcome and patient satisfaction in total knee patients over the age of 75. J Arthroplasty 1996; 11(7):831–40.

Anonymous. Analyzing functional status data helps hospital improve knee and hip replacements. Data Strateg Benchmarks 1998; 2(10):148–51.

Anouchi YS, McShane M, Kelly F Jr, Elting J, Stiehl J. Range of motion in total knee replacement. Clin Orthop 1996; (331):87–92.

Ansari S, Ackroyd CE, Newman JH. Kinematic posterior cruciate ligament-retaining total knee replacements. A 10-year survivorship study of 445 arthroplasties. Am J Knee Surg 1998; 11(1):9–14.

Ansari S, Newman JH, Ackroyd CE. St. Georg sledge for medial compartment knee replacement. 461 arthroplasties followed for 4 (1–17) years. Acta Orthop Scand 1997; 68(5):430–4.

Ansari S, Warwick D, Ackroyd CE, et al. Incidence of fatal pulmonary embolism after 1,390 knee arthroplasties without routine prophylactic anticoagulation, except in high-risk cases. J Arthroplasty 1997; 12(6):599–602.

Arnbjornsson AH, Ryd L. The use of isolated patellar prostheses in Sweden 1977–1986. Int Orthop 1998; 22(3):141–4.

Babis GC, Trousdale RT, Morrey BF. The effectiveness of isolated tibial insert exchange in revision total knee arthroplasty. J Bone Joint Surg Am 2002 Jan;84-A(1):64–8.

Bach CM, Nogler M, Steingruber IE, et al. Scoring systems in total knee arthroplasty. Clin Orthop 2002; (399):184–96.

Bach CM, Steingruber IE, Peer S, et al. Radiographic assessment in total knee arthroplasty. Clin Orthop 2001; (385):144–50.

Bachmeier C, March L, Cross M, et al. A comparison of outcomes in osteoarthritis patients undergoing total hip and knee replacement surgery. Osteoarthritis Cartilage 2001 Feb;9(2):137–46.

Back DL, Cannon SR, Hilton A, Bankes MJ, Briggs TW. The Kinemax total knee arthroplasty. Nine years' experience. J Bone Joint Surg Br 2001; 83(3):359–63.

Badhe N, Dewnany G, Livesley PJ. Should the patella be replaced in total knee replacement? Int Orthop 2001; 25(2):97–9.

Badner NH, Bourne RB, Rorabeck CH, et al. Intra-articular injection of bupivacaine in knee-replacement operations. Results of use for analgesia and for preemptive blockade. J Bone Joint Surg Am 1996; 78(5):734–8.

Baldwin J, El-Saied M, Rubinstein RJ. Uncemented total knee arthroplasty: report of 109 titanium knees with cancellous-structured porous coating. Orthopaedics 1996 Feb;19(2):123–30.

Baldwin J, Rubinstein RJ. The effect of bone quality on the outcome of ingrowth total knee arthroplasty. Am J Knee Surg 1996 Sp ring;9(2):45–9; discussion 9–50.

Baldwin JL, El-Saied MR, Rubinstein RA Jr. Uncemented total knee arthroplasty: report of 109 titanium knees with cancellous-structured porous coating. Orthopaedics 1996; 19(2):123–30.

Banks SA, Harman MK, Hodge WA. Mechanism of anterior impingement damage in total knee arthroplasty. J Bone Joint Surg Am 2002; 84-A Suppl 2:37–42.

Barck AL. Agreement among clinical assessment scales for knee replacement surgery. Knee 1997; 4(3):155–8.

Barck AL. Can the patient's memory of the timing of pain events replace chart notes? Acta Orthop Belg 1998; 64(1):1–3.

Barck AL. Measurement of clinical change caused by knee replacement. Conventional score or special change indexes? Arch Orthop Trauma Surg 1999; 119(1–2):76–8. Less than 100 knees in the study.

Barck AL. Minimize outcome measures after knee replacement. Arch Orthop Trauma Surg 1998; 117(8):461–3. Factors associated with outcome evaluation.

Barck AL. Pain and walking as outcome evaluation after knee replacement. Knee 1997; 4(4):193–5.

Barck AL. Patient's memory or repeated pain and function scores as index for major clinical change caused by knee replacement? Arch Orthop Trauma Surg 1997; 116(8):484–5.

Bardsley M, Cleary R. Assessing the outcomes of total knee replacement. J Eval Clin Pract 1999; 5(1):47–55. E

Barrack RL, Bertot AJ, Wolfe MW, Waldman DA, Milicic M, Myers L. Patellar resurfacing in total knee arthroplasty. A prospective, randomized, double-blind study with five to seven years of follow-up. J Bone Joint Surg Am 2001; 83–A(9):1376–81.

Barrack RL, Hoffman GJ, Tejeiro WV, et al. Surgeon work input and risk in primary versus revision total joint arthroplasty. J Arthroplasty 1995; 10(3):281–6.

Barrack RL, Schrader T, Bertot AJ, et al. Component rotation and anterior knee pain after total knee arthroplasty. Clin Orthop 2001; (392):46–55.

Barrack RL, Smith P, Munn B, et al. The Ranawat Award. Comparison of surgical approaches in total knee arthroplasty. Clin Orthop 1998; (356):16–21.

Barrack RL, Wolfe MW, Waldman DA, Milicic M, Bertot AJ, Myers L. Resurfacing of the patella in total knee arthroplasty. A prospective, randomized, double-blind study. J Bone Joint Surg Am 1997; 79(8):1121–31.

Barrett JP, Siviero P. Retrospective study of outcomes in Hyalgan(R)-treated patients with osteoarthritis of the knee. Clin Drug Invest 2002; 22(2):87–97.

Barwell J, Anderson G, Hassan A, et al. The effects of early tourniquet release during total knee arthroplasty: a prospective randomized double-blind study. J Bone Joint Surg Br 1997; 79(2):265–8.

Bassett RW. Results of 1,000 Performance knees: cementless versus cemented fixation. J Arthroplasty 1998; 13(4):409–13.

Bayley KB, London MR, Grunkemeier GL, Lansky DJ. Measuring the success of treatment in patient terms. Med Care 1995; 33(4 Suppl): AS226–35.

Beaupre L, Davies D, Jones C, et al. Exercise combined with continuous passive motion or slider board therapy compared with exercise only: a randomized controlled trial of patients following total knee arthroplasty. Phys Ther 2001 Apr;81(4):1029–37.

Bedi HS, Fletcher SF, Rush JH, et al. An audit of early hospital readmission after primary knee joint replacement. Aust NZ J Surg 1997; 67(6):340–2.

Bellamy N, Buchanan WW, Goldsmith CH, et al. Validation study of WOMAC: A health status instrument for measuring clinically important patient relevant outcomes to antirheumatic drug therapy in patients with osteoarthritis of the hip or knee. The Journal of Rheumatology 1988;15(12):1833–40.

Benezra VI. Electron microscopic investigation of interfaces in materials for orthopaedic applications. 1998.

Benjamin J, Engh G, Parsley B, et al. Morselized bone grafting of defects in revision total knee arthroplasty. Clin Orthop 2001 Nov;(392):62–7.

Benjamin J, Engh G, Parsley B, et al. Morselized bone grafting of defects in revision total knee arthroplasty. Clin Orthop 2001; (392):62–7.

Benoni G, Carlsson A, Petersson C, et al. Does tranexamic acid reduce blood loss in knee arthroplasty? Am J Knee Surg 1995; 8(3):88–92.

Benroth R, Gawande S. Patient-reported health status in total joint replacement. J Arthroplasty 1999; 14(5):576–80.

Bergenudd H, Sahlstrom A, Sanzen L. Total knee arthroplasty after failed proximal tibial valgus osteotomy. J Arthroplasty 1997; 12(6):635–8.

Berger RA, Lyon JH, Jacobs JJ, et al. Problems with cementless total knee arthroplasty at 11 years followup. Clin Orthop 2001; (392):196–207.

Berger RA, Rosenberg AG, Barden RM, Sheinkop MB, Jacobs JJ, Galante JO. Long-term follow-up of the Miller- Galante total knee replacement. Clin Orthop 2001; 388:58–67.

Berman AT, O'Brien JT, Israelite C. Use of the rotating hinge for salvage of the infected total knee arthroplasty. Orthopaedics 1996; 19(1):73–6.

Bert J, Gross M, Kline C. Outcome results after total knee arthroplasty: Does the patient's physical and mental health improve? Am J Knee Surg 2000 Fall;13(4):223–7.

Bert J, Gross M, Kline C. Patient demand matching in total knee arthroplasty: is it necessary? Am J Knee Surg 2001 Winter;14(1):39–42.

Bierbaum BE, Callaghan JJ, Galante JO, et al. An analysis of blood management in patients having a total hip or knee arthroplasty. J Bone Joint Surg Am 1999; 81(1):2–10. Comment in: J Bone Joint Surg Am. 2000 Jun;82(6):900–1.

Bierbaum BE, Meehan JP. Blood conservation in total joint arthroplasty. Orthopaedics 1998; 21(9):989–90.

Birdsall PD, Hayes JH, Cleary R, Pinder IM, Moran CG, Sher JL. Health outcome after total knee replacement in the very elderly. J Bone Joint Surg Br 1999; 81(4):660–2.

Blanchard J, Meuwly JY, Leyvraz PF, et al. Prevention of deep-vein thrombosis after total knee replacement. Randomised comparison between a low-molecular-weight heparin (nadroparin) and mechanical prophylaxis with a foot-pump system. J Bone Joint Surg Br 1999; 81(4):654–9.

Blanchard J, Meuwly JY, Leyvraz PF, et al. Prevention of deep-vein thrombosis after total knee replacement. Randomised comparison between a low-molecular-weight heparin (nadroparin) and mechanical prophylaxis with a foot-pump system. J Bone Joint Surg Br 1999; 81(4):654–9.

Boehm P, Holy T, Pietsch Breitfeld B, et al. Mortality after total knee arthroplasty in patients with osteoarthritis and rheumatoid arthritis. Arch Orthop Trauma Surg 2000; 120(1–2):75–8.

Bogoch ER, Henke M, Mackenzie T, et al. Lumbar paravertebral nerve block in the management of pain after total hip and knee arthroplasty: a randomized controlled clinical trial. J Arthroplasty 2002; 17(4):398–401.

Bohm P, Holy T, Pietsch-Breitfeld B, et al. Mortality after total knee arthroplasty in patients with osteoarthritis and rheumatoid arthritis. Arch Orthop Trauma Surg 2000; 120(1–2):75–8.

Bohm P, Holy T. Is there a future for hinged prostheses in primary total knee arthroplasty? A 20-year survivorship analysis of the Blauth prosthesis. J Bone Joint Surg Br 1998; 80(2):302–9.

Bombardier C, Melfi CA, Paul J, et al. Comparison of a generic and a disease-specific measure of pain and physical function after knee replacement surgery. Med Care 1995; 33(4 Suppl):AS131–44.91

Borenstein M, Rothstein H. Comprehensive Meta Analysis: A computer program for research synthesis. Englewood, NJ: Biostat, Inc.; 1999.

Bounameaux H, Miron MJ, Blanchard J, et al. Measurement of plasma D-dimer is not useful in the prediction or diagnosis of postoperative deep vein thrombosis in patients undergoing total knee arthroplasty. Blood Coagul Fibrinolysis 1998; 9(8):749–52.

Bourne R, Rorabeck C, Vaz M, et al. Resurfacing versus not resurfacing the patella during total knee replacement. Clin Orthop 1995 Dec;(321): 156–61.

Bourne RB, Sibbald WJ, Doig G, et al. The Southwestern Ontario Joint Replacement Pilot Project: electronic point-of-care data collection. Southwestern Ontario Study Group. Can J Surg 2001; 44(3):199–202. Comment in: Can J Surg. 2001 Jun;44(3):166.

Bourne RB, Whitewood CN. The role of rotating platform total knee replacements: design considerations, kinematics, and clinical results. J Knee Surg 2002; 15(4):247–53. Editorial/commentary/review article.

Braakman M, Verburg AD, Bronsema G, et al. The outcome of three methods of patellar resurfacing in total knee arthroplasty. Int Orthop 1995; 19(1):7–11.

Bradbury N, Borton D, Spoo G, Cross MJ. Participation in sports after total knee replacement. Am J Sports Med 1998; 26(4):530–5.

Brander VA, Malhotra S, Jet J, et al. Outcome of hip and knee arthroplasty in persons aged 80 years and older. Clin Orthop 1997; (345):67–78.

Brandis S, Murtagh S, Solia R. The Allied Health BONE (Best Orthopaedic New Enterprise) team: an interdisciplinary approach to orthopaedic early discharge and admission prevention. Aust Health Rev 1998; 21(3):211–22.

Brassard MF, Insall JN, Scuderi GR, Colizza W. Does modularity affect clinical success? A comparison with a minimum 10-year followup. Clin Orthop 2001; 388:26–32.

Brighton B, Tornetta P. Part I. Methodological issues in the design of orthopaedic studies: Hierarchy of evidence. From case reports to randomized controlled trials. Clinical Orthopaedics & Related Research 2003;413:19–24.

Brooks DH, Fehring TK, Griffin WL, et al. Polyethylene exchange only for prosthetic knee instability. Clin Orthop 2002 Dec;(405):182–8.

Brown T, Diduch D, Moskal J. Component size asymmetry in bilateral total knee arthroplasty. Am J Knee Surg 2001 Spring;14(2):81–4.

Buechel FF Sr, Buechel FF Jr, Pappas MJ, et al. Twenty-year evaluation of meniscal bearing and rotating platform knee replacements. Clin Orthop 2001; 388:41–50.

Buechel Sr FF. Long-term follow-up after mobile-bearing total knee replacement. Clin Orthop 2002; (404):40–50. Excluded outcomes scoring method.

Buehler KO, Venn-Watson E, D'Lima DD, Colwell CW Jr. The press-fit condylar total knee system: 8- to 10-year results with a posterior cruciate-retaining design. J Arthroplasty 2000; 15(6):698–701.

Bugbee WD, Ammeen DJ, Engh GA. Does implant selection affect outcome of revision knee arthroplasty? J Arthroplasty 2001; 16(5):581–5.

Bugbee WD, Ammeen DJ, Parks NL, Engh GA. 4- to 10-year results with the anatomic modular total knee. Clin Orthop 1998; 348:158–65.

Bullens P, van Loon C, de Waal Malefijt M, et al. Patient satisfaction after total knee arthroplasty: a comparison between subjective and objective outcome assessments. J Arthroplasty 2001 Sep;16(6): 740–7.

Byrne JM, Gage WH, Prentice SD. Bilateral lower limb strategies used during a step-up task in individuals who have undergone unilateral total knee arthroplasty. Clin Biomech (Bristol, Avon) 2002; 17(8):580–5.

Byrne JM, Prentice SD, Gage WH. A kinetic analysis of a stepping task following total knee arthroplasty. Arch Physiol Biochem 2000; 108 (1–2):4.

Calder JD, Ashwood N, Hollingdale JP. Survivorship analysis of the 'Performance' total knee replacement—7- year follow-up. Int Orthop 1999; 23(2):100–3.

Callaghan JJ, Squire MW, Goetz DD, Sullivan PM, Johnston RC. Cemented rotating-platform total knee replacement. A nine to twelve-year follow-up study. J Bone Joint Surg Am 2000; 82(5):705–11.

Callahan CM, Drake BG, Heck DA, et al. Patient outcomes following tricompartmental total knee replacement. A meta-analysis postoperative alignment of total knee replacement. Its effect on survival. JAMA 1994;271(17):1349–57.

Callahan CM, Drake BG, Heck DA, et al. Patient outcomes following unicompartmental or bicompartmental arthroplasty. A meta-analysis. J Arthroplasty 1995;10(2):141–50.

Cameron HU, Park YS. Total knee replacement following high tibial osteotomy and unicompartmental knee. Orthopaedics 1996; 19(9):807–8.

Cameron HU. Clinical and radiologic effects of diaphyseal stem extension in noncemented total knee replacement. Can J Surg 1995; 38(1):45–50.

Cameron HU. HA versus grit blast tibial components in total knee replacement. Acta Orthop Belg 1997; 63 Suppl 1:47–9.

Cameron U, Pedersen PU. Postoperative use of anti-embolism stockings-patient's use, practice and information. Vard I Norden Nurs Sci Res Nordic Countries 1999; 19(1):11–7.

Campbell DG, Mintz AD, Stevenson TM. Early patellofemoral revision following total knee arthroplasty. J Arthroplasty 1995; 10(3):287–91.

Campbell ML, Gregory AM, Mauerhan DR. Collection of surgical specimens in total joint arthroplasty. Is routine pathology cost effective? J Arthroplasty 1997; 12(1):60–3.

Capraro L. Transfusion practices in primary total joint replacements in Finland. Vox Sang 1998; 75(1):1–6.

Casha JN, Hadden WA. Suture reaction following skin closure with subcuticular polydioxanone in total knee arthroplasty. J Arthroplasty 1996; 11(7):859–61.

Caveney BJ, Caveney RA. Implications of patient selection and surgical technique for primary total knee arthroplasty. W V Med J 1996; 92(3):128–32.

CDC. Public health and aging: Projected prevalence of self-reported arthritis or chronic joint symptoms among persons aged 65 years-United States, 2005–2030. Morbidity and Mortality Weekly Report 2003;52(21, May 30, 2003):489.

Chen AL, Mujtaba M, Zuckerman JD, et al. Midterm clinical and radiographic results with the genesis I total knee prosthesis. J Arthroplasty 2001; 16(8):1055–62.

Chin KR, Dalury DF, Zurakowski D, et al. Intraoperative measurements of male and female distal femurs during primary total knee arthroplasty. J Knee Surg 2002; 15(4):213–7.

Chitnavis J, Sinsheimer JS, Clipsham K, et al. Genetic influences in end-stage osteoarthritis. Sibling risks of hip and knee replacement for idiopathic osteoarthritis. J Bone Joint Surg Br 1997; 79(4):660–4.

Chiu FY, Chen CM, Lin CF, et al. Cefuroxime- impregnated cement in primary total knee arthroplasty: a prospective, randomized study of three hundred and forty knees. J Bone Joint Surg Am 2002; 84-A(5):759–62. I

Chiu FY, Chen CM, Lin CF, et al. Cefuroxime-impregnated cement in primary total knee arthroplasty: a prospective, randomized study of three hundred and forty knees. J Bone Joint Surg Am 2002; 84-A(5): 759–62.

Chmell MJ, Scott RD. Balancing the posterior cruciate ligament during cruciate-retaining total knee arthroplasty: Description of the POLO test. J Orthop Tech 1996; 4(1):12–5.

Cho MK, Bero LA. Instruments for assessing the quality of drug studies published in the medical literature. JAMA 1994;272(2):101–4.

Cho S, Sakakibara J, Mori Y. Total knee arthroplasty in patients with rheumatoid arthritis: Results and complications. J Orthop Surg 1996; 4(1):23–9.

Chockalingam S, Scott G. The outcome of cemented vs. cementless fixation of a femoral component in total knee replacement (TKR) with the identification of radiological signs for the prediction of failure. Knee 2000; 7(4):233–8.

Christensen CP, Crawford JJ, Olin MD, et al. Revision of the stiff total knee arthroplasty. J Arthroplasty 2002 Jun;17(4):409–15.

Christie MJ, DeBoer DK, McQueen DA, et al. Salvage procedures for failed total knee arthroplasty. J Bone Joint Surg Am 2003; 85-A Suppl 1:S58–62.

Claeys M, Mosher C, Reesman D. The POP program: the patient education advantage ... progressive orthopaedic program. Orthop Nurs 1998; 17(4):37–47.

Clark C, Rorabeck C, MacDonald S, et al. Posterior-stabilised and cruciate-retaining total knee replacement: a randomized study. Clin Orthop 2001 Nov;(392):208–12.

Clarke HD, Scott WN. Mobile bearing total knee arthroplasty. J Knee Surg 2002; 15(4):235–9.

Clarke MT, Green JS, Harper WM , et al. Cement as a risk factor for deep-vein thrombosis. Comparison of cemented TKR, uncemented TKR and cemented THR. J Bone Joint Surg Br 1998; 80(4):611–3.

Clayton J. Arthritis and total knee replacement. Surg Technol 1995; 27(8):7–11.

Cloutier J, Sabouret P, Deghrar A. Total knee arthroplasty with re-tention of both cruciate ligaments. A 9- to 11-year follow-up study. Eur J Orthop Surg Traumatol 2001;11(1):41–6.

Cloutier JM, Sabouret P, Deghrar A. Total knee arthroplasty with re-tention of both cruciate ligaments. A nine to eleven-year follow-up study. J Bone Joint Surg Am 1999; 81(5):697–702.

Cohen R, Forrest C, Benjamin J. Safety and efficacy of bilateral total knee arthroplasty. J Arthroplasty 1997 Aug;12(5):497–502.

Colizza WA, Insall JN, Scuderi GR. The posterior stabilised total knee prosthesis. Assessment of polyethylene damage and osteolysis after a ten-year-minimum follow-up. J Bone Joint Surg Am 1995; 77(11):1713–20. Comment in: J Bone Joint Surg Am. 1996 Sep;78(9):1446–7. PMID: 8816665.

Collier JP, Sperling DK, Currier JH, et al. Impact of gamma sterili-zation on clinical performance of polyethylene in the knee. J Arthroplasty 1996; 11(4):377– 89.

Colwell CW Jr, Spiro TE, Trowbridge AA, et al. Efficacy and safety of enoxaparin versus unfractionated heparin for prevention of deep venous thrombosis after elective knee arthroplasty. Enoxaparin Clinical Trial Group. Clin Orthop 1995; (321):19–27.

Colwell CW Jr, Spiro TE, Trowbridge AA, et al. Efficacy and safety of enoxaparin versus unfractionated heparin for prevention of deep venous thrombosis after elective knee arthroplasty. Enoxaparin Clinical Trial Group. Clin Orthop 1995; (321):19–27.

Comparing compression bandaging and cold therapy in postoperative total knee replacement surgery. Perianesth Ambulatory Surg Nurs Update 2002; 10(4):51. Editorial/commentary/review article.

Concepts and clinical considerations in articular cartilage-Part 1. J Orthop Sports Phys Ther 1998; 28(4):191–261.

Controlling implant costs with ceiling prices. Or Manager 1998; 14(4): 11–5.

Corpe RS, Gallentine JW, Young TR, et al. Complications in total knee arthroplasty with and without surgical drainage. J South Orthop Assoc 2000; 9(3):207–12.

Coyte PC, Hawker G, Croxford R, et al. Rates of revision knee replacement in Ontario, Canada. J Bone Joint Surg Am 1999; 81 (6):773–82.

Coyte PC, Hawker G, Croxford R, et al. Variation in rheumatologists' and family physicians' perceptions of the indications for and outcomes of knee replacement surgery. J Rheumatol 1996 Apr;23(4):730–8.

Crutchfield J, Zimmerman L, Nieveen J, et al. Preoperative and postoperative pain in total knee replacement patients. Orthop Nurs 1996; 15(2):65–72.

Daltroy LH, Morlino CI, Eaton HM , et al. Preoperative education for total hip and knee replacement patients. Arthritis Care Res 1998; 11(6):469–78.

Dalury DF, Ewald FC, Christie MJ, Scott RD. Total knee arthroplasty in a group of patients less than 45 years of age. J Arthroplasty 1995; 10(5):598–602.

Davies AP. Rating systems for total knee replacement. Knee 2002; 9(4):261–6.

Dawson J, Fitzpatrick R, Murray D, et al. Questionnaire on the perceptions of patients about total knee replacement. J Bone Joint Surg Br 1998; 80(1):63–9.

De Leeuw JM, Villar RN. Obesity and quality of life after primary total knee replacement. Knee 1998; 5(2):119–23

Dejour D, Deschamps G, Garotta L, Dejour H. Laxity in posterior cruciate sparing and posterior stabilised total knee prostheses. Clin Orthop 1999; 364:182–93.

Dellon AL, Mont MA, Mullick T, et al. Partial denervation for persistent neuroma pain around the knee. Clin Orthop 1996; (329):216–22.

Deshmukh R, Hayes J, Pinder I. Does body weight influence outcome after total knee arthroplasty? A 1-year analysis. J Arthroplasty 2002 Apr;17(3):315–9.

Diduch D, Insall J, Scott W, et al. Total knee replacement in young, active patients. Long-term follow-up and functional outcome. J Bone Joint Surg Am 1997 Apr;79(4):575–82.

Dieppe P, Basler HD, Chard J, et al. Knee replacement surgery for osteoarthritis: Effectiveness, practice variations, indications and possible determinants of utilization. Rheumatology (Oxford) 1999;38(1):73–83.

Dieppe P, Chard J, Lohmander S, et al. Osteoarthritis. Clin Evid 2002; (7):1071–90.

Dorr LD. Fixation of the millennium: the knee. J Arthroplasty 2002; 17(4 Suppl 1):6–8.

Douketis JD, Eikelboom JW, Quinlan DJ, et al. Short-duration prophylaxis against venous thromboembolism after total hip or knee replacement: a meta-analysis of prospective studies investigating symptomatic outcomes. Arch Intern Med 2002; 162(13):1465–71.

Dowsey M M, Kilgour ML, Santamaria NM, et al. Clinical pathways in hip and knee arthroplasty: a prospective randomised controlled study. Med J Aust 1999; 170(2):59–62.

Drinkwater CJ, Neil MJ. Optimal timing of wound drain removal following total joint arthroplasty. J Arthroplasty 1995; 10(2):185–9.

Duffy G, Berry D, Rand J. Cement versus cementless fixation in total knee arthroplasty. Clin Orthop 1998 Nov;(356):66–72.

Dunbar MJ, Robertsson O, Ryd L, et al. Appropriate questionnaires for knee arthroplasty. Results of a survey of 3600 patients from The Swedish Knee Arthroplasty Registry. J Bone Joint Surg Br 2001; 83(3):339–44.

Dunbar MJ, Robertsson O, Ryd L, et al. Translation and validation of the Oxford-12 item knee score for use in Sweden. Acta Orthop Scand 2000; 71(3):268–74.

Dunbar MJ. Subjective outcomes after knee arthroplasty. Acta Orthop Scand Suppl 2001; 72(301):1–63.

Dunlop DD, Song J, Manheim LM, et al. Racial disparities in joint replacement use among older adults. Med Care 2003 Feb;41(2): 288–98.

Editorial/commentary/review article. Harner C. Musculoskeletal Q & A. Restoring mobility after knee arthroplasty. J Musculoskeletal Med 1999; 16(11):618.

Edwards TB, D'Ambrosia RD. Fracture of a three peg, nonmetal-backed, polyethylene patellar component. Orthopaedics 2002; 25(8):856–7.

Eggers KA, Jenkins BJ, Power I. Effect of oral and IV tenoxicam in postoperative pain after total knee replacement. Br J Anaesth 1999; 83(6):876–81. Anaesthesia/analgesia/pain study.

Elderly knee replacement patients fare better when treated in more experienced hospitals. Res Activities 1999; (224):6.

Elders MJ. The increasing impact of arthritis on public health. J Rheumatol Suppl 2000;60:6–8.

Elke R, Meier G, Warnke K, et al. Outcome analysis of total knee replacements in patients with rheumatoid arthritis versus osteoarthritis. Arch Orthop Trauma Surg 1995;114(6):330–4.

Emerson RH Jr, Ayers C, Head WC, et al. Surgical closing in primary total knee arthroplasties: flexion versus extension. Clin Orthop 1996; (331):74–80.

Emerson RH Jr, Ayers C, Higgins LL. Surgical closing in total knee arthroplasty: A series followup. Clin Orthop 1999; (368):176–81.

Emerson RH Jr, Higgins LL, Head WC. The AGC total knee prosthesis at average 11 years. J Arthroplasty 2000; 15(4):418–23.

Emmerson KP, Moran CG, Pinder IM. Survivorship analysis of the Kinematic Stabilizer total knee replacement: a 10- to 14-year follow-up. J Bone Joint Surg Br 1996; 78(3):441–5.

Engh GA, Ammeen D. Session II: Polyethylene wear. Clin Orthop 2002; (404):71–4.

Engh GA, Ammeen DJ. Periprosthetic fractures adjacent to total knee implants: Treatment and clinical results. J Bone Joint Surg Am 1997; 79(7):1100–13.

Engh GA, Holt BT, Parks NL. A midvastus muscle-splitting approach for total knee arthroplasty. J Arthroplasty 1997; 12(3):322–31.

Engh GA, Parks NL, Ammeen DJ. Influence of surgical approach on lateral retinacular releases in total knee arthroplasty. Clin Orthop 1996; (331):56–63. Comment in: Clin Orthop. 1997 Jul;(340):284.

Escarce JJ, Epstein KR, Colby DC, et al. Racial differences in the elderly's use of medical procedures and diagnostic tests. Am J Public Health. Jul 1993;83(7):948–54.

Espley AJ, Hill J, Hadden WA. A model for arthroplasty audit in a district general hospital. J R Coll Surg Edinburgh 1998; 43(3):209–10.

Etches RC, Warriner CB, Badner N, et al. Continuous intravenous administration of ketorolac reduces pain and morphine consumption after total hip or knee arthroplasty. Anesth Analg 1995; 81(6):1175–80.

Evanich C, Tkach T, von Glinski S, et al. 6- to 10-year experience using countersunk metal-backed patellas. J Arthroplasty 1997 Feb;12(2):149–54.

Ewald F, Wright R, Poss R, et al. Kinematic total knee arthroplasty: a 10- to 14-year prospective follow-up review. J Arthroplasty 1999 Jun;14(4):473–80.

Falatyn S, Lachiewicz PF, Wilson FC. Survivorship analysis of cemented total condylar knee arthroplasty. Clin Orthop 1995; (317):178–84.

Faraj AA, Nevelos AB, Nair A. A 4- to 10-year follow-up study of the Tricon-M noncemented total knee replacement. Orthopaedics 2001; 24(12):1151–4.

Faris PM, Ritter MA, Abels RI. The effects of recombinant human erythropoietin on perioperative transfusion requirements in patients having a major orthopaedic operation. The American Erythropoietin Study Group. J Bone Joint Surg Am 1996; 78(1):62–72.

Fehring TK, Odum S, Griffin WL, et al. Patella inversion method for exposure in revision total knee arthroplasty. J Arthroplasty 2002; 17(1):101–4.

Fehring TK. Rotational malalignment of the femoral component in total knee arthroplasty. Clin Orthop 2000; (380):72–9.

Felix NA, Stuart MJ, Hanssen AD. Periprosthetic fractures of the tibia associated with total knee arthroplasty. Clin Orthop 1997; (345): 113–24.

Fetzer GB, Callaghan JJ, Templeton JE, Goetz DD, Sullivan PM, Kelley SS. Posterior cruciate-retaining modular total knee arthroplasty: A 9- to 12-year follow-up investigation. J Arthroplasty 2002; 17(8): 961–6.

Fisher DA, Trimble S, Clapp B, et al. Effect of a patient management system on outcomes of total hip and knee arthroplasty. Clin Orthop 1997; (345):155–60.

Font-Rodriguez DE, Scuderi GR, Insall JN. Survivorship of cemented total knee arthroplasty. Clin Orthop 1997; (345):79–86.

Forrest G, Fuchs M, Gutierrez A, et al. Factors affecting length of stay and need for rehabilitation after hip and knee arthroplasty. J Arthroplasty 1998; 13(2):186–90.

Forster MC, Kothari P, Howard PW. Minimum 5–year follow-up and radiologic analysis of the all-polyethylene tibial component of the Kinemax Plus system. J Arthroplasty 2002; 17(2):196–200.

Fortin P, Clarke A, Joseph L, et al. Outcomes of total hip and knee replacement: preoperative functional status predicts outcomes at six months after surgery. Arthritis Rheum 1999 Aug;42(8):1722–8.

Fortin PR, Penrod JR, Clarke AE, et al. Timing of total joint replacement affects clinical outcomes among patients with osteoarthritis of the hip or knee. Arthritis Rheum 2002; 46(12):3327–30.

Francis CW, Pellegrini VD Jr, Leibert KM , et al. Comparison of two warfarin regimens in the prevention of venous thrombosis following total knee replacement. Thromb Haemost 1996; 75(5):706–11.

Francis CW, Pellegrini VD Jr, Leibert KM, et al. Comparison of two warfarin regimens in the prevention of venous thrombosis following total knee replacement. Thromb Haemost 1996; 75(5):706–11.

Freeman MA. The role of longitudinal tibial rotation in the replaced knee. Acta Orthop Belg 1998; 64 Suppl 2:64–9.

Fryzek JP, Ye W, Signorello LB, et al. Incidence of cancer among patients with knee implants in Sweden, 1980–1994. Cancer 2002; 94(11):3057–62.

Furnes O, Espehaug B, Lie SA, et al. Early failures among 7,174 primary total knee replacements: a follow-up study from the Norwegian Arthroplasty Register 1994–2000. Acta Orthop Scand 2002; 73(2):117–29.

Garino JP, Lotke PA, Kitziger KJ, et al. Deep venous thrombosis after total joint arthroplasty. The role of compression ultrasonography and the importance of the experience of the technician. J Bone Joint Surg Am 1996; 78(9):1359–65.

Gartland JJ. Orthopaedic clinical research. Deficiencies in experimental design and determinations of outcomes. Journal of Bone & Joint Surgery ?American Volume 1988;70(9):1357–64.

Gill G, Joshi A, Mills D. Total condylar knee arthroplasty. 16– to 21–year results. Clin Orthop 1999 Oct;(367):210–5.

Gill G, Joshi A. Long-term results of cemented, posterior cruciate ligament-retaining total knee arthroplasty in osteoarthritis . Am J Knee Surg 2001 Fall;14(4):209–14.

Gill GS, Joshi AB. Long-term results of Kinematic Condylar knee replacement. An analysis of 404 knees. J Bone Joint Surg Br 2001; 83(3):355–8.

Gioe T, Bowman K. A randomized comparison of all-polyethylene and metal-backed tibial components. Clin Orthop 2000 Nov;(380):108–15.

Glaser D, Lotke P. Cost-effectiveness of immediate postoperative radiographs after uncomplicated total knee arthroplasty: a retrospective and prospective study of 750 patients. J Arthroplasty 2000; 15(4):475–8.

Gofton WT, Tsigaras H, Butler RA, et al. Revision total knee arthroplasty: fixation with modular stems. Clin Orthop 2002 Nov;(404):158–68.

Goldstein WM, Branson JJ, Berland K. Posterior medial capsular release and external rotation of the tibia to enhance exposure during total knee arthroplasty. J Bone Joint Surg Am 2002; 84-A Suppl 2:105–8.

Golubtsov BV, Di Paola M, Baldwin E, et al. Pre-operative orthopaedic assessment clinic for major joint replacement operations: an assessment of value. Health Bull 1998; 56(3):648–52.

Green D, Lawler M, Rosen M, et al. Recombinant human erythropoietin: effect on the functional performance of anemic orthopaedic patients. Arch Phys Med Rehabil 1996; 77(3):242–6.

Greenfield MA, Insall JN, Case GC, et al. Instrumentation of the patellar osteotomy in total knee arthroplasty. The relationship of patellar thickness and lateral retinacular release. Am J Knee Surg 1996; 9(3):129–31.

Grelsamer RP. Patellofemoral arthroplasty. Tech Orthop 1997; 12(3):200–4.

Griffin F, Scuderi G, Insall J, et al. Total knee arthroplasty in patients who were obese with 10 years followup. Clin Orthop 1998 Nov;(356): 28–33.

Gross M. A critique of the methodologies used in clinical studies of hip-joint arthroplasty published in the English-language orthopaedic literature. Journal of Bone & Joint Surgery,American Volume 1988;70(9):1364–71.

Gruber G, Schlechta C, Sturz H. Ten-year follow-up of a bicondylar unlinked knee endoprosthesis with particular reference to mid-term results. Arch Orthop Trauma Surg 1998; 117(6–7):316–23.

Gunter N, Huang Y, Moore L, et al. Prophylactic antibiotic project. J S C Med Assoc 1997; 93(5):174–6.

Haas SB, Insall JN, Montgomery W III, et al. Revision total knee arthroplasty with use of modular components with stems inserted without cement. Journal of Bone & Joint Surgery, American Volume 1995;77(11):1700–7.

Hadorn DC, Holmes AC. The New Zealand priority criteria project. Part 1: Overview. BMJ 1997a;314(7074):131–4.

Hadorn DC, Holmes AC. The New Zealand priority criteria project. Part 2: Coronary artery bypass graft surgery. BMJ 1997b;314(7074):135–8.

Hamulyak K, Lensing AW, van der Meer J, et al. Subcutaneous low-molecular weight heparin or oral anticoagulants for the prevention of deep-vein thrombosis in elective hip and knee replacement? Fraxiparine Oral Anticoagulant Study Group. Thromb Haemost 1995; 74(6):1428–31.

Han CD, Shin DE. Postoperative blood salvage and reinfusion after total joint arthroplasty. J Arthroplasty 1997; 12(5):511–6.

Hanchett M, Enright C. Revising outcome measures for an established pathway. Hosp Case Manag 2000; 8(12):183–6, 178.

Hanssen AD, Osmon DR, Nelson CL. Prevention of deep periprosthetic joint infection . J Bone Joint Surg Am 1996; 78(3):458–71.

Hanssen AD. Bone-grafting for severe patellar bone loss during revision knee arthroplasty. J Bone Joint Surg Am 2001 Feb;83-A(2):171–6.

Harbour R, Miller J. A new system for grading recommendations in evidence based guidelines. BMJ 2001;323(7308):334–6.

Harry LE, Nolan JF, Elender F, et al. Who gets priority? Waiting list assessment using a scoring system. Ann R Coll Surg Engl 2000; 82(6 Suppl):186–8.

Hartford JM, Hunt T, Kaufer H. Low contact stress mobile bearing total knee arthroplasty: results at 5 to 13 years. J Arthroplasty 2001; 16(8):977–83.

Hartley RC, Barton-Hanson NG, Finley R, Parkinson RW. Early patient outcomes after primary and revision total knee arthroplasty. A prospective study. J Bone Joint Surg Br 2002; 84(7):994–9.

Harwin S. Patellofemoral complications in symmetrical total knee arthroplasty. J Arthroplasty 1998 Oct ;13(7):753–62.

Hasegawa M, Ohashi T, Uchida A. Heterotopic ossification around distal femur after total knee arthroplasty. Arch Orthop Trauma Surg 2002;122(5):274–8.

Hatzidakis AM, Mendlick RM, McKillip T, et al. Preoperative autologous donation for total joint arthroplasty. An analysis of risk factors for allogenic transfusion. J Bone Joint Surg Am 2000; 82(1):89–100.

Havelin L, Engesaeter LB, Espehaug B, et al. The Norwegian Arthroplasty Register: 11 years and 73,000 arthroplasties. Acta Orthop Scand 2000; 71(4):337–53.

Hawker G, Melfi C, Paul J, et al. Comparison of a generic (SF-36) and a disease specific (WOMAC) (Western Ontario and McMaster Universities Osteoarthritis Index) instrument in the measurement of outcomes after knee replacement surgery. J Rheumatol 1995; 22(6):1193–6.

Hawker G, Schemitsch E, Lineker S. Long-term care after knee replacement: the primary care physician's role. J Musculoskeletal Med 1997; 14(4):53–6, 59–60.

Hawker G, Wright J, Coyte P, et al. Health-related quality of life after knee replacement. J Bone Joint Surg Am 1998 Feb;80(2):163–73.

Hawker G. Total Knee Replacement PORT publishes recent findings. Res Activities 1996; (194):8–9.

Hawker GA, Coyte PC, Wright JG, et al. Accuracy of administrative data for assessing outcomes after knee replacement surgery. J Clin Epidemiol 1997; 50(3):265–73.

Hawker GA, Wright JG, Coyte PC, et al. Differences between men and women in the rate of use of hip and knee arthroplasty [comment]. New England Journal of Medicine 2000 Apr 6; 342(14):1016–22.

Healy W, Iorio R, Ko J, et al. Impact of cost reduction programs on short-term patient outcome and hospital cost of total knee arthroplasty. J Bone Joint Surg Am 2002 Mar;84-A(3):348–53.

Healy WL, Iorio R, Richards JA. Opportunities for control of hospital cost for total knee arthroplasty. Clin Orthop 1997; (345):140–7.

Healy WL, Wasilewski SA, Takei R, et al. Patellofemoral complications following total knee arthroplasty. Correlation with implant design and patient risk factors. J Arthroplasty 1995; 10(2):197–201.

Heck D, Robinson R, Partridge C, et al. Patient outcomes after knee replacement. Clin Orthop 1998 Nov;(356):93–110.

Heck DA, Melfi CA, Mamlin LA, et al. Revision rates after knee replacement in the United States. Med Care 1998; 36(5):661–9.

Heit JA, Berkowitz SD, Bona R, et al. Efficacy and safety of low molecular weight heparin (ardeparin sodium) compared to warfarin for the prevention of venous thromboembolism after total knee replacement surgery: a double-blind, dose-ranging study. Ardeparin Arthroplasty Study Group. Thromb Haemost 1997; 77(1):32–8.

Heit JA, Elliott CG, Trowbridge AA, et al. Ardeparin sodium for extended out-of-hospital prophylaxis against venous thromboembolism after total hip or knee replacement. A randomized, double-blind, placebo-controlled trial. Ann Intern Med 2000; 132(11):853–61.

Heit JA, Elliott CG, Trowbridge AA, et al. Ardeparin sodium for extended out-of-hospital prophylaxis against venous thromboembolism after total hip or knee replacement. A randomized, double-blind, placebo-controlled trial. Ann Intern Med 2000; 132(11):853–61. Comment in: Ann In-tern Med. 2000 Jun 6;132(11):914–5.

Hernandez-Vaquero D, Alvarez-Gonzalez UJ, Fernandez- Corona C, et al. Patellar complications after total knee arthroplasty. Int Orthop 1996; 20 (2):103–6.

Herrick IA, Ganapathy S, Komar W, et al. Postoperative cognitive impairment in the elderly. Choice of patient-controlled analgesia opioid. Anaesthesia 1996; 51(4):356–60.

Hewitt B, Shakespeare D. Flexion vs. extension: a comparison of postoperative total knee arthroplasty mobilization regimes. Knee 2001; 8(4):305–9.

Hofmann AA, Evanich JD, Ferguson RP, Camargo MP. Ten- to 14-year clinical follow-up of the cementless Natural Knee system. Clin Orthop 2001; 388:85–94.

Hofmann AA, Tkach TK, Evanich CJ, et al. Posterior stabilization in total knee arthroplasty with use of an ultracongruent polyethylene insert. J Arthroplasty 2000; 15(5):576–83.

Holt BT, Parks NL, Engh GA, et al. Comparison of closed-suction drainage and no drainage after primary total knee arthroplasty. Orthopaedics 1997; 20(12):1121–4.

Hsu R, Tsai Y, Huang T, et al. Hybrid total knee arthroplasty: a 3- to 6-year outcome analysis. J Formos Med Assoc 1998 Jun;97(6):410–5.

Hsu RW, Fan GF, Ho WP. A follow-up study of porous-coated anatomic knee arthroplasty. J Arthroplasty 1995; 10(1):29–36.

Huang CH, Cheng CK, Lee YT, et al. Muscle strength after successful total knee replacement: a 6- to 13-year follow-up. Clin Orthop 1996; (328):147–54.

Hubbard RC, Naumann TM, Traylor L, et al. Parecoxib sodium has opioid-sparing effects in patients undergoing total knee arthroplasty under spinal anaesthesia. Br J Anaesth 2003; 90(2):166–72.

Hube R, Sotereanos N, Reichel H. The midvastus approach for total knee arthroplasty. Orthop Traumatol 2002;10(3):235–44.

Hui AC, Heras-Palou C, Dunn I, et al. Graded compression stockings for prevention of deep-vein thrombosis after hip and knee replacement. J Bone Joint Surg Br 1996; 78(4):550–4.

Hull RD, Raskob GE, Pineo GF, et al. Subcutaneous low-molecular-weight heparin vs warfarin for prophylaxis of deep vein thrombosis after hip or knee implantation. An economic perspective. Arch Intern Med 1997; 157(3):298–303.

Ikejiani C, Leighton R, Petrie D. Comparison of patellar resurfacing versus nonresurfacing in total knee arthroplasty. Can J Surg 2000 Feb;43(1):35–8.

Indelli P, Aglietti P, Buzzi R, et al. The Insall-Burstein II prosthesis: A 5- to 9-year follow-up study in osteoarthritic knees. J Arthroplasty 2002;17(5):544– 9.

Insall JN, Dethmers DA. Revision of total knee arthroplasty. Clinical Orthopaedics & Related Research 1982;170:123–30.

Insall JN, Dorr LD, Scott RD, et al. Rationale of the Knee Society clinical rating system. Orthopaedics & Related Research 1989;248:13–4.

Iorio R, Healy WL, Kirven FM, et al. Knee implant standardization: an implant selection and cost reduction program. Am J Knee Surg 1998; 11(2):73–9.

Iorio R, Healy WL, Patch DA, et al. The role of bladder catheterization in total knee arthroplasty. Clin Orthop 2000; (380):80–4.

Iorio R, Healy WL, Richards JA. Comparison of the hospital cost of primary and revision total knee arthroplasty after cost containment. Orthopaedics 1999; 22(2):195–9.

Ip D, Wu WC, Tsang WL. Comparison of two total knee prostheses on the incidence of patella clunk syndrome. Int Orthop 2002; 26(1): 48–51.

Ireson CL. Critical pathways: effectiveness in achieving patient outcomes. J Nurs Adm 1997; 27(6):16–23.

Ishii Y, Ohmori G, Bechtold JE, et al. Extramedullary versus intramedullary alignment guides in total knee arthroplasty. Clin Orthop 1995; (318):167–75.

Itokazu M, Masuda K, Wada E, et al. Influence of anteroposterior and mediolateral instability on range of motion after total knee arthroplasty: an ultrasonographic study. Orthopaedics 2000; 23(1):49–52.

Jacobs JJ, Silverton C, Hallab NJ, et al. Metal release and excretion from cementless titanium alloy total knee replacements. Clin Orthop 1999; (358):173–80.

Jamison RN, Ross MJ, Hoopman P, et al. Assessment of postoperative pain management: patient satisfaction and perceived helpfulness. Clin J Pain 1997; 13(3):229–36. Less than 100 knees in the study.

Janecek M, Bucek P. PFC modular total knee replacement system: Middle term results. Ortop Traumatol Rehab 2002; 4(3):360–5.

Jarolem KL, Scott DF, Jaffe WL, et al. A comparison of blood loss and transfusion requirements in total knee arthroplasty with and without arterial tourniquet. Am J Orthop 1995; 24(12):906–9.

Jenny J, Jenny G. Preservation of anterior cruciate ligament in total knee arthroplasty. Arch Orthop Trauma Surg1998;118(3):145–8.

Jensen CH, Rofail S. Knee injury and obesity in patients undergoing total knee replacement: a retrospective study in 115 patients. J Orthop Sci 1999; 4(1):5–7.

Jessup DE, Worland RL, Clelland C, et al. Restoration of limb alignment in total knee arthroplasty: evaluation and methods. J South Orthop Assoc 1997; 6(1):37–47.

Jester R, Russell L, Fell S, Williams S, Prest C . A one hospital study of the effect of wound dressings and other related factors on skin blistering following total hip and knee arthroplasty. J Orthop Nurs 2000; 4(2):71–7.

Jones CA, Voaklander DC, Johnston DW, et al. The effect of age on pain, function, and quality of life after total hip and knee arthroplasty. Arch Intern Med 2001 Feb;161(3):454–60.

Jones CA, Voaklander DC, Johnston DW, Suarez-Almazor ME. Health related quality of life outcomes after total hip and knee arthroplasties in a community based population. J Rheumatol 2000; 27(7):1745–52.

Jones RE, Skedros JG, Chan AJ, et al. Total knee arthroplasty using the S-ROM mobile-bearing hinge prosthesis. J Arthroplasty 2001 Apr;16(3):279–87.

Jones RE. Management of complex revision problems with modular total knee system. Orthopaedics 1996; 19(9):802–4. Revision study.

Jordan L, Olivo J, Voorhorst P. Survivorship analysis of cementless meniscal bearing total knee arthroplasty. Clin Orthop 1997 May;(338):119–23.

Jordan LR, Dowd JE, Olivo JL, et al. The clinical history of mobile-bearing patella components in total knee arthroplasty. Orthopaedics 2002; 25(2 Suppl):s247–50.

Jordan LR, Siegel JL, Olivo JL. Early flexion routine. An alternative method of continuous passive motion. Clin Orthop 1995; (315):231–3.

Joshi AB, Gill G. Total knee arthroplasty in nonagenarians. J Arthroplasty 2002; 17(6):681–4.

Kageyama Y, Miyamoto S, Ozeki T, et al. Outcomes for patients undergoing one or more total hip and knee arthroplasties. Clin Rheumatol 1998; 17(2):130–4.

Kane RL, ed. Understanding Health Care Outcomes Research. Gaithersburg, MD: Aspen Publishers, Inc; 1997.

Kanekasu K, Yamakado K, Hayashi H. The clamp fixation method in cemented total knee arthroplasty. Dynamic experimental and radiographic studies of the tibial baseplate clamper. Bull Hosp Jt Dis 1997; 56(4):218–21. Clamp fixation study.

Kaper BP, Smith PN, Bourne RB, Rorabeck CH, Robertson D. Medium-term results of a mobile bearing total knee replacement. Clin Orthop 1999; 367:201–9.

Kaper BP, Woolfrey M, Bourne RB. The effect of built-in external femoral rotation on patellofemoral tracking in the genesis II total knee arthroplasty. J Arthroplasty 2000; 15(8):964–9.

Karst GM, Boonyawiroj EB, Hald RD, et al. Physical therapy intervention and functional ambulation outcomes for patients undergoing total knee arthroplasty. Issues Aging 1995; 18(1):5–9.

Katz B, Freund D, Heck D, et al. Demographic variation in the rate of knee replacement: a multi-year analysis. Health Serv Res 1996 Jun;31(2):125–40.

Katz BP, Freund DA, Heck DA, et al. Demographic variation in the rate of knee replacement: a multi-year analysis. Health Serv Res 1996; 31(2):125–40.

Kawakubo M, Matsumoto H, Otani T, et al. Radiographic changes in the patella after total knee arthroplasty without resurfacing the patella. Comparison of osteoarthritis and rheumatoid arthritis. Bull Hosp Jt Dis 1997; 56(4):237–44.

Keating EM, Faris PM, Meding JB, et al. Comparison of the midvastus muscle-splitting approach with the median parapatellar approach in total knee arthroplasty. J Arthroplasty 1999; 14(1):29–32.

Keating EM, Meding JB, Faris PM , et al. Predictors of transfusion risk in elective knee surgery. Clin Orthop 1998; (357):50–9.

Keating EM, Meding JB, Faris PM, et al. Long-term follow-up of nonmodular total knee replacements. Clin Orthop 2002; (404):34–9.

Kelly KD, Voaklander D, Kramer G, et al. The impact of health status on waiting time for major joint arthroplasty. Arthroplasty 2000; 15(7):877–83.

Kelly MA, Clarke HD. Long-term results of posterior cruciate-substituting total knee arthroplasty. Clin Orthop 2002; (404):51–7.

Kelly MH, Ackerman RM. Total joint arthroplasty: a comparison of postacute settings on patient functional outcomes. Orthop Nurs 1999; 18(5):75–84.

Kelly MH, Tilbury MS, Ackerman RM. Evaluation of fiscal and treatment outcomes in major joint replacement. Outcomes Manage Nurs Pract 2000; 4(1):46–50.

Kendall SJ, Singer GC, Briggs TW, et al. A functional analysis of massive knee replacement after extra-articular resections of primary bone tumors. J Arthroplasty 2000; 15(6):754–60.

Khan A, Emberson J, Dowd GS. Standardized mortality ratios and fatal pulmonary embolism rates following total knee replacement: a cohort of 936 consecutive cases. J Knee Surg 2002; 15(4):219–22.

Khaw FM, Kirk LM, Gregg PJ. Survival analysis of cemented Press-Fit Condylar total knee arthroplasty. J Arthroplasty 2001; 16(2):161–7.

Khaw FM, Kirk LM, Morris RW, et al. A randomised, controlled trial of cemented versus cementless press-fit condylar total knee replacement. Ten-year survival analysis. J Bone Joint Surg Br 2002; 84(5):658–66.

Kiebzak G, Campbell M, Mauerhan D. The SF-36 general health status survey documents the burden of osteoarthritis and the benefits of total joint arthroplasty: But why should we use it? Am J Managed Care 2002;8(5):463–74.

Kiebzak GM, Vain PA, Gregory AM , et al. SF-36 general health status survey to determine patient satisfaction at short-term follow-up after total hip and knee arthroplasty. J South Orthop Assoc 1997; 6(3): 169–72.

Kikuchi H, Tan A, Nonaka T, et al. Comparison of intravenous and subcutaneous erythropoietin therapy for preoperative acquisition of blood for autologous transfusion in patients undergoing total arthroplasty. J Ortop Sci 1997; 2(2):84–7.

Kim YH, Cho SH, Kim RS. Drainage versus nondrainage in simultaneous bilateral total knee arthroplasties. Clin Orthop 1998; (347): 188–93.

Kim YH, Kook HK, Kim JS. Comparison of fixed-bearing and mobile-bearing total knee arthroplasties. Clin Orthop 2001; 392:101–15.

Kirk Sanchez NJ, Roach KE. Relationship between duration of therapy services in a comprehensive rehabilitation program and mobility at discharge in patients with orthopaedic problems. Phys Ther 2001; 81(3):888–95.

Knight JL, Gorai PA, Atwater RD, et al. Tibial polyethylene failure after primary porous-coated anatomic total knee arthroplasty. Aids to diagnosis and revision. J Arthroplasty 1995; 10(6):748–57.

Knight JL, Sherer D, Guo J. Blood transfusion strategies for total knee arthroplasty: minimizing autologous blood wastage, risk of homologous blood transfusion, and transfusion cost. J Arthroplasty 1998; 13(1):70–6.

Knight RM, Pellegrini VD Jr. Bladder management after total joint arthroplasty. J Arthroplasty 1996; 11(8):882–8.

Ko PS, Tio MK, Tang YK, et al. Sealing the intramedullary femoral canal with autologous bone plug in total knee arthroplasty. J Arthroplasty 2003; 18(1):6–9.

Kocher MS, Erens G, Thornhill TS, et al. Cost and effectiveness of routine pathological examination of operative specimens obtained during primary total hip and knee replacement in patients with osteoarthritis. J Bone Joint Surg Am 2000; 82-A(11):1531–5.

Konig A, Kirschner S, Walther M, et al. Hybrid total knee arthroplasty. Arch Orthop Trauma Surg 1998;118(1–2):66–9.

Konig A, Scheidler M, Rader C, et al. The need for a dual rating system in total knee arthroplasty. Clin Orthop 1997 Dec;(345):161–7.

Konig A, Walther M, Kirschner S, et al. Balance sheets of knee and functional scores 5 years after total knee arthroplasty for osteoarthritis: a source for patient information. J Arthroplasty 2000 Apr;15(3): 289–94.

Kovacik MW, Singri P, Khanna S, et al. Medical and financial aspects of same-day bilateral total knee arthroplasties. Biomed Sci Instrum 1997; 33:429–34.

Kraay MJ, Darr OJ, Salata MJ, et al. Outcome of metal-backed cementless patellar components: the effect of implant design. Clin Orthop 2001; (392):239–44.

Kreder HJ, Williams JI, Jaglal S, et al. A population study in the Province of Ontario of the complications after conversion of hip or knee arthrodesis to total joint replacement. Can J Surg 1999; 42(6): 433–9.

Kreibich DN, Vaz M, Bourne RB, et al. What is the best way of assessing outcome after total knee replacement? Clin Orthop 1996; (331):221–5.

Kulkarni SK, Freeman MA, Poal-Manresa JC, et al. The patello-femoral joint in total knee arthroplasty: Is the design of the trochlea the critical factor? Knee Surg Sports Traumatol Arthrosc 2001; 9 Suppl 1:S8–12.

Kulkarni SK, Freeman MA, Poal-Manresa JC, et al. The patellofemoral joint in total knee arthroplasty: is the design of the trochlea the critical factor? J Arthroplasty 2000; 15(4):424–9.

Kumar N, Saleh J, Gardiner E, et al. Plugging the intramedullary canal of the femur in total knee arthroplasty: reduction in postoperative blood loss. J Arthroplasty 2000; 15(7):947–9.

Kurdy NM. Transfusion needs in hip and knee arthroplasty. Ann Chir Gynaecol 1996; 85(1):86–9.

Lachiewicz PF. The role of continuous passive motion after total knee arthroplasty. Clin Orthop 2000; (380):144–50. Continuous passive motion study.

Lane GJ, Hozack WJ, Shah S, et al. Simultaneous bilateral versus unilateral total knee arthroplasty. Outcomes analysis. Clin Orthop 1997; (345):106–12.

Lang CE. Comparison of 6– and 7–day physical therapy coverage on length of stay and discharge outcome for individuals with total hip and knee arthroplasty. J Orthop Sports Phys Ther 1998; 28(1):15–22.

Larcom PG, Lotke PA, Steinberg ME, et al. Magnetic resonance venography versus contrast venography to diagnose thrombosis after joint surgery. Clin Orthop 1996; (331):209–15.

Larson C, Lachiewicz P. Patellofemoral complications with the Insall-Burstein II posterior-stabilised total knee arthroplasty. J Arthroplasty 1999 Apr;14(3):288–92.

Larson C, McDowell C, Lachiewicz P. One-peg versus three-peg patella component fixation in total knee arthroplasty. Clin Orthop 2001 Nov;(392):94–100.

Larson CM, McDowell CM, Lachiewicz PF. One-peg versus three-peg patella component fixation in total knee arthroplasty. Clin Orthop 2001; (392):94–100.

Laskin RS, Maruyama Y, Villaneuva M, Bourne R. Deep-dish congruent tibial component use in total knee arthroplasty: a randomized prospective study. Clin Orthop 2000; 380:36–44.

Laskin RS, O'Flynn HM. The Insall Award. Total knee replacement with posterior cruciate ligament retention in rheumatoid arthritis. Problems and complications. Clin Orthop 1997; (345):24–8.

Laskin RS, van Steijn M. Total knee replacement for patients with patellofemoral arthritis. Clin Orthop 1999; (367):89–95.

Laskin RS. Cemented total knee replacement in patients with osteoarthritis: A five-year follow-up study using a prosthesis allowing both retention and resection of the posterior cruciate ligament. Knee 1997; 4(1):1–6.

Laskin RS. The genesis total knee prosthesis: a 10-year follow-up study. Clin Orthop 2001; 388:95–102.

Laskin RS. The Insall Award. Total knee replacement with posterior cruciate ligament retention in patients with a fixed varus deformity. Clin Orthop 1996; (331):29–34.

Lavernia CJ, Guzman JF, Gachupin-Garcia A. Cost effectiveness and quality of life in knee arthroplasty. Clin Orthop 1997; (345):134–9.

Lavernia CJ, Guzman JF. Relationship of surgical volume to short-term mortality, morbidity, and hospital charges in arthroplasty. J Arthroplasty 1995; 10(2):133–40.

Lavernia CJ, Sierra RJ, Baerga L. Nutritional parameters and short term outcome in arthroplasty. J Am Coll Nutr 1999; 18(3):274–8.

Leclerc JR, Geerts WH, Desjardins L, et al. Prevention of venous thromboembolism after knee arthroplasty. A randomized, double-blind trial comparing enoxaparin with warfarin. Ann Intern Med 1996; 124(7):619–26.

Leclerc JR, Geerts WH, Desjardins L, et al. Prevention of venous thromboembolism after knee arthroplasty. A randomized, double-blind trial comparing enoxaparin with warfarin. Ann Intern Med 1996; 124(7):619–26.

Leclerc JR, Gent M, Hirsh J, et al. The incidence of symptomatic venous thromboembolism during and after prophylaxis with enoxaparin: a multi-institutional cohort study of patients who underwent hip or knee arthroplasty. Canadian Collaborative Group. Arch Intern Med 1998; 158(8):873–8.

Leclerc JR, Gent M, Hirsh J, et al. The incidence of symptomatic venous thromboembolism after enoxaparin prophylaxis in lower extremity arthroplasty: a cohort study of 1,984 patients. Canadian Collaborative Group. Chest 1998; 114(2 Suppl Evidence):115S-8S.

Leclerc JR, Gent M, Hirsh J, et al. The incidence of symptomatic venous thromboembolism during and after prophylaxis with enoxaparin: a multi-institutional cohort study of patients who underwent hip or knee arthroplasty. Canadian Collaborative Group. Arch Intern Med 1998; 158(8):873–8.

Lee AS, Kelly AJ, Ansari S, et al. Flexion vs. extension suturing of Total Knee Replacement wounds: A randomised prospective study. Knee 1997; 4(2):65–7

Lee DC, Kim DH, Scott RD, et al. Intraoperative flexion against gravity as an indication of ultimate range of motion in individual cases after total knee arthroplasty. J Arthroplasty 1998; 13(5):500–3.

Leininger S. Quality circle of joint care. Orthop Nurs 1998; 17(5): 74–83.

Lensing AW, Doris CI, McGrath FP, et al. A comparison of compression ultrasound with color Doppler ultrasound for the diagnosis of symptomless postoperative deep vein thrombosis. Arch Intern Med 1997; 157(7):765–8.

Leonard M, Moore L, Algozzine R, et al. Recovery times from subarachnoid blocks using bupivacaine hydrochloride and tetracaine hydrochloride with and without epinephrine. AANA J 1997; 65(3): 260–4.

Leopold SS, McStay C, Klafeta K, et al. Primary repair of intraoperative disruption of the medial collateral ligament during total knee arthroplasty. J Bone Joint Surg Am 2001; 83A(1):86–91.

Leopold SS, Silverton CD, Barden RM, et al. Isolated revision of the patellar component in total knee arthroplasty. J Bone Joint Surg Am 2003 Jan;85-A(1):41–7.

Levi N. Incidence of total knee replacement in Copenhagen. Gazz Med Ital 1999; 158(2):41–3.

Levy O, Martinowitz U, Oran A, et al. The use of fibrin tissue adhesive to reduce blood loss and the need for blood transfusion after total knee arthroplasty. A prospective, randomized, multicentre study. J Bone Jt Surg Am 1999; 81(11):1580–8.

Lewis PL, Rorabeck CH, Bourne RB. Screw osteolysis after cementless total Knee Replacement. Clin Orthop 1995; (321):173–7.

Lewold S, Goodman S, Knutson K, et al. Oxford meniscal bearing knee versus the Marmor knee in unicompartmental arthroplasty for arthrosis. A Swedish multicentre survival study. J Arthroplasty 1995; 10(6):722–31.

Lewold S, Olsson H, Gustafson P, et al. Overall cancer incidence not increased after prosthetic knee replacement: 14,551 patients followed for 66,622 person-years. Int J Cancer 1996; 68(1):30–3.

Lewold S, Robertsson O, Knutson K, et al. Revision of unicompartmental knee arthroplasty: outcome in 1,135 cases from the Swedish Knee Arthroplasty study. Acta Orthop Sc 1998; 69(5):469–74.

Li E, Ritter MA, Moilanen T, et al. Total knee arthroplasty. J Arthroplasty 1995; 10(4):560–8; discussion 568–70.

Li PL, Zamora J, Bentley G. The results at ten years of the Insall-Burstein II total knee replacement. Clinical, radiological and survivorship studies. J Bone Jt Surg Br 1999; 81(4):647–53.

Liebergall M, Soskolne V, Mattan Y, et al. Preadmission screening of patients scheduled for hip and knee replacement: impact on length of stay. Clin Perform Qual Health Care 1999; 7(1):17–22.

Lin PC, Lin LC, Lin JJ. Comparing the effectiveness of different educational programs for patients with total knee arthroplasty. Orthop Nurs 1997; 16(5):43–9.

Lin Y, Su J, Lin G, et al. Impact of a clinical pathway for total knee arthroplasty. Kaohsiung J Med Sci 2002 Mar;18(3):134–40.

Lindahl TL, Lundahl TH, Nilsson L, et al. APC-resistance is a risk factor for postoperative thromboembolism in elective replacement of the hip or knee-a prospective study. Thromb Haemost 1999; 81(1):18–21.

Lindstrand A, Robertsson O, Lewold S, et al. The patella in total knee arthroplasty: resurfacing or nonresurfacing of patella. Knee Surg Sports Traumatol Arthrosc 2001; 9 Suppl 1:S21–3.

Lingard E, Hashimoto H, Sledge C. Development of outcome research for total joint arthroplasty. J Orthop Sci 2000; 5(2):175–7.

Lingard EA, Berven S, Katz JN, et al. Management and care of patients undergoing total knee arthroplasty: variations across different health care settings. Arthritis Care Res 2000; 13(3):129–36.

Lingard EA, Katz JN, Wright RJ, Wright EA, Sledge CB, Kinemax Outcomes Group. Validity and responsiveness of the Knee Society Clinical Rating System in comparison with the SF-36 and WOMAC. J Bone Jt Surg Am 2001; 83- A(12):1856–64.

Lingard EA, Wright EA, Sledge CB, The Kinemax Outcomes Group. Pitfalls of using patient recall to derive preoperative status in outcome studies of total knee arthroplasty. J Bone Jt Surg Am 2001; 83-A(8): 1149–56.

Liu T, Chen S. Simultaneous bilateral total knee arthroplasty in a single procedure. Int Orthop 1998;22(6):390–3.

Lofthouse RA, Boitano MA, Davis JR, et al. Preoperative administration of epoetin alfa to reduce transfusion requirements in elderly patients having primary total hip or knee reconstruction. J South Orthop Assoc 2000; 9(3):175–81.

Lombardi AV, Mallory TH, Fada RA, et al. Simultaneous bilateral total knee arthroplasties: who decides? Clin Orthop 2001; (392):319–29.

Lombardi Jr A, Mallory T, Fada R, et al. An algorithm for the posterior cruciate ligament in total knee arthroplasty. Clin Orthop 2001 Nov; (392):75–87.

Lonner JH, Beck TD Jr, Rees H, et al. Results of two-stage revision of the infected total knee arthroplasty. Am J Knee Surg 2001; 14(1):65–7.

Lonner JH, Desai P, Dicesare PE, et al. The reliability of analysis of intraoperative frozen sections for identifying active infection during revision hip or knee arthroplasty. J Bone Jt Surg Am 1996; 78(10): 1553–8.

Lonner JH, Lotke PA, Kim J, et al. Impaction grafting and wire mesh for uncontained defects in revision knee arthroplasty. Clin Orthop 2002 Nov;(404):145– 51.

Lonner JH, Siliski JM, Scott RD. Alternative surveillance after total knee arthroplasty: a viable option? Orthopaedics 1998; 21(9):1034–5.

Lonner JH, Siliski JM, Scott RD. Prodromes of failure in total knee arthroplasty. J Arthroplasty 1999; 14(4):488–92.

Lonner JH. Identifying ongoing infection after resection arthroplasty and before second-stage reimplantation. Am J Knee Surg 2001; 14(1):68–71.

Lonner JH. Thromboembolic disease in total knee arthroplasty. Am J Knee Surg 1999; 12(1):43–8.

Lotke PA, Palevsky H, Keenan AM , et al. Aspirin and warfarin for thromboembolic disease after total joint arthroplasty. Clin Orthop 1996; (324):251–8.

Lozano Gomez MR, Ruiz Fernandez J, Lopez Alonso A, et al. Long-term results of the treatment of severe osteoarthritis and rheumatoid arthritis with 193 total knee replacements. Knee Surg Sports Traumatol Arthrosc 1997; 5(2):102–12.

Mabrey JD, Toohey JS, Armstrong DA, et al. Clinical pathway management of total knee arthroplasty. Clin Orthop 1997; (345):125–33.

Macario A, Horne M, Goodman S, et al. The effect of a perioperative clinical pathway for knee replacement surgery on hospital costs. Anesth Analg 1998; 86(5):978–84.

Macario A, Vitez TS, Dunn B, et al. Hospital costs and severity of illness in three types of elective surgery. Anesthesiology 1997; 86(1): 92–100.

MacDermid JC, O'Callaghan C. Inpatient rehabilitation after total knee arthroplasty: risk factors for admission and effects of treatment. Physiother Can 2000; 52(1):45–9.

MacDonald SJ, Bourne RB, Rorabeck CH, McCalden RW, Kramer J, Vaz M. Prospective randomized clinical trial of continuous passive motion after total knee arthroplasty. Clin Orthop 2000; 380:30–5.

Maestro A, Harwin SF, Sandoval MG, et al. Influence of intramedullary versus extramedullary alignment guides on final total knee arthroplasty component position: a radiographic analysis. J Arthroplasty 1998; 13(5):552–8.

Mahomed NN, Koo Seen Lin MJ, Levesque J, et al. Determinants and outcomes of inpatient versus home based rehabilitation following elective hip and knee replacement. J Rheumatol 2000; 27(7): 1753–8.

Mahomed NN, Liang MH, Cook EF, et al. The importance of patient expectations in predicting functional outcomes after total joint arthroplasty. J Rheumatol 2002; 29(6):1273–9.

Mahoney OM, McClung CD, dela Rosa MA, et al. The effect of total knee arthroplasty design on extensor mechanism function. J Arthroplasty 2002; 17(4):416–21.

Malkani A, Rand J, Bryan R, et al. Total knee arthroplasty with the kinematic condylar prosthesis. A ten-year follow-up study. J Bone Jt Surg Am 1995 Mar;77(3):423–31.

Malmlin LA, Melfi CA, Parchman ML, et al. Management of osteoarthritis of the knee by primary care physicians. Arch Fam Med 1998;7:563–7.

Mancuso CA, Ranawat CS, Esdaile JM , et al. Indications for total hip and total knee arthroplasties. Results of orthopaedic surveys. J Arthroplasty 1996; 11(1):34–46.

Mancuso CA, Ranawat CS, Esdaile JM, et al. Indications for total hip and total knee arthroplasties. Results of orthopaedic surveys. J Arthroplasty 1996 Jan;11(1):34–46.

March LM, Cross MJ, Lapsley H, et al. Outcomes after hip or knee replacement surgery for osteoarthritis. A prospective cohort study comparing patients' quality of life before and after surgery with age-related population norms. Med J Aust 1999; 171(5):235–8.

Marks RM, Vaccaro AR, Balderston RA, et al. Postoperative blood salvage in total knee arthroplasty using the Solcotrans autotransfusion system. J Arthroplasty 1995; 10(4):433–7.

Martin S, McManus J, Scott R, et al. Press-fit condylar total knee arthroplasty. 5- to 9-year follow-up evaluation. J Arthroplasty 1997 Sep;12(6):603–14.

Mathias JM. A vertical pathway for total joint replacement. OR Manager 1999; 15(4):27, 29–30, 3.

Matsueda M, Gustilo R. Subvastus and medial parapatellar approaches in total knee arthroplasty. Clin Orthop 2000 Feb;(371):161–8.

Mauerhan DR, Campbell M, Miller JS, et al. Intra-articular morphine and/or bupivacaine in the management of pain after total knee arthroplasty. J Arthroplasty 1997; 12(5):546–52.

Mauerhan DR, Mokris JG, Ly A, et al. Relationship between length of stay and manipulation rate after total knee arthroplasty. J Arthroplasty 1998; 13(8):896–900.

Mauerhan DR, Nelson CL, Smith DL, et al. Prophylaxis against infection in total joint arthroplasty. One day of cefuroxime compared with three days of cefazolin. J Bone Joint Surg Am 1994 Jan;76(1): 39–45.

McBean AM, Gornick M. Differences by race in the rates of procedures performed in hospitals for Medicare beneficiaries. Health Care Financ Rev 1994 Summer;15(4):77–90.

McBeath DM, Shah J, Sebastian L, et al. The effect of patient controlled analgesia and continuous epidural infusion on length of hospital stay after total knee or total hip replacement. CRNA 1995; 6(1):31–6.

McCaskie AW, Deehan DJ, Green TP, et al. Randomised, prospective study comparing cemented and cementless total knee replacement: results of press-fit condylar total knee replacement at five years. J Bone Jt Surg Br 1998; 80(6):971–5.

Mcgrath D, Dennyson WG, Rolland M. Death rate from pulmonary embolism following joint replacement surgery. J R Coll Surg Edinb 1996; 41(4):265–6.

McGrory BJ, Morrey BF, Rand JA, et al. Correlation of patient questionnaire responses and physician history in grading clinical outcome following hip and knee arthroplasty. A prospective study of 201 joint arthroplasties. J Arthroplasty 1996; 11(1):47–57.

McGrory JE, Trousdale RT, Pagnano MW, et al. Preoperative hip to ankle radiographs in total knee arthroplasty. Clin Orthop 2002; (404):196–202.

McGuigan FX, Hozack WJ, Moriarty L, et al. Predicting quality-of-life outcomes following total joint arthroplasty. Limitations of the SF-36 Health Status Questionnaire. J Arthroplasty 1995; 10(6):742–7.

Meding J, Ritter M, Faris P, et al. Does the preoperative radiographic degree of osteoarthritis correlate to results in primary total knee arthroplasty? J Arthroplasty 2001 Jan;16(1):13–6.

Meding JB, Keating EM, Ritter MA, et al. Total knee replacement in patients with genu recurvatum. Clin Orthop 2001; (393):244–9.

Meding JB, Ritter MA, Faris PM. Total knee arthroplasty with 4.4 mm of tibial polyethylene: 10-year followup. Clin Orthop 2001; 388:112–7.

Meding JB, Ritter MA, Jones NL, et al. Determining the necessity for routine pathologic examinations in uncomplicated total hip and total knee arthroplasties. J Arthroplasty 2000; 15(1):69–71.

Melfi C, Holleman E, Arthur D, et al. Selecting a patient characteristics index for the prediction of medical outcomes using administrative claims data. J Clin Epidemiol 1995; 48(7):917–26.

Mendenhall S. Get the lowdown on orthopaedic implants. Mater Manag Health Care 1996;5(4):30–2.

Messieh M. Preoperative risk factors associated with symptomatic pulmonary embolism after total knee arthroplasty. Orthopaedics 1999; 22(12):1147–9.

Miebzak GM, Campbell M, Mauerhan DR. The SF-36 General Health Status Survey documents the burden of osteoarthritis and the benefits of total joint arthroplasty: but why should we use it? Am J Manage Care 2002; 8(5):463–74.

Mikkola H, Hakkinen U. The effects of case-based pricing on length of stay for common surgical procedures. J Health Serv Res Policy 2002; 7(2):90–7.

Miller CW, Pettygrow R. Long-term clinical and radiographic results of a pegged tibial baseplate in primary total knee arthroplasty. J Arthroplasty 2001; 16(1):70–5.

Miller M, Benjamin JB, Marson B, et al. The effect of implant constraint on results of conversion of unicompartmental knee arthroplasty to total knee arthroplasty. Orthopaedics 2002 Dec;25(12):1353–7; discussion 7.

Miller M, Benjamin JB, Marson B, Hollstein S. The effect of implant constraint on results of conversion of unicompartmental knee arthroplasty to total knee arthroplasty. Orthop edics 2002; 25(12): 1353–7.

Minter JE, Dorr LD. Indications for bilateral total knee replacement. Contemp Orthop 1995; 31(2):108–11.

Miric A, Lim M, Kahn B, et al. Perioperative morbidity following total knee arthroplasty among obese patients. J Knee Surg 2002; 15(2):77–83.

Miyasaka K, Ranawat C, Mullaji A. 10- to 20-year follow-up of total knee arthroplasty for valgus deformities. Clin Orthop 1997 Dec;(345):29–37.

Miyazaki T, Wada M, Kawahara H, et al. Dynamic load at baseline can predict radiographic disease progression in medial compartment knee osteoarthritis. Ann Rheum Dis 2002; 61(7):617–22.

Mokris J, Smith S, Anderson S. Primary total knee arthroplasty using the Genesis Total Knee Arthroplasty System: 3- to 6–year follow-up study of 105 knees. J Arthroplasty 1997 Jan;12(1):91–8.

Mont M, Yoon T, Krackow K, et al. Eliminating patellofemoral complications in total knee arthroplasty: clinical and radiographic results of 121 consecutive cases using the Duracon system. J Arthroplasty 1999 Jun;14(4):446–55.

Mont MA, Fairbank AC, Yammamoto V, et al. Radiographic characterization of aseptically loosened cementless total knee replacement. Clin Orthop 1995; (321):73–8.

Mont MA, Mathur SK, Krackow KA, Loewy JW, Hungerford DS. Cementless total knee arthroplasty in obese patients. A comparison with a matched control group. J Arthroplasty 1996; 11(2):153–6.

Mont MA, Mitzner DL, Jones LC, et al. History of the contralateral knee after primary knee arthroplasty for osteoarthritis. Clin Orthop 1995; (321):145–50.

Moon MS, Kim JM, Woo YK. Restoration of knee motion after total knee arthroplasty: subvastus approach and alternate flexion and extension splintage. Ryumachi 1997; 37(2):146.

Moore DJ, Freeman MA, Revell PA, et al. Can a total knee replacement prosthesis be made entirely of polymers? J Arthroplasty 1998; 13(4):388–95.

Morkis JG, Smith SW, Anderson SE. Primary total knee arthroplasty using the Genesis Total Knee Arthroplasty System: 3- to 6–year follow-up study of 105 knees. J Arthroplasty 1997; 12(1):91–8.

Moseley JB, O'Malley K, Petersen NJ, et al. A controlled trial of arthroscopic surgery for osteoarthritis of the knee. New Engl J Med 2002;347:81–8.

Moskal J, Diduch D. Postoperative radiographs after total knee arthroplasty: a cost-containment strategy. Am J Knee Surg 1998 Spring; 11(2):89–93.

Muller W, Wirz D. The patella in total knee replacement: does it matter? 750 LCS total knee replacements without resurfacing of the patella. Knee Surg Sports Traumatol Arthrosc 2001; 9 Suppl 1:S24–6.

Munin MC, Kwoh CK, Glynn N , et al. Predicting discharge outcome after elective hip and knee arthroplasty. Am J Phys Med Rehabil 1995; 74(4):294–301.

Munzinger UK, Petrich J, Boldt JG. Patella resurfacing in total knee arthroplasty using metal-backed rotating bearing components: a 2- to 10-year follow-up evaluation. Knee Surg Sports Traumatol Arthrosc 2001; 9 Suppl 1:S34–42

Murray DW, Frost SJ. Pain in the assessment of total knee replacement. J Bone Jt Surg Br 1998; 80(3):426–31.

Murray DW, Goodfellow JW, O'Connor JJ. The Oxford medial unicompartmental arthroplasty: a ten-year survival study. J Bone Jt Surg Br 1998; 80(6):983–9.

Nafei A, Kristensen O, Knudsen HM, et al. Survivorship analysis of cemented total condylar knee arthroplasty. A long-term follow-up report on 348 cases. J Arthroplasty 1996; 11(1):7–10.

Namba RS, Diao E. Tissue expansion for staged reimplantation of infected total knee arthroplasty. J Arthroplasty 1997; 12(4):471–4.

Nassif JM, Ritter MA, Meding JB, et al. The effect of intraoperative intravenous fixed-dose heparin during total joint arthroplasty on the incidence of fatal pulmonary emboli. J Arthroplasty 2000; 15(1): 16–21.

National Centre for Health Statistics. American Academy and American Association of Orthopaedic Surgeons Bulletin 1999;47(3):14.

Nayak KN, Rorabeck CH, Bourne RB, et al. Interpretation by radiologists of orthopaedic total joint radiographs: is it necessary or cost-effective? Can J Surg 1996; 39(5):393–6.

Naylor CD, Williams JI. Primary hip and knee replacement surgery: Ontario criteria for case selection and surgical priority. Qual Health Care 1996;5:20–30.

Nazarian DG, Mehta S, Booth Jr RE. A comparison of stemmed and unstemmed components in revision knee arthroplasty. Clin Orthop 2002 Nov;(404):256–62.

Nazarian DG, Mehta S, Booth Jr RE. A comparison of stemmed and unstemmed components in revision knee arthroplasty. Clin Orthop 2002; (404):256–62.

Nelson CL. Primary and delayed exchange for infected total knee arthroplasty. Am J Knee Surg 2001; 14(1):60–4.

Nendick M. Patient satisfaction with post-operative analgesia. Nurs St 2000; 14(22):32–7.

Nerurkar J, Wade WE, Martin BC. Cost/death averted with venous thromboembolism prophylaxis in patients undergoing total knee replacement or knee arthroplasty. PharmacoTher 2002; 22(8):990–1000.

Newman JH, Ackroyd CE, Shah NA, et al. Should the patella be resurfaced during total knee replacement? Knee 2000; 7(1):17–23.

Newman JH, Ackroyd CE, Shah NA. Unicompartmental or total knee replacement? Five-year results of a prospective, randomised trial of 102 osteoarthritic knees with unicompartmental arthritis. J Bone Jt Surg Br 1998; 80(5):862–5.

Newman JH, Bowers M, Murphy J. The clinical advantages of autologous transfusion. A randomized, controlled study after knee replacement. J Bone Jt Surg Br 1997; 79(4):630–2.

Ng SF, Oo CS, Loh KH, et al. A comparative study of three warming interventions to determine the most effective in maintaining perioperative normothermia. Anesth Analg 2003; 96(1):171–6.

Niskanen RO, Korkala O, Pammo H. Serum C-reactive protein levels after total hip and knee arthroplasty. J Bone Jt Surg Br 1996; 78(3): 431–3.

Nordentoft T, Schou J, Carstensen J. Changes in sexual behavior after orthopaedic replacement of hip or knee in elderly males-a prospective study. Int J Impot Res 2000; 12(3):143–6.

Norman-Taylor FH, Palmer CR, Villar RN. Quality-of-life improvement compared after hip and knee replacement. J Bone Jt Surg Br 1996; 78(1):74–7.

Norton E, Garfinkel S, McQuay L, et al. The effect of hospital volume on the in-hospital complication rate in knee replacement patients. Health Serv Res 1998 Dec 1998;33(5 Pt 1):1191–210. Comment in: Health Serv Res 1998 Dec;33(5 Pt 1):85–90. PMID: 9865216.

Norton EC, Garfinkel SA, McQuay LJ, et al. The effect of hospital volume on the in-hospital complication rate in knee replacement patients. Health Serv Res 1998; 33(5 Pt 1):1191–210.

Norton MR, Eyres KS. Irrigation and suction technique to ensure reliable cement penetration for total knee arthroplasty. J Arthroplasty 2000; 15(4):468–74.

Nozaki H, Banks SA, Suguro T, et al. Observations of femoral roll-back in cruciate-retaining knee arthroplasty. Clin Orthop 2002; (404):308–14.

O'Connor DP, Jackson AS. Predicting physical therapy visits needed to achieve minimal functional goals after arthroscopic knee surgery... including commentary by Irrgang JJ with author response. J Orthop Sports Phys Ther 2001; 31(7):340–52.

O'Rourke M, Callaghan J, Goetz D, et al. Osteolysis associated with a cemented modular posterior-cruciate-substituting total knee design: five to eight- year follow-up. J Bone Jt Surg Am 2002 Aug;84-A(8):1362–71.

Oberg U, Oberg T, Hagstedt B. Functional improvement after hip and knee arthroplasty: 6–month follow-up with a new functional assessment system. Physiother Theory Pract 1996; 12(1):3–13.

Olcott CW, Scott RD. A comparison of 4 intraoperative methods to determine femoral component rotation during total knee arthroplasty. J Arthroplasty 2000; 15(1):22–6.

Olcott CW, Scott RD. Determining proper femoral component rotational alignment during total knee arthroplasty. Am J Knee Surg 2000; 13(3):166–8.

Oldmeadow LB, McBurney H, Robertson VJ. Hospital stay and discharge outcomes after knee arthroplasty. J Qual Clin Pract 2001; 21(3):56–60.

Olsen JH, McLaughlin JK, Nyren O, et al. Hip and knee implantations among patients with osteoarthritis and risk of cancer: a record-linkage study from Denmark. Int J Cancer 1999; 81(5):719–22.

Onsten I, Nordqvist A, Carlsson AS, et al. Hydroxyapatite augmentation of the porous coating improves fixation of tibial components. A randomised RSA study in 116 patients. J Bone Jt Surg Br 1998; 80(3): 417–25.

Oonishi H, Murata N, Saito M , et al. 3- to 18-year clinical results of total knee replacement with ceramic components. Key Eng Mater 2001; 192–195:999–1002.

Orbell S, Espley A, Johnston M , et al. Health benefits of joint replacement surgery for patients with osteoarthritis: prospective evaluation using independent assessments in Scotland. J Epidemiol Community Health 1998; 52(9):564.

Orthopaedic Network News. 2002 hip and knee implant review. CMS MedPar (www.OrthopaedicNetworkNews.com). Accessed 9/8/03.

Ouellet D, Moffet H. Locomotor deficits before and two months after knee arthroplasty. Arthritis Rheum 2002; 47(5):484–93.

Paavolainen P, Pukkala E, Pulkkinen P, et al. Cancer incidence after total knee arthroplasty: a nationwide Finnish cohort from 1980 to 1996 involving 9,444 patients. Acta Orthop Sc 1999; 70(6):609–17.

Pagnano M, Cushner FD, Hansen A, et al. Blood management in two-stage revision knee arthroplasty for deep prosthetic infection. Clin Orthop 1999; (367):238–42.

Pagnano MW, Forero JH, Scuderi GR, et al. Is the routine examination of surgical specimens worthwhile in primary total knee arthroplasty? Clin Orthop 1998; (356):79–84.

Pagnano MW, Trousdale RT. Asymmetric patella resurfacing in total knee arthroplasty. Am J Knee Surg 2000; 13(4):228–33.

Pap G, Meyer M, Weiler HT, et al. Proprioception after total knee arthroplasty: a comparison with clinical outcome. Acta Orthop Sc 2000; 71(2):153–9.

Papanikolaou A, Droulias K, Nikolaides A, Polyzoides AJ. Results of a single total knee prosthesis compared with multiple joint replacement in the lower limb. Int Orthop 2000; 24(2):80–2. 105

Parker DA, Rorabeck CH, Bourne RB. Long-term follow-up of cementless versus hybrid fixation for total knee arthroplasty. Clin Orthop 2001; 388:68–76.

Partio E, Wirta J. Comparison of patellar resurfacing and nonresurfacing in total knee arthroplasty: A prospective randomized study. J Orthop Rheumatol 1995; 8(2):69–74.

Parvizi J, Seel MJ, Hanssen AD, et al. Patellar component resection arthroplasty for the severely compromised patella. Clin Orthop 2002 Apr;(397):356–61.

Pavone V, Boettner F, Fickert S, et al. Total condylar knee arthroplasty: a long-term follow-up. Clin Orthop 2001; 388:18–25.

Pearson S, Moraw I, Maddern GJ. Clinical pathway management of total knee arthroplasty: a retrospective comparative study. Aust N Z J Surg 2000; 70(5):351–4.

Pecina M, Djapic T, Haspl M. Survival of cementless and cemented porous-coated anatomic knee replacements: retrospective cohort study. Croat Med J 2000; 41(2):168–72.

Pence CD, Spencer S. Complications of intravenous heparin therapy for treatment of thromboembolic disease in joint arthroplasty patients. Kans Med 1996; 97(1):16–8.

Pereira D, Jaffe F, Ortiguera C. Posterior cruciate ligament-sparing versus posterior cruciate ligament-sacrificing arthroplasty. Functional results using the same prosthesis. J Arthroplasty 1998 Feb;13(2): 138–44.

Perhoniemi V, Vuorinen J, Myllynen P, et al. The effect of enoxaparin in prevention of deep venous thrombosis in hip and knee surgery-a comparison with the dihydroergo tamine-heparin combination. Ann Chir Gynaecol 1996; 85(4):359–63.

Perhoniemi V, Vuorinen J, Myllynen P, et al. The effect of enoxaparin in prevention of deep venous thrombosis in hip and knee surgery-a comparison with the dihydroergotamine-heparin combination. Ann Chir Gynaecol 1996; 85(4):359–63.

Periti P, Stringa G, Mini E. Comparative multicentre trial of teicoplanin versus cefazolin for antimicrobial prophylaxis in prosthetic joint implant surgery. Italian Study Group for Antimicrobial Prophylaxis in Orthopaedic Surgery. Eur J Clin Microbiol Infect Dis 1999; 18(2): 113–9.

Periti P, Stringa G, Mini E. Comparative multicentre trial of teicoplanin versus cefazolin for antimicrobial prophylaxis in prosthetic joint implant surgery. Italian Study Group for Antimicrobial Prophylaxis in Orthopaedic Surgery. Eur J Clin Microbiol Infect Dis 1999; 18(2): 113–9.

Perka C, Arnold U, Buttgereit F. Influencing factors on perioperative morbidity in knee arthroplasty. Clin Orthop 2000; (378):183–91.

Perseghin P, Beverina I, Bongiorno U, et al. Blood transfusion and deep venous thrombosis in primary total hip and knee replacement surgery: a retrospective analysis of 339 patients. Transfus Sci 1996; 17(3):397–406.

Petrie RS, Hanssen AD, Osmon DR, et al. Metal-backed patellar component failure in total knee arthroplasty: a possible risk for late infection. Am J Orthop 1998; 27(3):172–6.

Peyron JG. Osteoarthritis. The epidemiologic viewpoint. Clin Orthop 1986;213:13–9.

Pollock DC, Ammeen DJ, Engh GA. Synovial entrapment: a complication of posterior stabilised total knee arthroplasty. J Bone Joint Surg Am 2002; 84-A(12):2174–8.

Polyzoides AJ, Dendrinos GK, Tsakonas H. The Rotaglide total knee arthroplasty. Prosthesis design and early results. J Arthroplasty 1996; 11(4):453–9.

Pomeroy DL, Schaper LA, Badenhausen WE, et al. Results of all-polyethylene tibial components as a cost-saving technique. Clin Orthop 2000; 380:140–3.

Price AJ, Rees JL, Beard D, et al. A mobile-bearing total knee prosthesis compared with a fixed-bearing prosthesis. A multicentre single-blind randomised controlled trial. J Bone Joint Surg Br 2003; 85(1): 62–7.

Procicchiani D, Bianchini D, La Bruna S, et al. The functional independence measure in the rehabilitation of elderly patients after orthopaedic surgery. Eur Medicophys 1998; 34(3):111–9.

Rader CP, Barthel T, Haase M, et al. Heterotopic ossification after total knee arthroplasty. 54/615 cases after 1–6 years' follow-up. Acta Orthop Sc 1997; 68(1):46–50 Ossification study.

Rader CP, Kramer C, Konig A, et al. Low-molecular-weight heparin and partial thromboplastin time-adjusted unfractionated heparin in thromboprophylaxis after total knee and total hip arthroplasty. J Arthroplasty 1998; 13(2):180–5.

Ranawat C, Luessenhop C, Rodriguez J. The press-fit condylar modular total knee system. Four-to-six-year results with a posterior-cruciate-substituting design. J Bone Jt Surg Am 1997 Mar;79(3):342–8.

Ranawat CS. Results of cemented cruciate substituting and sacrificing total knee arthroplasty. Orthopaedics 1996; 19(9):787–8.

Rand J, Gustilo R. Comparison of inset and resurfacing patellar prostheses in total knee arthroplasty. J Orthop Surg 1996;4(1):13–22.

Rand JA, Gustilo B. Comparison of inset and resurfacing patellar prostheses in total knee arthroplasty. Acta Orthop Belg 1996; 62 Suppl 1:154–63.

Rasmussen GL, Steckner K, Hogue C, et al. Intravenous parecoxib sodium foracute pain after orthopaedic knee surgery. Am J Orthop 2002; 31(6):336–43.

Reed MR, Bliss W, Sher JL, et al. Extramedullary or intramedullary tibial alignment guides: a randomised, prospective trial of radiological alignment. J Bone Jt Surg Br 2002; 84(6):858–60.

Rees JL, Price AJ, Lynskey TG, et al. Medial unicompartmental arthroplasty after failed high tibial osteotomy. J Bone Jt Surg Br 2001; 83(7): 1034–6.

Regner L, Carlsson L, Karrholm J, et al. Clinical and radiologic survivorship of cementless tibial components fixed with finned polyethylene pegs. J Arthroplasty 1997 Oct ;12(7):751–8.

Reisch JS, Tyson JE, Mize SG. Aid to the evaluation of therapeutic studies. Pediatrics 1989;84(5):815–27.

Reuben SS, Fingeroth R, Krushell R, et al. Evaluation of the safety and efficacy of the perioperative administration of rofecoxib for total knee arthroplasty. J Arthroplasty 2002; 17(1):26–31.

Reynolds LW, Hoo RK, Brill RJ, et al. The COX-2 Specific Inhibitor, Valdecoxib, Is An Effective, Opioid- Sparing Analgesic in Patients Undergoing Total Knee Arthroplasty. J Pain Symptom Manage 2003; 25(2):133–41.

Rinta-Kiikka I, Savilahti S, Pajamaki J, et al. A five to seven years follow-up of 102 cementless Synatomic knee arthroplasties. Ann Chir Gynaecol 1996;85(1):77–85.

Rinta-Kiikka I, Savilahti S, Pajamaki J, Lindholm TS. Intermediate-term clinical and radiographic results of Synatomic and AGC knee prostheses. Orthopaedics 1999; 22(3):295–9.

Rinta-Kiikka I. Clinical and radiographic outcome of total knee arthroplasty-factors related to loosening. Ann Chir Gynaecol 2000; 89(2): 147.

Rissanen P, Aro S, Paavolainen P. Hospital- and patient- related characteristics determining length of hospital stay for hip and knee replacements. Int J Technol Assess Health Care 1996; 12(2):325–35.

Rissanen P, Aro S, Sintonen H, et al. Costs and cost-effectiveness in hip and knee replacements. A prospective study. Int J Technol Assess Health Care 1997; 13(4):575–88.

Rissanen P, Aro S, Sintonen H, Slatis P, Paavolainen P. Quality of life and functional ability in hip and knee replacements: a prospective study. Qual Life Res 1996; 5(1):56–64.

Rissanen P, Aro S, Slatis P, et al. Health and quality of life before and after hip or knee arthroplasty. J Arthroplasty 1995; 10(2):169–75.

Rissanen P, Sogaard J, Sintonen H. Do QOL instruments agree? A comparison of the 15D (Health-Related Quality of Life) and NHP (Nottingham Health Profile) in hip and knee replacements. Int J Technol Assess Health Care 2000; 16(2):696–705.

Ritter M, Berend M, Meding J, et al. Long-term follow-up of anatomic graduated components posterior cruciate-retaining total knee replacement. Clin Orthop 2001 Jul;388:51–7.

Ritter M, Mamlin LA, Melfi CA, et al. Outcome implications for the timing of bilateral total knee arthroplasties. Clin Orthop 1997; (345):99–105.

Ritter M, Worland R, Saliski J, et al. Flat-on-flat, nonconstrained, compression molded polyethylene total knee replacement. Clin Orthop 1995 Dec;(321):79–85.

Ritter MA, Albohm MJ, Keating EM , et al. Comparative outcomes of total joint arthroplasty. J Arthroplasty 1995; 10(6):737–41.

Ritter MA, Berend ME, Meding JB, et al. Long-term follow-up of anatomic graduated components posterior cruciate-retaining total knee replacement. Clin Orthop 2001; 388:51–7.

Ritter MA, Eizember L, Keating EM, et al. The influence of age and gender on the outcome of total knee arthroplasty. Todays OR Nurse 1995; 17(4):10–5.

Ritter MA, Faris PN, Carr KD, et al. Revision total joint arthroplasty: Does Medicare reimbursement justify time spent? Orthopaedics 1996; 19(2):137–40.

Ritter MA, Herbst SA, Keating EM, et al. Patellofemoral complications following total knee arthroplasty. Effect of a lateral release and sacrifice of the superior lateral geniculate artery. J Arthroplasty 1996; 11(4):368–72.

Ritter MA, Koehler M, Keating EM , et al. Intra-articular morphine and/or bupivacaine after total knee replacement. J Bone Jt Surg Br 1999; 81(2):301–3.

Ritter MA, Montgomery TJ, Zhou H , et al. The clinical significance of proximal tibial resection level in total knee arthroplasty. Clin Orthop 1999; (360):174–81.

Ritter MA. Session I: Long-term follow-up after total knee arthroplasty. Clin Orthop 2002; (404):32–3.

Robertsson O, Borgquist L, Knutson K, et al. Use of unicompartmental instead of tricompartmental prostheses for unicompartmental arthrosis in the knee is a cost-effective alternative. 15,437 primary tricompartmental prostheses were compared with 10,624 primary medial or lateral unicompartmental prostheses. Acta Orthop Sc 1999; 70(2):170–5.

Robertsson O, Dunbar M, Knutson K, et al. Validation of the Swedish Knee Arthroplasty Register: a postal survey regarding 30,376 knees operated on between 1975 and 1995. Acta Orthop Sc 1999; 70(5):467–72.

Robertsson O, Dunbar M, Pehrsson T, et al. Patient satisfaction after knee arthroplasty: a report on 27,372 knees operated on between 1981 and 1995 in Sweden. Acta Orthop Sc 2000; 71(3):262–7.

Robertsson O, Dunbar MJ, Knutson K, et al. The Swedish Knee Arthroplasty Register. 25 years experience. Bull Hosp Jt Dis 1999; 58(3):133–8.

Robertsson O, Dunbar MJ. Patient satisfaction compared with general health and disease-specific questionnaires in knee arthroplasty patients. J Arthroplasty 2001; 16(4):476– 82.

Robertsson O, Knutson K, Lewold S, et al. Knee arthroplasty in rheumatoid arthritis. A report from the Swedish Knee Arthroplasty Register on 4,381 primary operations 1985–1995. Acta Orthop Sc 1997; 68(6):545–53.

Robertsson O, Knutson K, Lewold S, et al. The routine of surgical management reduces failure after unicompartmental knee arthroplasty. J Bone Jt Surg Br 2001; 83(1):45–9.

Robertsson O, Knutson K, Lewold S, et al. The Swedish Knee Arthroplasty Register 1975–1997: an update with special emphasis on 41,223 knees operated on in 1988–1997. Acta Orthop Sc 2001; 72(5):503–13.

Robertsson O, Scott G, Freeman MA. Ten-year survival of the cemented Freeman-Samuelson primary knee arthroplasty. Data from the Swedish Knee Arthroplasty Register and the Royal London Hospital. J Bone Jt Surg Br 2000; 82(4):506–7.

Robertsson O. Unicompartmental arthroplasty. Results in Sweden 1986–1995. Orthopade 2000; 29 Suppl 1:S6–8. No post-operative outcomes scores.

Robinson KS, Anderson DR, Gross M, et al. Ultrasonographic screening before hospital discharge for deep venous thrombosis after arthroplasty: the post-arthroplasty screening study. A randomized, controlled trial. Ann Intern Med 1997; 127(6):439–45.

Robinson KS, Anderson DR, Gross M, et al. Ultrasonographic screening before hospital discharge for deep venous thrombosis after arthroplasty: the post-arthroplasty screening study. A randomized, controlled trial. Ann Intern Med 1997; 127(6):439–45.

Rodriguez J, Saddler S, Edelman S, et al. Long-term results of total knee arthroplasty in class 3 and 4 rheumatoid arthritis. J Arthroplasty 1996 Feb;11(2):141–5.

Rodriguez JA, Baez N, Rasquinha V, Ranawat CS. Metal-backed and all-polyethylene tibial components in total knee replacement. Clin Orthop 2001; 392:174–83.

Rodriguez JA, Bhende H, Ranawat CS. Total condylar knee replacement: a 20-year follow-up study. Clin Orthop 2001; 388:10–7.

Rorabeck CH. Mechanisms of knee implant failure. Orthopaedics 1995; 18(9):915–8.

Rorabeck CH. Total knee replacement: should it be cemented or hybrid? Can J Surg 1999; 42(1):21–6.

Rosenbaum CC, Woods SE, Hasselfeld KA. Correlation of the change in the International Normalized Ratio and decreasing the coumadin dosage following total joint arthroplasty. Orthopaedics 2002; 25(12):1359–63.

Rosenberg AG. TKA salvage: when reimplantation won't work. Orthopaedics 1997; 20(9):851–4.

Rowley DI, McGurty DW. A seven-year experience of data collection on the Insall-Burstein II total knee arthroplasty. A prospective study. J Bone Jt Surg Br 2001; 83(2):185–90.

Rubash HE, Miller MC. Orthopaedics. Knee implants. Rehabil R D Prog Rep 1997; 34:219–20.

Ryd L, Albrektsson BE, Carlsson L, et al. Roentgen stereophotogrammetric analysis as a predictor of mechanical loosening of knee prostheses. J Bone Jt Surg Br 1995; 77(3):377–83.

Ryu J, Sakamoto A, Honda T, et al. The postoperative drain-clamping method for hemostasis in total knee arthroplasty. Reducing postoperative bleeding in total knee arthroplasty. Bull Hosp Jt Dis 1997; 56(4):251–4.

Saleh KJ, Clark CR, Rand JA, et al. Modes of failure and preoperative evaluation. J Bone Joint Surg Am 2003; 85–A Suppl 1:S21–5.

Saleh KJ, Dykes DC, Tweedie RL, et al. Functional outcome after total knee arthroplasty revision: a meta-analysis. J Arthroplasty 2002 Dec;17(8):967–77.

Saleh KJ, Radosevich DM, Kassim RA, et al. Comparison of commonly used orthopaedic outcome measures using palm-top computers and paper surveys. J Orthop Res 2002;20(6):1146–51.

Sanchez-Sotelo J, Ordonez JM, Prats SB. Results and complications of the low contact stress knee prosthesis. J Art hroplasty 1999; 14(7): 815–21.

Sanzen L, Sahlstrom A, Gentz CF, et al. Radiographic wear assessment in a total knee prosthesis. 5– to 9–year follow-up study of 158 knees. J Arthroplasty 1996; 11(6):738–42. 108

Schai PA, Thornhill TS, Scott RD. Total knee arthroplasty with the PFC system. Results at a minimum of ten years and survivorship analysis. J Bone Jt Surg Br 1998; 80(5):850–8.

Scherb CA. Outcomes research: making a difference in practice. Outcomes Manag 2002; 6(1):22–6.

Schroder H, Berthelsen A, Hassani G, et al. Cementless porous-coated total knee arthroplasty: 10-year results in a consecutive series. J Arthroplasty 2001 Aug;16(5):559–67.

Schroder HM, Kristensen PW, Petersen MB, et al. Patient survival after total knee arthroplasty. 5–year data in 926 patients. Acta Orthop Sc 1998; 69(1):35–8.

Schurman DJ, Matityahu A, Goodman SB, et al. Prediction of post-operative knee flexion in Insall-Burstein II total knee arthroplasty. Clin Orthop 1998; (353):175–84.

Schwagerl W. Application of ODH-titanium in total knee arthroplasty. Acta Orthop Belg 1997; 63 Suppl 1:56–8.

Scott RD. The incidence and causes of re-operation after press-fit condylar (PFC) total knee arthroplasty. J Ortop Sci 1997; 2(1):46–52.

Scriven MW, Fligelstone LJ, Oshodi TO, et al. The influence of total knee arthroplasty on lower limb blood flow. J R Coll Surg Edinb 1996; 41(5):323–4.

Scuderi GR. Revision total knee arthroplasty: how much constraint is enough? Clin Orthop 2001; (392):300–5.

Sculco TP, Gallina J. Blood management experience: relationship between autologous blood donation and transfusion in orthopaedic surgery. Orthopaedics 1999; 22(1 Suppl):s129–34.

Sculco TP. The economic impact of infected joint arthroplasty. Orthopaedics 1995; 18(9):871–3.

Sextro G, Berry D, Rand J. Total knee arthroplasty using cruciate-retaining kinematic condylar prosthesis. Clin Orthop 2001 Jul;388: 33–40.

Sextro GS, Berry DJ, Rand JA. Total knee arthroplasty using cruciate-retaining kinematic condylar prosthesis. Clin Orthop 2001; 388:33–40.

Shakoor N, Block JA, Shott S, et al. Nonrandom evolution of end-stage osteoarthritis of the lower limbs. Arthritis Rheum 2002; 46(12):3185–9.

Sharma L, Sinacore J, Daugherty C, et al. Prognostic factors for functional outcome of total knee replacement: a prospective study. J Gerontol A Biol Sci Med Sci 1996; 51(4):M152–7.

Sharma L, Sinacore J, Stulberg SD, et al. Role of growth hormone status in the outcome of total knee replacement. Clin Orthop 1997; (336): 177–85.

Sharrock NE, Cazan MG, Hargett M J, et al. Changes in mortality after total hip and knee arthroplasty over a ten-year period. Anesth Analg 1995; 80(2):242–8.

Shenolikar A, Wareham K, Newington D, et al. Cell salvage auto transfusion in total knee replacement surgery. Transfus Med 1997; 7(4):277–80.

Shepperd S, Harwood D, Gray A, et al. Randomised controlled trial comparing hospital at home care with inpatient hospital care. II: cost minimisation analysis. BMJ 1998; 316(7147):1791–6.

Shepperd S, Harwood D, Jenkinson C, et al. Randomised controlled trial comparing hospital at home care with inpatient hospital care. I: three month follow-up of health outcomes. BMJ 1998; 316(7147): 1786–91.

Shiga H, Yoshino S, Nakamura H, Nagashima M. Long-term results of Yoshino total knee arthroplasties in rheumatoid arthritis. Arch Orthop Trauma Surg 1998; 117(1–2):15–7.

Shoji H, Shimozaki E. Patellar clunk syndrome in total knee arthroplasty without patellar resurfacing. J Arthroplasty 1996; 11(2):198–201.

Simmons S, Lephart S, Rubash H, et al. Proprioception following total knee arthroplasty with and without the posterior cruciate ligament. J Arthroplasty 1996; 11(7):763–8. Less than 100 knees in the study.

Smith J, Stevens J, Taylor M, et al. A randomized, controlled trial comparing compression bandaging and cold therapy in postoperative total knee replacement surgery. Orthop Nurs 2002; 21(2):61–6.

Smith JS, Watts HG. Methods for locating missing patients for the purpose of long-term clinical studies. Journal of Bone & Joint Surgery?American Volume 1998;80(3):431–8.

Smith S, Naima VS, Freeman MA. The natural history of tibial radiolucent lines in a proximally cemented stemmed total knee arthroplasty. J Arthroplasty 1999; 14(1):3–8.

Sorrells RB, Stiehl JB, Voorhorst PE. Midterm results of mobile-bearing total knee arthroplasty in patients younger than 65 years. Clin Orthop 2001; (390):182–9.

Sorrells RB. The rotating platform mobile bearing TKA. Orthopaedics 1996; 19(9):793–6.

Spicer DD, Pomeroy DL, Badenhausen WE, et al. Body mass index as predictor of outcome in total knee replacement. Int Orthop 2001; 25(4):246–9.

Springer BD, Hanssen AD, Sim FH, et al. The kinematic rotating hinge prosthesis for complex knee arthroplasty. Clin Orthop 2001 Nov;(392): 283–91.

Squire MW, Callaghan JJ, Goetz DD, et al. Unicompartmental knee replacement. A minimum 15 year followup study. Clin Orthop 1999; (367):61–72.

Stern SH, Wixson RL, O'Connor D. Evaluation of the safety and efficacy of enoxaparin and warfarin for prevention of deep vein thrombosis after total knee arthroplasty. J Arthroplasty 2000; 15(2):153–8.

Stickles B, Phillips L, Brox W, et al. Defining the relationship between obesity and total joint arthroplasty. Obes Res 2001 Mar;9(3):219–23.

Stiehl JB, Cherveny PM. Femoral rotational alignment using the tibial shaft axis in total knee arthroplasty. Clin Orthop 1996; (331):47–55.

Stiehl JB, Voorhorst PE, Keblish P, et al. Comparison of range of motion after posterior cruciate ligament retention or sacrifice with a mobile bearing total knee arthroplasty. Am J Knee Surg 1997; 10(4): 216–20.

Stiehl JB, Voorhorst PE. Total knee arthroplasty with a mobile-bearing prosthesis: comparison of retention and sacrifice of the posterior cruciate ligament in cementless implants. Am J Orthop 1999; 28(4): 223–8.

Stowell CP, Chandler H, Jove M, et al. An open-label, randomized study to compare the safety and efficacy of perioperative epoetin alfa with preoperative autologous blood donation in total joint arthroplasty. Orthopaedics 1999; 22(SUPPL.):s105–s112.

Stratton MA, Anderson FA, Bussey HI, et al. Prevention of venous thromboembolism: adherence to the 1995 American College of Chest Physicians consensus guidelines for surgical patients. Arch Intern M ed 2000; 160(3):334–40.

Study documents savings from total knee pathway. OR Manager 1998; 14(7):1, 6–7, 9.

Stulberg SD. Extensor mechanism complications after total knee arthroplasty. Orthopaedics 1995; 18(9):919–20.

Sturmer T, Gunther KP, Brenner H. Obesity, overweight and patterns of osteoarthritis: the Ulm Osteoarthritis Study. J Clin Epidemiol 2000; 53(3):307–13.

Svard UC, Price AJ. Oxford medial unicompartmental knee arthroplasty. A survival analysis of an independent series. J Bone Jt Surg Br 2001; 83(2):191–4.

Taylor HD, Dennis DA, Crane HS. Relationship between mortality rates and hospital patient volume for Medicare patients undergoing major orthopaedic surgery of the hip, knee, spine, and femur. J Arthroplasty 1997; 12(3):235–42.

Tayot O, Ait Si Selmi T, Neyret P. Results at 11.5 years of a series of 376 posterior stabilised HLS1 total knee replacements. Survivorship analysis, and risk factors for failure. Knee 2001; 8(3):195–205.

Teller RE, Christie MJ, Martin W, et al. Sequential indium-labeled leukocyte and bone scans to diagnose prosthetic joint infection. Clin Orthop 2000; (373):241–7.

Teter KE, Bregman D, Colwell CW Jr. Accuracy of intramedullary versus extramedullary tibial alignment cutting systems in total knee arthroplasty. Clin Orthop 1995; (321):106–10.

Thadani PJ, Spitzer AI. Primary total knee arthroplasty: Indications and long-term results. Curr Opin Orthop 2000; 11(1):41–8.

Thadani PJ, Vince KG, Ortaaslan SG, Blackburn DC, Cudiamat CV. Ten- to 12-year follow-up of the Insall-Burstein I total knee prosthesis. Clin Orthop 2000; 380:17–29.

Tierney WM, Fitzgerald JF, Heck D, et al. Tricompartmental knee replacement: A comparison of orthopaedic surgeons' self reported performance rates with surgical indications, intraindications, and expected outcomes. Clinical Orthopaedics 1994;305:209–17.

Title C, Rodriguez J, Ranawat C. Posterior cruciate-sacrificing versus posterior cruciate-substituting total knee arthroplasty: a study of clinical and functional outcomes in matched patients. J Arthroplasty 2001 Jun;16(4):409–14.

Toksvig-Larsen S, Ryd L, Stentstrom A, et al. The Porous-Coated Anatomic total knee experience. Special emphasis on complications and wear. J Arthroplasty 1996; 11(1):11–7. No post-operative outcomes scores.

Tooma GS, Kobs JK, Thomason HC 3rd, et al. Results of knee arthroplasty using the cemented press-fit condylar prosthesis. Based on a preliminary report. Am J Orthop 1995; 24(11):831–4.

Turner G, Blake D, Buckland M, et al. Continuous extradural infusion of ropivacaine for prevention of postoperative pain after major orthopaedic surgery. Br J Anaesth 1996; 76(5):606–10.

Unnanantana A. Press-fit-condylar total knee replacement: experience in 465 Thai patients. J Med Assoc Thai 1997; 80(9):565–9.

Vaczi G, Udvarhelyi I, Sarungi M. Comparison of results of different types of knee arthroplasties. Arch Orthop Trauma Surg 1997; 116(3):177–80.

Vail TP, Callaghan JJ. Total knee replacement with patella magna and pagetoid patella. Orthopaedics 1995; 18(12):1174–7.

Valdivia GG, Dunbar MJ, Jenkinson RJ, et al. Press-fit versus cemented all-polyethylene patellar component: midterm results. J Arthroplasty 2002; 17(1):20–5.

van Essen GJ, Chipchase LS, O'Connor D, et al. Primary total knee replacement: short-term outcomes in an Australian population. J Qual Clin Pract 1998; 18(2):135–42.

Van Walraven Carl, Paterson Michael, Kapral Moira, et al. Appropriateness of primary total hip and knee replacements in regions of Ontario with high and low utilization rates. Can Med Assoc J 1996; 155(6):697–706.

Vazquez-Vela Johnson G, Worland RL, Keenan J, et al. Patient demographics as a predictor of the ten-year survival rate in primary total knee replacement. J Bone Joint Surg Br 2003; 85(1):52–6.

Ververeli P, Sutton D, Hearn S, et al. Continuous passive motion after total knee arthroplasty. Analysis of cost and benefits. Clin Orthop 1995 Dec;(321):208– 15.

Ververeli PA, Masonis JL, Booth RE, et al. Radiographic cost reduction strategy in total joint arthroplasty. A prospective analysis. J Arthroplasty 1996; 11(3):277–80

Ververeli PA, Sutton DC, Hearn SL, et al. Continuous passive motion after total knee arthroplasty. Analysis of cost and benefits. Clin Orthop 1995; (321):208–15.

Vince KG. Fixation for primary total knee arthroplasty: cemented. J Arthroplasty 1996; 11(2):123–5.

Vresilovic EJ, Hozack WJ, Booth RE Jr, et al. Comparative risk of early postoperative pulmonary embolism after cemented total knee versus total hip arthroplasty with low-dose warfarin prophylaxis. Am J Knee Surg 1996; 9(1):2–6.

Vrettou I, Voyagis GS. Intravenous regional infusion of imipenem for antimicrobial chemoprophylaxis in orthopaedic surgery. Eur J Anaesthesiol 1998; 15(6):801–2.

Waikakul S, Un-Nanuntana A, Jaisue N. Recovery of joint position sense after total knee replacement: the effects of soft tissue dissection. J Med Assoc Thai 1999; 82(12):1187–92.

Wakankar HM, Nicholl JE, Koka R, et al. The tourniquet in total knee arthroplasty. A prospective, randomised study. J Bone Jt Surg Br 1999; 81(1):30–3.

Wakankar HM, Nicholl JE, Koka R, et al. The tourniquet in total knee arthroplasty. A prospective, randomised study. J Bone Jt Surg Br 1999; 81(1):30–3.

Wakitani S, Kuwata K, Imoto K, et al. Knee and/or hip joint destruction in rheumatoid arthritis is associated with HLA-DRB1*0405 in Japanese patients. Clin Rheumatol 1998; 17(6):485–8.

Waldman BJ, Mont MA, Hungerford DS. Total knee arthroplasty infections associated with dental procedures. Clin Orthop 1997; (343):164–72.

Walker PS, Ambarek MS, Morris JR, et al. Anterior-posterior stabil-ity in partially conforming condylar knee replacement. Clin Orthop 1995; (310):87–97.

Walker PS, Manktelow AR. Comparison between a Constrained Condylar and a Rotating Hinge in revision knee surgery. Knee 2001; 8(4):269–79.

Walsh M, Kennedy D, Stratford PW, et al. Perioperative functional performance of women and men following total knee arthroplasty. Physiother Can 2001; 53(2):92–100.

Wammack L, Mabrey JD. Outcomes assessment of total hip and total knee arthroplasty: critical pathways, variance analysis, and continuous quality improvement. Clin Nurse Spec 1998; 12(3):122–9.

Wang ST, Hsu HC, Wu JJ, et al. Patellar dislocation after total knee arthroplasty. Zhonghua Yi Xue Za Zhi (Taipei) 1996; 57(5):348–54.

WangCJ, Wang HE. Descriptive analysis of the factors associated with patellar fracture after total knee arthroplasty. Medscape Orthop Sports Med New York 1997; 1(9).

Warwick DJ, Whitehouse S. Symptomatic venous thromboembolism after total knee replacement. J Bone Jt Surg Br 1997; 79(5):780–6.

Wasielewski RC, Weed H, Prezioso C, et al. Patient comorbidity: relationship to outcomes of total knee arthroplasty. Clin Orthop 1998; (356):85–92.

Waters TS, Bentley G. Patellar resurfacing in total knee arthroplasty: a prospective, randomized study. J Bone Joint Surg Am 2003; 85–A(2):212–7.

Weale AE, Halabi OA, Jones PW, et al. Perceptions of outcomes after unicompartmental and total knee replacements. Clin Orthop 2001; (382):143–53.

Weale AE, Murray DW, Newman JH, et al. The length of the patellar tendon after unicompartmental and total knee replacement. J Bone Jt Surg Br 1999; 81(5):790–5.

Weber AB, Worland RL, Keenan J, Van Bowen J. A study of polyethylene and modularity issues in >1,000 posterior cruciate-retaining knees at 5 to 11 years. J Arthroplasty 2002; 17(8):987–91.

Weingarten S, Riedinger MS, Sandhu M, et al. Can practice guidelines safely reduce hospital length of stay? Results from a multicentre interventional study. Am J Med 1998; 105(1):33–40.

Weingarten SR, Conner L, Riedinger M, et al. Total knee replacement. A guideline to reduce postoperative length of stay. West J Med 1995; 163(1):26–30.

Werkmeister JA, White JF, Edwards GA, et al. Early performance appraisal of the omniflow II vascular prosthesis as an indicator of long-term function. J Long Term Eff Med Implants 1995; 5(1):1–10.

Werle JR, Goodman SB, Imrie SN. Revision total knee arthroplasty using large distal femoral augments for severe metaphyseal bone deficiency: a preliminary study. Orthopaedics 2002 Mar;25(3):325–7.

Westrich GH, Allen ML, Tarantino SJ, et al. Ultrasound screening for deep venous thrombosis after total knee arthroplasty. 2-year reassessment. Clin Orthop 1998; (356):125–33.

Westrich GH, Sculco TP. Prophylaxis against deep venous thrombosis after total knee arthroplasty: Pneumatic plantar compression and aspirin compared with aspirin alone. J Bone Jt Surg Am 1996; 78(6): 826–34.

Westrich GH, Sculco TP. Prophylaxis against deep venous thrombosis after total knee arthroplasty: Pneumatic plantar compression and aspirin compared with aspirin alone. J Bone Jt Surg Am 1996; 78(6): 826–34.

Wheeler EC. The CNS's impact on process and outcome of patients with total knee replacement. Clin Nurse Spec 2000; 14(4):159–69.

White RE Jr, Allman JK, Trauger JA, et al. Clinical comparison of the midvastus and medial parapatellar surgical approaches. Clin Orthop 1999; (367):117–22.

Whiteside LA, Bicalho PS. Radiologic and histologic analysis of morselized allograft in revision total knee replacement. Clinical Orthopaedics & Related Research 1998;357:149–56.

Whiteside LA, Mihalko WM. Surgical procedure for flexion contracture and recurvatum in total knee arthroplasty. Clin Orthop 2002; (404):189–95.

Whiteside LA. Effect of porous-coating configuration on tibial osteolysis after total knee arthroplasty. Clin Orthop 1995; (321):92–7.

Whiteside LA. Fixation for primary total knee arthroplasty: cementless. J Arthroplasty 1996; 11(2):125–7; discussion 128–9.

Whiteside LA. Long-term follow-up of the bone ingrowth Ortholoc knee system without a metal-backed patella. Clin Orthop 2001; 388: 77–84.

Whiteside LA. Selective ligament release in total knee arthroplasty of the knee in valgus. Clin Orthop 1999; (367):130–40.

Williams HR, Macdonald DA. Audit of thromboembolic prophylaxis in hip and knee surgery. Ann R Coll Surg Engl 1997; 79(1):55–7.

Williams JI, Llewellyn Thomas H, Arshinoff R, et al. The burden of waiting for hip and knee replacements in Ontario. Ontario Hip and Knee Replacement Project Team. J Eval Clin Pract 1997; 3(1):59–68.

Williams-Russo P, Sharrock NE, Haas SB, et al. Randomized trial of epidural versus general anaesthesia: outcomes after primary total knee replacement. Clin Orthop 1996; (331):199–208.

Williams-Russo P, Sharrock NE, Mattis S, et al. Cognitive effects after epidural vs general anaesthesia in older adults. A randomized trial. JAMA 1995; 274(1):44–50.

Wilson MG, May DS, Kelly JJ. Racial differences in the use of total knee arthroplasty for osteoarthritis among older Americans. Ethn Dis 1994 Winter;4(1):57–67.

Wood DJ, Smith AJ, Collopy D, White B, Brankov B, Bulsara MK. Patellar resurfacing in total knee arthroplasty: a prospective, randomized trial. J Bone Jt Surg Am 2002; 84-A(2):187–93. 1

Woolson ST, Robinson RK, Khan NQ, et al. Deep venous thrombosis prophylaxis for knee replacement: warfarin and pneumatic compression. Am J Orthop 1998; 27(4):299–304.

Worland R, Arredondo J, Angles F, et al. Home continuous passive motion machine versus professional physical therapy following total knee replacement. J Arthroplasty 1998 Oct ;13(7):784–7.

Worland RL, Jessup DE, Clelland C. Simultaneous bilateral total knee replacement versus unilateral replacement. Am J Orthop 1996; 25(4):292–5.

Worland RL, Jessup DE, Vazquez-Vela Johnson G, et al. The effect of femoral component rotation and asymmetry in total knee replacements. Orthopaedics 2002; 25(10):1045–8.

Worland RL, Jessup DE, Warburton KJ, Clelland C. Total knee arthroplasty in the octogenarian. The patients' perspective. Va Med Q 1997; 124(3):188–9.

Wright JG, Coyte P, Hawker G, et al. Variation in orthopaedic surgeons' perceptions for and outcomes of knee replacement. Can Med Assoc J 1995;152:687–97.

Wright JG, Hawker GA, Bombardier C, et al. Physician enthusiasm as an explanation for area variation in the utilization of knee replacement surgery. Med Care 1999 Sep;37(9):946–56.

Wu CL, Perkins FM. Oral anticoagulant prophylaxis and epidural catheter removal. Reg Anesth 1996; 21(6):517–24. Comment in: Reg Anesth. 1996 Nov-Dec;21(6):503–7.

Wulff W, Incavo SJ. The effect of patella preparation for total knee arthroplasty on patellar strain: a comparison of resurfacing versus inset implants. J Arthroplasty 2000; 15(6):778–82.

Xenakis TA, Malizos KN, Dailiana Z, et al. Blood salvage after total hip and total knee arthroplasty. Acta Orthop Sc Suppl 1997; 275:135–8.

Yamazaki J, Ishigami S, Nagashima M, Yoshino S. Hy-Flex II total knee system and range of motion. Arch Orthop Trauma Surg 2002; 122(3):156–60.

Yang K, Yeo S, Lee B, et al. Total knee arthroplasty in diabetic patients: a study of 109 consecutive cases. J Arthroplasty 2001 Jan;16(1):102–6.

Yang SH, Liu TK. Intramedullary versus extramedullary tibial alignment guides in total knee arthroplasty. J Formos Med Assoc 1998; 97(8):564–8.

Yashar AA, Venn-Watson E, Welsh T, et al. Continuous passive motion with accelerated flexion after total knee arthroplasty. Clin Orthop 1997; (345):38–43.

Yokoyama Y, Inoue H, Ohta Y, Hayashi T, Koura H. Relationship between retention of the posterior cruciate ligament and postoperative flexion in total knee arthroplasty. Acta Med Okayama 1995; 49(6): 295–300.

Yoshino S, Nakamura H, Shiga H, et al. Recovery of full flexion after total knee replacement in rheumatoid arthritis-a follow-up study. Int Orthop 1997; 21(2):98–100.

Younger AS, Beauchamp CP, Duncan CP, et al. Position of the knee joint after total joint arthroplasty. J Arthroplasty 1995; 10(1):53–61.

Zahiri CA, Schmalzried TP, Szuszczewicz ES, et al. Assessing activity in joint replacement patients. J Arthroplasty 1998; 13(8):890–5.

Zamora-Navas P, Collado-Torres F, de la Torre-Solis F. Closed suction drainage after knee arthroplasty. A prospective study of the effectiveness of the operation and of bacterial contamination. Acta Orthop Belg 1999; 65(1):44–7.

Zenios M, Wykes P, Johnson DS, et al. The use of knee splints after total knee replacements. Knee 2002; 9(3):225–8. No post-operative outcomes scores.

group; here these 'homogeneous' parts are already noncompact. We take up the group $\mathcal{P}$ later. All three, $SO(3,1)$, $SL(2,\mathbb{C})$ and $\mathcal{P}$, are crucial for special relativistic physics.

In this part we study $SO(3,1)$ first, $SL(2,\mathbb{C})$ second, and then their relationship, via their defining representations. Their Lie algebras are the same (as with $SO(3)$ and $SU(2)$), and are simple as they have no invariant subalgebras. Then we survey their finite dimensional irreducible representations, which when nontrivial are nonunitary. At the end, we make some comments on their UIR's as well as on their infinite dimensional nonunitary irreducible representations.

10.4.1 The group $SO(3,1)$

We set $c = 1$, and begin with metric conventions for Minkowski spacetime:

$$\text{Metric choice}: g_{00} = -1,\ g_{11} = g_{22} = g_{33} = 1;\ \mu,\nu,\lambda,\cdots = 0,1,2,3;$$

$$g^{\mu\nu}g_{\nu\lambda} = \delta^{\mu}_{\lambda};$$

$$x^{\mu} = \text{four-vector} \Rightarrow x^{\mu}x_{\mu} = x \cdot x = g_{\mu\nu}x^{\mu}x^{\nu}$$

$$= \boldsymbol{x}^2 - (x^0)^2. \tag{10.87}$$

A homogeneous Lorentz transformation is a linear transformation x^{μ} to $x'^{\mu} = \Lambda^{\mu}_{\nu}x^{\nu}$, Λ a real 4×4 matrix, such that $x' \cdot x' = x \cdot x$; so we have the defining representation

$$O(3,1) = \{\Lambda = (\Lambda^{\mu}_{\nu}) = 4 \times 4 \text{ real matrix}|\Lambda^{T}g\Lambda = g\}. \tag{10.88}$$

Here the left index μ is a row index, the right index ν is a column index. Indices are raised and lowered using the metric tensors $g^{\mu\nu}$, $g_{\mu\nu}$; so in detail the 'pseudo-orthogonality' condition in (10.88) reads:

$$\Lambda^{T}g\Lambda = g \Leftrightarrow \Lambda^{\rho}_{\mu}g_{\rho\nu}\Lambda^{\nu}_{\lambda} = g_{\mu\lambda}$$

$$\Leftrightarrow \Lambda_{\nu\mu}\Lambda^{\nu}_{\lambda} = \Lambda^{\rho}_{\mu}\Lambda_{\rho\lambda} = g_{\mu\lambda}. \tag{10.89}$$

Group composition is given by matrix multiplication, and we have the rules:

$$\text{Composition law}:\ (\Lambda'\Lambda)^{\mu}_{\nu} = \Lambda'^{\mu}_{\rho}\Lambda^{\rho}_{\nu};$$

$$\text{Identity}:\ \Lambda^{\mu}_{\nu} = \delta^{\mu}_{\nu},\ \Lambda_{\mu\nu} = g_{\mu\nu};$$

$$\text{Inverses}:\ (\Lambda^{-1})^{\mu}_{\nu} = g^{\mu\rho}g_{\nu\sigma}\Lambda^{\sigma}_{\rho} = \Lambda^{\mu}_{\nu};$$

$$\Lambda^{-1} = g^{-1}\Lambda^{T}g. \tag{10.90}$$

It is easily seen from (10.89) that

$$\Lambda \in O(3,1) \Rightarrow \det \Lambda = \pm 1, \ (\Lambda^0{}_0)^2 = 1 + \Lambda_{j0}\Lambda_{j0} \geq 1. \qquad (10.91)$$

This leads to $O(3,1)$ breaking up into four disjoint components, each of them connected, with associated physical meanings:

$$\Lambda^0{}_0 \geq 1, \ \det \Lambda = +1 \ : \ \text{no space reflection } \mathcal{P}, \ \text{no time reversal } T;$$

$$\Lambda^0{}_0 \geq 1, \ \det \Lambda = -1 \ : \ \text{space reflection } \mathcal{P}, \text{no time reversal } T;$$

$$\Lambda^0{}_0 \leq -1, \det \Lambda = -1 \ : \ \text{no } \mathcal{P}, \text{ but } T,$$

$$\Lambda^0{}_0 \leq -1, \ \det \Lambda = +1 \ : \ \text{both } \mathcal{P} \text{ and } T \text{ included.} \qquad (10.92)$$

The first component is the one connected to the identity and is sometimes indicated by $SO(3,1)^{\uparrow}_{+}$ and called the proper orthochronous homogeneous Lorentz group. We denote it by $SO(3,1)$ with the defining representation

$$SO(3,1) = \{\Lambda = (\Lambda^{\mu}{}_{\nu}) = 4 \times 4 \text{ real matrix} \,|\, \Lambda^T g \Lambda = g,$$

$$\Lambda^0{}_0 \geq 1, \ \det \Lambda = 1\} \subset O(3,1). \qquad (10.93)$$

It is clear that $SO(3,1)$ is an invariant subgroup of $O(3,1)$; we study this (doubly) connected Lie group. From special relativity many of its properties are familiar, and we recall some important ones.

Proper spatial rotations form an $SO(3)$ subgroup of $SO(3,1)$ but not an invariant one:

$$SO(3) = \{\Lambda \in SO(3,1) : \Lambda^0{}_0 = 1, \ \Lambda^j{}_0 = \Lambda^0{}_j = 0, \ \Lambda_{jk} = A_{jk}(\boldsymbol{\alpha}),$$

$$A(\boldsymbol{\alpha}) \in SO(3)\} \subset SO(3,1),$$

$$\text{i.e., } \Lambda(\boldsymbol{\alpha}) = \begin{pmatrix} 1 & 0 & 0 & 0 \\ 0 & & & \\ 0 & & A(\boldsymbol{\alpha}) & \\ 0 & & & \end{pmatrix} \in SO(3) \text{ subgroup.} \qquad (10.94)$$

This is a three parameter maximal compact subgroup of the noncompact $SO(3,1)$. There are also subgroups having the structures of $SO(2,1)$ and $E(2)$ important for the unitary representation theory of $\mathcal{P}$. We identify them later.

Pure Lorentz transformations form a *subset* of $SO(3,1)$, *not* a subgroup. Each such Lorentz transformation is determined by a rapidity vector $\boldsymbol{\zeta} \in \mathbb{R}^3$, a real three dimensional vector, and we write the corresponding $SO(3, 1)$ element as $L(\boldsymbol{\zeta})$:

$$\boldsymbol{\zeta} \in \mathbb{R}^3 \to L(\boldsymbol{\zeta}) \in SO(3, 1) \; : \; L^0{}_0(\boldsymbol{\zeta}) = \cosh \zeta,$$

$$L^j{}_0(\boldsymbol{\zeta}) = L^0{}_j(\boldsymbol{\zeta}) = -\zeta_j \frac{\sinh \zeta}{\zeta},$$

$$L_{jk}(\boldsymbol{\zeta}) = \delta_{jk} + \zeta_j \zeta_k \frac{\cosh \zeta - 1}{\zeta^2}, \; \zeta = |\boldsymbol{\zeta}|. \tag{10.95}$$

The usual relative velocity vector is, reinstating c,

$$\boldsymbol{v} = c \, \boldsymbol{\zeta} \, \frac{\tanh \zeta}{\zeta} = c \hat{\boldsymbol{\zeta}} \tanh \zeta,$$

$$|\boldsymbol{v}| < c. \tag{10.96}$$

It is a fact that any $\Lambda \in SO(3, 1)$ is uniquely expressible as the product of an $SO(3)$ element and a pure Lorentz transformation in a definite order:

$$\Lambda \in SO(3, 1) \; : \; \Lambda = L(\boldsymbol{\zeta})\Lambda(\boldsymbol{\alpha})$$

$$= \Lambda(\boldsymbol{\alpha})L(A(\boldsymbol{\alpha})^{-1}\boldsymbol{\zeta}). \tag{10.97}$$

This is also the polar decomposition of Λ since $L(\boldsymbol{\zeta})$ is symmetric positive definite and $\Lambda(\boldsymbol{\alpha})$ is proper orthogonal. We see that each $L(\boldsymbol{\zeta})$ is a representative element from one $SO(3)$ coset in $SO(3, 1)$. This defining four dimensional representation of $SO(3, 1)$ is nonunitary, and cannot be made unitary by any similarity transformation. We have a noncompact six parameter Lie group here, with $\boldsymbol{\alpha}$ and $\boldsymbol{\zeta}$ as convenient parameters. Topologically, $SO(3, 1) \sim SO(3) \times \mathbb{R}^3$, so like $SO(3)$ it is doubly connected.

To obtain the independent generators and commutation relations in the defining representation, we consider the form of an infinitesimal element:

$$\Lambda^\mu{}_\nu \simeq \delta^\mu{}_\nu + \omega^\mu{}_\nu, \; \Lambda \in SO(3, 1) \Leftrightarrow \omega_{\mu\nu} = -\omega_{\nu\mu}. \tag{10.98}$$

Since the ω's are real, we have as expected six independent real parameters here. If we extract a factor of i and write this Λ as

$$\Lambda \simeq \mathbb{1} + \frac{i}{2}\omega^{\mu\nu} J^{(0)}_{\mu\nu}, \tag{10.99}$$

the superscript (0) indicating that we are working in the defining representation, we have the (pure imaginary) generator matrices and commutation relations:

$$J_{\mu\nu}^{(0)} = -J_{\nu\mu}^{(0)},$$

$$(J_{\mu\nu}^{(0)})^{\rho}{}_{\sigma} = i(\delta^{\rho}{}_{\nu}g_{\mu\sigma} - \delta^{\rho}{}_{\mu}g_{\nu\sigma}),$$

$$[J_{\mu\nu}^{(0)}, J_{\rho\sigma}^{(0)}] = -i(g_{\nu\rho}J_{\mu\sigma}^{(0)} - g_{\mu\rho}J_{\nu\sigma}^{(0)} + g_{\nu\sigma}J_{\rho\mu}^{(0)} - g_{\mu\sigma}J_{\rho\nu}^{(0)}) \qquad (10.100)$$

We see the similarity to the $SO(2l)$, $SO(2l + 1)$ Lie algebra relations in Eq. (5.27), with the Kronecker symbol δ replaced by the Minkowski metric g corresponding to pseudo-orthogonality. These same commutation relations (10.100) are obeyed by the generators $J_{\mu\nu}$ of any reducible or irreducible unitary or nonunitary representation of $SO(3, 1)$. In finite dimensional representations, which are necessarily nonunitary, the $J_{\mu\nu}$ cannot all be hermitian. In UIR's and UR's, necessarily infinite dimensional, the $J_{\mu\nu}$ can all be made hermitian.

The split 3+1 form of the commutation relations (10.100) reads:

$$J_{23}, J_{31}, J_{12} = J_1, J_2, J_3; \ J_{01}, J_{02}, J_{03} = K_1, K_2, K_3:$$

$$[J_j, J_k] = -[K_j, K_k] = i\epsilon_{jkl}J_l,$$

$$[J_j, K_k] = i\epsilon_{jkl}K_l. \qquad (10.101)$$

These commutation relations do not admit any nontrivial neutral elements! Arguments similar to those used for $E(3)$ show that they can be transformed away in the $[J, J]$ and $[J, K]$ relations. Then

$$[K_j, K_k] = -i\epsilon_{jkl}J_l + id_{jk} \Rightarrow$$

$$d_{jk} = -d_{kj} \Rightarrow$$

$$d_{jk} = \epsilon_{jkl}d_l \Rightarrow d_j = 0 \qquad (10.102)$$

as d_j is a numerically invariant three-vector.

The connection to the factorisation (10.97) is that in any representation,

$$\Lambda(\boldsymbol{\alpha}) \rightarrow e^{-i\boldsymbol{\alpha}\cdot\boldsymbol{J}}, L(\boldsymbol{\zeta}) \rightarrow e^{-i\boldsymbol{\zeta}\cdot\boldsymbol{K}}. \qquad (10.103)$$

It happens that in all finite dimensional representations we can arrange to have $\boldsymbol{J}^{\dagger} = \boldsymbol{J}$, $\boldsymbol{K}^{\dagger} = -\boldsymbol{K}$, so $\Lambda(\boldsymbol{\alpha})$ and $L(\boldsymbol{\zeta})$ are represented by unitary and hermitian positive definite matrices, respectively. But before looking for all solutions to (10.101) in finite dimensions, we look at the group $SL(2,\mathbb{C})$ and its relation to $SO(3,1)$ as their Lie algebras are the same.

10.4.2 The group $SL(2,\mathbb{C})$ and the connection to $SO(3,1)$

This is very similar to the $SU(2)$-$SO(3)$ relationship, $SL(2,\mathbb{C})$ being the simply connected double covering of $SO(3,1)$. We begin with notations, for the three Pauli matrices and the unit matrix:

$$\sigma_\mu : \sigma_0 = \mathbb{1}, \ \sigma_j = \text{usual Pauli triplet};$$

$$\tilde{\sigma}_\mu : \tilde{\sigma}_0 = -\mathbb{1}, \ \tilde{\sigma}_j = \sigma_j;$$

$$\text{Tr}(\sigma_\mu \tilde{\sigma}_\nu) = 2g_{\mu\nu} = 2 \times \text{Minkowski metric}. \tag{10.104}$$

Now we associate with each real four-vector x^μ a hermitian 2×2 matrix $H(x)$ in this way:

$$H(x) = x^\mu \sigma_\mu = x^0 \cdot \mathbb{1} + x_j \sigma_j = \begin{pmatrix} x^0 + x^3 & x^1 - ix^2 \\ x^1 + ix^2 & x^0 - x^3 \end{pmatrix},$$

$$H(x)^\dagger = H(x), \ \det H(x) = -x \cdot x = -g_{\mu\nu} x^\mu x^\nu. \tag{10.105}$$

If now a is any complex 2×2 matrix, $aH(x)a^\dagger$ is evidently hermitian, so we have:

$$aH(x)a^\dagger = H(x'), \ x'^\mu = \text{real linear in } x^\nu,$$

$$x' \cdot x' = |\det a|^2 x \cdot x. \tag{10.106}$$

(Clearly every hermitian 2×2 matrix is $H(x')$ for some real x'^μ.) If we arrange $\det a = 1$, then $x' \cdot x' = x \cdot x$ and the relation between x' and x is via some homogeneous Lorentz transformation. This leads to the definition of the group $SL(2,\mathbb{C})$:

$$SL(2,\mathbb{C}) = \{ a = \begin{pmatrix} \alpha & \beta \\ \gamma & \delta \end{pmatrix} = \text{complex } 2 \times 2 \text{ matrix} \mid \det a = \alpha\delta - \beta\gamma = 1 \}. \tag{10.107}$$

Group composition is given by matrix multiplication, and $a^{-1} = \begin{pmatrix} \delta & -\beta \\ -\gamma & \alpha \end{pmatrix}$. We can now combine $(10.104, 10.106)$ to see that each $a \in SL(2,\mathbb{C})$ determines uniquely some $\Lambda(a) \in SO(3,1)$ by,

$$aH(x)a^\dagger = H(\Lambda(a)x),$$

$$\text{i.e.,} \quad ax^\mu \sigma_\mu a^\dagger = \Lambda(a)^\mu{}_\nu x^\nu \sigma_\mu,$$

$$\text{i.e.,} \quad a\sigma_\mu a^\dagger = \Lambda(a)^\nu{}_\mu \sigma_\nu,$$

$$\text{i.e.,} \quad \Lambda(a)^\nu{}_\mu = \frac{1}{2} Tr(a\sigma_\mu a^\dagger \tilde{\sigma}^\nu), \quad \tilde{\sigma}^\nu = g^{\nu\rho}\tilde{\sigma}_\rho. \tag{10.108}$$

One can check by repeated use of Eq. (10.106) that we have a homomorphism $SL(2,\mathbb{C}) \rightarrow SO(3,1)$, two to one as in the $SU(2) \rightarrow SO(3)$ case, with kernel consisting of $\pm \mathbb{1}_{2\times2}$. For unitary a, we recover $SU(2)$ as a subgroup of $SL(2,\mathbb{C})$. The $SL(2,\mathbb{C})$ elements that map onto the pure Lorentz transformations $L(\boldsymbol{\zeta})$ in $SO(3,1)$ are hermitian (positive or negative definite) matrics $a \in SL(2,\mathbb{C})$: referring to Eqs. (10.94, 10.95) we find:

$$a = u(\boldsymbol{\alpha}) \in SU(2) \subset SL(2,\mathbb{C}) \; : \; \Lambda(u(\boldsymbol{\alpha})) = \Lambda(\boldsymbol{\alpha}) \text{ of } (10.94);$$

$$a = h(\boldsymbol{\zeta}) = \cosh\frac{\zeta}{2} \cdot \mathbb{1} + \hat{\boldsymbol{\zeta}} \cdot \sigma \sinh\frac{\zeta}{2} \in SL(2,\mathbb{C}) \; : \; \Lambda(\pm h(\boldsymbol{\zeta})) = L(\boldsymbol{\zeta}) \text{ of } (10.95).$$
$$\tag{10.109}$$

So with the 2×2 polar decomposition we have:

$$a = h(\boldsymbol{\zeta})u(\boldsymbol{\alpha}) \rightarrow \Lambda(a) = L(\boldsymbol{\zeta})\Lambda(\boldsymbol{\alpha}). \tag{10.110}$$

The Lie algebra $\boldsymbol{SL(2,\mathbb{C})}$ can be studied in the defining representation (10.107) by taking a close to the unit matrix:

$$a \simeq \mathbb{1} - i\epsilon J \in SL(2,\mathbb{C}) \; : \; \det a = 1 \Leftrightarrow Tr\, J = 0$$

$$\Leftrightarrow J = \text{complex linear combination of } \sigma_j$$

$$= \text{real linear combination of } \frac{1}{2}\sigma_j \text{ and } -\frac{i}{2}\sigma_j. \tag{10.111}$$

As expected, $\boldsymbol{SL(2,\mathbb{C})}$ is a real six dimensional Lie algebra, and if in the defining representation we take the basis in the notation (10.101) to be

$$J_j \rightarrow \frac{1}{2}\sigma_j, \; K_j \rightarrow -\frac{i}{2}\sigma_j, \tag{10.112}$$

then the commutation relations (10.101) are obeyed. Thus we have identified the generators in this representation, matching with the $\boldsymbol{SO(3,1)}$ structure.

Now to construct all the finite dimensional irreps of $SL(2, \mathbb{C})$ and $SO(3,1)$, we must find all finite dimensional irreps of generators $\boldsymbol{J}, \boldsymbol{K}$ obeying the commutation relations (10.101), then exponentiate them as in (10.103), and see what happens globally. Here the following trick helps, since $\boldsymbol{J}, \boldsymbol{K}$ lead to two mutually commuting 'angular momenta':

$$\boldsymbol{J}^{(1)} = \frac{1}{2}(\boldsymbol{J} + i\boldsymbol{K}), \boldsymbol{J}^{(2)} = \frac{1}{2}(\boldsymbol{J} - i\boldsymbol{K}):$$

$$\boldsymbol{J} = \boldsymbol{J}^{(1)} + \boldsymbol{J}^{(2)}, \boldsymbol{K} = -i(\boldsymbol{J}^{(1)} - \boldsymbol{J}^{(2)});$$

$$[J_j^{(1)}, J_k^{(1)}] = i\epsilon_{jkl}J_l^{(1)},$$

$$[J_j^{(2)}, J_k^{(2)}] = i\epsilon_{jkl}J_l^{(2)},$$

$$[J_j^{(1)}, J_k^{(2)}] = 0. \tag{10.113}$$

Thus the most general irreducible finite dimensional solution to (10.101) is obtained by choosing some spin j_1 hermitian irrep for $\boldsymbol{J}^{(1)}$ and some spin j_2 hermitian irrep for $\boldsymbol{J}^{(2)}$, which are known to us from $SU(2)$ and $SO(3)$ representation theory. We denote the resulting irrep of $SL(2, \mathbb{C})$ (possibly double valued irrep of $SO(3,1)$) by the pair (j_1, j_2) with $j_1, j_2 = 0, \frac{1}{2}, 1, \cdots$, independently. The dimension of (j_1, j_2) is $(2j_1 + 1)(2j_2 + 1)$, the 'true' generators $\boldsymbol{J}, \boldsymbol{K}$ are, respectively, hermitian and antihermitian if as usual we take $\boldsymbol{J}^{(1)}$ and $\boldsymbol{J}^{(2)}$ to be hermitian.

There are two Casimir invariants with definitions and values as under in (j_1, j_2):

$$\mathcal{C}_1 = \boldsymbol{J}^2 - \boldsymbol{K}^2 = 2\{j_1(j_1 + 1) + j_2(j_2 + 1)\},$$

$$\mathcal{C}_2 = \boldsymbol{J} \cdot \boldsymbol{K} = -i\{j_1(j_1 + 1) - j_2(j_2 + 1)\},$$

$$= -i(j_1 - j_2)(j_1 + j_2 + 1). \tag{10.114}$$

Changing $\boldsymbol{K}$ to $-\boldsymbol{K}$ preserves the commutation relations (10.101), and carries (j_1, j_2) to (j_2, j_1). In the irrep (j_1, j_2), $SO(3)$ or $SU(2)$ elements are represented by unitary matrices, while pure Lorentz transformations are represented by hermitian (positive/negative definite) matrices. (Here we ignore the trivial irrep $j_1 = j_2 = 0$). The latter statement is consistent with the fact that pure Lorentz transformations are a subset and not a subgroup of $SO(3,1)$.

The 'spectrum of spin values', or irreps of the $SO(3)/SU(2)$ subgroup of $SO(3,1)/SL(2,\mathbb{C})$, is determined by the addition rules for angular momentum :

$$(j_1, j_2): j = j_1 + j_2, \ j_1 + j_2 - 1, \ j_1 + j_2 - 2, \cdots, |j_1 - j_2|, \text{ once each.} \tag{10.115}$$

So this spectrum is the same for (j_1, j_2) and (j_2, j_1), and the value of C_2 distinguishes between these two irreps.

The irreps (j_1, j_2) and (j_1', j_2') are equivalent if and only if $j_1' = j_1$ and $j_2' = j_2$. Other useful properties which can be shown using what we know from the quantum theory of angular momentum are, using the definitions in Eq. (1.38):

$$\text{each } (j_1, j_2) \text{ is self contragredient};$$
$$\text{complex conjugate of } (j_1, j_2) \text{ is } (j_2, j_1);$$
$$\text{adjoint of } (j_1, j_2) \text{ is } (j_2, j_1). \tag{10.116}$$

From the 'spin spectrum' (10.115) it is clear that:

$$j_1 + j_2 = \text{integer} \; : \; (j_1, j_2) = \text{irrep of } SO(3, 1),$$
$$\text{nonfaithful irrep of } SL(2, \mathbb{C});$$
$$j_1 + j_2 = \text{half odd integer} \; : \; (j_1, j_2) = \text{faithful irrep of } SL(2, \mathbb{C}),$$
$$\text{double-valued irrep of } SO(3, 1). \tag{10.117}$$

Here are some familiar examples of these $SO(3, 1)$ and $SL(2, \mathbb{C})$ representations:

$(0, 0)$: scalar, trivial irrep;

$\left(\dfrac{1}{2}, 0\right)$: defining irrep of $SL(2, \mathbb{C})$ with $\boldsymbol{J} = \dfrac{1}{2}\boldsymbol{\sigma}$, $\boldsymbol{K} = -\dfrac{i}{2}\boldsymbol{\sigma}$,

two-component Weyl spinor;

$\left(0, \dfrac{1}{2}\right)$: complex conjugate of $(1/2, 0)$, with $\boldsymbol{J} = \dfrac{1}{2}\boldsymbol{\sigma}$, $\boldsymbol{K} = \dfrac{i}{2}\boldsymbol{\sigma}$,

two-component Weyl spinor;

$\left(\dfrac{1}{2}, 0\right) \oplus \left(0, \dfrac{1}{2}\right)$: reducible four-component Dirac spinor;

$\left(\dfrac{1}{2}, \dfrac{1}{2}\right)$: defining four-vector irrep of $SO(3,1)$;

$(1, 0)$: self dual antisymmetric second rank tensors like $\boldsymbol{E} + i\boldsymbol{B}$,

ie., $F_{\mu\nu} = -F_{\nu\mu}$ and $\epsilon_{\mu\nu\rho\sigma} F^{\rho\sigma} = 2iF_{\mu\nu}$, transforming

by the matrices of $SO(3, \mathbb{C})$;

$(0,1)$: Complex conjugate of $(1,0)$, antiself dual antisymmetric second rank tensors like $\boldsymbol{E} - i\boldsymbol{B}$, ie., $F_{\mu\nu} = -F_{\nu\mu}$ and $\epsilon_{\mu\nu\rho\sigma} F^{\rho\sigma} = -2iF_{\mu\nu};$

$(1,1)$: 9 dim. irrep of $SO(3,1)$ corresponding to symmetric trace free second rank tensors;

$\left(1,\dfrac{1}{2}\right), \left(\dfrac{1}{2},1\right)$: Rarita-Schwinger fields. $\hspace{2cm}$ (10.118)

In connection with the irreps $(1,0)$ and $(0,1)$, we note that $\epsilon_{0123} = +1$ by convention; and $SO(3,\mathbb{C})$ matrices are of the form $e^{-i\boldsymbol{\alpha}\cdot\boldsymbol{S}}$, where $\boldsymbol{\alpha}$ is a complex 3-vector and S_j are the generators of the defining spin one representation of $SO(3)$. So $SO(3,\mathbb{C})$ is the group of all complex orthogonal unimodular matrices in three dimensions.

We conclude this discussion of the irreducible representations of $SO(3,1)$ and $SL(2,\mathbb{C})$ with a few comments on their infinite dimensional unitary representations. Two very special UIR's of $SL(2,\mathbb{C})$ were known to and used by Majorana as early as 1932 [Majorana, 1932] while constructing his two infinite component relativistic wave equations. The next major step forward came in 1945 when Dirac [Dirac 1945] constructed his unitary expansor representations of $SO(3,1)$, but these were very 'bulky' and 'highly' reducible. The construction of all the UIR's of $SO(3,1)$ and of $SL(2,\mathbb{C})$ was carried out independently by Harish Chandra and by Gelfand and Naimark around 1945–1946 and published in 1947. There is a so-called Principal Series of UIR's labelled $\{j_0, \rho\}$ where $j_0 = 0, \frac{1}{2}, 1, \cdots$ is the lowest spin present in the UIR, and ρ is a real continuous parameter in the range $-\infty < \rho < \infty$. The Casimir invariants of Eq. (10.114) have the values $\mathcal{C}_1 = j_0^2 - \rho^2 - 1$, $\mathcal{C}_2 = -\rho j_0$. The spectrum of spin values in $\{j_0, \rho\}$ is $j = j_0, j_0+1, j_0+2, \cdots$, once each. Then there is the so-called Supplementary Series of UIR's labelled $\{0, i\rho\}$ with lowest spin $j_0 = 0$ (spin spectrum $j = 0, 1, 2, \cdots$, once each), and $0 < \rho < 1$. Now we have $\mathcal{C}_1 = \rho^2 - 1$, $\mathcal{C}_2 = 0$. These latter UIR's are not needed for the expansion of square integrable functions on $SO(3,1)$ or $SL(2,\mathbb{C})$ in terms of the matrix elements of the representation matrices in the various UIR's. For this purpose the Principal Series suffices.

Apart from all these infinite dimensional UIR's, there are also infinite dimensional nonunitary irreducible representations. These were also found by Harish Chandra and by Gelfand and Naimark, and a complete discussion may be found in the classic monograph by Naimark [Naimark, 1964].

10.5 The Poincaré Group $\mathcal{P}$

To conclude this chapter, we study the proper Poincaré group $\mathcal{P}$, leaving out space and time reflections (except for some comments on the parity operator at the end). The group $\mathcal{P}$ combines the homogeneous Lorentz group $SO(3,1)$ and the abelian spacetime translations T_4 in a semidirect product. The action of a general element of $\mathcal{P}$ on a spacetime point with Minkowski coordinates x^μ is

$$x^\mu \to x'^\mu = \Lambda^\mu{}_\nu x^\nu + a^\mu,$$

$$\Lambda \in SO(3,1), \, a \in \mathbb{R}^4. \tag{10.119}$$

Thus an element of $\mathcal{P}$ is an ordered pair $g = (\Lambda, a)$. The composition law is read off from the action (10.119) on spacetime:

$$(\Lambda', a')(\Lambda, a) = (\Lambda'\Lambda, a' + \Lambda'a). \tag{10.120}$$

The similarity to the $E(3)$ composition law (10.9) is evident: We have here a generalisation from three dimensional space to four dimensional spacetime, with the Euclidean metric replaced by the indefinite Minkowski metric. Clearly the order of $\mathcal{P}$ is ten, as it is for the Galilei group $\mathcal{G}$: six parameters in Λ, four in the translations a^μ. The associative law is easily checked. As for the identity and inverses, similar to (10.10) for $E(3)$:

$$e \to (\delta^\mu{}_\nu, 0); \; (\Lambda, a)^{-1} = (\Lambda^{-1}, -\Lambda^{-1}a). \tag{10.121}$$

Two important subgroups are:

$$SO(3,1) = \{(\Lambda, 0) \mid \Lambda \in SO(3,1)\},$$

$$T_4 = \{(\mathbb{1}, a^\mu) \mid a^\mu \in \mathbb{R}^4\}, \tag{10.122}$$

the latter both abelian and invariant. Clearly $\mathcal{P}$ is the semidirect product

$$\mathcal{P} = SO(3,1) \rtimes T_4, \tag{10.123}$$

to be compared with (10.12) for $E(3)$. Compared to $\mathcal{G}$, the structure of $\mathcal{P}$ seems much more elegant and appealing. Topologically, $\mathcal{P} \sim SO(3) \times \mathbb{R}^3 \times \mathbb{R}^4$. The quotient $\mathcal{P}/T_4$ is isomorphic to $SO(3,1)$.

Our main concern will be with the UIR's of $\overline{\mathcal{P}}$, the two-fold universal covering group of $\mathcal{P}$, which will be defined in the sequel. We will aim only for the physicist's level of mathematical rigour. In the terminology used by Wigner in his classic paper [Wigner, 1939], UIR's of $\overline{\mathcal{P}}$ describe 'elementary systems'.

We begin by considering the Lie algebra of $\mathcal{P}$, and the possibility of occurrence of neutral elements. In a general UR of $\mathcal{P}$ we have unitary operators representing group elements, on some Hilbert space $\mathcal{H}$, as follows:

$$(\Lambda, a) = (\mathbb{1}, a)(\Lambda, 0) \rightarrow \overline{U}(\Lambda, a) = \overline{U}(\mathbb{1}, a)\overline{U}(\Lambda, 0)$$
$$\equiv \overline{U}(\mathbb{1}, a)\overline{U}(\Lambda), \qquad (10.124)$$

where $\overline{U}(\Lambda)$ is a UR of $SO(3, 1)$. We write the translation operator as

$$\overline{U}(\mathbb{1}, a) = e^{-ia^\mu P_\mu}, \qquad (10.125)$$

and then the relations to be obeyed can be expressed in a partly finite and partly infinitesimal form:

$$\Lambda', \Lambda \in SO(3, 1) \ : \ \overline{U}(\Lambda')\overline{U}(\Lambda) = \overline{U}(\Lambda'\Lambda);$$
$$\overline{U}(\Lambda)e^{-ia\cdot\mathcal{P}}\overline{U}(\Lambda)^{-1} = e^{-i(\Lambda a)\cdot\mathcal{P}},$$
$$e^{-ia'\cdot\mathcal{P}}e^{-ia\cdot\mathcal{P}} = e^{-i(a'+a)\cdot\mathcal{P}}. \qquad (10.126)$$

These then amount to

$$\overline{U}(\Lambda')\overline{U}(\Lambda) = \overline{U}(\Lambda'\Lambda),$$
$$\overline{U}(\Lambda)P_\mu\overline{U}(\Lambda)^{-1} = \Lambda^\nu{}_\mu P_\nu,$$
$$[P_\mu, P_\nu] = 0, \qquad (10.127)$$

to be compared with Eq. (10.28) for $E(3)$. In fully infinitesimal form, we bring in the generators $J_{\mu\nu}$ of $\overline{U}(\Lambda)$ as in (10.100); the Poincaré commutation relations are:

$$[J_{\mu\nu}, J_{\lambda\rho}] = i(g_{\mu\lambda}J_{\nu\rho} - g_{\nu\lambda}J_{\mu\rho} + g_{\mu\rho}J_{\lambda\nu} - g_{\nu\rho}J_{\lambda\mu}),$$
$$[J_{\mu\nu}, P_\lambda] = i(g_{\mu\lambda}P_\nu - g_{\nu\lambda}P_\mu),$$
$$[P_\mu, P_\lambda] = 0. \qquad (10.128)$$

So a UR of $\mathcal{P}$ is given by unitary $\overline{U}(\Lambda)$ and hermitian P_μ obeying (10.127), or hermitian $J_{\mu\nu}$ and P_μ obeying (10.128).

In contrast to $\mathcal{G}$, these relations do not admit any neutrals in a nontrivial manner. We already know that the $SO(3, 1)$ relations can be adjusted so that there are no neutrals in them. The only extension needed is from $SO(3, 1)$ to $SL(2, \mathbb{C})$ but we come to that later. To examine possible neutrals, let us write the commutation relations (10.128) in three dimensional form: with $P^0 = H$,

$$[J_j, J_k] = i\epsilon_{jkl}J_l, \; [J_j, K_k] = i\epsilon_{jkl}K_l, \; [K_j, K_k] = -i\epsilon_{jkl}J_l;$$

$$[J_j, P_k] = i\epsilon_{jkl}P_l, \; [J_j, H] = 0;$$

$$[K_j, P_k] = i\delta_{jk}H, \; [K_j, H] = iP_j;$$

$$[P_j, P_k] = 0, \; [P_j, H] = 0. \tag{10.129}$$

From the $E(3)$ and $SO(3,1)$ cases we know there are no neutrals in the $[J, J], [J, K], [K, K], [J, P], [P, P]$ relations; and in the further analysis none of $\boldsymbol{J}, \boldsymbol{K}, \boldsymbol{P}$ may be shifted by neutrals, while H can be shifted. Next we check the four remaining relations:

$$[J_j, H] = id_j: [J_k, [J_j, H]] + [J_j, [H, J_k]] + [H, [J_k, J_j]] = 0 \Rightarrow$$

$$\epsilon_{jkl}d_l = 0 \Rightarrow d_j = 0. \tag{10.130}$$

Then $[P_j, H]$ cannot involve any neutrals as the Jacobi identity with J_k shows. Continuing:

$$[K_j, P_k] = i(\delta_{jk}H + d_{jk}) \Rightarrow \text{ for any } A \in SO(3), \overline{U}(A) \text{ generated by } \boldsymbol{J},$$

$$\overline{U}(A)[K_j, P_k]\overline{U}(A)^{-1} = i(\delta_{jk}H + d_{jk}) \Rightarrow$$

$$A_{lj}A_{mk}[K_l, P_m] = i(\delta_{jk}H + d_{jk}) \Rightarrow$$

$$A_{lj}A_{mk}(\delta_{lm}H + d_{lm}) = \delta_{jk}H + d_{jk} \Rightarrow$$

$$A_{lj}A_{mk}d_{lm} = d_{jk} \Rightarrow d_{jk} = c\delta_{jk}, \tag{10.131}$$

for some neutral c. Now we redefine $H \to H - c$ which does not disturb $[J_j, H] = 0$ or $[P_j, H] = 0$, and we have

$$[K_j, P_k] = i\delta_{jk}H. \tag{10.132}$$

There is no more freedom to shift H, i.e., the zero point of energy is fixed, unlike in the case of $\mathcal{G}$. Now with such generators the final commutation relation cannot have any neutrals:

$$[K_j, H] = i(P_j + d_j) \Rightarrow A_{kj}[K_k, H] = i(A_{kj}P_k + d_j)$$

$$\Rightarrow A_{kj}d_k = d_j \Rightarrow d_j = 0. \tag{10.133}$$

So, again in contrast to $\mathcal{G}$, the Lie algebra $\mathcal{P}$ of $\mathcal{P}$ does not admit any nontrivial neutral elements. We need only contend with the global relation between $SO(3,1)$

and $SL(2, \mathbb{C})$, i.e., for quantum mechanical purposes we must allow double-valued representations of $SO(3, 1)$. That is, we have to look for true UR's of the two-fold covering group $\overline{\mathcal{P}}$ of $\mathcal{P}$, also the universal covering group of $\mathcal{P}$, which is the semidirect product of $SL(2, \mathbb{C})$ and T_4. Permitting some overuse of the letter a:

$$\overline{\mathcal{P}} = SL(2, \mathbb{C}) \rtimes T_4 \colon a \in SL(2, \mathbb{C}), \ a^\mu \in T_4 \to g = (a, a^\mu) \in \overline{\mathcal{P}};$$

$$g'g = (a', a'^\mu)(a, a^\mu) = (a'a, a'^\mu + \Lambda(a')^\mu{}_\nu a^\nu). \tag{10.134}$$

Topologically, $\overline{\mathcal{P}} \sim \mathbb{S}^3 \times \mathbb{R}^3 \times \mathbb{R}^4$.

Clearly at the Lie algebra level, there is no change in $(10.128, 10.129)$, but in (10.127) we must allow for a two-valuedness in the composition law among $\overline{U}(\Lambda)$.

We will be somewhat simple minded in studying the UIR's of $\overline{\mathcal{P}}$, which are in any case infinite dimensional and involve unbounded generators. In case $P_\mu = 0$, we have a UIR of $SO(3, 1)$ or of $SL(2, \mathbb{C})$ appearing as a nonfaithful UIR of $\overline{\mathcal{P}}$. Thus while strictly speaking these are UIR's of $\overline{\mathcal{P}}$, we ignore them. Hereafter we assume P^μ does not vanish identically. There are two algebraic Casimir invariants: one is the invariant 'norm squared' of the energy momentum P^μ which generates translations and is quadratic:

$$\mathcal{C}_1 = -P^\mu P_\mu. \tag{10.135}$$

To construct the second, we define the Pauli–Lubanski four-vector:

$$W_\mu = \frac{1}{2} \epsilon_{\mu\nu\lambda\rho} P^\nu J^{\lambda\rho} \colon$$

$$W_0 = \boldsymbol{P} \cdot \boldsymbol{J} = \boldsymbol{J} \cdot \boldsymbol{P},$$

$$\boldsymbol{W} = -P^0 \boldsymbol{J} - \boldsymbol{P} \wedge \boldsymbol{K};$$

$$P^\mu W_\mu = 0, \quad [P_\lambda, W_\mu] = 0. \tag{10.136}$$

The component W_0 is an $E(3)$ invariant, the helicity times the magnitude of momentum. The components W_μ do not mutually commute. The second Casimir invariant is

$$\mathcal{C}_2 = W^\mu W_\mu. \tag{10.137}$$

That this is an invariant follows from the translation invariance of W_μ and the Lorentz invariance of $\mathcal{C}_2$. Later in specific UIR's of $\overline{\mathcal{P}}$ we will find other nonalgebraic invariants. Notice that unlike $\mathcal{C}_1$, $\mathcal{C}_2$ is quartic in the generators.

Now to the UIR's, their structures and constructions. Since the P^μ are hermitian and mutually commuting, as in the $E(3)$ case we make them part of some complete commuting set and write their idealised eigenvectors as

$$|p;\alpha\rangle : P^\mu|p;\alpha\rangle = p^\mu|p;\alpha\rangle,$$

$$p^\mu = \text{four-vector eigenvalue.} \qquad (10.138)$$

So in a UIR a certain set of p's will occur, and we characterise it presently. The label α is to accommodate any other quantum numbers that may be needed to represent the eigenvalues of a complete commuting set of (hermitian) operators which include P^μ. We handle the problems of (continuum) normalisation later. Now from the second line of (10.127) we easily find:

$$P^\mu\overline{U}(\Lambda)|p;\alpha\rangle = \overline{U}(\Lambda)\overline{U}(\Lambda)^{-1}P^\mu\overline{U}(\Lambda)|p;\alpha\rangle$$

$$= \overline{U}(\Lambda)\Lambda^\mu{}_\nu P^\nu|p;\alpha\rangle$$

$$= (\Lambda^\mu{}_\nu p^\nu)\overline{U}(\Lambda)|p;\alpha\rangle,$$

$$\text{i.e., } \overline{U}(\Lambda)|p;\alpha\rangle \sim |\Lambda p;\beta\rangle. \qquad (10.139)$$

Then if a particular p^μ occurs in a UIR, so will Λp for all $\Lambda \in SO(3,1)$. Irreducibility then means the set of all p's present is of this form: some p^μ and all $SO(3,1)$ transforms of it, and nothing more. We therefore define the important concept of the $SO(3,1)$-orbit of a numerical energy-momentum four-vector p:

$$\vartheta_p = \text{orbit of } p = \{\Lambda p | p \text{ fixed, } \Lambda \in SO(3,1)\}. \qquad (10.140)$$

Thus an orbit is a 'homogeneous space' with respect to $SO(3,1)$: given any two points p, p' on it, there are in general infinitely many $\Lambda \in SO(3,1)$ such that $p' = \Lambda p$. From the properties of four-vectors, we can list all possible orbits and display a convenient representative point on each one as well as the associated invariants:

Type of orbit	Representative point $p^{(0)}$	Invariants	
Timelike positive	$(m_0,\mathbf{0}), m_0 > 0$	$p^\mu p_\mu = -m_0^2,$ Sign p^0 positive	
Timelike negative	$(-m_0,\mathbf{0}), m_0 > 0$	$p^\mu p_\mu = -m_0^2,$ Sign p^0 negative	(10.141)
Lightlike positive	$(1,0,0,1)$	Sign p^0 positive	
Lightlike negative	$(-1,0,0,-1)$	Sign p^0 negative	
Spacelike	$(0,0,0,\kappa), \kappa > 0$	$p^\mu p_\mu = \kappa^2.$	

So each orbit may be written as $\vartheta_{p^{(0)}}$ for some choice of $p^{(0)}$. In the language of four-vectors we see that each orbit is a three dimensional connected manifold with corresponding features:

Timelike cases: ϑ_p = positive or negative branch of timelike hyperboloid;

Lightlike cases: ϑ_p = positive or negative light cone without tip;

Spacelike cases: ϑ_p = single sheeted space like hyperboloid.   (10.142)

To proceed, and to understand the additional labels α in $|p; \alpha\rangle$, we ask: Given some orbit $\vartheta_{p^{(0)}}$, and choosing some $p \in \vartheta_{p^{(0)}}$, how much freedom is there in the choice of $\Lambda \in SO(3, 1)$ such that $\Lambda p^{(0)} = p$? This in turn depends on the answer to the question: what are the elements Λ such that $\Lambda p^{(0)} = p^{(0)}$? We formulate the latter by introducing the notion of the stability or little group of a given p, and in terms of $SL(2, \mathbb{C})$ rather than $SO(3, 1)$:

$$G_p = \text{stability group of } p$$
$$= \text{subgroup of } SL(2, \mathbb{C}) \text{ determined by } p$$
$$= \{a \in SL(2, \mathbb{C}) | \Lambda(a)p = p\}. \qquad (10.143)$$

For each (nonzero) p, G_p is a three parameter subgroup of $SL(2, \mathbb{C})$. (Of course for $p^\mu = 0$, $G_p = SL(2, \mathbb{C})$). Using Eq. (10.108), we can easily find them and their generators for each $p^{(0)}$ appearing in (10.141), working in the defining irreducible representation $(\frac{1}{2}, 0)$ of $SL(2, \mathbb{C})$ in which we have:

$$a \in SL(2, \mathbb{C}) : ap^\mu \sigma_\mu a^\dagger = p'^\mu \sigma_\mu, \ p' = \Lambda(a)p;$$

$$J = \frac{1}{2}\sigma, \ K = -\frac{i}{2}\sigma. \qquad (10.144)$$

Then we find the following pattern of results:

Time like cases $p^{(0)} = \pm(m_0, \mathbf{0})$:

$$G_{p^{(0)}} = \left\{ \begin{pmatrix} \alpha & \beta \\ -\beta^* & \alpha^* \end{pmatrix} \middle| |\alpha|^2 + |\beta|^2 = 1 \right\} = SU(2) \subset SL(2, \mathbb{C}),$$

generators $J = \frac{1}{2}\sigma$;   (10.145a)

Light like cases $p^{(0)} = \pm(1, 0, 0, 1)$:

$$G_{p^{(0)}} = \left\{ \begin{pmatrix} e^{-i\varphi/2} & (ia_2 - a_1)e^{-i\varphi/2} \\ 0 & e^{i\varphi/2} \end{pmatrix} = \begin{pmatrix} e^{-i\varphi/2} & 0 \\ 0 & e^{i\varphi/2} \end{pmatrix} \begin{pmatrix} 1 & ia_2 - a_1 \\ 0 & 1 \end{pmatrix} \right| $$

$$0 \le \varphi < 4\pi, \; -\infty < a_1, a_2 < \infty \} = E(2) \subset SL(2, \mathbb{C}),$$

generators $J_3 = \dfrac{1}{2}\sigma_3, \; K_1 + J_2 = \begin{pmatrix} 0 & -i \\ 0 & 0 \end{pmatrix}, \; K_2 - J_1 = \begin{pmatrix} 0 & -1 \\ 0 & 0 \end{pmatrix}$ obeying

$$[J_3, K_1 + J_2] = i(K_2 - J_1), \; [J_3, K_2 - J_1] = -i(K_1 + J_2),$$

$$[K_1 + J_2, \; K_2 - J_1] = 0; \tag{10.145b}$$

Spacelike Cases $p^{(0)} = (0, 0, 0, \kappa)$:

$$G_{p^{(0)}} = \left\{ \begin{pmatrix} \alpha & \beta \\ \beta^* & \alpha^* \end{pmatrix} \middle| |\alpha|^2 - |\beta|^2 = 1 \right\} = SU(1, 1) \subset SL(2, \mathbb{C}),$$

generators $J_3 = \dfrac{1}{2}\sigma_3, \; K_1 = -\dfrac{i}{2}\sigma_1, \; K_2 = -\dfrac{i}{2}\sigma_2$ obeying

$$[J_3, K_1] = iK_2, \; [J_3, K_2] = -iK_1, \; [K_1, K_2] = -iJ_3. \tag{10.145c}$$

(We note that $E(2)$ in the lightlike case is isomorphic to the Euclidean group in the $x - y$ plane in physical space, and $SU(1, 1)$ in the spacelike case is isomorphic to $Sp(2, \mathbb{R})$ which in turn is isomorphic to $SL(2, \mathbb{R})$). So for each 'standard configuration' $p^{(0)}$ in the list (10.141), the corresponding little group $G_{p^{(0)}}$ is some three parameter subgroup, $SU(2)$ or $E(2)$ or $SU(1, 1)$, in $SL(2, \mathbb{C})$. The first is compact, the other two noncompact. $SU(2)$ and $SU(1, 1)$ are simple at the Lie algebra level, but $E(2)$ has an invariant abelian subgroup of 'translations' T_2' generated by $K_1 + J_2, K_2 - J_1$. These are called 'screw-type' generators and $E(2)$ is the semidirect product $SO(2) \ltimes T_2'$.

For general $p \in \vartheta_{p^{(0)}}$, G_p is a subgroup in $SL(2, \mathbb{C})$ conjugate to $G_{p^{(0)}}$. Each orbit $\vartheta_{p^{(0)}}$ is a coset space, $SL(2, \mathbb{C})/SU(2)$ or $SL(2, \mathbb{C})/E(2)$ or $SL(2, \mathbb{C})/SU(1, 1)$ as the case may be. (These are not quotients but coset spaces).

Now we return to the construction of the UIR's of $\overline{\mathcal{P}}$. Having chosen $p^{(0)}$ and determined $G_{p^{(0)}}$, we look at the (ideal) basis vectors $|p^{(0)}; \alpha\rangle$ and realise that from Eq. (10.139):

$$a \in G_{p^{(0)}} \; : \; \overline{U}(a)|p^{(0)}; \alpha\rangle = \text{linear combination of } |p^{(0)}; \beta\rangle \tag{10.146}$$

Thus the state labels α must refer to the rows and columns of some UIR of $G_{p^{(0)}}$. Denote this by D, so we have

$$a \in G_{p^{(0)}} : \quad \overline{U}(a)|p^{(0)};\alpha\rangle = \sum_{\beta} D_{\beta\alpha}(a)|p^{(0)};\beta\rangle. \qquad (10.147)$$

We see that we are building up the UIR of $\overline{\mathcal{P}}$ 'brick by brick'. The next step is to choose for each $p \in \vartheta_{p^{(0)}}$ some element $l(p) \in SL(2,\mathbb{C})$ which 'carries' $p^{(0)}$ to p:

$$p \in \vartheta_{p^{(0)}} \rightarrow l(p) \in SL(2,\mathbb{C}) : \quad p = \Lambda(l(p))\, p^{(0)} \qquad (10.148)$$

(Of course, we choose $l(p^{(0)})$ to be the identity element in $SL(2,\mathbb{C})$.) Such $l(p)$ can always be found, they are coset representatives. But $l(p)$ is nonunique to the extent of an arbitrary element of $G_{p^{(0)}}$ on the right. Subject to this, we make some convenient choice of $l(p)$, as far as possible varying smoothly with p. These elements are called 'Wigner boosts'. We then define the general basis vectors $|p;\alpha\rangle$ by

$$|p;\alpha\rangle = \overline{U}(l(p))|p^{(0)};\alpha\rangle, \quad P^{\mu}|p;\alpha\rangle = p^{\mu}|p;\alpha\rangle, \qquad (10.149)$$

thus fixing the 'meaning' of the label α in general. Apart from normalisation of these basis vectors the other crucial ingredient is the effect of $\overline{U}(\Lambda)$ on $|p;\alpha\rangle$ for general Λ and p. This is obtained by a computation similar to what we used in the case of $E(3)$, Eq. (10.37). Working at the $SL(2,\mathbb{C})$ level as we should, we have:

$$a \in SL(2,\mathbb{C}), \quad p \in \vartheta_{p^{(0)}}$$

$$\begin{aligned}
\overline{U}(a)|p;\alpha\rangle &= \overline{U}(a)\overline{U}(l(p))|p^{(0)};\alpha\rangle \\
&= \overline{U}(l(\Lambda(a)p))\overline{U}(l(\Lambda(a)p))^{-1}\overline{U}(a)\overline{U}(l(p))|p^{(0)};\alpha\rangle \\
&= \overline{U}(l(\Lambda(a)p))\overline{U}(l(\Lambda(a)p)^{-1}al(p))|p^{(0)};\alpha\rangle \\
&= \sum_{\beta} D(w(p,a))_{\beta\alpha}|p';\beta\rangle,
\end{aligned}$$

$$p' = \Lambda(a)p, \quad w(p,a) = l(\Lambda(a)p)^{-1}al(p) \in G_{p^{(0)}}. \qquad (10.150)$$

By construction, the 'Wigner rotation' $w(p,a) \in SL(2,\mathbb{C})$ is an element of the little group of $p^{(0)}$. Finally the normalisation is defined symbolically by

$$p', p \in \vartheta_{p^{(0)}} : \quad \langle p';\beta|p;\alpha\rangle = \delta_{\alpha\beta}\delta^{(3)}(p',p), \qquad (10.151)$$

where $\delta^{(3)}(p',p)$ is a suitable (possibly Lorentz invariant) three dimensional Dirac delta function appropriate for $\vartheta_{p^{(0)}}$. We will see an example later.

The strategy for constructing UIR's of $\overline{\mathcal{P}}$ is now clear, and it has involved these steps:

(i) Choose a momentum space orbit and representative four-momentum $p^{(0)}$, i.e., choose $\vartheta_{p^{(0)}}$, with associated invariants.

(ii) Determine the stability group $G_{p^{(0)}}$, choose some UIR $D(\,\cdot\,)$ of it.

(iii) For each $p \in \vartheta_{p^{(0)}}$, choose a Wigner boost $l(p) \in SL(2,\mathbb{C})$ in any convenient manner.

After these steps, all things are in place, the UIR being obtained by putting together Eqs. (10.138, 10.146, 10.149, 10.150, 10.151).

Now we look at the three major cases and possible choices of the UIR D of the little group, in a general way, then return to the physically more interesting cases.

Table 10.1   Pattern of UIR's of the Poincaré Group

	Nature of p^μ	Possible choices of D	Comments on UIR of $\overline{\mathcal{P}}$
a)	Timelike positive/ negative	Spin s UIR of $SU(2)$, $s = 0, \frac{1}{2}, 1, \cdots$, dim $(2s+1)$	Finite mass finite spin UIR $[m_0, s]_\pm$, $p^0 > 0$ or $p^0 < 0$.
b)	Lightlike positive/ negative	(i) Fixed finite helicity $J_3 = \lambda = 0, \pm\frac{1}{2}, \pm 1, \cdots$, $K_1 + J_2 = K_2 - J_1 = 0$.	Lightlike UIR $[0, \lambda]_\pm$, fixed Lorentz invariant helicity, $p^0 > 0$ or $p^0 < 0$.
		(ii) $K_1 + J_2, K_2 - J_1 \neq 0$: spectrum of $J_3 =$ $\{0, \pm 1, \pm 2, \cdots\}$ or $\{\pm\frac{1}{2}, \pm\frac{3}{2}, \cdots\}$.	Lightlike 'Continuous spin' UIR, infinitely many helicity states for each p.
c)	Spacelike	(i) Trivial UIR of $SU(1,1)$	'Spinless' spacelike UIR characterised by κ.
		(ii) Nontrivial UIR of $SU(1,1)$, Spectrum of J_3 as in (b(ii)) above, or semi-infinite as in UIR's $D_k^{(\pm)}$ of $SU(1,1)$	'Continuous spin' spacelike UIR, infinitely many helicities for each p

We add some comments:

(i) Only the positive timelike finite spin UIR's $[m_0, s]_+$ and the positive lightlike fixed helicity UIR's $[0, \lambda]_+$ are regarded as physically relevant.

(ii) The problem of constructing the spacelike UIR's (c) was left incomplete by Wigner [Wigner, 1939] and had to await Bargmann's construction [Bargmann, 1947] of all the UIR's of $SU(1, 1)$.

We now study the two physical cases in some detail, with comments and statements of interesting properties.

Timelike UIR's $[m_0, s]_+$

For fixed m_0 and $p^0 > 0$, the points on the orbit $\vartheta_{p^{(0)}}$ can be smoothly and globally parametrised by the three-momentum $\boldsymbol{p}$:

$$\vartheta_{p^{(0)}} = \left\{ p^\mu = \left(\sqrt{m_0^2 + \boldsymbol{p}^2} \,, \, \boldsymbol{p} \right) | \boldsymbol{p} \in \mathbb{R}^3 \right\}, \qquad (10.152)$$

and the orbit is topologically trivial. The Wigner boost $l(\boldsymbol{p})$ is usually chosen to be a pure Lorentz transformation, varying smoothly with $\boldsymbol{p}$:

$$l(\boldsymbol{p}) = \{2 m_0 (m_0 + p^0)\}^{-1/2} (m_0 + p^\mu \sigma_\mu) = l(\boldsymbol{p})^\dagger \in SL(2, \mathbb{C}),$$
$$l(\boldsymbol{p}) p^{(0)\mu} \sigma_\mu l(\boldsymbol{p})^\dagger = m_0 l(\boldsymbol{p})^2 = p^\mu \sigma_\mu. \qquad (10.153)$$

The ideal momentum basis vectors are $|\boldsymbol{p}, m\rangle$ where according to the spin s UIR of $SU(2)$ the magnetic quantum number $m = s, s - 1, \cdots, -s$. An explicitly Lorentz invariant normalisation rule is to set

$$\langle \boldsymbol{p}', m' | \boldsymbol{p}, m \rangle = \delta_{m'm} p^0 \delta^{(3)}(\boldsymbol{p}' - \boldsymbol{p}). \qquad (10.154)$$

In terms of momentum space wave functions we have the Hilbert space $\mathcal{H}$ for the UIR $[m_0, s]_+$ built up as follows:

$$\mathcal{H} = \left\{ f_m(\boldsymbol{p}) = (2s + 1)\text{-component complex column vector } | \right.$$

$$\left. \|f\|^2 = \sum_{m=-s}^s \int \frac{d^3 p}{p^0} f(\boldsymbol{p})^\dagger f(\boldsymbol{p}) < \infty \right\}. \qquad (10.155)$$

In this description after some algebra we find the ten generators of $\overline{\mathcal{P}}$ to be:

$$P^\mu = p^\mu \; : \; \text{multiplicative:}$$

$$\boldsymbol{J} = -i\boldsymbol{p} \wedge \frac{\partial}{\partial \boldsymbol{p}} + \boldsymbol{S}, \; \text{sum of orbital and spin parts,}$$

$$\boldsymbol{S} = \text{generators of spin } s \text{ UIR of } SU(2);$$

$$\boldsymbol{K} = ip^0 \frac{\partial}{\partial \boldsymbol{p}} + (m_0 + p^0)^{-1} \boldsymbol{p} \wedge \boldsymbol{S}. \tag{10.156}$$

An equivalent form via a similarity transformation uses an ordinary three dimensional non Lorentz invariant expression for the inner product, and this leads to a change only in $\boldsymbol{K}$:

$$\psi_m(\boldsymbol{p}) = \frac{1}{\sqrt{p^0}} f_m(\boldsymbol{p}) \; : \; \|\psi\|^2 = \int d^3 p \, \psi(\boldsymbol{p})^\dagger \psi(\boldsymbol{p}),$$

$$P^\mu = p^\mu, \, \boldsymbol{J} = \boldsymbol{q} \wedge \boldsymbol{p} + \boldsymbol{S}, \, \boldsymbol{K} = \frac{1}{2}\{p^0, \boldsymbol{q}\} + \frac{\boldsymbol{p} \wedge \boldsymbol{S}}{m_0 + p^0},$$

$$\boldsymbol{q} = i\frac{\partial}{\partial \boldsymbol{p}}. \tag{10.157}$$

This is called the Shirokov–Foldy form [Shirokov, 1954; Foldy, 1956] for the Hilbert space and generators of the UIR $[m_0, s]_+$ describing a point particle with fixed mass and spin. Here one sees that a natural position operator $\boldsymbol{q}$ has appeared. In fact in these UIR's of $\overline{\mathcal{P}}$ one can construct $\boldsymbol{q}$ or express it explicitly in terms of the generators of $\overline{\mathcal{P}}$. We return to this in a moment.

The two algebraic Casimir invariants have values

$$[m_0, s]_+ \; : \; \mathcal{C}_1 = m_0^2, \, \mathcal{C}_2 = m_0^2 s(s+1). \tag{10.158}$$

so they determine the UIR uniquely.

The Heisenberg canonical commutation relations among $\boldsymbol{q}$ and $\boldsymbol{p}$ are not obtainable from the Lie algebra $\mathcal{P}$ of $\overline{\mathcal{P}}$ in as simple a way as they arise from $\mathcal{G}$ in the Galilean case. Indeed the existence of a physically reasonable position operator $\boldsymbol{q}$ is not guaranteed in a general UIR of $\overline{\mathcal{P}}$. In fact in the lightlike UIR's $[0, \lambda]_+$ (for $\lambda \neq 0$) and the spacelike UIR's, no 'reasonable' $\boldsymbol{q}$ or position exists. By 'reasonable' we mean: having commuting components and behaving as expected under $E(3)$. Thus we would like to have operators q_j obeying:

$$q_j^\dagger = q_j, \ [q_j, q_k] = 0, \ [q_j, P_k] = i\delta_{jk}, \ [J_j, q_k] = i\epsilon_{jkl} q_l. \tag{10.159}$$

This problem was first examined by Newton and Wigner [Newton and Wigner, 1949]. In the UIR's $[m_0, s]_\pm$, position q does exist, as Eq. (10.157) show. Thus the total angular momentum J is indeed the sum of kinematically independent orbital and spin parts. One can see that starting with the primitive independent operators q, p, S obeying (10.83) and specifying m_0, one can build up as in Eq. (10.157) the hermitian generators of the UIR $[m_0, s]_+$ of $\overline{\mathcal{P}}$. However, from the same 'building blocks' one can also build up the generators of the irreducible ray representation of $\overline{\mathcal{G}}$ for mass M and spin s, as in Eq. (10.84).

Here is an interesting fact: this UIR $[m_0, s]_+$ of $\overline{\mathcal{P}}$ is equivalent by a similarity transformation to the tensor product of the spin zero UIR $[m_0, 0]_+$ of $\mathcal{P}$ and the nonunitary irreducible representation $(s, 0)$ or $(0, s)$ of $SL(2, \mathbb{C})$. The Shirokov–Foldy generators are similarity-equivalent to

$$P^\mu, J = q \times p + S, \ K = \frac{1}{2}\{p^0, q\} - iS. \tag{10.160}$$

In words: $[m_0, 0]_+$ of $\mathcal{P} \times (s, 0)$ of $SL(2, \mathbb{C})$ is irreducible, essentially unitary, and 'is' $[m_0, s]_+$ of $\overline{\mathcal{P}}$!

Lightlike UIR's $[0, \lambda]_+$

We present a few remarks. The Hilbert space consists of single component complex momentum space wave functions:

$$\mathcal{H} = \left\{ f(k) \Big| \ \|f\|^2 = \int \frac{d^3 k}{|k|} \ |f(k)|^2 < \infty , \ k^0 = |k| \right\}. \tag{10.161}$$

Points on the orbit $\vartheta_{p^{(0)}}$, $p^{(0)} = (1, 0, 0, 1)$, are labelled by k:

$$\vartheta_{p^{(0)}} = \{ k^\mu = (k^0, k), \ k^0 = |k|, \ k \neq 0 \}, \tag{10.162}$$

so the domain of definition of $f(k)$ is the positive light cone omitting the vertex or tip, but this makes no contribution in the integration in (10.161). There is no way to choose the Wigner boosts $l(k)$ for all $k \neq 0$ in a globally smooth manner – this is in contrast to the timelike UIR's. The behaviour of $f(k)$ under $SU(2)$ (or $SO(3)$) is as it was in the $E(3)$ case in Eq. (10.39). Under general elements of $SL(2, \mathbb{C})$ we have to follow the rules recounted earlier to see how the vectors $|k\rangle$ behave. It is a fact that in these UIR's

$$W^\mu = -\lambda P^\mu, \quad \mathcal{C}_1 = \mathcal{C}_2 = 0, \tag{10.163}$$

so the Casimir invariants do not reveal the value of the helicity.

For nonzero λ, in particular for photons with $\lambda = \pm 1$, there is no reasonable position operator $\boldsymbol{q}$ in the Newton–Wigner sense. This is why photons cannot be localised. Here is an easy argument. If there existed a position operator $\boldsymbol{q}$ in the space of the UIR $[0, \lambda]_+$, Eq. (10.159), we could define an orbital angular momentum and would find:

$$\boldsymbol{L} = \boldsymbol{q} \wedge \boldsymbol{P} = \text{orbital angular momentum};$$

$$[J_j, L_k] = i\epsilon_{jkl} L_l;$$

$$\therefore \boldsymbol{J} - \boldsymbol{L} = \boldsymbol{S} \text{ obeys } [J_j, S_k] = i\epsilon_{jkl} S_l,$$

$$[L_j, S_k] = 0, [P_j, S_k] = 0, \ [S_j, S_k] = i\epsilon_{jkl} S_l. \tag{10.164}$$

Then $\boldsymbol{J} = \boldsymbol{L} + \boldsymbol{S}$ is the sum of two kinematically independent angular momenta, and $\boldsymbol{P} \cdot \boldsymbol{J} = \boldsymbol{P} \cdot \boldsymbol{S}$ cannot be limited to the single value $\lambda|\boldsymbol{P}|$.

In spacelike UIR's too position $\boldsymbol{q}$ cannot be defined since $\boldsymbol{p}$ does not range over all of $\mathbb{R}^3$ but is limited to the exterior of the sphere of radius κ.

The inclusion of parity

As a final item for this chapter, we consider briefly the condition for being able to define a parity – space reflection – operator in an acceptable manner in the context of the UIR's and UR's of $\overline{\mathcal{P}}$. In the timelike (positive or negative) UIR $[m_0, s]_\pm$, we can construct an operator P, unitary and determined up to a phase, such that

$$P\{P^0, \boldsymbol{P}, \boldsymbol{J}, \boldsymbol{K}\}P^{-1} = \{P^0, -\boldsymbol{P}, \boldsymbol{J}, -\boldsymbol{K}\}, \ P^2 = \mathbb{1}. \tag{10.165}$$

So, in passing, we note that parity is not Lorentz invariant. For instance, we can choose (apart from a phase)

$$P = e^{i\frac{\pi}{2}(\boldsymbol{q}^2 + \boldsymbol{p}^2)}, \tag{10.166}$$

since $\boldsymbol{q}$ is available, and on the primitive operators the action is as expected:

$$P\{\boldsymbol{q}, \boldsymbol{p}, \boldsymbol{S}\}P^{-1} = \{-\boldsymbol{q}, -\boldsymbol{p}, \boldsymbol{S}\}. \tag{10.167}$$

But in the lightlike finite helicity UIR's $[0, \lambda]_+$ we cannot construct such P. This is so for $\lambda \neq 0$. This is clear from the relation (10.163) and the fact that if P could be constructed, then W^μ would be a pseudovector while P^μ is a true vector. We also see that the construction (10.166) fails as there is no position vector q with reasonable properties within such a UIR. Helicity changes sign under parity, so to define the latter we need to operate with the direct sum of two UIR's, $[0, \lambda]_+$ and $[0, -\lambda]_+$; then P will exchange these two UIR's.

Problems

P10.1 In the Euclidean group $E(3)$ which is a semidirect product, for each $A \in SO(3)$ identify the outer automorphism acting on the translation subgroup T_3.

P10.2 Show that the $SO(3,1)$ Lie algebra relations, Eq. (10.101), lead to the two Casimir invariants $\mathcal{C}_1 = J^2 - K^2$ and $\mathcal{C}_2 = J \cdot K$.

P10.3 Construct a nonunitary momentum and spin dependent similarity transformation that converts the set of Poincaré generators Eq. (10.157) into the set Eq. (10.160).

P10.4 For the light like finite helicity UIR's of $\mathcal{P}$, construct an argument to show that the Wigner boost $l(k) \in SL(2, \mathbb{C})$, $k \neq 0$, cannot be chosen to be globally smooth as a function of k. (This problem has been analysed in [Dutta and Mukunda, 1987]).

Bibliography

Bargmann, V. (1947). Irreducible Unitary Representations of the Lorentz Group. *Annals of Mathematics*. 48: 568.

Dirac, P. A. M. (1945). Unitary Representations of the Lorentz Group. *Proc. Roy. Soc. London*. A 183: 284.

Dutta, B. and Mukunda, N. (1987). Group Representations and the Method of Sections. *Pramana - Journal of Physics*. 29: 437.

Dyson, F. J. (1966). *Symmetry Groups in Nuclear and Particle Physics. A Lecture Note and Reprint Volume*. New York: W. A. Benjamin.

Foldy, L. L. (1956). Synthesis of Covariant Particle Equations. *Phys. Rev.* 102: 568.

Inonu, E. and Wigner, E. P. (1956). Representations of the Galilei Group. *Il Nuovo Cimento*. 9: 705.

Majorana, E. (1932). Relativistic Theory of Particles with Arbitrary Intrinsic Angular Momentum. *Il Nuovo Cimento*. 9: 335.

Naimark, M. A. (1964). *Linear Representations of the Lorentz Group*. New York: MacMillan.

Newton, T. D. and Wigner, E. P. (1949). Localized States for Elementary Systems. *Revs. Mod. Phys.* 21: 400.

Shirokov, Iu. M. (1954). On a New Class of Relativistic Equations for Elementary Particles. *Dokl. Akad. Nauk. SSSR*. 94: 857; 97: 737.

Sudarshan, E. C. G. and Mukunda, N. (1974). *Classical Dynamics {A Modern Perspective}*. New York: Wiley. Reprinted (2015). New Delhi: Hindustan Book Agency.

Wigner, E. P. (1939). On Unitary Representations of the Inhomogeneous Lorentz Group. *Annals of Mathematics*. 40: 149.

Index